Radiology Study Guide

Radiology Study Guide

Terry R. Yochum, B.S., D.C., D.A.C.B.R., F.C.C.R. (C), F.I.C.C., Fellow, A.C.C.R.
Director, Rocky Mountain Chiropractic Radiological Center, Denver, Colorado
Adjunct Professor of Radiology, Los Angeles College of Chiropractic
Instructor, Skeletal Radiology, Department of Radiology, University of Colorado School of Medicine, Denver, Colorado
Formerly:
Senior Lecturer, Department of Diagnostic Sciences, Division Head, Department of Radiology, Phillip Institute of Technology—School of Chiropractic, Melbourne, Australia
Professor and Chairman, Department of Radiology, Logan College of Chiropractic, St. Louis, Missouri
Assistant Professor of Radiology, National College of Chiropractic, Lombard, Illinois

Jolie V. Haug, B.S., D.C.
Private Practice, Beijing, China

Lindsay J. Rowe, M. App. Sc. (Chiropractic), M.D., D.A.C.B.R., F.C.C.R. (C), F.A.C.C.R. (AUS), F.I.C.C.
Adjunct Faculty, School of Chiropractic, Royal Melbourne Institute of Technology University, Melbourne, Australia
Lecturer and Tutor, Faculty of Medicine, University of Newcastle, Newcastle, Australia
Senior Radiology Registrar, Department of Medical Imaging, John Hunter Hospital, Newcastle, Australia
Post Graduate Faculty, Northwestern Chiropractic College, Minneapolis, Minnesota, Canadian Memorial Chiropractic College, Toronto, Canada
Formerly:
Associate Professor and Chairman, Department of Radiology, Northwestern Chiropractic College, Minneapolis, Minnesota
Associate Professor and Chairman, Department of Radiology, Canadian Memorial Chiropractic College, Toronto, Canada

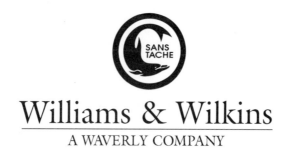

Williams & Wilkins
A WAVERLY COMPANY

BALTIMORE • PHILADELPHIA • LONDON • PARIS • BANGKOK
BUENOS AIRES • HONG KONG • MUNICH • SYDNEY • TOKYO • WROCLAW

Editor: Rina Steinhauer
Managing Editor: Susan Kimner
Marketing Manager: Christine Kushner
Production Coordinator: Carol Eckhart
Project Editor: Kathy Gilbert
Designer: Artech Graphics II
Illustration Planner: Wayne Hubbel
Cover Designer: Artech Graphics II
Typesetter: Bi-Comp, Inc.
Printer and Binder: Mack Printing Group

Copyright © 1998 Williams & Wilkins

351 West Camden Street
Baltimore, Maryland 21201-2436 USA

Rose Tree Corporate Center
1400 North Providence Road
Building II, Suite 5025
Media, Pennsylvania 19063-2043 USA

Accurate indications, adverse reactions and dosage schedules for drugs are provided in this book, but it is possible that they may change. The reader is urged to review the package information data of the manufacturers of the medications mentioned.

Printed in the United States of America

Library of Congress Cataloging-in-Publication Data

Yochum, Terry R.
    Radiology study guide / Terry R. Yochum, Jolie V. Haug, Lindsay J. Rowe.
       p.   cm.
    Companion v. to: Essentials of skeletal radiology / Terry R. Yochum, Lindsay J. Rowe. 2nd ed. c1996.
    Includes bibliographical references and index.
    ISBN 0-683-30139-X
    1. Radiography, Medical. 2. Radiography, Medical—Examinations, questions, etc. 3. Human skeleton—Radiography. 4. Human skeleton—Radiography—Examinations, questions, etc. I. Rowe, Lindsay J. II. Haug, Jolie V. III. Yochum, Terry R. Essentials of skeletal radiology, IV. Title.
    [DNLM: 1. Bone and Bones—pathology—examination questions. 2. Bone Diseases—diagnosis—examination questions. 3. Diagnostic Imaging—examination questions. WE 18.2 Y54r 1998]
    RC78.Y63 1998
    616.7'107572—dc21
    DNLM/DLC
    for Library of Congress   97-42362
                                            CIP

The publishers have made every effort to trace the copyright holders for borrowed material. If they have inadvertently overlooked any, they will be pleased to make the necessary arrangements at the first opportunity.

To purchase additional copies of this book, call our customer service department at **(800) 638-0672** or fax orders to **(800) 447-8438.** For other book services, including chapter reprints and large quantity sales, ask for the Special Sales department.

Canadian customers should call **(800) 665-1148,** or fax **(800) 665-0103.** For all other calls originating outside of the United States, please call **(410) 528-4223** or fax us at **(410) 528-8550.**

Visit Williams & Wilkins on the Internet **http://www.wwilkins.com** or contact our customer service department at **custserv@wwilkins.com**. Williams & Wilkins customer service representatives are available from 8:30 am to 6:00 pm, EST, Monday through Friday, for telephone access.

98 99 00 01 02
1 2 3 4 5 6 7 8 9 10

Picture 1 on front cover reprinted with permission from Freundlich. Radiologic Approach to Diseases of the Chest, 1st ed. Baltimore: Williams & Wilkins, 1997:2.

Picture 2 on front cover reprinted with permission from Yochum TR, Rowe LJ. Essentials of Skeletal Radiology, 2nd ed. Baltimore: Williams & Wilkins, 1996:756.

Picture on back cover reprinted with permission from Daffner. Clinical Radiology: The Essentials, 1st ed. Baltimore: Williams & Wilkins, 1993:170.

Dedication

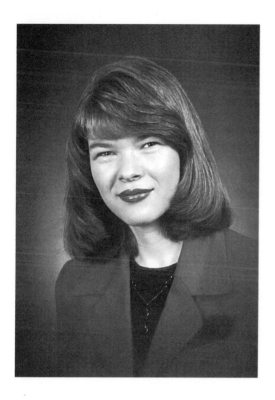

Kimberley Ann Yochum is a rare young woman. Despite living in a society that undervalues the art of gracious interaction among its people, Kimberley exhibits a dignity and gentle courtesy that is immediately apparent and tremendously attractive. She has internalized the social graces her mother and father, Inge and Terry R. Yochum, have taught her, and she reflects them naturally.

Whether describing the background of each of her individually-created dolls, or explaining the samples in her impressive collection of semi-precious stones and minerals, Kimberley's quiet delight is contagious. As the day-to-day work on this book progressed, the thought of her lively interest was an inspiration. Her kind and radiant spirit served to encourage me through the long hours of organizing, writing, re-writing, and re-organizing. It is with warm appreciation that I dedicate this book to her.

Jolie V. Haug, B.S., D.C.

O Son of Spirit!
My first counsel is this: Possess a pure, kindly and radiant heart, that thine may be a sovereignty ancient, imperishable and everlasting.

Bahá'u'lláh

Foreword

I am proud to say I have been able to call the authors my friends and colleagues for many years, and I am pleased to have the opportunity to write this foreword. I am particularly proud that one of my stellar former students, Dr. Jolie V. Haug, has performed so beautifully in the creation of this text and that she has written this with two of the more prominent and prolific authors in the field of radiology and chiropractic, Drs. Terry R. Yochum and Lindsay J. Rowe. I am pleased with the inclusion of material on the chest and abdomen because a person concentrating on skeletal studies must never overlook the subtle and important soft tissue findings on their plain films.

This text would have been a great help if it had been available during my four decades of teaching radiology to undergraduate students at Western States Chiropractic College and a very good review for the radiology residents.

I find it to be an exceptional self-testing review of radiology for all those in preparation for boards and those staying on top of essential information in the field of radiology.

The inclusion of test-yourself questions adds the opportunity for immediate feedback and encouragement to continue—for studying should always be a life-long pursuit.

Appa L. Anderson, D.C., D.A.C.B.R., F.I.C.C., Fellow, A.C.C.R.
Professor Emeritus and Past Chairman
Department of Radiology
Western States Chiropractic College
Portland, Oregon

Preface

When the second edition of *Essentials of Skeletal Radiology* was published, it met with instant, enthusiastic acceptance. Dr. Terry R. Yochum, one of the primary authors of that text, asked Dr. Jolie V. Haug, who had edited the book in preparation for the second edition, to proofread its first printing. When that task was completed, the publishers suggested creating a study guide to accompany the two-volume reference work. Since Dr. Haug was already intimately familiar with the original text, Dr. Yochum suggested her as the logical author to work with him on the study guide.

As work progressed, questions arose about the scope of the study guide. Should it include greater detail on x-ray physics? Should it cover soft-tissue radiology, specifically chest and abdomen imaging? The authors ultimately decided to include these topics, but with less emphasis than was given to skeletal radiology. What has emerged is a general study outline designed to serve as a quick basic reference for practitioners and a review manual for state and national board examinations in radiology.

The majority of material is taken directly from *Essentials of Skeletal Radiology* by Terry R. Yochum and Lindsay J. Rowe, (second edition, 1996; Williams & Wilkins). Information on diagnostic imaging and x-ray physics was gleaned primarily from *Essentials of Diagnostic Imaging* by Gary M. Guebert, Othel L. Pirtle, and Terry R. Yochum (1995; Mosby-Year Book, Inc.). Chapter 9, on imaging the chest and abdomen, represents a compendium of information, most of which was drawn from six texts:

1. Stephen R. Baker, Milton Elkin. Plain film approach to abdominal calcifications. WB Saunders, 1983.
2. Benjamin Felson. Chest roentgenology. WB Saunders, 1973.
3. Benjamin Felson, Aaron S. Weinstein, Harold B. Spitz. Principles of chest roentgenology. WB Saunders, 1965.
4. John V. Forrest, David S. Feigin. Essentials of chest radiology. WB Saunders, 1982.
5. Irwin M. Freundlich, David G. Bragg. A radiologic approach to diseases of the chest, 2nd ed. Williams & Wilkins, 1997.
6. Lester W. Paul, John H. Juhl. The essentials of roentgen interpretation, 3rd ed. Harper & Row, 1972.

In addition, for many of the disease entities discussed in Chapter 9, clinical and laboratory findings came from *The Merck Manual of Diagnosis and Therapy*, 16th ed; Merck Research Laboratories, 1992. In cases in which these sources conflicted, we used information from the most recent text.

The basic premise behind this text is that orderly organization of information is conducive to better understanding and memorization. To facilitate efficient and effective recall, study questions appear at 10- to 20-page intervals, for a total of about 600 questions. Wherever possible, these questions are inserted at a logical break point: usually following discussion of a specific pathologic entity. However, in the interest of keeping these "bites" of information more readily digestible, questions were occasionally inserted in the middle of a discussion. We debated including answers to these questions, but decided that, since they covered so few pages, and since the information was in easily accessible outline form, repeating it after the questions would be redundant. We suggest that the student preparing for an examination take the time to test herself or himself on these study questions, and if the answers are not readily apparent, re-read the relevant sections.

A small pointing finger "icon" has been inserted at the start of any section or sub-heading that may be particularly essential for board review. Some icons indicate a complete pathologic entity. For example, one should know all one can about multiple myeloma. In other cases, an icon may appear only at a sub-heading, or an additional icon may appear within a section, indicating special emphasis on certain details. There is no guarantee that your examinations will contain questions about this material or that you will not be questioned about other material. The key simply indicates that any physician could reasonably be expected to be familiar with that material, so it would be wise for the student to pay particular attention to it.

Each chapter is followed by a practice test of 100 multiple-choice questions. A 600-question multiple-choice test over all nine chapters follows the chapters, and a 225-question test also is included for additional practice. The material is weighted heavily toward neoplasms, arthritides, and trauma, with fewer questions over the other topics. Answer keys follow at the end of the tests.

It is the sincere hope of the authors that this text may fill the need for a comprehensive and accessible radiologic review for students and physicians alike.

Terry R. Yochum
Jolie V. Haug
Lindsay J. Rowe

Acknowledgments

As is the case with most technical or professional texts, the creation of this one entailed the combined efforts of many people. Although a few words on this page cannot adequately convey our thanks to them, it is appropriate that we attempt to acknowledge their contributions to the finished product.

Striving for accuracy, as well as readability, we enlisted the aid of knowledgeable colleagues. Michael S. Barry, D.C., D.A.C.B.R, and Jeffrey R. Thompson, D.C., D.A.C.B.R., both agreed to read through the manuscript and offer comments and suggestions. Gary M. Guebert, D.C., D.A.C.B.R., twice reviewed and amended Chapter 2, ensuring that it accurately reflected the material in his book. The finished product is much the better for their input, and we appreciate their contributions of time and expertise.

Peter T. Haug, M.S., Ph.D, Jolie's husband, offered invaluable assistance in editing the manuscript. His experience as a writer and editor makes him eminently qualified to function as an advisor, and Jolie took shameless advantage of his willingness to assist. He also endured (uncomplainingly, most of the time) the evenings, weekends, and holidays when she was immersed in working on the book.

Terry's devoted wife, Inge, once more supported him through the seemingly endless hours of work on this text. His children, Kimberley Ann, Philip Andrew, and Alicia Marie, continued through their patience and love to enable him to devote time to yet another monumental project.

The staff at Williams & Wilkins, especially our editors, Rina Steinhauer and Sue Kimner, gave assistance unstintingly. Sue is affectionately known in the Haug household as "Skimner," because of the frequency of e-mail that flowed between us. We appreciate the bounty of having such responsive and accommodating coworkers.

Finally, we have discovered an unexpected bonus in working together. We share a passion for perfection and a commitment to high quality. The growth of friendship based on mutual trust and admiration was an additional gift, which has made the working relationship a joy.

Terry R. Yochum
Jolie V. Haug
August 1997

Contents

Chapter 1

NORMAL ANATOMY
Views, Positioning, Mensuration

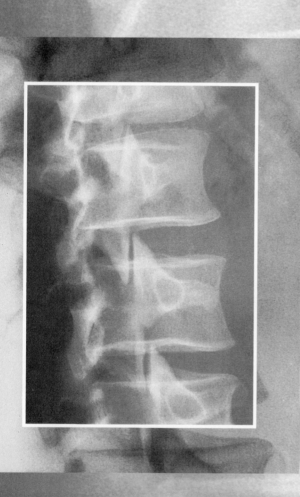

A. SKULL

1. **Lateral Projection**

   a) Demonstrates sella turcica, sinuses, calvarium, IOP, EOP, occipitocervical junction

   b) Mensuration
   - Sella turcica size: measure AP and vertical diameter
     1) significance: enlarged by pituitary neoplasm (normals: AP 5–16 mm; vertical 4–12 mm)
   - Basilar angle (sphenobasilar angle): (Fig. 1.1) two lines drawn from the midpoint between the clinoid processes: one to the anterior margin of the foramen magnum (basion), one to the frontal-nasal junction (nasion)
     1) normal = 123–152°
     2) significance: enlarged in platybasia
   - McGregor's line (basal line): (Fig. 1.2) line from posterosuperior margin of hard palate to most inferior surface of occiput
     1) normal: odontoid apex < 10 mm above line
     2) significance: > 10 mm above line in basilar impression
     3) causes of basilar invagination
   - Chamberlain's line: (Fig. 1.3) line from posterosuperior hard palate to posterior margin of foramen magnum (opisthion)
     1) normal: odontoid apex < 3 mm above line
     2) significance: > 3 mm above line in basilar impression
   - Macrae's line: (Fig. 1.4) line between basion and opisthion
     1) normal: odontoid apex beneath the anterior quarter of the line, inferior margin of the occiput below the line

Causes of Basiliar Invagination

"COOP"

Congenital

Osteogenesis imperfecta

Osteomalacia

Paget's disease

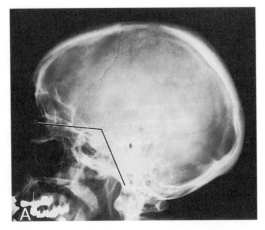

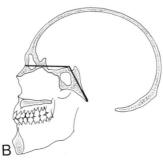

Figure 1.1.

Basilar angle (sphenobasilar angle). Reprinted with permission from Yochum TR, Rowe LJ. Essentials of Skeletal Radiology, 2nd ed. Baltimore: Williams & Wilkins, 1996:142.

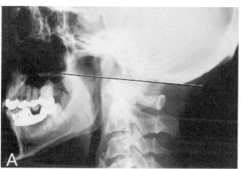
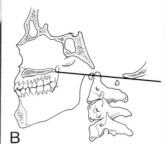
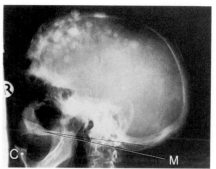

Figure 1.2.

*McGregor's line (basal line). **A** and **B**. Normal McGregor's line. **C**. Abnormal McGregor's line. Reprinted with permission from Yochum TR, Rowe LJ. Essentials of Skeletal Radiology, 2nd ed. Baltimore: Williams & Wilkins, 1996:143.*

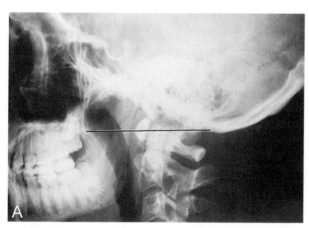
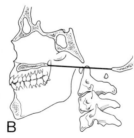

Figure 1.3.

Chamberlain's Line. Reprinted with permission from Yochum TR, Rowe LJ. Essentials of Skeletal Radiology, 2nd ed. Baltimore: Williams & Wilkins, 1996:144.

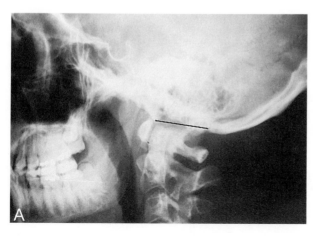
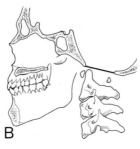

Figure 1.4.

Macrae's line. Reprinted with permission from Yochum TR, Rowe LJ. Essentials of Skeletal Radiology, 2nd ed. Baltimore: Williams & Wilkins, 1996:144.

2) significance: inferior occiput above line in basilar impression; posterior odontoid may indicate dislocation, fracture, or dysplasia of the dens

2. **Caldwell Projection (Posteroanterior)**

   a) Position with forehead and nose tip against bucky (cervical flexion)

   b) 15° caudal tube tilt

   c) Demonstrates: sinuses, orbits, sphenoid wings, petrous ridges

   d) Optimal projection for facial bones

3. **Towne's Projection (Anteroposterior)**

   a) Position with base of occiput against bucky (chin tucked in flexion)

   b) 35° caudal tube tilt

   c) Demonstrates: foramen magnum, petrous pyramids, dorsum sellae

   d) Occipital projection

 4. **Water's Projection (Posteroanterior)**

   a) Position with chin and nose tip against bucky (slight cervical extension)

   b) Demonstrates: sinuses (optimal view for frontal and maxillary sinuses), orbits, zygomatic arches; open mouth to visualize sphenoid sinuses

B. CERVICAL SPINE

1. **AP Lower Cervical Spine (APLC)**

    a) 15° cephalad tube tilt

   b) Demonstrates: C3–7 vertebral bodies, facet lateral margins, von Luschka joints, spinous processes; T1–3 vertebral bodies, spinous processes; posterior ribs 1–3; medial clavicles; lung apices; trachea shadow

2. **AP Open Mouth Projection (APOM)**

   a) Demonstrates atlas arches, lateral masses and transverse processes; axis body, odontoid process, spinous process, transverse processes; styloid processes, mastoid processes

   b) mAs must be increased by 50–100% over APLC setting

   c) Mensuration
   - alignment of lateral margins of atlas lateral masses with axis body
     1) normal = lateral margins match smoothly
     2) significance: atlas margins lateral to axis may indicate atlas fracture, dens lesion, or rotational malposition
   - digastric line (biventer line): line connecting left and right digastric groove

1) normal = tip of odontoid is 1–21 mm below line; atlanto-occipital joint is from 4–20 mm below line

2) significance: distances decreased in platybasia, occipitalization, basilar invagination

☞ **3. Neutral Lateral Cervical Projection**

a) Demonstrates: AP cervical alignment, cervico-occipital relationships; atlas' anterior and posterior tubercles; odontoid process; cervical bodies, laminae, spinous processes; IVDs; EOP, sella turcica; retropharyngeal and retrotracheal interspace

b) Taken non-bucky, TFD 72

c) If C7 cannot be seen clearly:
- increase exposure; take a spot projection
- patient holds weights to pull down the shoulders
- take a "swimmer's lateral" to demonstrate C7-T2 more clearly
- may require a CT to demonstrate the area adequately

d) To evaluate function, take flexion lateral and extension lateral

☞ e) Mensuration
- cervical lordosis measurements
  1) depth of lordosis: 7–17 mm normal
  2) Method of Jochumsen: 1–9 mm normal
  3) angle of cervical curve: 35–45° normal
  4) Method of Drexler: 16–60° normal
- cervical stress lines: (Fig. 1.5) (evaluated in neutral, flexion and extension): normals

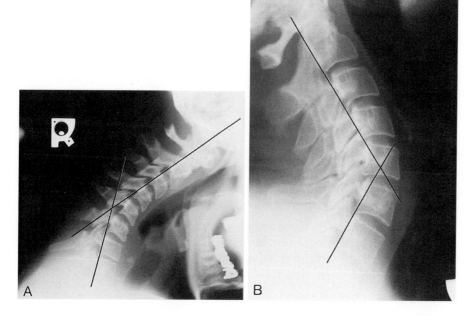

Figure 1.5.

Cervical stress lines. **A**. *Flexion.* **B**. *Extension. Reprinted with permission from Yochum TR, Rowe LJ. Essentials of Skeletal Radiology, 2nd ed. Baltimore: Williams & Wilkins, 1996:1454.*

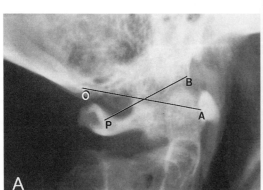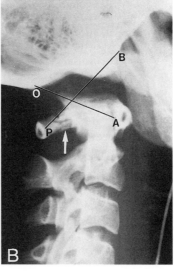

Figure 1.6.

*Atlanto-occipital dislocation (Power's index). **A**. Normal atlanto-occipital relationship. **B**. Anterior atlanto-occipital dislocation. Reprinted with permission from Yochum TR, Rowe LJ. Essentials of Skeletal Radiology, 2nd ed. Baltimore: Williams & Wilkins, 1996:147.*

intersect at C5, C5–6 interspace, C4–5 interspace, respectively

- prevertebral soft tissue evaluation (pharyngeal and laryngeal spaces): normals should be < 7 mm in pharyngeal (at C2) and < 20 mm in laryngeal (at C5 or 6) areas
- atlanto-occipital dislocation (Power's Index): (Fig. 1.6) ratio of B-P:O-A = < 1
- atlanto-dental interval (ADI), in neutral, flexion and extension: in adult normal is < 3 mm, in child normal is < 5 mm
- Method of Bull: for odontoid malposition—posterior angle of intersection 13° or less is normal
- George's Line (posterior body line): should be smooth, uninterrupted
- posterior cervical line (spinolaminar junction line): should be smooth
- sagittal cervical canal dimension: stenosis indicated by dimensions < 12 mm at C4–7; < 13 mm at C3; < 14 mm at C2; < 16 mm at C1
- cervical gravity line: should pass through C7 vertebral body

☞ **4. Flexion and Extension Lateral Cervical Projections**

    a) Taken to evaluate atlanto-axial stability and intersegmental motion

    b) Flexion: first tuck the chin, then flex the neck; marker is behind the head

    c) Extension: first lift the chin, then extend the neck; marker is below the chin

    d) Contraindications for these views: odontoid lesions, fracture/dislocations in cervical spine; postural vertigo; vertebrobasilar ischemia or significant neurologic deficits

    e) Non-bucky; TFD 72"

5. **Oblique Cervical Projection**

- **a)** Demonstrates von Luschka joints, pedicles, facets, intervertebral foramina (IVFs)
  - anterior oblique shows ipsilateral IVFs
  - posterior oblique shows contralateral IVFs
- **b)** Body at 45° angle to bucky, head parallel to bucky
- **c)** Marker placement:
  - anterior oblique: marker behind spine
  - posterior oblique: marker under mandible
- **d)** 15° tube tilt: caudal for anterior, cephalad for posterior oblique

6. **Articular Pillars Projection (PA) (Pillar View)**

- **a)** Demonstrates articular pillars, facet joints
- **b)** 35° cephalad tube tilt (tilt caudal if taken AP)
- **c)** Patient facing bucky, with head turned 45–50° away from side of interest
- **d)** Marker behind spine on side of interest

   7. **Davis Series**

- **a)** Seven views: AP lower cervical; AP open mouth; right and left obliques; neutral, flexion and extension lateral cervical spine

C. THORACIC SPINE

1. **Anteroposterior Projection (AP Thoracic Spine)**

- **a)** Demonstrates vertebral bodies, spinous processes, transverse processes, posterior rib articulations, lung fields, mediastinum, medial clavicles, sternum, scoliosis
- **b)** Taken on suspended full inspiration
-    **c)** Filtration on upper half to two-thirds of thoracic spine

2. **Lateral Projection**

- **a)** Demonstrates vertebral bodies, intervertebral discs (IVDs), ribs, heart, lung fields, kyphosis
- **b)** Taken on suspended full inspiration to depress the diaphragm
-    **c)** Filtration on lower half of thoracic spine
- **d)** Mensuration
  - thoracic cage dimension: anterior T8 body to posterior sternal surface
    1) average 12 cm females, 14 cm males
    2) significance: reduced space may indicate straight back syndrome
  - thoracic kyphosis
    1) lines tangential to superior endplate of T1 and inferior endplate of T12

2) perpendiculars constructed, angle of intersection measured

3) norms vary with age and gender

☞   **3. Swimmer's Lateral (Cervicothoracic) Projection**

    a) Demonstrates lower cervical and upper thoracic vertebral bodies and discs

    b) Patient positioned lateral to bucky, rotated backwards toward bucky about 20°, arm closest to bucky flexed with hand cupping occiput, arm farthest from bucky extended at shoulder, with hand on hip

D. LUMBAR SPINE

   1. Anteroposterior Lumbopelvic Projection

    a) Demonstrates lumbar vertebral bodies, transverse processes, spinous processes, pedicle shadows, ilia, acetabular joints

    b) Taken upon suspended expiration

☞   **c)** Obese patient filmed supine to compress abdomen, or upright with belly compression band

☞   **d)** Mensuration

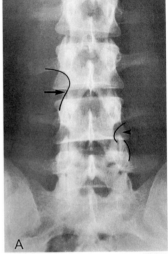

    • Hadley's "S" curve: (Fig. 1.7A and B) also used with oblique projection

      1) follow inferior margin of transverse process, inferior articular process, across joint space to outer edge of superior articular process

      2) line should form a smooth curve, should not be interrupted

      3) interruptions caused by facet imbrication, disc derangement

    • interpediculate distance

      1) normals vary segment to segment

      2) reduced in spinal stenosis, congenital malformation

      3) increased by intraspinal neoplasms

    • canal/body ratio: requires AP and lateral projections

      1) interpediculate distance × sagittal canal width, divided by transverse body diameter × sagittal body diameter

      2) normal should be ≥ 1:3

      3) significance: higher ratio may indicate spinal stenosis

      4) not considered a very reliable indicator

    • intercrestal line

      1) predicts lumbar stress patterns

      2) crests at L4 level: L4–5 degeneration more likely, especially if coupled with long L5 transverse processes, hypoplastic ribs, transitional vertebra

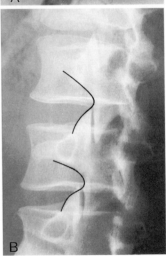

Figure 1.7.

*Hadley's "S" curve. **A**. Anteroposterior normal (arrow), anteroposterior abnormal (arrowhead). **B**. Oblique normal. Reprinted with permission from Yochum TR, Rowe LJ. Essentials of Skeletal Radiology, 2nd ed. Baltimore: Williams & Wilkins, 1996:164.*

    3) crests at L5 level: lumbosacral degeneration more likely, especially if coupled with short L5 transverse processes, no other lumbar anomalies

- lumbar transverse process evaluation
  1) construct bilateral vertical lines tangential to distal tip of L3 transverse processes
  2) assess comparative length of L5 transverse processes
  3) significance: longer transverse processes at L5 may enhance lumbosacral stability

2. Lateral Lumbosacral Projection

a) Demonstrates lumbar vertebral bodies, disc spaces, articular processes, IVFs, pedicles, sacral base, thoracolumbar and lumbosacral junctions

b) Taken on suspended expiration

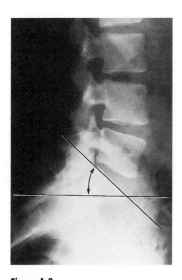

c) Soft tissues should be examined carefully; search for evidence of aneurysm

d) Mensuration
- Hurxthal IVD height = mid-disc vertical height
- Farfan IVD height = anterior disc height/ disc diameter divided by posterior disc height/disc diameter
  1) significant segmental rotation or lateral flexion render these measurements meaningless
- IVD angles: normals average L1 - 8°; L2 - 10°; L3 - 12°; L4 and L5 - 14°
- lumbar lordosis
  1) lines constructed tangential to L5 inferior endplate or sacral base, L1 superior endplate
  2) perpendiculars constructed to these lines and their angles of intersection measured
  3) average is 50–60°
  4) significance: increased angle may be implicated in low back pain
- lumbosacral lordosis
  1) body centers of L3, L5, and S1 located via diagonals
  2) body centers connected and angle at L5 measured
  3) average is 146°, wide range of "normals"
- lumbosacral angle (sacral base angle; Ferguson's angle) (Fig. 1.8)
  1) line made tangential to sacral base
  2) true horizontal drawn to intersect tangential line
  3) angle of intersection should average around 40° (27–57° range)

Figure 1.8.

Lumbosacral angle. Reprinted with permission from Yochum TR, Rowe LJ. Essentials of Skeletal Radiology, 2nd ed. Baltimore: Williams & Wilkins, 1996:161.

☞

- lumbosacral disc angle (sacrovertebral disc angle) (Fig. 1.9)
    1) lines tangential to inferior L5 endplate and sacral base
    2) angle of intersection should average 10–15°
- sacral inclination angle
    1) line tangential to posterior margin of S1
    2) true vertical constructed to intersect with it
    3) average angle of intersection: 46° (range: 30–72°)

☞

- gravitational line from L3 (lumbar gravity line, Ferguson's gravitational line, Ferguson's weight-bearing line)
    1) diagonals locate L3 vertebral body center
    2) true vertical dropped through it should pass through or close to sacral promontory
    3) > 10 mm (½") anterior may indicate increased shearing stress
    4) significance: posterior alignment may indicate increased weight-bearing stress on facet joints and pars interarticularis

☞

- Macnab's line (Fig. 1.10)
    1) line tangential to inferior anterior and posterior endplate margins should not intersect subadjacent superior articular process
    2) significance: intersection may indicate facet imbrication

☞

- Ullmann's line (right-angle test line, Garland-Thomas line) (Fig. 1.11)
    1) line tangential to superior anterior and posterior S1 endplates
    2) perpendicular constructed to it at the anterosuperior margin
    3) anteroinferior L5 body should not intersect this line
    4) significance: anterolisthesis
    5) N.B., intersection may be caused by loss of lumbar lordosis rather than listhesis

☞

- Meyerding's spondylolisthesis grading: (Fig. 1.12)
    1) superior endplate subadjacent to listhesis is marked off in quarters
    2) posteroinferior endplate will align above one of these quarters
    3) grade 1, posterior quarter; grade 2, posterior half; grade 3, anterior half; grade 4, anterior quarter; grade 5, totally anterior to subadjacent segment

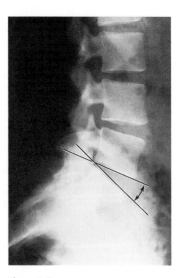

Figure 1.9.

Lumbosacral disc angle. Reprinted with permission from Yochum TR, Rowe LJ. Essentials of Skeletal Radiology, 2nd ed. Baltimore: Williams & Wilkins, 1996:161.

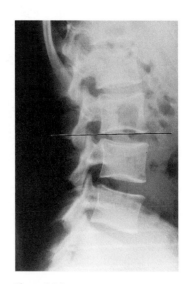

Figure 1.10.

Macnab's line. Reprinted with permission from Yochum TR, Rowe LJ. Essentials of Skeletal Radiology, 2nd ed. Baltimore: Williams & Wilkins, 1996:163.

- Eisenstein's sagittal canal measurement (Fig. 1.13)
  1) construct articular process line, connecting tips of articulating superior and inferior facet joints
  2) measure between midpoint of posterior vertebral body margin and articular process line
  3) < 15 mm may indicate spinal stenosis

3. Oblique Lumbar Projection

   a) Demonstrates pars interarticularis, facet joints, pedicles, transverse processes, superior and inferior articular processes, and disc space (Scotty dog image)
- posterior oblique displays ipsilateral facets and pars
- anterior oblique displays contralateral facets and pars

   b) Side marker placement
- posterior oblique - in front of spine
- anterior oblique - behind the spine

   c) Taken on suspended full expiration

   d) Patient rotated about 45° from AP or PA position

   e) Mensuration
- Hadley's "S" curve: used with AP and oblique projections
  1) line follows inferior margin of transverse process, along inferior facet margin, crossing joint space to outer edge of superior facet

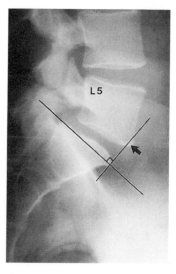

Figure 1.11.

Ullmann's line. Spondylolisthesis of the fifth lumbar segment demonstrated by the intersection of the line with the fifth lumbar body (arrow). Reprinted with permission from Yochum TR, Rowe LJ. Essentials of Skeletal Radiology, 2nd ed. Baltimore: Williams & Wilkins, 1996:167.

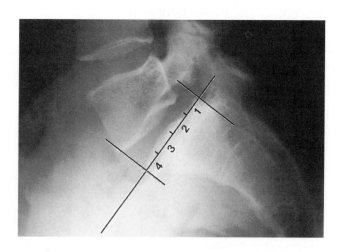

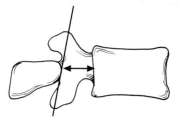

Figure 1.12.

Meyerding's classification of spondylolisthesis. Reprinted with permission from Yochum TR, Rowe LJ. Essentials of Skeletal Radiology, 2nd ed. Baltimore: Williams & Wilkins, 1996:167.

Figure 1.13.

Eisenstein's sagittal canal measurement. Reprinted with permission from Yochum TR, Rowe LJ. Essentials of Skeletal Radiology, 2nd ed. Baltimore: Williams & Wilkins, 1996:169.

2) transition across facet joint should be smooth

3) significance: break in line may indicate facet imbrication, DJD

4. **Anteroposterior Tilt-up Lumbosacral Spot**

a) Demonstrates sacroiliac and lumbosacral joints, upper sacral segments, and L5

b) Tube tilt cephalad, matching sacral base angle, or (generic) about 20°

c) N.B., similar visualization obtained by flattening sacral base: seat patient, or have lumbar lordosis flattened by flexing at hips and knees

d) If projection is performed PA, tube tilt is caudal

5. **Lateral Lumbosacral Spot Projection**

a) Supplemental film to demonstrate L5, S1, or the lumbosacral joint more definitively

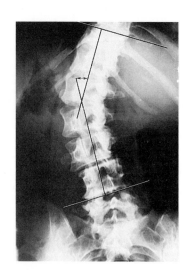

Figure 1.14.

Cobb method of scoliosis evaluation. Reprinted with permission from Yochum TR, Rowe LJ. Essentials of Skeletal Radiology, 2nd ed. Baltimore: Williams & Wilkins, 1996:156.

E. SCOLIOSIS EVALUATION

1. **Projections**

a) Upright AP spine for mensuration

b) Upright lateral with curve convexity adjacent to bucky

2. **Mensurations**

a) Cobb method, Risser-Ferguson method

b) Cobb method generally preferred: with a 40° curve, yields numbers as much as 10° greater than those given by the Risser-Ferguson method

• Cobb method: (Fig. 1.14)

1) line tangential to superior endplate of uppermost vertebral body that tilts to the concavity

2) line tangential to inferior endplate of lowest vertebral body that tilts to the concavity

3) perpendiculars constructed to these lines and their angle of intersection measured

• Risser-Ferguson method: (Fig. 1.15)

1) diagonals locate vertebral body centers of uppermost and lowest vertebral body that tilt to the concavity

2) diagonals locate vertebral body center of apical vertebra

3) these three centers are connected, and the angle of intersection at the apical vertebra is measured (may be up to 25% lower than the value found with the Cobb method)

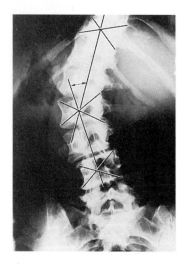

Figure 1.15.

Risser-Ferguson method of scoliosis evaluation. Reprinted with permission from Yochum TR, Rowe LJ. Essentials of Skeletal Radiology, 2nd ed. Baltimore: Williams & Wilkins, 1996:156.

☞

    c) Protocols
- baseline films taken are upright AP and lateral views, which include both upper and lower extremes of the scoliosis
- with double curves, each component is measured separately
- during growth years (around puberty) patient should be monitored with an AP film every 3 months
  1) same landmarks must be used in each evaluation to minimize error
- curves < 20° do not require bracing
- curves between 20° and 40° should be braced (still controversial)
- progression > 5° in a 3-month period may indicate need for bracing
- surgery may be required with curvature > 40°
- other indications for surgery include underlying anomaly, rapid progression of curve in an immature spine, or cosmetic reasons

F. PELVIS

1. Anteroposterior Sacral Projection

    a) Demonstrates sacrum, lumbosacral, and sacroiliac joints; sacrococcygeal junction

    b) Tube tilt about 15° cephalad, but best to check lateral projection and set tilt to make central ray perpendicular to the body of the sacrum

2. Lateral Sacral Projection

    a) Demonstrates sacral body, sacral crest, sacrococcygeal and lumbosacral joints

    b) Mensuration
- in adults, presacral space > 2 cm may indicate soft tissue mass
- in children, normal presacral space approximately 0.5 cm

3. Anteroposterior Coccyx Projection

    a) Demonstrates inferior portion of sacrum, sacral foramina, sacrococcygeal junction, coccygeal cornu

    b) Tilt tube so central ray is perpendicular to ventral surface of coccyx (usually about 10° caudal tilt)

4. Lateral Coccygeal Projection

    a) Central ray through sacrococcygeal junction

    b) Compare two views (seated and recumbent) to show mobility

    c) Significance: hypermobility may be linked to coccygodynia

5. Anteroposterior Pelvis

    a) Demonstrates entire pelvic girdle, including proximal femora

☞   **b)**   Internally rotate feet about 15° to display femoral necks and trochanters

     c)   Mensurations
- symphysis pubis width
  1) measure width midway between superior and inferior margins
  2) normal varies; average approximately 6 mm

☞
- Y-Y line measurements
  1) Y-Y line is a horizontal (transverse) line across the pelvis through the left and right cotyloid notches
  2) this is through the triradiate cartilage at the pelvic brim
  3) gives the baseline for the following measurements
     - acetabular angle: (Fig. 1.16A)
       a. construct Y-Y line
       b. construct line connecting lateral and medial margins of the acetabulum
       c. measure the angles formed by their intersection
       d. average 20° (infants)
     - iliac angle: (Fig. 1.16B)
       a. construct Y-Y line
       b. on each side, make a line tangential to the lateral iliac wing and iliac body margin
       c. measure angle of intersection with Y-Y line

Figure 1.16.

A. Acetabular angle. **B**. Iliac angle. **C**. Epiphyseal relationships. **D**. Diaphyseal interval. **E**. Vertical line of Ombredanne. Reprinted with permission from Yochum TR, Rowe LJ. Essentials of Skeletal Radiology, 2nd ed. Baltimore: Williams & Wilkins, 1996:175–176.

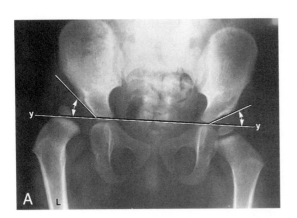

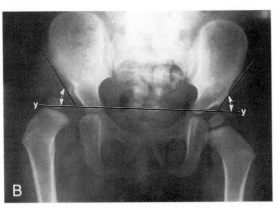

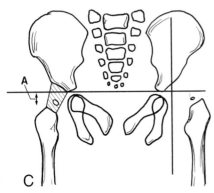

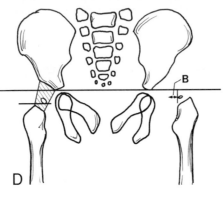

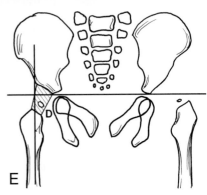

d. normal average in infant: 45–55°

☞ • iliac index:

a. measure iliac angle and acetabular angle (see above)

b. add these four angles together, and divide by 2

c. average in infant: 68–80°

d. < 60°, probable Down's syndrome; 60–68°, possible Down's syndrome; > 68°, Down's syndrome unlikely

• epiphyseal relationships: (Fig. 1.16C)

a. left and right epiphyseal apices should be equally below the Y-Y line

• diaphyseal interval: (Fig. 1.16D)

a. tops of femoral diaphyses should be equally below the Y-Y line, and not < 6 cm below it

• vertical line of Ombredanne: (Fig. 1.16E)

a. construct Y-Y line

b. construct a perpendicular to it through the lateral acetabular margin

c. epiphyseal center should lie medial to the vertical line and below the Y-Y Line

REVIEW—STUDY QUESTIONS

1. Name four skull projections and explain what criteria you would use to take each one.

2. What views comprise a Davis series?

3. What oblique views would you take to demonstrate the left cervical IVFs?

4. List as many mensurations as you can that would be derived from a neutral lateral cervical film.

5. What are the possible contraindications for flexion and extension lateral cervical films?

6. Which cervical films require tube tilt, and what is the tilt required (direction and degree)?

7. Which films are taken on full inspiration, and which are taken on full expiration?

8. Describe patient positioning for a Swimmer's lateral projection.

9. What mensurations may be used to evaluate for lumbar facet imbrication? For hip dysplasia?

10. List as many mensurations as you can that might be derived from a lateral lumbar film.

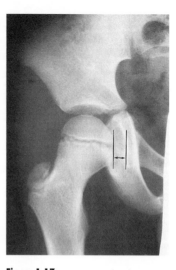

11. Describe the Cobb method of scoliosis measurement and tell why it is preferred.

12. Explain the uses of the Y-Y line in evaluation of the infant hip.

G. FULL SPINE

1. Anteroposterior Full Spine Projection

a) Used for postural evaluation, not assessment for pathology

b) Optimum TFD = 84" (200 cm)

c) Filtration of upper third of film essential

d) Gonadal shielding required

2. Lateral Full Spine Projection

a) For postural assessment only

H. ACETABULAR JOINT

 ### 1. Anteroposterior Hip Projection

a) Demonstrates acetabular joint and proximal femur, especially femoral neck and greater trochanter

b) Foot is internally rotated 15° (as for AP Pelvis)

c) Children under 12: do both hips and compare

d) Mensuration

  • teardrop distance (Fig. 1.17)
    1) medial margin of femoral head should not be > 11 mm from lateral pelvic teardrop margin
    2) teardrop distance should be bilaterally nearly equal, not > 2 mm larger on one side than on the other

  • hip joint space width: (Fig. 1.18)
    1) three distances measured: acetabular surface to femoral head surface at the superior joint, the medial joint, and the acetabular notch (axial space)
    2) superior and axial spaces average about 4 mm; medial space about twice as wide

  • acetabular depth: (Fig. 1.19)
    1) construct a straight line from superior-medial angle of the pubis to the lateral acetabular margin
    2) measure the greatest height from this to the acetabulum
    3) average is about 12 mm: < 9 mm is dysplastic and may lead to DJD of the hip

Figure 1.17.

Teardrop distance, normal. Reprinted with permission from Yochum TR, Rowe LJ. Essentials of Skeletal Radiology, 2nd ed. Baltimore: Williams & Wilkins, 1996:172.

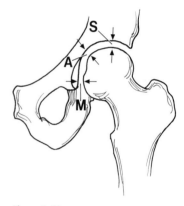

Figure 1.18.

Hip joint space widths. S = Superior, A = Axial, M = Medial. Reprinted with permission from Yochum TR, Rowe LJ. Essentials of Skeletal Radiology, 2nd ed. Baltimore: Williams & Wilkins, 1996:173.

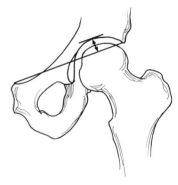

Figure 1.19.

Acetabular depth. Reprinted with permission from Yochum TR, Rowe LJ. Essentials of Skeletal Radiology, 2nd ed. Baltimore: Williams & Wilkins, 1996:173.

- center-edge (CE) angle (of Wiberg): (Fig. 1.20)
    1) construct a vertical line through the center of the femoral head
    2) construct a second line from the femoral head center to the lateral acetabular margin
    3) measure the resulting angle
    4) average is about 36°: shallow angle may indicate acetabular dysplasia, predisposing to hip DJD

- parallelogram of Kopitz
    1) four points are connected horizontally and vertically to form a parallelogram: the lateral and medial acetabular margins, and the lateral and medial margins of the proximal femoral diaphysis
    2) normally, the corners form approximately 90° angles

- pivot point interval
    1) the apex of the epiphysis should not be > 16 mm from the floor of the acetabulum

- Kohler's line: (Fig. 1.21)
    1) construct a straight line tangential to the lateral margin of the obturator foramen and the cortical margin of the pelvic inlet
    2) acetabular floor should not cross this line, should lie lateral to it
    3) significance: protrusio acetabuli assessment

- Shenton's line: (Fig. 1.22)
    1) curvilinear line follows inferior margin of superior pubic ramus and inferomedial surface of femoral neck
    2) disruption of smooth, unbroken curve may indicate slipped femoral capital epiphysis, femoral dislocation, or fracture

- iliofemoral line: (Fig. 1.23)
    1) trace the lateral margins of the ilium and femoral neck
    2) should be smooth (small bulge for femoral head is normal) and bilaterally symmetrical
    3) same assessments and significance as with Shenton's line

- femoral (neck) angle (of incidence): (Fig. 1.24)
    1) also called Mikulicz's angle
    2) straight lines constructed along the long axis of the femoral neck and long axis of the femoral shaft

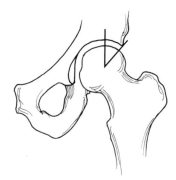

Figure 1.20.

Center-edge angle (CE angle of Wiberg). Reprinted with permission from Yochum TR, Rowe LJ. Essentials of Skeletal Radiology, 2nd ed. Baltimore: Williams & Wilkins, 1996:174.

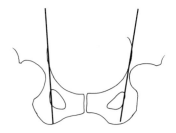

Figure 1.21.

Kohler's line. Reprinted with permission from Yochum TR, Rowe LJ. Essentials of Skeletal Radiology, 2nd ed. Baltimore: Williams & Wilkins, 1996:177.

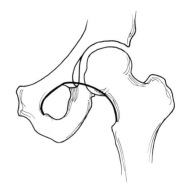

Figure 1.22.

Shenton's line. Reprinted with permission from Yochum TR, Rowe LJ. Essentials of Skeletal Radiology, 2nd ed. Baltimore: Williams & Wilkins, 1996:177.

3) their angle of intersection measured

4) normal: 120–130°

5) significance: < 120° indicates coxa vara; > 130° indicates coxa valga

6) N.B., films taken without 15° internal rotation of the limb (toes in) give an inaccurate angle

☞ • Skinner's line: (Fig. 1.25)

1) first line is constructed along the long axis of the femoral shaft

2) a true perpendicular to this line is constructed tangential to the superior margin of the greater trochanter

3) normally, this second line intersects the acetabular rim at or below the fovea capitus (screens for fracture, or coxa vara of any etiology)

☞ • Klein's line: (Fig. 1.26)

1) line tangential to superolateral femoral neck margin should intersect a small portion of the femoral head

2) degree of overlap should be bilaterally equal

3) significance: slipped femoral capital epiphysis assessment

☞ **2. Frog-Leg Projection**

a) Demonstrates acetabular joint, proximal femur, lesser trochanter

b) Hip flexed 90° and fully abducted; or **Appa's view:** standing frog leg

c) Mensurations

• Shenton's line and Klein's line are evaluated in this view (see AP hip mensurations)

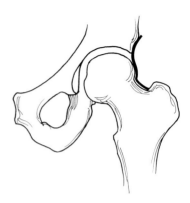

Figure 1.23.

Iliofemoral line. Reprinted with permission from Yochum TR, Rowe LJ. Essentials of Skeletal Radiology, 2nd ed. Baltimore: Williams & Wilkins, 1996:178.

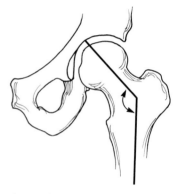

Figure 1.24.

Femoral neck angle. Reprinted with permission from Yochum TR, Rowe LJ. Essentials of Skeletal Radiology, 2nd ed. Baltimore: Williams & Wilkins, 1996:178.

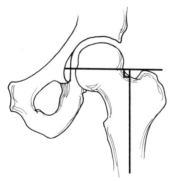

Figure 1.25.

Skinner's line. Reprinted with permission from Yochum TR, Rowe LJ. Essentials of Skeletal Radiology, 2nd ed. Baltimore: Williams & Wilkins, 1996:179.

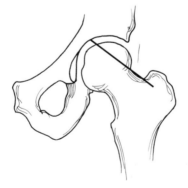

Figure 1.26.

Klein's line. Reprinted with permission from Yochum TR, Rowe LJ. Essentials of Skeletal Radiology, 2nd ed. Baltimore: Williams & Wilkins, 1996:179.

I. KNEE

☞ **1. Anteroposterior Knee Projection**

  a) Demonstrates femorotibial joint, patella

  b) 5° cephalad tube tilt to make central ray tangential to superior tibial surface

  c) Leg should be in slight internal rotation for true anteroposterior knee position

  d) For evaluation of joint narrowing/instability: take PA upright film with knee flexed about 45° and a caudal tube tilt of about 10°

  e) Mensurations
   • femoral angle of the knee: (Fig. 1.27)
    1) angle formed by intersection of femoral shaft long axis and a line tangential to both femoral condyles' articular surfaces
    2) normal is between 75–85°
   • tibial angle: (Fig. 1.28)
    1) angle formed by intersection of tibial shaft long axis line and a line tangential to the anterosuperior margins of both tibial plateaus
    2) normal is between 85–100°
   • "Q" angle: (Fig. 1.29)
    1) angle formed by intersection of a line from the ASIS to the center of the patella, and a line from the tibial tubercle to the center of the patella
    2) normal range: 15–20°; > 20° is patellar malalignment

☞ **2. Lateral Knee Projection**

  a) Demonstrates patellofemoral joint, femoral condyles, tibial tuberosity, patellar fat pads

  b) To superimpose femoral condyles use 5° cephalic tube tilt

  c) Lateral knee is against film, and knee is flexed about 45°

  d) For true lateral, posterior surface of buttocks must be perpendicular to film

  e) Mensuration
   • patellar position (patella alta evaluation)
    1) length of patella from superoposterior pole to anteroinferior pole should be roughly equal to distance from inferior surface of patella to tibial tuberosity (length of infrapatellar tendon)
    2) if tendon is > 20% longer, it indicates patella alta, which predisposes to chondromalacia patellae

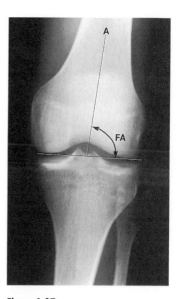

Figure 1.27.
Femoral angle of the knee. Reprinted with permission from Yochum TR, Rowe LJ. Essentials of Skeletal Radiology, 2nd ed. Baltimore: Williams & Wilkins, 1996:180.

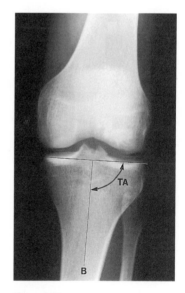

Figure 1.28.
Tibial angle. Reprinted with permission from Yochum TR, Rowe LJ. Essentials of Skeletal Radiology, 2nd ed. Baltimore: Williams & Wilkins, 1996:180.

3)   if tendon is shortened, it indicates patella baja, which occurs in achondroplasia, polio, JRA, tibia tubercle transposition

 3. Tunnel Knee Projection (Intercondylar Projection)

a)   Demonstrates femorotibial joint

b)   Knee flexed about 45° (this is a PA projection, performed two ways)

- patient prone with thigh on table, support leg to maintain 45° flexion; 45° caudal tube tilt

- patient kneeling with leg on table, leaning forward until anterior thigh is at about 45° angle from horizontal; no tube tilt; central ray enters at approximately 45° caudal angle

 4. Tangential Knee Projection (Skyline or Sunrise Projection)

a)   Demonstrates patellar position, patellofemoral joint, retropatellar surface

b)   Patient prone with knee in full flexion

c)   Tube tilt 10° cephalad

d)   Central ray forms a 45° angle with long axis of the tibia

e)   Mensurations

- patellar apex

1)   apex should align directly above lowest point of intercondylar sulcus

- sulcus angle: (Fig. 1.30)

1)   intersecting angle of lines from the center of the sulcus to highest point on lateral and medial surfaces of groove

2)   angle should be between 132–144°

3)   shallow groove indicates instability

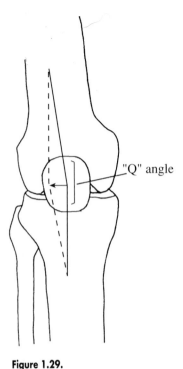

Figure 1.29.

"Q" angle. Modified from Kessler JA. Management of Common Musculoskeletal Disorders. New York: Harper & Rowe, 1983:440.

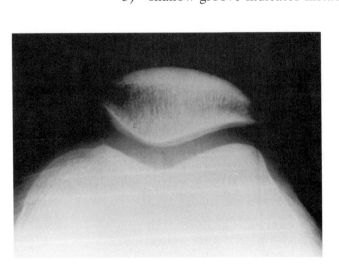

Figure 1.30.

Sulcus angle. Reprinted with permission from Yochum TR, Rowe LJ. Essentials of Skeletal Radiology, 2nd ed. Baltimore: Williams & Wilkins, 1996:181.

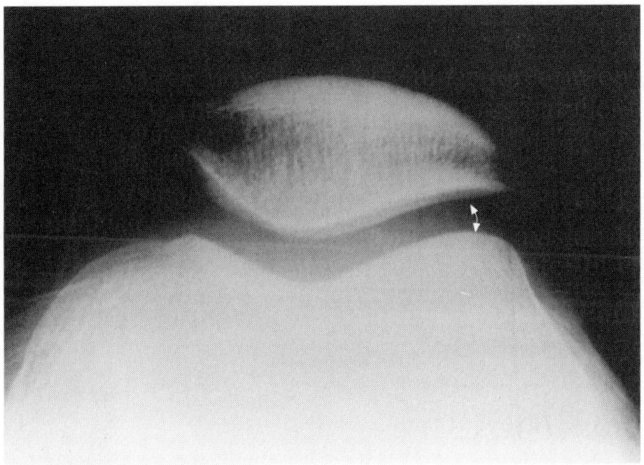

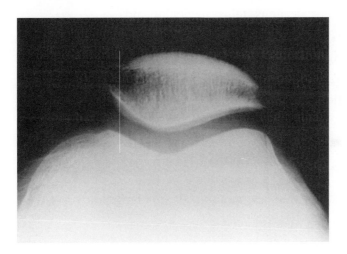

Figure 1.31.
Lateral patellofemoral angle. Reprinted with permission from Yochum TR, Rowe LJ. Essentials of Skeletal Radiology, 2nd ed. Baltimore: Williams & Wilkins, 1996:181.

- lateral patellofemoral joint index
    1) narrowest medial joint width should be smaller than or equal to the narrowest lateral joint width
    2) significance: medial width enlarged in chondromalacia
- lateral patellofemoral angle: (Fig. 1.31)
    1) line tangential to lateral patellar facet intersects line tangential to highest margins of femoral condyles
    2) angle should open laterally
- lateral patellar displacement: (Fig. 1.32)
    1) line drawn tangential to highest margins of femoral condyles
    2) line perpendicular to this is constructed at medial lip of the intercondylar sulcus: should be 1 mm or less medial to medial patellar margin

Figure 1.32.
Lateral patellar displacement. Reprinted with permission from Yochum TR, Rowe LJ. Essentials of Skeletal Radiology, 2nd ed. Baltimore: Williams & Wilkins, 1996:181.

J. ANKLE

 1. Anteroposterior Ankle Projection

    a) Demonstrates talar mortise joint, lateral and medial malleoli

    b) Foot in slight dorsiflexion, slight internal rotation, to have plantar surface perpendicular to film and intermalleolar line parallel to film

    c) Mensurations

      • tibial angle: (Fig. 1.33)

        1) formed by intersection of a line tangential to the talar dome's articular surface, and a line tangential to the articular surface of the medial malleolus

        2) should be between 45° and 65°

      • fibular angle: (Fig. 1.34)

        1) formed by intersection of a line tangential to articular surface of the talar dome and one tangential to the articular surface of the lateral malleolus

        2) should be between 43° and 63°

 2. Medial Oblique Ankle Projection

    a) Demonstrates talar dome and head, sinus tarsi, calcaneus' anterior tubercle, fifth metatarsal base, talonavicular joint, distal fibula, distal posterior tibia

    b) Foot is in slight dorsiflexion and internal rotation to produce about 45° angle between intermalleolar line and film surface

3. Lateral Ankle Projection

    a) Demonstrates tibiotalar joint, posterior tibial malleolus, calcaneus, talus, navicular and cuboid

    b) Foot slightly dorsiflexed

    c) Mensurations (see lateral calcaneus projection)

K. FOOT

1. Dorsiplantar Foot Projection

    a) Demonstrates tarsals, metatarsals, phalanges

    b) 10° cephalic tube tilt

    c) Compensatory filter for distal foot

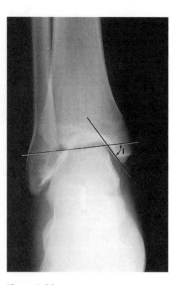

Figure 1.33.
Tibial angle. Reprinted with permission from Yochum TR, Rowe LJ. Essentials of Skeletal Radiology, 2nd ed. Baltimore: Williams & Wilkins, 1996:182.

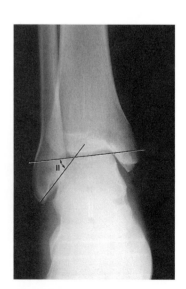

Figure 1.34.
Fibular angle. Reprinted with permission from Yochum TR, Rowe LJ. Essentials of Skeletal Radiology, 2nd ed. Baltimore: Williams & Wilkins, 1996:182.

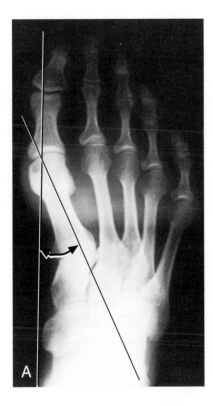 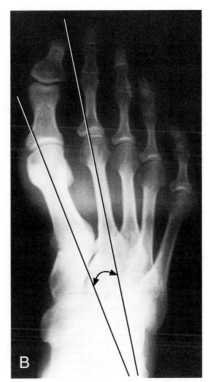 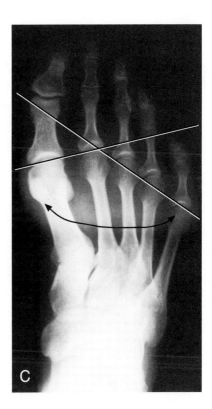

d) Mensurations
- hallux abductus angle: (Fig. 1.35A)
  1) angle at junction of axial shaft of first metatarsal and axial shaft of proximal phalanx of first digit
  2) should not be > 15°
- intermetatarsal angle: (Fig. 1.35B)
  1) angle between axial shafts of first and second metatarsals
  2) should not be > 14°
- metatarsal angle: (Fig. 1.35C)
  1) line constructed tangential to distal articular surfaces of first and second metatarsals
  2) second line tangential to distal articular surfaces of second and fifth metatarsals
  3) angle of intersection should be around 140°

Figure 1.35.

A. Hallux abductus angle. *B*. Inter-metatarsal angle. *C*. Metatarsal angle. Reprinted with permission from Yochum TR, Rowe LJ. Essentials of Skeletal Radiology, 2nd ed. Baltimore: Williams & Wilkins, 1996:79.

2. **Medial Oblique Foot Projection**
   a) Demonstrates tarsals, calcaneocuboid joint, metatarsal bases, tarso-metatarsal joints, phalanges, intertarsal joints
   b) 10° cephalad tube tilt
   c) Foot tilted medially so plantar surface forms about 35° angle with film surface

3. **Lateral Foot Projection**
   a) Demonstrates calcaneus, talus, navicular, cuboid, fifth metatarsal and their interarticulations

b) Plantar surface should be perpendicular to film, lateral foot abuts film

c) Mensurations
- heel pad thickness
    1) distance from most inferior point of calcaneus to skin surface directly below it
    2) average 19 mm
    3) > 25 mm may indicate acromegaly
- Achilles tendon thickness
    1) measure thickness of tendon 1–2 cm above calcaneus
    2) normally 4–8 mm
    3) thickened by edema or inflammation
- Boehler's angle (tuber angle): (Fig. 1.36)
    1) connect highest point of calcaneus with superoanterior margin, extending the line posteriorly
    2) connect highest point of calcaneus with its superoposterior margin
    3) posterior angle of intersection averages 30–35°
    4) < 28° is abnormal: usually indicates fractured calcaneus

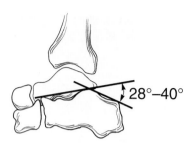

Figure 1.36.
Boehler's angle. Reprinted with permission from Yochum TR, Rowe LJ. Essentials of Skeletal Radiology, 2nd ed. Baltimore: Williams & Wilkins, 1996:183.

L. TOES

1. Dorsiplantar Toes Projection

a) Displays interphalangeal and metatarsophalangeal joints

b) Improved detail for specific site evaluation

2. Oblique Toes Projection

a) Displays metatarsophalangeal joints with improved detail

b) Pronate foot so plantar surface is at about 45° angle to film surface

c) For detail of lateral digits, supinate to about 45°

M. CALCANEUS

1. Axial Calcaneus Projection

a) Demonstrates body and posterior margins of calcaneus

b) Posterior heel against film, slight dorsiflexion brings plantar surface perpendicular to film surface

c) About 35–40° cephalad tube tilt

2. Lateral Calcaneus Projection

a) Demonstrates subtalar joints, Achilles tendon

b) Mensurations: see lateral foot projection

N. SHOULDER

☞ **1. Anteroposterior Internal Rotation Projection**

    a) Displays proximal humerus, anterior glenohumeral and acromioclavicular joints

    b) Patient rotated to 30° angle with bucky, so shoulder is flush with film surface

    c) With elbow extended, rotate internally to have intraepicondylar line perpendicular to film

    d) alternatively: with elbow flexed 90°, rest forearm over abdomen

☞ **2. Anteroposterior External Rotation Projection**

    a) Displays greater tuberosity, glenohumeral and acromioclavicular joints

    b) Patient's back is at about 30° angle to bucky

    c) Arm externally rotated so interepicondylar line is perpendicular to film

    d) Mensurations

      • acromiohumeral joint space

        1) measure space between inferior margin of acromion and apex of humerus

        2) normal is 7–11 mm

        3) decreased in rotator cuff tear or tendinitis

        4) increased in stroke, brachial plexus lesions, dislocation

      • acromioclavicular joint space: (Fig. 1.37)

        1) measure AC joint space at superior and inferior margins and average the two numbers

        2) males average 2.5–4.1 mm; females average 2.1–3.7 mm

        3) decreased in DJD

        4) increased in trauma, osteolysis (caused by RA, hyperparathyroid)

        5) compare right to left and weighted to nonweighted

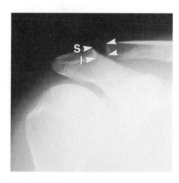

Figure 1.37.

Acromioclavicular joint space. Reprinted with permission from Yochum TR, Rowe LJ. Essentials of Skeletal Radiology, 2nd ed. Baltimore: Williams & Wilkins, 1996:185.

3. Anteroposterior Abduction Shoulder Projection (Baby Arm Projection)

    a) Demonstrates coracoid and acromion, acromioclavicular joint, distal clavicle

    b) Arm is abducted 90°, elbow flexed 90°

4. Posteroanterior Clavicle Projection

    a) Demonstrates clavicle, upper ribs

    b) PA: 10° caudal tube tilt, head rotated to contralateral side

    c) AP: 10° cephalad tube tilt

5. **Anteroposterior Acromioclavicular Projection**

   a) Demonstrates acromioclavicular joint in detail for evaluation of acromioclavicular and coracoclavicular ligament integrity

   b) Two films taken: with and without weights

   c) 5° cephalad tube tilt

   d) Mensuration: see External Shoulder Rotation Projection

O. ELBOW

1. **Anteroposterior Elbow Projection**

   a) Demonstrates radiohumeral, humeroulnar, and proximal radioulnar joints

   b) If arm cannot be fully extended, requires 2 AP views: one with humerus lying on film and one with forearm lying on film

   c) Decrease radiation to patient by having lead vinyl beneath cassette

   d) Mensurations
   • carrying angle: (Fig. 1.38)
     1) line along axial shaft of humerus (humeral shaft line) intersects line along axial shaft of ulna (ulnar shaft line)
     2) the lateral angle of their intersection is measured
     3) norms: 154–178°
   • humeral angle: (Fig. 1.39)
     1) humeral shaft line intersects a transverse line tangential to the most distal surfaces of the capitellum and trochlea (humeral articular line)
     2) their proximal medial angle of intersection is measured
     3) norms: 72–95°
   • ulnar angle: (Fig. 1.40)
     1) distal medial angle of intersection of humeral articular line and ulnar shaft line is measured
     2) norms: 72–99°

2. **Medial Oblique Elbow Projection**

   a) Demonstrates radial head, ulnar coronoid process, medial epicondyle

   b) Arm extended, forearm pronated on the film

3. **Lateral Elbow Projection**

   a) Demonstrates proximal radius, ulna; distal humerus; pericapsular and supinator fat lines

   b) Best visualization of radial head, capitellum, and coronoid process: tilt tube 45 degrees toward radial head

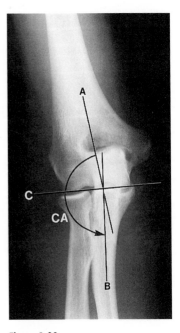

Figure 1.38.
Carrying angle. Reprinted with permission from Yochum TR, Rowe LJ. Essentials of Skeletal Radiology, 2nd ed. Baltimore: Williams & Wilkins, 1996:186.

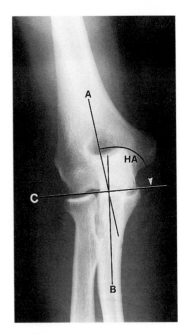

Figure 1.39.
Humeral angle. Reprinted with permission from Yochum TR, Rowe LJ. Essentials of Skeletal Radiology, 2nd ed. Baltimore: Williams & Wilkins, 1996:186.

c) Elbow flexed 90°, ulnar forearm on film (hand pronated), humerus parallel to film

d) Mensuration
- radiocapitellar line
  1) line through long axis of radius should intersect center of capitellum

4. Tangential Elbow Projection (Jones Projection)

a) Demonstrates radial head, olecranon, trochlea, ulnar groove, olecranon-trochanteric joint

b) Humerus parallel to film, elbow in full flexion

c) Central ray perpendicular to humerus, 2 inches proximal to olecranon tip

P. WRIST

 1. Posteroanterior Wrist Projection

a) Displays carpal joints, distal radio-ulnar joint, radiocarpal and ulnocarpal joints

b) Wrist pronated flat on film, fist loosely closed

c) Better view of scapholunate joint with 10° lateral tube tilt toward radius

d) Relatively smooth arcs should be seen at:
- proximal scaphoid, lunate, triquetrum surface
- distal scaphoid, lunate, triquetrum surface
- proximal capitate, hamate surface

e) Mensuration
- radioulnar angle: (Fig. 1.41)
  1) line through axial shaft of radius intersects line from distal radial styloid tip to ulnar styloid base
  2) proximal lateral angle formed should be 72–95°

 2. Posteroanterior Ulnar Flexion Wrist Projection

a) Demonstrates scaphoid for optimal fracture evaluation

b) Wrist pronated on film in full ulnar deviation

3. Medial Oblique Wrist Projection

a) Demonstrates radiocarpal, ulnocarpal joints

b) Semipronated wrist; dorsum at 45° angle to film

4. Lateral Wrist Projection

a) Displays carpal (particularly lunate) alignment, especially in relationship to distal radius

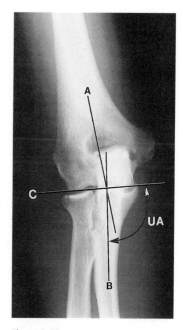

Figure 1.40.

Ulnar angle. Reprinted with permission from Yochum TR, Rowe LJ. Essentials of Skeletal Radiology, 2nd ed. Baltimore: Williams & Wilkins, 1996:186.

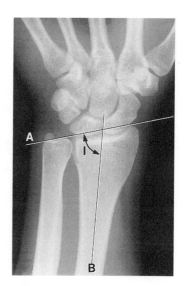

Figure 1.41.

Radioulnar angle. Reprinted with permission from Yochum TR, Rowe LJ. Essentials of Skeletal Radiology, 2nd ed. Baltimore: Williams & Wilkins, 1996:187.

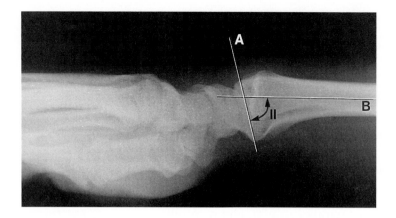

Figure 1.42.

Lateral radius angle. Reprinted with permission from Yochum TR, Rowe LJ. Essentials of Skeletal Radiology, 2nd ed. Baltimore: Williams & Wilkins, 1996:187.

    b)   Mensuration
- lateral radius angle: (Fig. 1.42)
    1) a line tangential to most distal radial cortex (Radius Articular Line)
    2) a line along axial radial shaft (Radial Shaft Line)
    3) the palmar proximal angle formed by their intersection is measured
    4) norms: 79–94°

Q. HAND

1. Posteroanterior Hand Projection

    a)   Displays carpals, metacarpals, phalanges

    b)   Mensuration
- metacarpal sign
    1) a straight line tangential to both fourth and fifth metacarpal heads
    2) line should touch or pass distal to third metacarpal head
    3) significance: intersection of third metacarpal head occurs in Turner syndrome (gonadal dysgenesis) or in traumatic injury

2. Oblique Hand Projection

    a)   Depicts traumatic lesions of metacarpals

    b)   Hand semipronated to 45°, fingers lightly flexed

3. Lateral Finger Projection

    a)   PA, oblique, and lateral films done as for hands, with central ray and collimation adjusted

R. THUMB

1. Anteroposterior Thumb

    a)   Displays phalanges, first metacarpal, trapezium, and scaphoid and their articulations

    b)   Patient sits with back to film, rotates arm internally until posterior surface of thumb lies on horizontal film

    2. Lateral Thumb

        a) Displays first metacarpophalangeal joint

        b) Hand prone with metacarpophalangeal joints slightly flexed to bring thumb to true lateral position

        c) Oblique projection is optional

S. RIBS

1. Anteroposterior Rib Projection

    a) Demonstrates posterior rib lesion

2. Posteroanterior Rib Projection

    a) Demonstrates anterior rib lesion

3. Anterior or Posterior Oblique Rib Projection

    a) Lesion should be centered against bucky

    b) On all rib projections: for lesions above diaphragm, film should be taken on suspended full inspiration, for lesions below diaphragm, suspended full exhalation

T. CHEST

1. Posteroanterior Chest Projection

    a) Depicts lung fields, heart, great vessels, ribs, diaphragms

    b) Full inspiration

    c) Should display 10 posterior and seven anterior ribs

    d) Full exhalation useful for visualizing pneumothorax

2. Lateral Chest Projection

    a) Depicts retrosternal space

    b) Left lateral is standard, to minimize cardiac magnification

3. Lordotic Projection

    a) Displays lung apices, middle lobe and lingula

    b) Patient fully upright: tube tilt 30° cephalad

    c) Patient standing about a foot in front of bucky, leaning back to press head, neck and upper thoracic spine against bucky; no tube tilt

U. ABDOMEN

1. Anteroposterior Projection; Kidneys, Ureter, Bladder (KUB)

    a) Scout film, to display soft tissue shadows of abdominal organs and look for evidence of stone formation.

    b) With very obese patients, PA works better to compress fat mass

REVIEW—STUDY QUESTIONS

1. Explain patient positioning for an AP Hip Projection, and why it must be done accurately.

2. What is the optimal view when a scaphoid fracture is suspected?

3. Describe the views taken to rule out damaged acromioclavicular ligaments.

4. Explain positioning and breathing instructions for films examining rib trauma.

5. List four basic elbow projections, explain the positioning for each.

6. What modification is necessary for an AP Elbow projection if the patient cannot extend the elbow?

7. Name and describe four projections for examining the knee, and the what each of these best displays.

8. How is the clavicle best viewed? (Describe two alternatives.)

9. Name and describe at least six mensurations that can be derived from an AP Hip film.

10. Describe two ways to take a "Lordotic" Chest Projection.

1. All the following are true about an AP full spine projection except:

    a) Gonadal shielding is required.
    b) The film must be taken non-bucky.
    c) There must be filtration of the upper third of the film.
    d) This projection is not suitable for assessment for pathology.

2. All the following are used in evaluating for slipped femoral capital epiphysis except:

    a) Klein's line.
    b) Skinner's line.
    c) iliofemoral line.
    d) Shenton's line.

3. The angle formed by the intersection of the femoral shaft's long axis and a line tangential to the articular surfaces of both femoral condyles is the:

    a) "Q" angle.
    b) tibial angle.
    c) femoral angle of the knee.
    d) condylar angle.

4. Evaluation of the acromioclavicular joint is optimal with:

    a) bilateral, weighted and non-weighted AP acromioclavicular projections.
    b) weighted PA clavicle projections.
    c) an anteroposterior abduction shoulder projection.
    d) weighted and non-weighted AP internal rotation shoulder projections.

5. The dorsiplantar foot projection requires:

    a) 10° caudal tube tilt.
    b) no tube tilt.
    c) 10° cephalic tube tilt.
    d) 20° cephalic tube tilt.

6. In the lumbar spine, the normal canal/body ratio should be equal to or greater than:

    a) 1:2
    b) 1:4
    c) 2:3
    d) 1:3

7. A right posterior oblique lumbar projection will display:

    a) left pars interarticularis and the right facets.
    b) left pars interarticularis and the left facets.
    c) right pars interarticularis and the right facets.
    d) right pars interarticularis and the left facets.

8. The Method of Bull is a means of evaluating:

    a) the lumbar lordosis.
    b) scoliosis.
    c) the cervical curve.
    d) odontoid malposition.

9. The best way to see the lumbosacral joint clearly in a coronal plane is:

    a) via an AP sacral projection with 15° caudal tube tilt.
    b) via an AP sacral projection with 45° cephalic tube tilt.
    c) via an AP projection with a caudal tube tilt set to make the central ray perpendicular to the sacral body.
    d) via an AP projection with a cephalad tube tilt set to make the central ray perpendicular to the sacral body.

10. The preferred method for measuring a scoliosis is:

    a) the Risser-Ferguson method.
    b) the method of Jochumsen.
    c) Drexler's method.
    d) the Cobb-Libman method.

11. For a full spine AP projection, the optimum TFD is:

    a) 200 centimeters.
    b) 82 inches.
    c) 72 inches.
    d) 300 centimeters.

12. On an AP hip projection, Shenton's line is useful in evaluating for all of the following except:

    a) fracture.
    b) slipped femoral capital epiphysis.
    c) degenerative arthritis of the hip.
    d) femoral dislocation.

13. The normal femoral angle of the knee should be:

    a) between 75 and 85°.
    b) between 90 and 100°.
    c) between 60 and 75°.
    d) between 56 and 60°.

14. A posteroanterior clavicle projection is not:

    a) taken with a 10° caudal tube tilt.
    b) sometimes taken as an AP, with a 10° cephalad tube tilt.
    c) taken with the head rotated to the contralateral side.
    d) taken during active respiration.

15. In addition to an AP projection, a study of the ankle requires a medial oblique projection to:

    a) better visualize the medial malleolus.
    b) better visualize the mortise joint.
    c) better visualize the talar dome and head.
    d) better visualize the metatarsal heads.

16. Interpediculate distance may be increased by:

    a) intraspinal neoplasms.
    b) spinal stenosis.
    c) congenital malformations.
    d) arthritides.

17. Using Eisenstein's sagittal canal measurement, spinal stenosis may be indicated by a measurement of:

    a) < 25 mm.
    b) < 20 mm.
    c) < 18 mm.
    d) < 15 mm.

18. When evaluating a lateral cervical projection, pharyngeal prevertebral soft tissue at the C2 level should be no wider than:

    a) 20 mm.
    b) 7 mm.
    c) 4 mm.
    d) 10 mm.

19. All the following statements about scoliosis are true except:

    a) Any curves > 40° must be braced.
    b) When there is a double curve, each component must be measured separately.
    c) It is important to use the same landmarks each time the curve is evaluated.
    d) Baseline films must include both the upper and lower extremities of the curve.

20. A decreased Boehler's angle indicates:

    a) impaction fracture of the calcaneus.
    b) platybasia.
    c) genu varum.
    d) genu valgum.

21. There is a strong likelihood of Down's syndrome if the iliac index of an infant is:

    a) < 60°.
    b) > 60°.
    c) > 68°.
    d) Down's syndrome is apparent at birth, and the iliac index has no relationship to its diagnosis.

22. Kohler's line is constructed:

    a) along the inferior margin of the superior pubic ramus and inferomedial femoral neck.
    b) tangential to the superolateral and inferolateral acetabular margins.
    c) tangential to the superior margin of the femoral neck.
    d) tangential to the lateral obturator foramen and the cortical margin of the pelvic inlet.

23. The AP knee projection is modified by taking it upright, with the knee flexed 45° and with a 10° caudal tube tilt, to evaluate for:

    a) chondromalacia patella.
    b) osteochondritis dissecans.
    c) joint instability.
    d) ochronosis.

24. The " baby arm projection" is:

    a) performed with the arm abducted 90° and the elbow flexed 90°.

    b) taken to demonstrate the complex interconnections of the elbow.
    c) another name for an AP internal rotation shoulder projection.
    d) another name for a lateral elbow projection.

25. At the ankle, the tibial angle and the fibular angle should each measure:

    a) between 60 and 80°.
    b) between 10 and 15°.
    c) between 23 and 45°.
    d) between 43 and 65°.

26. The structures that form the Hadley's "S" curve are:

    a) the transverse process, inferior articular process, and superior articular process.
    b) the transverse process, inferior articular process, and mammillary process.
    c) the inferior articular process, mammillary process, and superior articular process.
    d) the transverse process, mammillary process, and superior articular process.

27. Meyerding's spondylolisthesis grading is reported with reference to:

    a) quarters of the subadjacent vertebral body endplate.
    b) percentages of the subadjacent vertebral body endplate.
    c) millimeters of anterior translation.
    d) inches of anterior translation.

28. Towne's projection requires a:

    a) 35° caudal tube tilt.
    b) 15° caudal tube tilt.
    c) 35° cephalad tube tilt.
    d) 15° cephalad tube tilt.

29. A patient with scoliosis should be monitored:

    a) every 6 months until age 40, because the curve can continue to progress after the growth years.
    b) with an AP film done every 3 months during the years of rapid growth.
    c) every 3 months, until age 18.
    d) at least once a year, with upright AP and lateral views.

30. Macnab's line:

    a) is usually applied on lateral lumbar films.
    b) requires oblique views.
    c) is used to evaluate lumbar stenosis.
    d) is used to evaluate discogenic spondylosis.

31. On an AP pelvis projection, the iliac angle is measured by the intersection of:

    a) the Y-Y line and a vertical line tangential to the inner acetabular margin.
    b) the Y-Y line and the vertical line of Ombredanne.

c) the Y-Y line and a line tangential to the lateral iliac wing and iliac body margin.

d) the vertical line of Ombredanne and a line tangential to the lateral iliac body margin.

32. Kohler's line is used for the assessment of:

a) retrolisthesis.
b) hip dysplasia.
c) slipped femoral capital epiphysis.
d) protrusio acetabuli.

33. The AP knee projection requires:

a) a cephalad tube tilt of 5°.
b) a 10° cephalad tube tilt.
c) a caudal tube tilt of 5°.
d) no tube tilt.

34. An increased acromioclavicular joint space is likely to be caused by any of the following except:

a) rheumatoid arthritis.
b) degenerative arthritis.
c) hyperparathyroidism.
d) trauma.

35. The sunrise projection allows good evaluation of:

a) patella alta.
b) genu varum.
c) genu valgum.
d) lateral displacement of the patella.

36. Filtration should be used on the lower half of the thoracic spine in a:

a) Swimmer's lateral projection.
b) AP thoracic spine projection.
c) PA chest film.
d) lateral thoracic spine projection.

37. Macnab's line is drawn:

a) through the superior margin of the superior facet and the inferior margin of the inferior facet.
b) tangential to the superior anterior and posterior S1 endplate margins.
c) tangential to the inferior anterior and posterior vertebral endplate margins.
d) tangential to the L5 posterior vertebral body margin.

38. The AP open mouth projection (APOM) best demonstrates:

a) the maxillary sinuses.
b) the integrity of the C1 spinous process.
c) the alignment of the atlas lateral margins with the axis body.
d) a C1 anterolisthesis.

39. Scoliosis may require surgical stabilization if the curve:

a) shows progression within a 6-month period.
b) is at least 15° and progressing.
c) is greater than 40°.
d) is between 20–30°.

40. The most accurate radiographic measurement for evaluating lumbar spinal canal stenosis is:

a) Eisenstein's method.
b) the canal/body ratio.
c) the interpediculate distance.
d) Van Akkerveeken's measurement.

41. The normal acetabular angle for infants averages around:

a) 20°.
b) 10°.
c) 30°.
d) 45°.

42. Acetabular dysplasia may be indicated by:

a) acetabular depth < 9 mm, or a Center-Edge angle < 36°.
b) an iliac index > 68°.
c) an iliac index < 60°.
d) an acetabular angle of 20°, or an iliac angle of 50°.

43. On a frog-leg projection, one can evaluate:

a) Kohler's line and Klein's line.
b) Shenton's line and Kohler's line.
c) Klein's line and Shenton's line.
d) Kohler's line and Skinner's line.

44. Normal acromiohumeral joint space is:

a) 1.5–2.0 cm.
b) 1.0–1.5 cm.
c) 7–11 mm.
d) 12–16 mm.

45. The intercondylar projection is:

a) an AP projection.
b) a lateral projection.
c) a PA projection.
d) done as either a PA or an AP projection.

46. For optimal clarity, an AP projection of the thoracic spine should be made with:

a) filtration on the upper half to two-thirds of the thoracic spine.
b) filtration on the upper third of the thoracic spine.
c) filtration on the lower half of the thoracic spine.
d) filtration of the lower two-thirds of the thoracic spine.

47. The gravitational line from L3 should not:

a) pass through the sacral promontory.
b) pass more than 5 mm anterior to the sacral promontory.
c) pass posterior to the sacral promontory.
d) pass more than 10 mm anterior to the sacral promontory.

48. When preparing to take an AP lower cervical spine (APLC) projection:

a) tilt the tube 15° caudad.
b) tilt the tube 30° cephalad.
c) tilt the tube 15° cephalad.
d) do not tilt the tube.

49. The Cobb (Cobb-Libman) method of scoliosis evaluation requires:
    a) location of the uppermost vertebra that tilts toward the concavity.
    b) location of the vertebra at the apex of the scoliotic curve.
    c) location of the center of the vertebral body at the apex of the scoliotic curve.
    d) location of the center of the lowest vertebral body that is tilted toward the concavity.

50. The left posterior oblique projection of the cervical spine:
    a) shows the right intervertebral foramina.
    b) shows the left intervertebral foramina.
    c) is positioned with the anterior right shoulder against the bucky.
    d) is positioned with the posterior right shoulder against the bucky.

51. Decreased acromiohumeral joint space may indicate:
    a) rotator cuff tear.
    b) stroke.
    c) glenohumeral joint effusion.
    d) brachial plexus lesions.

52. Skinner's line would not be a good indicator of:
    a) femoral neck fracture.
    b) coxa vara.
    c) slipped femoral capital epiphysis.
    d) rheumatoid arthritis of the hip.

53. The Center-Edge (CE) angle is also called:
    a) the Angle of Kopitz.
    b) the Angle of Wiberg.
    c) the iliac angle.
    d) the acetabular angle.

54. The "Y-Y" line (on an AP pelvis projection) is drawn:
    a) horizontally, through both left and right upper, outer, acetabular margins.
    b) horizontally, through the left and right cotyloid notches.
    c) horizontally, above both left and right triradiate cartilages.
    d) horizontally, through the superior margin of the "teardrop."

55. When performing a lateral film of a scoliosis patient, one should:
    a) take a cross-table lateral with the curve concavity adjacent to the bucky.
    b) take a cross-table lateral with the curve convexity adjacent to the bucky.
    c) take an upright lateral with the curve concavity adjacent to the bucky.
    d) take an upright lateral with the curve convexity adjacent to the bucky.

56. Ferguson's gravitational line has not been called:
    a) the gravitational line from L3.
    b) Ferguson's weight-bearing line.
    c) the lumbar gravity line.
    d) Ferguson's vertical line.

57. The articular pillars projection is taken with:
    a) the patient facing the bucky, and the head turned 45–50° away from the side of interest.
    b) the marker beneath the mandible on the side of interest.
    c) a 15° cephalad tube tilt.
    d) a 15° caudal tube tilt.

58. The intercondylar projection is also known as:
    a) the sunrise projection.
    b) the tangential knee projection.
    c) the skyline projection.
    d) the tunnel knee projection.

59. The optimal projection for evaluation of the frontal and maxillary sinuses is:
    a) Towne's projection.
    b) AP open mouth projection.
    c) Water's projection.
    d) Caldwell's projection.

60. PA chest films taken on full exhalation are helpful in visualizing:
    a) atelectasis.
    b) pleural effusions.
    c) apical lesions.
    d) pneumothorax.

61. For AP shoulder projections, either internal or external rotation, the patient should:
    a) have the elbow flexed 90°, with the forearm resting on the abdomen.
    b) stand rotated about 45°, so the shoulder is almost parallel to the surface of the bucky.
    c) maintain the intraepicondylar line in a position perpendicular to the film surface.
    d) maintain the intraepicondylar line in a position parallel to the film surface.

62. The angle of incidence is used in evaluations for:
    a) malum coxae senilis.
    b) protrusio acetabuli.
    c) coxa vara or coxa valga.
    d) Legg-Calvé-Perthes disease.

63. When the acetabular depth of an infant's hip is:
    a) 12 mm, it is considered average.
    b) > 9 mm, it is considered anomalous.
    c) < 9 mm, it is considered average.
    d) 15 mm, it is considered average.

64. Although the range of normal is fairly wide, the symphysis pubis width should average:
    a) about 6 mm.
    b) about 3 cm.
    c) about 6 cm.
    d) about 1 inch.

65. To obtain a clearer view of a questionable area involving sacroiliac joint, one may take:

    a) an AP tilt-up lumbosacral spot projection.
    b) a lateral lumbosacral spot projection.
    c) an oblique sacroiliac joint projection.
    d) a frog-leg projection.

66. A normal sacral base angle might be:

    a) about 45°.
    b) about 15°.
    c) about 145°.
    d) about 120°.

67. When taking a cervical posterior oblique projection, place the marker:

    a) behind the spine.
    b) at the top left corner of the film.
    c) under the mandible.
    d) at the top right corner of the film.

68. Patella alta is evaluated on the:

    a) AP knee projection.
    b) sunrise projection.
    c) lateral knee projection.
    d) tunnel knee projection.

69. Radiographic evaluation for platybasia may involve all the following except:

    a) Ullmann's line.
    b) Macrae's line.
    c) Chamberlain's line.
    d) digastric (biventer) line.

70. For rib projections:

    a) respiration should always be suspended with full inspiration.
    b) respiration should always be suspended with full expiration.
    c) for lesions below the diaphragm, respiration should be suspended on full inspiration.
    d) for lesions above the diaphragm, respiration should be suspended on full inspiration.

71. Boehler's angle helps to rule out:

    a) heel spurs.
    b) calcaneal fracture.
    c) occult fracture of the talar dome.
    d) occult fracture of the distal fibula.

72. On an AP hip projection, constructing lines along the axis of the femoral neck and shaft will provide:

    a) the angle of Wiberg.
    b) Mikulicz's angle.
    c) the "Q" angle.
    d) the acetabular angle.

73. When hip joint space is measured, the distance from the acetabular surface to the acetabular notch is:

    a) called the superior joint space.
    b) called the medial joint space.
    c) called the axial joint space.
    d) not measured.

74. To adequately demonstrate the femoral neck and trochanters on an AP pelvis projection:

    a) internally rotate the feet about 15°.
    b) externally rotate the feet about 15°.
    c) internally rotate the feet about 30°.
    d) externally rotate the feet about 30°.

75. A break in the normally smooth Hadley's "S" curve may indicate:

    a) osteomalacia.
    b) osteoporosis.
    c) facet imbrication.
    d) fibrous dysplasia.

76. Ferguson's angle is:

    a) the sacral base angle.
    b) the sacrovertebral angle.
    c) the lumbosacral disc angle.
    d) the sacrovertebral disc angle.

77. Oblique cervical projections are used to demonstrate all of the following except:

    a) integrity of the cervical pillars.
    b) integrity of the intervertebral foramina.
    c) degeneration of the facet joints.
    d) degeneration of the neurocentral joints.

78. Patellar malalignment can be evaluated with the:

    a) carrying angle.
    b) "Q" angle.
    c) femoral angle of the knee.
    d) tibial angle.

79. Steele's Rule of Thirds is helpful in the evaluation of:

    a) lumbar intervertebral disc diminution.
    b) lumbar stenosis caused by retrolisthesis.
    c) prevertebral soft tissue swellings.
    d) atlantoaxial subluxation.

80. The metacarpal sign is positive when a straight line tangential to both fourth and fifth metacarpal heads:

    a) passes distal to the third metacarpal head.
    b) passes < 3 mm distal to the third metacarpal head.
    c) passes through or proximal to the third metacarpal head.
    d) passes tangential to the third metacarpal head.

81. The average normal heel pad thickness is about:

    a) 2.5 cm.
    b) 19 mm.
    c) 1 cm.
    d) 5 mm.

82. Mikulicz's angle:

    a) must be derived from films taken without internal rotation of the lower limb.
    b) is normally < 120°.
    c) may indicate coxa valga or coxa vara.
    d) is also called the "Q" angle.

83. The bilateral variation in teardrop distance should not exceed:

    a) 5 mm.
    b) 2 mm.
    c) 11 mm.
    d) 1 cm.

84. The lateral coccygeal projection should be taken both seated and recumbent, and the views should be compared:

    a) to show hypermobility.
    b) to show hypomobility.
    c) to demonstrate the appearance of a vacuum phenomenon when flexion stress occurs.
    d) to compress soft tissue around the bone, especially in the obese patient.

85. The "Scotty dog" seen on the lumbar oblique projection is formed by:

    a) the transverse process, pedicle, mammillary process, superior articular process, and pars interarticularis.
    b) the transverse process, pedicle, superior articular process, pars interarticularis, and inferior articular process.
    c) the pedicle, superior articular process, pars interarticularis, spinous process, and inferior articular process.
    d) the transverse process, pedicle, spinous process, pars interarticularis, and inferior articular process.

86. Lumbar intervertebral disc height measurements may be meaningless if there is:

    a) a central, contained herniation.
    b) an abdominal aortic aneurysm.
    c) a significant anterolisthesis.
    d) significant segmental rotation.

87. The oblique cervical projection demonstrates:

    a) intervertebral disc spaces.
    b) the cervical pillars.
    c) the von Luschka joints.
    d) alterations in the cervical curve.

88. The normal range of the "Q" angle is:

    a) between 85 and 100°.
    b) between 75 and 85°.
    c) between 15 and 20°.
    d) between 30 and 40°.

89. The cervical lordosis may be evaluated by all except:

    a) Hadley's curve.
    b) method of Jochumsen.
    c) angle of cervical curve.
    d) depth of cervical curve.

90. The PA ulnar flexion wrist projection is the optimal view for:

    a) evaluation for lunate subluxation.
    b) evaluation of the scaphoid.
    c) evaluation of the radioulnar angle.
    d) evaluation of the ulnocarpal joints.

91. To obtain a medial oblique projection of the foot, the foot should be tilted:

    a) laterally to form an approximately 35° angle with the film surface.
    b) medially to form an approximately 35° angle with the film surface.
    c) laterally to form an approximately 15° angle with the film surface.
    d) medially to form an approximately 15° angle with the film surface.

92. All of the following are true of the iliofemoral line except:

    a) it simply traces the lateral margins of the ilium and femoral neck.
    b) it should be smooth and bilaterally symmetrical.
    c) it normally has a bulge for the femoral head.
    d) it traces the margins of the medial femoral head and the lateral teardrop.

93. On an AP hip projection, the normal teardrop distance should be:

    a) no more than 2 mm from the lateral pelvic margin of the teardrop.
    b) no less than 11 mm from the lateral pelvic margin of the teardrop.
    c) no more than 11 mm from the lateral pelvic margin of the teardrop.
    d) no less than 2 mm from the medial margin of the teardrop.

94. In an adult, the presacral space (as measured on a lateral sacral projection) should:

    a) be around 0.5 cm.
    b) not exceed 2 cm.
    c) be around 5 cm.
    d) be between 5 and 8 cm.

95. In an anterior oblique lumbar projection, the side marker should be placed:

    a) in the lower left-hand corner.
    b) in the upper left-hand corner.
    c) in front of the spine.
    d) behind the spine.

96. A lumbar canal/body ratio that is higher than normal may indicate:

    a) spina bifida occulta.
    b) an increased interpediculate distance.
    c) spinal stenosis.
    d) spinal dysraphism.

97. Contraindications to cervical flexion or extension lateral projections include all the following except:

    a) postural vertigo.
    b) a loss of strength in muscles innervated by the right median nerve.
    c) cervical strain or sprain without neurologic symptoms.
    d) signs of vertebrobasilar ischemia.

98. The angle formed by the intersection of the tibial shaft's long axis and a line tangential to the tibial plateaus' anterosuperior margins is the:

    a) "Q" angle.
    b) tibial angle.
    c) femoral angle of the knee.
    d) condylar angle.

99. The subtle shift of a femoral capital epiphysis is best detected by:

    a) Macnab's line.
    b) Klein's line.
    c) Shenton's line.
    d) Skinner's line.

100. A synonym for George's line is:

    a) posterior body line.
    b) spinolaminar junction line.
    c) posterior cervical line.
    d) cervical gravity line.

PRACTICE TEST CHAPTER 1—ANSWER KEY

1.	b	11.	a	21.	a	31.	c	41.	a	51.	a	61.	c	71.	b	81.	b	91.	b
2.	b	12.	c	22.	d	32.	d	42.	a	52.	d	62.	c	72.	b	82.	c	92.	d
3.	c	13.	a	23.	c	33.	a	43.	c	53.	b	63.	a	73.	c	83.	b	93.	c
4.	a	14.	d	24.	a	34.	b	44.	c	54.	b	64.	a	74.	a	84.	a	94.	b
5.	c	15.	c	25.	d	35.	d	45.	a	55.	d	65.	a	75.	c	85.	b	95.	d
6.	d	16.	a	26.	a	36.	d	46.	a	56.	d	66.	a	76.	a	86.	d	96.	c
7.	c	17.	d	27.	a	37.	c	47.	d	57.	a	67.	c	77.	a	87.	c	97.	c
8.	d	18.	b	28.	a	38.	c	48.	c	58.	d	68.	c	78.	b	88.	c	98.	b
9.	d	19.	a	29.	b	39.	c	49.	a	59.	c	69.	a	79.	d	89.	a	99.	b
10.	d	20.	a	30.	a	40.	b	50.	a	60.	d	70.	d	80.	c	90.	b	100.	a

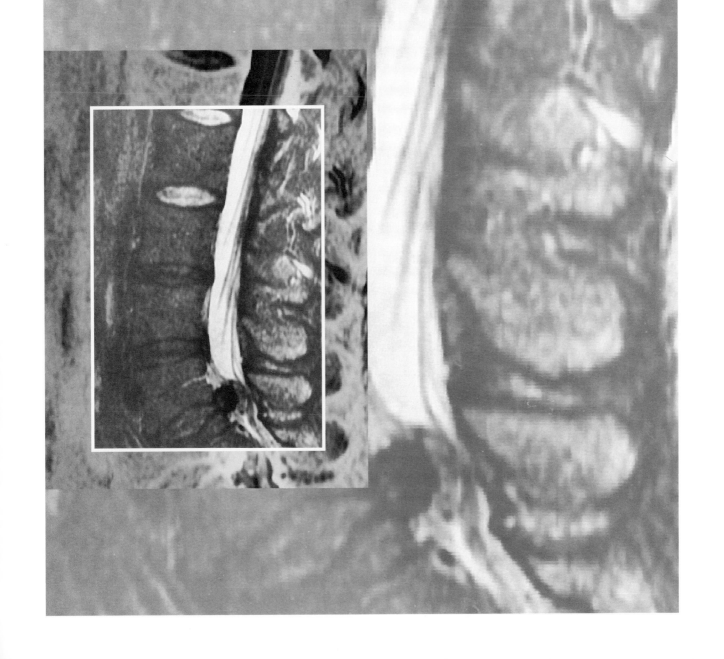

Chapter 2

DIAGNOSTIC IMAGING MODALITIES
Techniques, Equipment, Interpretation, Reporting

A.   X-RAY

☞   **1.   Equipment**

    a)   Cathode $(-)$ ray ejects electrons toward anode $(+)$

    b)   Grid function: absorb scatter radiation
- optimum ratio 12:1; 103 lines per inch
- a stationary grid is preferable

    c)   Cassettes: hold intensifying screens and film in uniform close contact

☞   **2.   X-ray Production**

    a)   Energy: 99% heat production and 1% x-rays

    b)   Number of electrons ejected depends upon milliamperage seconds **(mAs)**

    c)   Amount of thrust or force generated by the x-ray beam is directly related to kilovolts peaked **(kVp)**

    d)   85% of x-ray photons in the beam are bremsstrahlung ("braking radiation"): create the image on the film

    e)   15% of the photons are characteristic radiation: do not contribute to image formation ($<$70 kVp)

    f)   Increasing energy (raising kVp) leads to shorter wavelength, higher frequency

☞   **g)**   Anode heel effect: beam is weaker at anode end; anode should be at the **TOP** of horizontal beam

☞   **3.   X-ray Effects**

    a)   Classic (coherent) scattering: high energy rays, no change in wavelength or energy

    b)   Compton scatter (incoherent)
- predominant effect: energy reduced, wavelength increased; fogs the film
- effects minimized via grid, adequate collimation, shielding

    c)   Photoelectric interaction: little effect on film; significant contribution to radiation dose

    d)   Pair production and photodisintegration: do not occur with diagnostic x-ray

    e)   Absorption: energy deposited in matter

    f)   Attenuation: loss or redirection of energy from the beam
- HVL (half value layer) = thickness of filtering material that will absorb 50% of energy; standard reference material is aluminum or one cm of water
- TVL (tenth value layer) = thickness of filtering material that will absorb 90% of energy; standard reference material is lead

    g)   Beam hardening: after attenuation, average

intensity of remaining photons in beam is higher, so beam is considered "harder"

4. **Radiation Protection**

a) **ALARA** = **A**s **L**ow **A**s **R**easonably **A**chievable: the concept of aiming for minimal radiation dose with each exposure

b) Radiation dose
- exposure in air: coulombs/Kg (C/Kg = R)
- absorbed in tissue: Gray (1 Gy = 100 Rad)
- biologic effect equivalent: Sievert (1 Sv = 100 Rem)

c) MPD = maximum permissible dose

d) mA: inversely proportional to exposure time
- yields milliamperage seconds (mAs) for a given exposure

e) Current MPD for whole body exposure: 5 Rems/year (0.05 Sv/Yr)

f) GSD = genetically significant dose

g) Exposure limited by control of time and distance:
- **inverse square law**: radiation varies *inversely* with the square of distance from beam source (distance *increase* squared = decreased radiation)

h) Shield personnel and bystanders from primary radiation; shield patient (and everyone else) from secondary and scatter radiation

i) Reduce time: faster times with rare earth film-screen systems, high frequency generators

j) Reduce patient dose: collimation, shields and protective apparel, tube housing

k) Reduce need for repeat exposures: good stabilization of patients (compression bands for upright films), use of grids (to control scatter and increase film contrast)

l) Considerations in pregnancy:
- fetus' exposure can be calculated by x-ray physicist
- Bergonie-Tribondeau law: x-rays in the first trimester are most hazardous to fetus
- 10-day rule: film during first 10 days after onset of last menses

 5. **Radiation Effects**

a) Stochastic effects: the RISK is proportional to dose received by the affected tissue
- e.g., carcinogenesis, genetic aberrations

b) Nonstochastic effects: direct threshold effect—actual damage rather than risk
- e.g., radiation burns, cataracts

    c) Acute radiation syndrome (nonstochastic)
- LD 50/30 = lethal within 30 days to 50% of exposed experimental animals
- especially sensitive tissues include: hematopoietic, gastrointestinal, eyes, gonads, CNS

6. Films, Screens, Cassettes

    a) Intensifying screens fluoresce, producing visible light; helps to create the image

    b) Film may have single emulsion (one side only) or both sides may have emulsion

    c) Duplicating film: single side emulsion only

    d) Film consists of base and emulsion

    e) Emulsion: silver halides and sensitivity specks (silver sulfite) in a crystal lattice formation

    f) Long scale = more shades of gray

    g) Latent image is present on undeveloped film

    h) Film may be fogged by x-rays, light, pressure, heat, humidity

    i) Intensifying screens luminesce in various spectra—green or blue: match with film

    j) Useful screen life is about 7 years

7. Processing

    a) Wetting agents swell the emulsion; allow developing chemicals to penetrate

    b) Developer: starts reduction-oxidation reaction, maintains alkalinity, controls extent of silver reduction and prevents its own oxidation; controls emulsion swelling

    c) Manual developing: a stop bath drops the pH

    d) Automatic processor: the fixer drops the pH

    e) Fixing agent: clears emulsion of undeveloped silver halide, hardens emulsion, prevents image degradation by light

    f) Water bath: prevents unwanted chemical reactions

    g) Drying: clean, dry air prevents degradation of image

8. Technique Basics

    a) Kilovoltage
- too high yields **black** film, poor contrast, high amounts of Compton scatter
- too low yields white film, poor contrast, demands higher mAs (longer times)
- fixed kVp (variable mAs) preferred: as kVp rises, Compton scatter increases and contrast is lost
- **contrast**: primarily a **function of kVp** (Table 2.1): higher kVp yields longer scale

TABLE 2.1	
Suggested kVp Chart (Single Phase)	
50–65	upper or lower extremities
65–75	clavicle; abdomen (KUB)
70–80	shoulder
75–85	ribs (75 kVp above diaphragm, 85 kVp below), cervicals, AP thoracics, oblique lumbars, pelvis, hip
80–90	skull, AP lumbar
85–95	lateral thoracic, lateral lumbar, full spine
100–120	chest, PA abdomen

N.B., kVp settings are lower for high frequency generators to maintain contrast seen on single phase.

of contrast; lower kVp yields shorter scale of contrast

b) Milliamperage (mA)
- higher mA requires shorter time for same mAs
- larger focal spot needs higher mA, shorter time
- moving bucky: grid lines may show at less than 0.1 seconds
- rule of thumb: with children, or with osteopenia—reduce mAs 30% (minimum) with heavy muscle or large-boned patient—raise mAs 50% (minimum)

 c) Detail improved by SHORT object-film distance, LONG focal-film distance, SHORT exposure time, SMALL focal spot, SLOW film-screen combination
- factors must be balanced in a compromise

9. Quality Control

a) Automatic processor: fresh chemicals, monitored water temperature, adequate washing and drying
- 30-minute warm-up before use each day
- clean crossover racks
- developer temperature between 88–96° F
- monitor drying temperature
- regular monthly cleaning, chemical replacement

b) Darkroom: no light leaks, safelight check, no fluorescent lighting
- do semi-annual "fog-test" on sensitized film

c) Cassette, film/screen combinations
- ID each cassette: artifact caused by specific cassette can be traced
- Check spectral match between film and screen

- Ensure uniform film/screen contact
- Clean screens quarterly
- Screen life: 5–7 years—replace as needed
- Check for light leaks on cassettes (e.g., sprung hinges or worn felt on old-style cassettes)

d) X-ray machine
- power adequate and uniform
- beam quality: should exceed minimum HVL standard
- linear relationship between mA stations at a single kVp setting
- CR perpendicular to image plane (with no tube tilt) within 2°
- collimator alignment accurate within 2%
- timer accurate within 10%

e) Patient exposure ALARA concept (*As Low As Reasonably Achievable*)
- no "safe" minimum radiation exposure

f) Viewing equipment
- clean diffuser on viewbox
- uniform color, unflickering, strong lights
- individual panel controls
- variable intensity hot lights
- no extraneous light in viewing room

10. Site Considerations

a) State regulates shielding requirements

b) Interlock system: film bin cannot open while white light is on or darkroom door is unlocked

c) No carpet: reduce static electricity

d) Floor drain for darkroom

e) No black paint

f) Large fiberglass utility sink for cleaning processor

g) Site as close as possible to power and water sources

h) No fluorescent lights in darkroom (afterglow fogs film)

i) Variable light intensity in X-ray room (easier to see collimator light on patient)

REVIEW—STUDY QUESTIONS

1. What components of the x-ray system must be monitored for quality control and how?
2. How is radiation dose to the patient quantified?
3. What is anode heel effect and how is it compensated for?
4. What factors improve detail in a film?
5. Describe the steps in film processing.
6. Describe the function and effects of kVp and mAs.

7. How is mAs modified for filming smaller or larger than average patients, osteopenic, heavily boned, or muscular patients?

8. Describe the various kinds of scatter radiation and their effects.

9. Define and explain ALARA and the MPD.

10. List some factors that reduce patient radiation dose.

11. Explain and give examples of stochastic and nonstochastic radiation effects.

12. To what does LD50/30 relate?

13. What body tissues are most sensitive to radiation effects?

14. Explain the composition and function of film emulsions.

15. What factors may cause film "fogging?"

B. COMPUTED TOMOGRAPHY (CT)

1. Equipment

    a) Rotating x-ray tube with stationary detector ring (tube rotates around patient)

    b) Data displayed on monitor after computer correlates image

2. Principles of Interpretation

    a) Initial CT image is axial; reformatted into other planes by computer

    b) May obtain 1 mm to 5 mm slice thickness

    c) Original sagittal images may be obtained in small body parts

    d) Helical/spiral scanners faster, reduce scan time, reduce motion artifacts, improve resolution

    e) CT contrast studies: intravenous, intra-arterial, intrathecal, intradiscal, gastrointestinal

    f) Pixel: 1×1 mm two-dimensional area

    g) Voxel: three-dimensional area 1–10 mm deep, 1 mm wide, 1 mm high

    h) Hounsfield Unit: density measurement
- 0 = water density
- $-$ 1000 = air
- $+$ 1000 = metal or cortical bone

    i) Bone window or soft tissue window

3. Capabilities and Applications

    a) Traumatic lesions, pathology, or anomalies: well demonstrated in areas of complex anatomy that are difficult to display on plain film
- e.g., skull, facial bones, spine, pelvis

    b) CT shows soft tissue contrast 10 times better than plain film

c) Occult fractures, bone fragment location, intraarticular fractures shown clearly

d) CT: modality of choice for **calcified** soft tissue lesions, hematomas, myositis ossificans

e) CT: good for displaying discitis, osteomyelitis, Brodie's abscess

f) Aneurysms (especially intracranial): well demonstrated by CT

- shows intra-abdominal well, but diagnostic ultrasound (US) is more economical and less invasive

g) Often the modality of choice for evaluating both soft tissue and osseous neoplasms: osseous effects, calcifications well demonstrated

h) Bony malformations well depicted: spina bifida occulta (SBO) or manifesta, spondylolysis (especially cervical), facet planes, spinal stenosis, lateral recess stenosis; assessment of cortical bone is excellent; may be enhanced with intravenous (IV) contrast studies

i) Accurate assessment of degenerative changes, including ligamentum flavum hypertrophy and disc lesions; may be best evaluated with CT

j) QCT (quantitative computed tomography): used to evaluate bone mineral density (BMD) to determine risk factors for fracture in osteoporotic patients

☞ **4. Limitations and Contraindications**

a) Radiation dose is a serious consideration

b) Contrast infusion may be contraindicated by hypersensitivity to contrast media (iodine); congestive heart failure; diabetes; compromised renal clearance

c) BUN and creatinine must be evaluated and be normal before contrast studies are safe to perform

d) Image artifacts may result from metallic objects in area of interest

e) Occasionally, claustrophobia or physical size of patient may be a limiting factor

C. MAGNETIC RESONANCE IMAGING (MRI)

1. Equipment

a) Superconducting magnets—supercooled with liquid cryogens, kept near absolute zero

b) Magnet is in gantry

c) Surface coils may be used

d) Radiofrequency emitted to deflect proton orientation

        e) Computer evaluates patterns of energy emitted by reorientation of polar protons; produces image

2. Physics and Mechanical Principles of Operation

        a) Polar protons have nuclei with odd number of particles and will align in a magnetic field (^{1}H, ^{13}C, ^{23}Na, ^{31}P, ^{39}K)

        b) Resonance factor (RF pulse): energy required to shift nuclei from parallel to antiparallel state

        c) Nuclei returning to parallel state emit energy at a specific radio-frequency

        d) Larmor frequency: frequency of precession (wobble/rotation) for the resonating nuclei

        e) Relaxation times (T1 and T2): longitudinal or spin-lattice relaxation; spin-spin relaxation

        f) T1: short time to echo (TE) and short time to repetition (TR); fat density is brightest

        g) T2: longer TE and TR; water density is brightest

        h) Proton density weighted: short TE with longer TR

3. Capabilities and Applications

        a) Provides optimal visualization of spatial relationships and distinct soft tissue contrast, to view IVD, spinal cord and meninges, bone marrow, paravertebral soft tissue, brain

        b) MRI shows soft tissue contrast 100 times better than CT

        c) Multiplanar imaging (axial, sagittal, and coronal): excellent with MRI, no loss of clarity as with CT

        d) Non-ionizing: there is no radiation dose

        e) Contrast-enhanced (with gadolinium) views for vascular lesions (e.g., vascularized cord lesions, neoplasms)

        f) Congenital conditions best visualized via MRI include: tethered cord syndrome, diastematomyelia, syrinx, Arnold-Chiari malformations (Types I, II, and III), perineural (Tarlov's) sacral cyst

        g) Traumatic lesions best evaluated by MRI include: soft tissue components
           • e.g., spinal cord or nerve root lesions, hemorrhage, bone marrow edema, "aging" of lesion by stage of edema or hemorrhage, epidural hematoma, Schmorl's nodes, cord contusion

        h) Infections, such as infectious spondylitis or epidural abscess: detected earlier via MRI than possible with CT

i) MRI: most sensitive modality for detecting osseous spinal metastasis; with primary tumors, best at showing the extent of invasion within the marrow cavity and cortical breakthrough into adjacent soft tissue

j) Gold standard for visualizing spinal cord tumors and accurately locating them

k) IVD pathology: MRI is optimum imaging modality for all IVD disorders; can demonstrate spinal DJD much earlier than possible with plain film or CT

- **Modic classification** of marrow changes adjacent to degenerating discs:
    1) Type I: endplate disruption and fissuring by vascularized fibrous tissue that invades the marrow
    2) Type II: endplate disruption with fatty marrow replacement in adjacent vertebral body
    3) Type III: dense, woven fibrous or compact bone deposition replacing the marrow

l) Best imaging of ligamentum flavum hypertrophy; exiting nerve roots, dorsal root ganglion, and cauda equina

m) Synovial cysts well visualized, best with T2 images

n) Postoperative evaluations: avoids metal artifact image distortions, provides good distinction between epidural scarring and recurrent disc herniation

- gadolinium enhances well-vascularized scar quickly; disc has little or no blood supply and thus no early enhancement but may "light up" 30 to 45 minutes later

o) Arachnoiditis: difficult to diagnose; MRI, especially with enhancement, can image characteristic signs, especially in mid-development or advanced stages

p) MRI can demonstrate MS plaques in the brain and spinal cord

q) Hip lesions

- best for detecting osteonecrosis, bone marrow edema, soft tissue hip lesions (iliopsoas bursitis; malignant fibrous histiocytoma, aneurysmal bone cyst, chondrosarcoma)
- limited MRI used to scan for occult hip fracture

r) Knee lesions

- MRI is considered optimum for meniscal lesions, ligament damage, articular cartilage imaging, chondromalacia patellae evaluation, tendon lesions (Osgood-Schlatter's disease, Jumper's knee), occult knee fractures, myositis ossificans, osteonecrosis, osteochondritis dissecans, bone infarcts, Baker's cysts, popliteal artery aneurysm, pigmented villonodular synovitis (PVNS), osteosarcoma

s) Ankle lesions

- ligament and tendon lesions easily visualized, as are ganglions, stress fractures, and talar osteochondritis dissecans

t) Shoulder lesions

- lesions of tendons or bursae, such as shoulder impingement; rotator cuff tears or tendinitis; and bursitis or bicipital tendinitis can be demonstrated clearly
- lesions of the glenoid labrum or humeral head occurring with dislocations, such as Hill-Sachs (hatchet) defect, Bankart lesions, and SLAP lesions, are shown well
- MRI detects osteonecrosis early

u) Elbow lesions

- elbow cartilage, marrow, and periarticular soft tissues well delineated; MRI is useful for imaging tendinitis, ligament injuries, post-traumatic osteochondritis dissecans

v) Wrist lesions

- occult fractures (most frequently scaphoid) and osteonecrosis (usually scaphoid or lunate) clearly displayed
- carpal ligament tears, damage to the triangular fibrocartilage
- with carpal tunnel syndrome, MRI may show edema, swelling, deformation of median nerve

w) Temporomandibular joint (TMJ) lesions

- MRI: ideal modality for imaging TMJ disc tears, displacement and/or meniscal derangements

☞ **4. Limitations and Contraindications**

a) Very large patients do not fit into scanner

b) Claustrophobia or long immobility may make patient too uncomfortable

c) Ferromagnetic objects in patient's body are contraindication: pacemaker, cochlear implant, certain heart valves, aneurysm clips, intraocular fragments (seen in welders), metal shards or shrapnel, tattooed eyeliner, body piercing

d) Not done during pregnancy unless mother's life is at risk, because risks are unknown

D. MYELOGRAPHY

1. Equipment

a) X-ray of the spine with contrast material injected into the subarachnoid space; may be performed with CT as well (CTM = CT myelography)

b) Water-soluble contrast agents now used: iohexol (Omnipaque) or iopamidol (Isovue)

c) Injected into subarachnoid space under fluoroscopy

2. **Procedures**

a) Lumbar or cervical puncture to inject contrast medium into subarachnoid space, under fluoroscopy

b) Analysis of CSF sample (sample taken during original puncture)

c) X-rays: PA (prone), lateral decubitus, oblique for lumbars; AP, lateral, oblique and Swimmer's lateral for cervicals

3. **Capabilities and Indications**

a) Outlines margins of space-occupying lesions within spinal canal and at dural sleeves

 b) Indicates locale of lesion (Fig. 2.1)
- extradural: in spinal canal but outside thecal sac, e.g., IVD herniation
- intradural extramedullary: within thecal sac but outside spinal cord, e.g., neurofibroma, meningioma
- intradural intramedullary: within the spinal cord proper, e.g., astrocytoma, ependymoma, lipoma, syrinx

 c) CTM (computed tomographic myelography) plus MRI: the modality of choice for diagnosis of arachnoiditis (difficult to diagnose and often missed)

Figure 2.1.

Lesion locale (under capabilities and indications for myelography).
A. Extradural. B. Intradural extramedullary. C. Intradural intramedullar. Reprinted with permission from Yochum TR, Rowe LJ. Essentials of Skeletal Radiology, 2nd ed. Baltimore: Williams & Wilkins, 1996:410,412, 406.

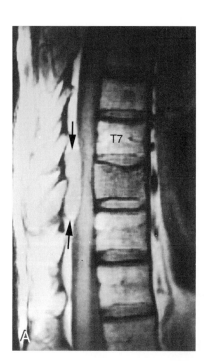

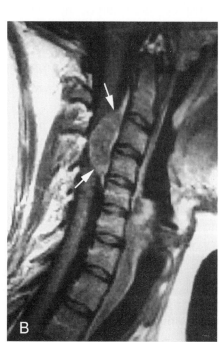

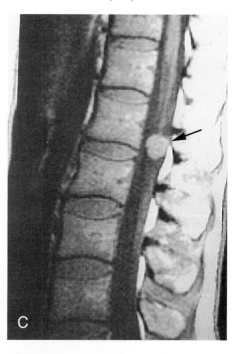

☞   **4. Limitations and Contraindications**

    a) Very invasive; has significant side-effects (radiculitis, hyperreflexia, seizures, CNS ischemia, visual or auditory problems, meningitis symptoms, headaches, nausea, dizziness, vomiting) that mainly are neurotoxic reactions to contrast agents

    b) Contraindicated for patients sensitive to iodine

    c) Problems arise with patients with a history of seizures

    d) Patients must be well hydrated

    e) Contraindicated if patient is on tricyclic antidepressants, monoamine oxidase inhibitors, phenothiazine compounds

    f) Errors in injection lead to nerve root injury, arachnoiditis, pulmonary oil emboli, epidermoid formation, disc perforation with subsequent herniation

E. DISCOGRAPHY (WITH X-RAY OR CT)

1. Equipment and Procedures

    a) Fluoroscopic examination

    b) Contrast medium inserted into nucleus of disc under fluoroscopy

    c) Large-bore needle inserted first, smaller needle inserted through it, and specific amount of normal saline injected, followed by contrast agent

2. Capabilities and Indications

    a) Displays herniation routes

    b) Aids in localization of pain source

    c) Aids in establishing the spinal level of a symptomatic lesion:

☞   • **provocational discogram**: saline injected into disc, to recreate (*provoke*) patient's pain; then anesthetic agent injected into disc to stop pain.

☞   **3. Contraindications**

    a) Iodine sensitivity

F. NUCLEAR SCANNING

☞   **1. Equipment and Procedures**

    a) Usually a 3-phase procedure:
    • Phase 1. Radionuclide angiogram = flow phase
      1) first 2–4 minutes: follows vascular flow of injected radionuclide tracer
    • Phase 2. Blood-pool phase
      1) 5 minutes after injection: tracer is followed in extravascular space

- Phase 3. Bone-scan phase (delayed)
    1) static images taken 4 hours post-injection; images bone uptake of tracer
    2) osteomyelitis evaluation via 24-hour scan

b) Radiopharmaceutical: injected, ingested, or inhaled

c) Gamma rays emitted by radionuclide detected, used to generate a computer image

d) Equipment required
- radiopharmaceutical: pharmacologic "carrier" that is metabolized by organ or tissue of interest, carrying a radionuclide of relatively short half-life and high enough energy to emit detectable gamma rays
- gamma camera to detect gamma rays
- computer to process them, then produce and record images

e) For aseptic inflammations and infections: Gallium-67 or Indium-111; show affinity for bacterial and cellular debris and leukocytes

f) For bone imaging: diphosphonate compounds labeled with ^{99m}Tc-MDP most often used, preferentially taken up at sites of new bone formation

2. **Capabilities and Indications**

a) Very sensitive to early bone growth

b) **SPECT** = **s**ingle **p**hoton **e**mission **c**omputed **t**omography
- permits accurate localization; offers improved resolution and spatial orientation
- excellent for musculoskeletal lesions (e.g., occult spondylolysis), heart, brain, or abdominal evaluations
- multi-planar imaging

c) **PET** = **p**ositron **e**mission **t**omography (Table 2.2)
- still investigational
- positively charged electrons (antimatter) emitted
- highest uptake in high-grade malignant soft-tissue lesions, aiding DDX
- also used for brain, heart physiologic evaluations

3. **Contraindications and Limitations**

a) Low specificity

b) Radiation to patient: bladder is the critical or target organ because of concentration of cleared radionuclide in pooled urine

c) Pregnancy or lactation are contraindications

TABLE 2.2
Applications for Bone Scan

Arthritides	inflammatory (e.g., RA), hypertrophic (e.g., osteoarthropathy)
Clinical	monitor response to treatment, monitor course of disease, other imaging normal
Infections	cellulitis, osteomyelitis, septic arthritis
Tumor-like Processes	fibrous dysplasia, Paget's disease
Neoplasms	benign: detect, monitor for recurrence or malignant transformation malignant: detect, monitor for recurrence or metastasis
Prosthesis	infection, loosening
Traumatic injuries	occult fracture, stress or insufficiency fracture, fracture "aging" bone bruise, acute spondylolysis, soft tissue injuries
Vascular lesions	infarction, hyperemia, osteonecrosis, reflex sympathetic dystrophy

REVIEW—STUDY QUESTIONS

1. What are the basic principles upon which MRI operates?
2. What is precession?
3. What tissue gives the brightest signal in T1 weighted MRI sequences? With T2 weighting?
4. List contraindications for MRI.
5. List contraindications for CT.
6. Explain the basic principles upon which CT operates.
7. Describe the three phases of a nuclear bone scan.
8. What are the indications and contraindications for myelography?
9. Describe the procedure for discography, its uses, and its disadvantages.
10. For what suspected pathology would you order a nuclear scan? A CT scan? An MRI study?

G. PRINCIPLES OF INTERPRETATION

1. Plain Film Analysis

    a) Viewer must know what normals look like

    b) **ABCS** : note **A**lignment; **B**one quality (trabecular patterns, density, medullary cavities and cortical integrity and thickness); **C**artilage (joint space and its symmetry); **S**oft tissues

    c) Note number of lesions:

- monostotic lesions are characteristic of osteoid osteoma, osteosarcoma, staph infections, Perthes disease
- polyostotic lesions are characteristic of battered child, RA, multiple myeloma, metastasis, rickets, sickle cell anemia, hyperparathyroidism

d) Note symmetry of lesions:
- asymmetrical distribution suggests metastasis, Paget's disease, psoriasis
- symmetrical distribution is characteristic of metabolic processes such as osteomalacia, osteoporosis, leukemia, hyperparathyroidism

e) Analyze bone lesion as to:
- position in bone, site of origin, location on skeleton, shape, size, margination, cortical effect, behavior, appearance of matrix, effect on periosteum

TABLE 2.3
Preferential Long Bone Sites

Epiphysis	chondroblastoma (giant cell tumor prefers bone end, but after closure of physis)
Epiphysis/metaphysis	aneurysmal bone cyst, giant cell tumor, metastasis
Metaphysis	bone island, enchondroma, fibrous cortical defect, nonossifying fibroma, osteoid osteoma, osteochondroma, simple bone cyst, chondrosarcoma, fibrosarcoma, metastasis, osteosarcoma
Metaphysis/diaphysis	chondromyxoid fibroma, nonossifying fibroma, osteoid osteoma, chondrosarcoma, metastasis, osteosarcoma, multiple myeloma
Diaphysis	osteoid osteoma, latent bone cyst, adamantinoma, Ewing's sarcoma, metastasis, multiple myeloma, non-Hodgkin's lymphoma

TABLE 2.4
Site of Origin

Medullary origin	fibrous or cartilaginous lesions; may scallop or thin endosteal cortex
Cortical origin	eccentric location; may destroy, distort, or expand cortex
Periosteal origin	little bony abnormality; mostly separated from underlying bone
Extraosseous origin	separated by cleft from cortical surface

Bone Tumors and Diseases Favoring Vertebral Bodies

"CALL HOME"

Chordoma
Aneurysmal bone cyst
Leukemia
Lymphoma
Hemangioma
Osteoid osteoma, Osteoblastoma
Myeloma, Metastasis
Eosinophilic granuloma

TABLE 2.5
Preferential Tumor Skeletal Locations

Skeletal Site	Tumor	Character	Skeletal Site	Tumor	Character
		Malignant/ Benign			Malignant/ Benign
Skull	chordoma	M	Tibia	adamantinoma	M
	hemangioma	B		fibrosarcoma	M
Skull, sinus	osteoma	B		osteosarcoma	M
Mandible	adamantinoma	M		giant cell tumor	Quasi-M
Spine (cervical)	chordoma (C2 body)	M		aneurysmal bone cyst	B
Spine (general)	multiple myeloma	M		chondromyxoid fibroma	B
	non-Hodgkin's lymphoma	M		fibrous cortical defect	B
	hemangioma	B		nonossifying fibroma	B
Spine (neural arch)	aneurysmal bone cyst	B		osteochondroma	B
	osteoblastoma	B		osteoid osteoma	B
	osteoid osteoma	B	Scapula	chondrosarcoma	M
	neurofibroma	B	Sternum	chondrosarcoma	M
Pelvis	chondrosarcoma	M		multiple myeloma	M
	Ewing's sarcoma	M	Humerus	chondrosarcoma	M
	multiple myeloma	M		Ewing's sarcoma	M
	non-Hodgkin's lymphoma	M		multiple myeloma	M
	bone island	B		osteosarcoma	M
Sacrum/coccyx	chordoma	M		non-Hodgkin's lymphoma	M
Femur	chondrosarcoma	M		aneurysmal bone cyst	B
	Ewing's sarcoma	M		chondroblastoma	B
	fibrosarcoma	M		osteoblastoma	B
	multiple myeloma	M		osteochondroma	B
	osteosarcoma	M		simple bone cyst	B
	parosteal sarcoma	M	Radius	giant cell tumor	99%M
	non-Hodgkin's lymphoma	M	Ulna	chondromyxoid fibroma	B
	giant cell tumor	quasi-M			
	aneurysmal bone cyst	B			
	bone island	B			
	chondroblastoma	B			
	enchondroma	B			
	fibrous cortical defect	B			
	nonossifying fibroma	B			
	osteoblastoma	B			
	osteochondroma	B			
	osteoid osteoma	B			
	simple bone cyst	B			

TABLE 2.6
Lesion Matrix

Fat matrix	may have central calcifications; difficult to identify on plain film; often show only with CT
Cartilage	a) stippled calcification—spotty, small densities; e.g. enchondroma b) flocculent calcification—confluent stippling (often, both seen in one lesion) c) arc and ring calcification—eggshell-like curvilinear fragments at periphery of cartilage lobules ("rings and broken rings"); e.g., chondrosarcoma
Osseous	may be diffuse, hazy, or dense (ivory)
Fibrous	"smoky," *ground glass* look; e.g., fibrous dysplasia

TABLE 2.7
Lesion Behaviors

Osteolytic lesions: patterns of bone destruction	a) **Geographic:**	(circumscribed, or uniformly lytic) usually solitary, > 1 cm, sharply marginated may have a sclerotic, encapsulated border may be septated usually slow-growing, benign may expand bone
	b) **Moth-eaten:**	multiple, poorly marginated, 2–5 mm ragged, irregular margins, may be confluent usually an aggressive lesion (lytic metastasis, osteomyelitis) no sclerotic border usually does not expand bone
	c) **Permeative:**	multiple holes in bone, <1 mm, wide zone of transition no sclerotic border usually does not expand bone indicates the most aggressive tumors (myeloma, lytic metastases, Ewing's tumor)

TABLE 2.8
Lesion Differentiation

	Margination	Cortical Involvement	Periosteal Response
Benign	sharply marginated	cortical expansion or preservation	solid periosteal response
Malignant	imperceptible margins	cortical disruption	laminated, spiculated

---

Blow-out Lesions of Posterior Spinal Elements

"GO APE"

Giant cell tumor
Osteoblastoma
Aneurysmal bone cyst
Plasmacytoma
Eosinophilic granuloma

Ivory Vertebra

"MY ONLY SISTER LEFT HOME ON FRIDAY PAST"

Myelosclerosis
Osteoblastic metastasis
Sickle-cell disease
Lymphoma
Hemangioma
Osteoporosis
Fluorosis
Paget's disease

TABLE 2.9
Cortical Effects

Cortical thinning	all cortices: osteoporosis localized thinning: tumor or infection endosteal scalloping: medullary tumors (MM, enchondroma, fibrous dysplasia)
Cortical thickening	generalized: Paget's disease localized: osteoid osteoma, fracture repair, stress fracture, Brodie's abscess
Cortical expansion	bulging shows slow tumor growth: benign or slow-growing malignancy
Cortical destruction	aggressive bone disease; osteolytic tumor or infection

Solitary Lytic Skull Defects

"M T HOLE"

Multiple myeloma, Metastasis

Tuberculosis, Trauma

Histiocytosis X

Osteomyelitis

Leptomeningeal cyst

Epidermoid/dermoid, Enigma (fibrous dysplasia)

TABLE 2.10
Patterns of Periosteal Response

Solid	continuous layer, attached to outer cortex; may be undulating; slowly formed; e.g., osteoid osteoma, stress fracture, venous stasis, degenerative arthritis (buttress formation at the hip)
Laminated	(a.k.a. *layered, lamellated, onion-skin*) alternating thin layers of lucency and opacity; may indicate cyclical irritations, slow or aggressive tumors, infections; e.g., Ewing's sarcoma
Spiculated	(a.k.a. *perpendicular, sunburst, brushed whiskers, hair-on-end*) very aggressive lesion; usually a primary malignant bone tumor; e.g., osteosarcoma (most common cause)
Codman's Triangle	(a.k.a. *Codman's angle, periosteal cuff, periosteal buttress, periosteal collar*), periosteal new bone triangle at periphery of lesion/cortex junction; most common with osteosarcoma, but can be found with other tumors, infection, traumatic periostitis

TABLE 2.11
Tumor Size and Shape

Benign	usually < 6 cm	elongated along long axis of bone
	exceptions that may be very large:	ABC, SBC, giant cell tumor, fibrous dysplasia
Malignant	often > 6 cm	pleomorphic

f) Clinical data: age, gender and sometimes ethnicity, history, signs and symptoms, and laboratory results if available

g) Analyze articular effects
  - infection invades the joint
  - most tumors do not destroy articular cortices or cross joints (however, CT sometimes demonstrates tumor crossing joints)
  - nonuniform loss of joint space is most indicative of DJD or trauma
  - uniform loss of joint space suggests inflammatory arthritis; e.g., RA

h) Note soft tissue changes
  - myofascial planes
  - fat pads
  - skin lines
  - masses
  - alterations in density

TABLE 2.12
Age Predilections

Disease Category	(birth–20)	(20–40)	(> 40)
Arthritides	JRA	AS osteitis condensans ilii lupus erythematosus psoriatic arthritis Reiter's syndrome RA scleroderma synoviochondrometaplasia	DJD DISH Gout CPPD (pseudogout)
Neoplasms	osteosarcoma Ewing's sarcoma fibrosarcoma craniocerv. chordoma osteochondroma osteoid osteoma enchondroma NOF/FCD SBC/UBC ABC fibrous dysplasia neurofibromatosis	osteosarcoma parosteal sarcoma non-Hodgkin's lymphoma fibrosarcoma giant cell tumor enchondroma	multiple myeloma parosteal sarcoma chondrosarcoma fibrosarcoma lumbosacral chordoma hemangioma Paget's disease
Hematologic/ vascular	acute leukemia osteochondritis dissecans Legg-Calvé-Perthes Osgood-Schlatter's Scheuermann's	chronic leukemia	spontaneous osteonecrosis of the knee (SONK)

TABLE 2.13
Pathologies with Laboratory Test Value Indicators

Pathologies	Laboratory Indications
Rheumatoid arthritis	RA factor; present in 3% of the population
Seronegative arthritis	HLA B27; present in 6 to 8% of the population
Gout	uric acid levels > 6 mg/100 ml; normal = 3–6 mg/100 ml
Prostate metastasis	elevated acid phosphatase; normal = 0.5–2 (Bodansky)
Liver, bone disease	elevated alkaline phosphatase; normal = 2–4.5 (Bodansky)
Infection	CBC: elevated WBC (total); normal = 4500—11,000 mm^3
Anemia	CBC: hematocrit, hemoglobin, RBC and WBC totals Counts will be low, but levels vary with different types of anemia
Multiple myeloma	anemia, thrombocytopenia inverted A/G ratio (normal 2:1–3:1 with Globulin < 3 gm/100 ml) marked elevation of serum calcium (normal 8.5–10.5 mg/100 ml) Bence Jones proteinuria (40% of patients)
Bone destruction	elevated serum calcium (> 8.5–0.5 mg/100 ml)—not always reliable elevated serum phosphorus (normal = 2–4.5 mg/100 ml)
Inflammation	presence of C-reactive protein (CRP): normally absent elevated erythrocyte sedimentation rate (ESR); very low specificity norms = males: 0–15 mm/hr; females: 0–20 mm/hr
Tumor	elevated serum calcium (> 8.5–10.5 mg/100 ml) elevated serum phosphorus (> 2–4.5 mg/100 ml) elevated total protein (normal = 6–8 gm/100 ml) elevated ESR presence of CRP

2. **Supplemental examinations add information not available on standard plain films**

   a) Contrast examinations
   - arthrography: sometimes combined air/ contrast media for double contrast; excellent for assessment of joint component integrity
   - angiography: arterial or venous evaluation; assessment of tumor vascularity

- lymphangiography: lymphatic system assessed for obstruction, metastasis, or lymphoma
- myelography: contrast in subarachnoid space helps locate cord or canal space-occupying lesions
- discography: disc pathology and pain patterns evaluated

b) Radionuclide imaging
- highly sensitive
- amount and rate of tracer uptake can localize lesion

c) Ultrasound
- most often used to assess size, contours, and location of soft-tissue lesions
- can differentiate between cystic and solid masses

d) Videofluoroscopy
- motion studies
- evaluate joint mechanics, integrity or failure of arthrodesis
- radiation dose is generally higher than plain film of same area

e) Tomography
- selective view of thin slice of a structure
- high radiation dose

f) Computed tomography (CT)
- evaluation of soft tissues and bone lesions; CNS lesions
- used with or without contrast agents

g) Magnetic resonance imaging (MRI)
- almost photographic-quality images of anatomical structures and tissues
- greatest disadvantage is expense

h) Laboratory studies (see previous chart)

i) Biopsy
- needle aspiration
- incision
- sometimes the only method for reaching definitive diagnosis

H. BIOCHEMISTRY OF BONE

 1. Minerals

a) Calcium and phosphorus (2:1)

b) Main mineral complex is hydroxyapatite

c) Calcium deposition is affected by
- stress vectors
- vitamin D availability
- parathormone
- alkaline phosphatase
- trace minerals

d) Phosphorus allows calcium to precipitate at the bone crystal surface

☞   **2. Hormones**

    a) Parathormone (PTH)
- from parathyroid glands
- promotes calcium resorption, causing subperiosteal resorption of bone
- increased serum PTH levels cause increased osteoclastic activity
- high serum PTH levels correlate with decreased serum phosphorus

    b) Calcitonin
- PTH antagonist

    c) Estrogen
- stimulates bone production
- induces protein anabolism; important in bone maturation

    d) Androgen
- functions in the male like estrogens in the female

    e) Growth hormone (GH)
- produced in anterior pituitary
- governs chondrocyte proliferation and hypertrophy at growth plates

    f) Glucocorticoids
- encourage osteoclasis by inducing phosphorus excretion and protein catabolism

I. LESION LOCATION WITHIN BONE

☞   **1. Skeletal Development**

    a) Intramembranous ossification
- fibrous membrane hosts developing membranous bones
- flat bones, e.g., skull, mandible, scapula
- clavicles are membranous at first, later develop cartilaginous centers
- long tubular bone *width* develops via membranous growth

    b) Endochondral (or *enchondral*) ossification
- cartilage model forms first, then calcifies and eventually ossifies
- this growth is along the long axis of the bone and within epiphyseal centers

    c) Primary growth centers demonstrate calcification at birth

    d) Secondary growth centers develop calcification after birth

☞   **2. Long Bone Structure**

    a) Epiphysis
- end of a long bone
- produces and supports articular cartilage
- spinal analogue: apophysis

☞
- epiphyseal lesions: dysplasias, ischemic necrosis, arthritides, tumors (chondroblastoma, giant cell tumor)

b) Apophysis
- separated by physis from parent bone, but does not contribute to lengthening of bone
- functions as point of attachment for tendons and ligaments

c) Physis (growth plate, epiphyseal plate)
- growth zone
- layers of cartilage in process of maturation and developing into bone
- produces lengthwise growth of bones
- seen as radiolucent band until bone growth is completed

d) Zone of provisional calcification (ZPC)
- at junction of physis and metaphysis
- calcified but not yet ossified
- seen as a thin line of increased density
- ☞ **ZPC lesions:** calcium disorders, such as rickets

e) Metaphysis
- most metabolically active area of long bones; area of greatest blood supply
- area of trabecular formation
- normal periosteal resorption of bone creates characteristic tubulation here
- ☞ **metaphyseal lesions:** numerous tumors, infections, nutritional/metabolic/endocrine aberrations; e.g., Gaucher's disease (causes Erlenmeyer flask deformity)

f) Diaphysis
- long shaft of bone
- thick cortex around medullary space
- provides strength, rigidity
- houses red marrow
- ☞ **diaphyseal lesions:** leukemia, multiple myeloma, Ewing's sarcoma, non-Hodgkin's lymphoma, infections, Engelmann's disease

g) Cortex
- dense, outer rind of bone
- compact lamellar bone with interconnecting Haversian canals

h) Medulla
- internal cavity containing trabecular bone (spongiosa) and marrow

i) Periosteum
- thin membrane enclosing the diaphysis and metaphysis; can produce three patterns of new bone formation (solid, laminated, spiculated)
- fibrous outer layer with Sharpey's fibers attaching tendons and ligaments to bone
- cambium (inner layer): single layer that houses metabolic activity, mediating osteoblastic or osteoclastic functions (bone production and resorption) as needed

- no intra-articular periosteum
- blends with ligamentous tissue to form part of joint capsule

    j) Endosteum
- inner cortex

J. MNEMONIC FOR BONE DISEASE CATEGORIES

1. Screen diagnostic possibilities by disease category

2. *Congenital*
- spinal segmentation defects
- congenital dysplasias
- polydactyly
- achondroplasia
- osteopetrosis

3. *Arthritides*
- alignment disturbances
- juxtaarticular osteopenia or sclerosis
- loss of joint space (uniform vs. nonuniform)
- soft tissue swelling, masses or calcifications

4. *Trauma*
- fractures
- dislocations
- subluxations
- soft tissue swelling or calcification (myositis ossificans)

5. *Blood (Hematologic Pathologies)*
- anemias
- osteonecrosis

6. *Infection*
- osteomyelitis
- septic arthritis

7. *Tumor*
- lytic and blastic lesions
- cortical erosion
- periosteal reactions

8. *Endocrine, Nutritional and Metabolic Conditions*
- nutritional osteopenias
- hormonal effects on bone
- parathyroid pathology

9. *Soft tissue lesions*
- calcifications
- displacement
- swelling
- compression

> **Bone Disease Categories**
>
> ## "CAT BITES"
>
> **C**ongenital
> **A**rthritis
> **T**rauma
> **B**lood (hematologic)
> **I**nfection
> **T**umor
> **E**ndocrine (plus nutritional and metabolic etiologies; commonly referred to as "NME")
> **S**oft Tissue lesions

K. REPORTING

1. Viewing Conventions
- A-P studies: conventionally placed with patient's right on viewer's left; this is reversed for spinal examination

- Lateral studies: placed as patient was positioned; e.g., left lateral is placed with patient facing reading right
- Obliques: those displaying right-sided structures placed on left, and vice versa; with all oblique films side by side:

  - N.B., cervical obliques: RAO displays right neural foramina, RPO displays left neural foramina and vice versa
  - Lumbar obliques: RAO displays left pars and facets, RPO displays right pars and facets and vice versa

- Chest and abdomen: films viewed with patient's right on viewer's left
- Distal extremities viewed with digits pointing up and as if looking at the dorsal surface

2. **Introductory information should include:**
   - Clinic and physician name and address
   - Patient's name, address, date of birth, gender
   - File identification (file number, or patient number for clinic records)
   - Date films were taken
   - Views taken
   - Technique factors are reported optionally

3. **Report**
   - Relevant history: chief complaint; clinical findings (biomechanical and pathologic); rationale (reason for study)
   - Findings (narrative style)

4. **Conclusion or Impression**
   - Listed summary of findings

5. **Recommendations**
   - Follow-up studies indicated
   - Treatment indications or contraindications

6. **Dated signature of evaluator, with qualifying degree, e.g., D.C., M.D.**

L. VIEWING AIDS

1. **Systematic search pattern**
   - Sequential ABCS evaluation

2. **Reexamine hard-to-see areas minutely**
   - Complex anatomy (e.g., skull, lung apices, or through the heart)
   - Darker areas of film
   - Around film holder clips, ID marker, film edges

3. **Re-check each film with hot light to limit field of view and better visualize overexposed areas (if hot light is not available, roll a 14 × 17 film into a cylinder and look through it)**

4. **Use film envelope to cover up film, slowly slide it down, allowing the eye to notice individual details as they are uncovered**
5. **Other "tricks" to enhance viewing acuity:**
     - Tilt film slightly
     - Look for finger prints on film (areas of particular interest to other viewers)
     - Hand-held magnifying lens
     - Expose and process two 14 × 17 films, cut them in half lengthwise, and use blackened film to block viewbox lights around the 8 × 10 or 10 × 12 films being examined

M. COMMON REPORT TERMINOLOGY FOR MUSCULOSKELETAL FINDINGS

1. **Congenital Conditions**
     - Agenesis, dysplasia, hyperplasia, hypoplasia, overdevelopment, underdevelopment
2. **Arthritides**
     - Alignment, ankylosis, articular margin, disc height, entheses, joint space, osteophytes, sclerosis, subchondral bone, syndesmophytes
3. **Trauma**
     - Alignment, apposition, callus, comminution, dislocation, displacement, fracture
4. **Blood (hematologic)**
     - Avascular necrosis, curvilinear calcification, fragmentation, ischemic necrosis, joint effusions, medullary infarcts, myelofibrosis, myeloproliferative, osteonecrosis, osteopenia, phleboliths, pseudotumor, rarefaction, subchondral bone cysts
5. **Infection**
     - Articular cortex, cloaca (cortex), geographic lesions, involucrum (solid, laminated), moth-eaten lesions, periostitis, sequestrum, soft tissue planes
6. **Tumors and Tumor-like Processes**
     - Cortical integrity, lesions (geographic, moth-eaten, permeative), location (centric, eccentric, diaphysis, epiphysis, metaphysis), periosteal response, periostitis (laminated, solid, spiculated), soft tissue mass, zone of transition
7. **Endocrine, metabolic, nutritional (conventionally referred to as "NME")**
     - Accentuated trabecular pattern, cortical thinning, decreased bone density, osteopenia, osteoporosis, osteomalacia
8. **Biomechanical**
     - Ankylosis, fixation, hypermobility, hypomobility, intersegmental instability, malposition, misalignment, subluxation

REVIEW—STUDY QUESTIONS

1. What laboratory findings would be indicative of bone destruction?

2. What is the difference between alignment and apposition?

3. List at least five malignant tumors that preferentially locate in the femur.

4. In what age group, and in what areas of the body, would you be most likely to see a Ewing's sarcoma?

5. What group of patients are most apt to have multiple myeloma, and what laboratory indications would you see?

6. What lesions are most commonly found in the metaphysis?

7. In what part of the long bones are giant cell tumors most often found?

8. Describe the manner of growth of intramembranous and endochondral bone.

9. What minerals and hormones are most prominent in the healthy growth, remodeling, and repair of bone?

10. Describe the anatomy of a typical long bone.

11. What are the radiologic keys for differentiating inflammatory versus degenerative arthritis?

12. What elements should be present in a professionally prepared report of radiographic findings?

1. Monostotic lesions are most characteristic of:

    a) rickets.
    b) sickle cell anemia.
    c) Perthes disease.
    d) hyperparathyroidism.

2. A "smoky" or "ground glass" appearance indicates:

    a) a fibrous lesion.
    b) a cartilaginous lesion.
    c) a fatty lesion.
    d) an osseous lesion.

3. A neoplasm that may be expected to occur in patients younger than 20 years old is:

    a) lumbosacral chordoma.
    b) hemangioma.
    c) fibrosarcoma.
    d) chondrosarcoma.

4. All of the following are intradural intramedullary lesions except:

    a) astrocytoma.
    b) neurofibroma.
    c) ependymoma.
    d) lipoma.

5. The periosteum is a:

    a) thin membrane enclosing the epiphysis and diaphysis of a long bone.
    b) thin membrane enclosing the diaphysis of a long bone.
    c) thin membrane with a fibrous outer layer into which Sharpey's fibers insert.
    d) thin membrane enclosing the epiphysis and metaphysis of a long bone.

6. When the kilovolt setting is too high, the film will:

    a) appear too white.
    b) require longer exposure time.
    c) show poor contrast.
    d) demand higher mAs settings.

7. The Hounsfield unit is:

    a) a measure of density used for CT.
    b) a measure of density used for MRI.
    c) a measure of depth of the slice of a single CT image.
    d) a measure of thickness of shielding required.

8. Rare earth film-screen systems enable the technician to:

    a) use less shielding for the patient.
    b) dispense with narrow collimation.
    c) reduce the exposure time.
    d) reduce the kVp.

9. Meningioma is considered to be:

    a) an intradural intramedullary lesion.
    b) an extradural lesion.
    c) an intradural extramedullary lesion.
    d) an intramedullary lesion.

10. The kVp setting determines all of the following except:

    a) the force with which electrons are ejected.
    b) the wavelength of the ejected electrons.
    c) the frequency.
    d) the number of electrons ejected.

11. Nuclear scans are:

    a) very sensitive diagnostic tests.
    b) very specific diagnostic tests.
    c) very specific only if SPECT scanning is used.
    d) very specific only if PET scanning is used.

12. A tumor with an osseous matrix:

    a) may appear homogeneously dense on x-rays.
    b) may show stippled calcification.
    c) may show flocculent calcification.
    d) may show "eggshell" calcification.

13. Arthritides that are typically seen in younger patients (younger than 40 years) include:

    a) DISH.
    b) CPPD.
    c) Reiter's syndrome.
    d) pseudogout.

14. Contraindications to MRI include all of the following except:

    a) breast enhancement implants.
    b) tattooed eyeliner.
    c) shrapnel shards.
    d) pacemakers.

15. The most metabolically active area of a long bone is the:

    a) epiphysis.
    b) physis.
    c) zone of provisional calcification.
    d) metaphysis.

16. The function of wetting agents in film processing is to:

    a) swell the emulsion.
    b) drop the pH of the solution.
    c) rinse the emulsion of undeveloped silver halide.
    d) maintain the alkalinity of the developing solution.

17. The initial CT image:

    a) is on a sagittal plane, but is reformatted by computer into other planes.
    b) is on an axial plane, but is reformatted by computer into other planes.
    c) is always collimated to a 1-mm slice.
    d) is always collimated to a 2-mm slice.

18. The inverse square law deals with:

    a) the amount of exposure to radiation.
    b) the amount of time of the exposure.

c) the tube/film distance.

d) the kVp setting.

19. Infectious spondylitis or epidural abscess are detected earlier:

a) by MRI than by CT.

b) by CT than by MRI.

c) by myelography than by MRI.

d) by myelography than by CT.

20. In setting technique factors for taking x-rays, remember that mAs:

a) governs the number of electrons ejected.

b) governs the speed at which electrons are ejected.

c) governs the force with which electrons are ejected.

d) governs the number of electrons that reach the screen.

21. Nuclear bone scans require the detection of:

a) x-rays.

b) gamma rays.

c) Larmor frequencies.

d) beta rays.

22. Tumors that show a predilection for the spine include:

a) adamantinoma.

b) chordoma.

c) osteosarcoma.

d) Ewing's sarcoma.

23. The onset of gout usually is in patients:

a) more than 40 years old.

b) between 20 and 40 years old.

c) more than 70 years old.

d) less than 20 years old.

24. The optimal imaging modality for accurate location of spinal cord tumors is:

a) bone scan.

b) CT.

c) myelography.

d) MRI.

25. The physis:

a) is a thin layer of bone that is calcified, but not ossified.

b) is seen on x-rays as a thin line of increased density.

c) is associated with lengthwise bone growth.

d) is also known as the zone of provisional calcification.

26. X-ray film may be "fogged" by all of the following except:

a) pressure.

b) humidity.

c) excessive cold.

d) light.

27. Fluorescent lights are not suitable for a darkroom because:

a) they flicker too much.

b) they do not give a full spectrum of light.

c) they have an afterglow when they are extinguished.

d) they do not give off any heat.

28. The current MPD for whole body exposure is:

a) 10 Rems/year.

b) 5 Rads/year.

c) 5 Rems/year.

d) 10 Rads/year.

29. In cases of trauma, MRI is the modality of choice for evaluating:

a) spinal fractures.

b) muscle spasm contracture.

c) spinal cord contusion.

d) fractures in areas of complex anatomy, such as cranial bones.

30. Because of the anode heel effect:

a) filtration must always be used.

b) the anode must be at the bottom of the tube.

c) the anode should be at the top of the horizontal beam.

d) the kVp must be greater than 80.

31. Nuclear scans involve three phases which, in chronological order, are:

a) blood-pool phase, angiogram phase, bone-scan phase.

b) blood-pool phase, flow phase, delayed phase.

c) angiogram phase, blood-pool phase, delayed phase.

d) angiogram phase, bone-scan phase, delayed phase.

32. Multiple myeloma is preferentially found in:

a) the radius.

b) the scapula.

c) the femur.

d) the fibula.

33. A periosteal cuff of new bone at the periphery of the cortex/lesion junction is not known as:

a) a periosteal collar.

b) Codman's triangle.

c) a periosteal buttress.

d) an involucrum.

34. Taking x-rays with the kilovolt setting too low:

a) results in increased amounts of Compton scatter.

b) results in a black film.

c) results in a need for very low mAs settings.

d) results in a film with poor contrast.

35. Epiphyseal lesions commonly include all of the following except:

a) Gaucher's disease.

b) ischemic necrosis.

c) chondroblastoma.

d) Legg-Calvé-Perthes disease.

36. Intensifying screens:

a) always have double emulsion.

b) have single emulsion only.

c) fluoresce when struck by photons.
d) screen out scatter radiation.

37. All of the following may contribute to poor quality of films except:

a) poor or uneven contact between the film and the intensifying screen.
b) a miss-match of spectra between the film and the intensifying screen.
c) intensifying screens that are more than 7 years old.
d) developer temperature greater than 88°.

38. A factor in radiation protection is the fact that:

a) mA is directly proportional to exposure time.
b) mA is directly proportional to distance.
c) mA is inversely proportional to exposure time.
d) mA is inversely proportional to distance.

39. On a T2-weighted MRI study:

a) the brightest signal will be emitted by fat.
b) the brightest signal will be emitted by cortical bone.
c) the brightest signal will be emitted by water.
d) the brightest signal will be emitted by arterial blood.

40. The greatest majority of the energy from an x-ray tube is:

a) bremsstrahlung radiation.
b) heat.
c) x-rays.
d) characteristic radiation.

41. Myelography involves all of the following except:

a) Swimmer's lateral projection for cervical studies.
b) oblique projections for lumbar studies.
c) lateral decubitus projections.
d) AP open mouth projection.

42. Ewing's sarcoma shows a predilection for:

a) the epiphysis.
b) the metaphysis.
c) the diaphysis.
d) the metaphysis/diaphysis.

43. A solid periosteal response might be expected with all of the following lesions except:

a) venous stasis.
b) osteoid osteoma.
c) degenerative arthritis.
d) osteosarcoma.

44. During x-ray film developing, the fixing agent serves all of the following functions except:

a) hardening the emulsion.
b) rinsing undeveloped silver halide from the emulsion.
c) preventing the image from being degraded by light.
d) reducing the pH.

45. The availability of parathormone, vitamin D, and alkaline phosphatase all affect:

a) renal clearance.
b) bilirubin clearance.
c) thyroid function.
d) calcium deposition in bone.

46. Body tissues especially sensitive to radiation damage include all of the following except:

a) hematopoietic tissue.
b) myofascial tissue.
c) gastrointestinal tissue.
d) gonadal tissue.

47. To improve the detail on the film:

a) use the longest object-film distance possible.
b) lengthen the focal-film distance.
c) use a fast film-screen combination.
d) use a larger focal spot.

48. Sievert (Sv) is the unit sometimes used to express:

a) exposure in air.
b) Rads.
c) Rems.
d) absorption by tissue.

49. On a T1 weighted MRI study:

a) the brightest signal will be emitted by fat.
b) the brightest signal will be emitted by cortical bone.
c) the brightest signal will be emitted by water.
d) the brightest signal will be emitted by arterial blood.

50. The function of a grid is to:

a) enhance film/screen contact.
b) absorb scatter radiation.
c) prevent excess motion.
d) make the film appear lighter.

51. Intensifying screens:

a) should be selected in a green or blue spectrum to match the film used.
b) have a useful screen life of about 10 years.
c) always have emulsion on both sides.
d) always luminesce in a green spectrum.

52. A stress fracture is most likely to produce:

a) a solid periosteal response.
b) an onion-skin periosteal response.
c) a lamellated periosteal response.
d) Codman's triangle.

53. Adamantinoma is:

a) a benign tumor that may be found in the mandible.
b) a benign tumor that may be found in the tibia.
c) a malignant tumor that may be found in the tibia.
d) a malignant tumor that is most often found in the sacrum.

54. In myelography, contrast material is injected into the:

    a) subarachnoid space.
    b) subdural space.
    c) epidural space.
    d) neural canal.

55. Before contrast studies are initiated, the patient must be screened for:

    a) elevated BUN and creatinine.
    b) elevated white cell count.
    c) elevated ESR.
    d) elevated leukocyte count.

56. When filming a patient with known severe osteopenia:

    a) raise the mAs about 50%.
    b) raise the mAs about 30%.
    c) lower the mAs about 50%.
    d) lower the mAs about 30%.

57. The following choices are true of acute radiation syndrome except:

    a) it is especially destructive to eyes, gonads, and the central nervous system.
    b) it is nonstochastic in nature.
    c) it is lethal to 50% of exposed experimental animals within 30 days of exposure.
    d) it consists of stochastic effects.

58. In normal bone, the calcium:phosphorus ratio is:

    a) 3:1.
    b) 2:1.
    c) 1:2.
    d) 1:3.

59. When discussing the amount of radiation absorbed in tissue, the units are expressed as:

    a) Rads.
    b) Sieverts.
    c) Rems.
    d) coulombs/Kg.

60. Benign lesions usually are characterized by:

    a) cortical disruption.
    b) cortical expansion or thickening.
    c) imperceptible margins.
    d) laminated periosteal response.

61. Compton scatter radiation does all of the following except:

    a) reduces the energy of the photons.
    b) increases the wavelength of the photons.
    c) fogs the film.
    d) reduces the wavelength of the photons.

62. Cortical thickening is an indication of:

    a) a slow-growing malignancy.
    b) osteoporosis.
    c) Paget's disease.
    d) medullary tumors.

63. Fibrous lesions of bone usually originate in:

    a) outer cortex.
    b) medullary bone.
    c) periosteal tissue.
    d) inner cortex.

64. MRI studies:

    a) are contraindicated in pregnancy, although the risks are very low.
    b) are contraindicated in pregnancy because of high risk of fetal damage.
    c) are contraindicated in pregnancy because the risks are unknown.
    d) are not contraindicated in pregnancy.

65. Infusion of contrast material for a CT scan is contraindicated in patients with:

    a) claustrophobia.
    b) metallic implants.
    c) diabetes.
    d) metastatic disease of hematogenous spread.

66. When filming a patient who is particularly large-boned or heavily muscled:

    a) you should consider raising the mAs by about 50%.
    b) you should consider raising the mAs by about 30%.
    c) you should consider raising the kVp to about 100.
    d) you should consider reducing the mAs by about 30%.

67. Nonstochastic effects of radiation include:

    a) genetic aberrations.
    b) cataracts.
    c) carcinogenesis.
    d) leukemia.

68. The main mineral complex in bone is:

    a) calcium diphosphate.
    b) calcium phosphate.
    c) hydroxyapatite.
    d) calcium chloride.

69. "Beam hardening" refers to:

    a) the lower average intensity of remaining photons after attenuation.
    b) the higher average intensity of remaining photons after attenuation.
    c) the longer wavelength of remaining photons after attenuation.
    d) the lower frequency of photons after attenuation.

70. A tumor that shows a predilection for the scapula includes:

    a) chondrosarcoma.
    b) osteochondroma.
    c) osteosarcoma.
    d) chondroblastoma.

71. The image on the film is created by:

    a) scatter radiation.
    b) characteristic radiation.
    c) bremsstrahlung radiation.
    d) pair production.

72. A benign neoplasm characteristically has:

    a) a laminated periosteal response.
    b) a solid periosteal response.
    c) an "onion skin" periosteal response.
    d) a spiculated periosteal response.

73. Metastases are not commonly found in the:

    a) metaphysis.
    b) diaphysis.
    c) epiphysis.
    d) epiphysis/metaphysis.

74. Although difficult to diagnose, arachnoiditis may be detected by:

    a) CT.
    b) discography.
    c) CT myelography.
    d) myelography.

75. Bone mineral density (BMD) is evaluated most effectively by:

    a) bone scan.
    b) QCT (quantitative computed tomography).
    c) MRI.
    d) CT.

76. PA chest or abdomen films are usually taken:

    a) at a slightly lower kVp than that used for AP thoracic or lumbar films.
    b) at a slightly lower kVp than that used for lateral thoracic films.
    c) at a higher kVp than that used for spinal studies.
    d) at about the same kVp as that used for AP thoracic or lumbar studies.

77. Radiation burns and cataracts are both examples of:

    a) stochastic effects.
    b) nonstochastic effects.
    c) effects for which the risk is proportional to dose received.
    d) effects that do not become apparent for several years after exposure.

78. Elevated acid phosphatase may be a warning sign of:

    a) RA.
    b) prostate metastasis.
    c) gout.
    d) multiple myeloma.

79. Half value layer (HVL) is a measure of:

    a) attenuation, or absorption of energy from the x-ray beam.
    b) photoelectric interaction.
    c) pair production.
    d) photodisintegration.

80. Tumors of extraosseous origin:

    a) are separated from the cortical surface by a cleft that may be visible on x-ray.
    b) tend to expand the cortex.
    c) thin the endosteal cortex.
    d) may scallop the endosteal cortex.

81. Involucrum, sequestrum, and periostitis are all commonly associated with:

    a) arthritides.
    b) infections.
    c) tumors.
    d) endocrine disorders.

82. Permeative lesions are characterized by:

    a) a wide zone of transition.
    b) clear septation.
    c) slow growth.
    d) sharp margination.

83. An epiphyseal tumor suggests a diagnosis of:

    a) chondroblastoma.
    b) nonossifying fibroma.
    c) osteosarcoma.
    d) Ewing's sarcoma.

84. MRI limitations include:

    a) large dose of ionizing radiation.
    b) allergy to iodine-based contrast media.
    c) long immobility required.
    d) None of the above.

85. The modality of choice for visualization of calcified soft tissue lesions is:

    a) contrast CT.
    b) MRI.
    c) plain film.
    d) CT.

86. Extremity films should be taken:

    a) with a kVp between 80 and 90.
    b) with a kVp between 70 and 80.
    c) with a kVp between 50 and 65.
    d) with a kVp between 65 and 75.

87. Stochastic effects of radiation are those:

    a) that show the actual damage of radiation at the time the patient is exposed.
    b) called direct threshold effects.
    c) are those for which the patient is at risk, and the risk is proportional to dose received.
    d) are those that become apparent within 30 days of exposure.

88. HLA B27 is likely to be present with:

    a) RA.
    b) gout.
    c) seronegative arthritis.
    d) DJD.

89. The major effect of photoelectric interaction is:

    a) fogging of the film.
    b) creating the image on the film.
    c) increasing radiation dose.
    d) blurring the film image.

90. Polyostotic lesions might suggest a diagnosis of:

    a) Paget's disease.
    b) eosinophic granuloma.
    c) staph infection.
    d) osteoid osteoma.

91. Alignment, apposition, and comminution are all terms one might use in a report concerning:

    a) an arthritic patient.
    b) a patient with a hematologic disorder.
    c) a trauma patient.
    d) a metabolic disorder.

92. A solitary, sharply marginated lytic lesion might be described as:

    a) an aggressive lesion.
    b) a moth-eaten lesion.
    c) a permeative lesion.
    d) a geographic lesion.

93. Lesions tend to be fairly symmetrically distributed in:

    a) Paget's disease.
    b) psoriasis.
    c) metastasis.
    d) leukemia.

94. Nausea and vomiting, radiculitis, meningitis symptoms, CNS ischemia are possible side-effects of:

    a) MRI.
    b) myelography.
    c) bone scan.
    d) CT.

95. CT contrast studies are used to visualize all of the following except:

    a) intrathecal lesions.
    b) intradiscal lesions.
    c) occult fractures.
    d) gastrointestinal lesions.

96. Compton scatter increases when:

    a) mAs is increased.
    b) mAs is reduced.
    c) kVp is reduced.
    d) kVp is increased.

97. The Bergonie-Tribondeau law refers to:

    a) the genetically significant dose.
    b) the inverse square law.
    c) the maximum permissible dose.
    d) the fetus' exposure during the first trimester.

98. Elevated alkaline phosphatase is an indication of the presence of:

    a) bone disease.
    b) kidney disease.
    c) pancreatic disease.
    d) ovarian disease.

99. Classic scatter radiation on an x-ray is also called:

    a) coherent scatter.
    b) incoherent scatter.
    c) compton scatter.
    d) bremsstrahlung.

100. Patients may be protected from excessive irradiation by all of the following except:

    a) using grids.
    b) using close collimation.
    c) using rare earth film-screen systems.
    d) using high frequency generators.

PRACTICE TEST CHAPTER 2—ANSWER KEY

1. c	11. a	21. b	31. c	41. d	51. a	61. d	71. c	81. b	91. c
2. a	12. a	22. b	32. c	42. c	52. a	62. c	72. b	82. a	92. d
3. c	13. c	23. a	33. d	43. d	53. c	63. b	73. c	83. a	93. d
4. b	14. a	24. d	34. d	44. d	54. a	64. c	74. c	84. c	94. b
5. c	15. d	25. c	35. a	45. d	55. a	65. c	75. b	85. d	95. c
6. c	16. a	26. c	36. c	46. b	56. d	66. a	76. c	86. c	96. d
7. a	17. b	27. c	37. d	47. b	57. d	67. b	77. b	87. c	97. d
8. c	18. a	28. c	38. c	48. c	58. b	68. c	78. b	88. c	98. a
9. c	19. a	29. c	39. c	49. a	59. a	69. b	79. a	89. c	99. a
10. d	20. a	30. c	40. b	50. b	60. b	70. a	80. a	90. a	100. a

Chapter 3

DYSPLASIAS, COMMON SKELETAL ANOMALIES, AND VARIANTS

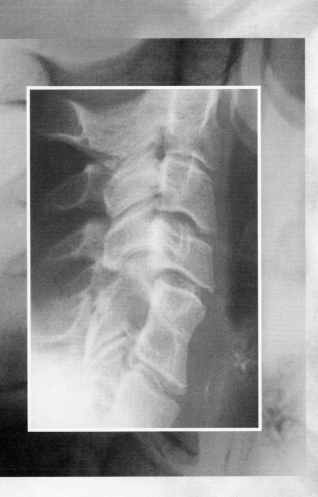

A. DYSPLASIAS

 1. **Achondroplasia (synonyms: chondrodystrophia fetalis; chondrodystrophic dwarfism, micromelia)**

    a) **General features**
- most common congenital dwarf
- autosomal dominant transmission

    b) **Clinical features**
- normal mentation
- rhizomelia: markedly shortened long bones
- large brachiocephalic cranium, prominent forehead, depressed nasal bridge

    c) **Radiologic features**
- cranial
    1) constricted skull base with small foramen magnum
    2) basilar impression
- thoracic: angular thoracolumbar kyphosis
- lumbar/lumbosacral
    1) hyperlordotic lumbar spine
    2) horizontally oriented sacrum
    3) short, thick lumbar pedicles, with decreased interpedicular distance
- vertebrae
    1) *"bullet-nosed"* vertebrae (Fig. 3.1)
    2) posteriorly scalloped vertebral bodies
    3) intervertebral disc height = vertebral body height
- appendicular skeleton
    1) scapulae squared inferiorly
    2) short ribs
    3) short, flat ilia
    4) proximal long bones most affected
    5) metaphyseal cupping
    6) short, thick tubular bones in hands and feet
    7) characteristic trident hand: widely spaced third and fourth digits

    d) **Neurologic consequences**
- sleep apnea
- hydrocephalus, which may lead to cord compression
- spinal or foraminal stenosis, with consequent
    1) intermittent cauda equina claudication
    2) nerve root compression
    3) chronic transverse myelopathy (due to severe kyphosis)
    4) acute traumatic transverse myelopathy with paraplegia
- complications caused by disc herniation and/or osteophytic stenosis

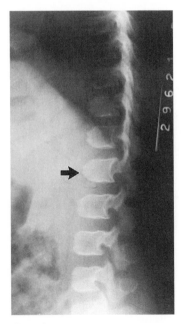

Figure 3.1.

"Bullet-nosed" vertebra, posterior scalloped body. Reprinted with permission from Yochum TR, Rowe LJ. Essentials of Skeletal Radiology, 2nd ed. Baltimore: Williams & Wilkins, 1996:1515.

2. **Cleidocranial Dysplasia (synonyms: cleidocranial dysostosis, spondylo-megaepiphyseal-metaphyseal dysplasia)**

   a) **General features**
   - faulty intramembranous bone ossification
   - recessive inheritance

   b) **Clinical features**
   - normal mentation
   - large head with small face
   - abnormal dentition: periodontitis and severe caries
   - sometimes hearing loss due to ossicle abnormalities
   - drooping, hypermobile shoulders
   - narrow, cone-shaped chest

   c) **Radiologic features**
   - skull
      1) platybasia
      2) large, deformed foramen magnum
      3) multiple wormian bones
      4) persistent metopic suture
      5) "hot cross bun" look caused by wide sagittal and coronal sutures
      6) thickened supraorbital, temporal squama, occipital bone
      7) brachiocephalic (enlarged width)
   - thorax
      1) agenesis or hypoplasia of clavicles
      2) anomalous development of clavicles
      3) scapulae small; may be winged or elevated
   - pelvis
      1) small, underdeveloped pelvic bones
      2) midline defect at pubic symphysis
      3) early coxa valgus, changing with age to coxa varus
   - spine
      1) biconvex vertebrae
      2) SBO, most often in cervical and upper dorsal segments
      3) hemivertebrae
      4) lumbar spondylolysis
      5) abnormal curvatures
   - extremities
      1) elongated second metacarpal caused by accessory epiphysis
      2) pointed, hypoplastic distal phalanges
      3) radius occasionally shortened

   d) **Complications**
   - hearing loss
   - dental lesions
   - shoulder, hip dislocations
   - severe scoliosis

3. **Epiphyseal Dysplasias**

I. **Chondrodysplasia Punctata (synonyms: stippled epiphyses; dysplasia epiphysealis punctata; chondrodystrophia fetalis calcificans; chondrodystrophia calcificans congenita)**

   a) **General features**
   - Conradi-Hunermann syndrome: dominant transmission
   - rhizomelic form: recessive transmission (lethal)

   b) **Clinical features**
   - appearance similar to achondroplastic dwarf, short limbs
   - rhizomelic form: mental retardation, death usually in first year
   - Conradi-Hunermann syndrome: normal mentation
     1) ichthyosiform skin lesions
     2) cataracts
     3) linear areas of alopecia
     4) nail abnormalities
   - One rare, recessive x-linked form of Conradi-Hunermann syndrome more severe, with retardation, asymmetric limb shortening, small distal phalanges

   c) **Radiologic features**
   - epiphyseal stippling (disappears after first year of life)
   - rhizomelic lethal recessive form
     1) epiphyseal stippling in hips, shoulders, knees, wrists
     2) symmetrically shortened limbs (proximal bones especially)
     3) flared metaphyses
     4) bowed long bones
     5) coronally cleft vertebrae
   - Conradi-Hunermann syndrome
     1) stippling at ends of long bones, in short tubular bones
     2) occasionally, asymmetric limb shortening
     3) normal metaphyses, diaphyses
     4) may be stippled vertebrae
     5) may have kyphoscoliosis
     6) may stipple ribs, hyoid bone, thyroid cartilage, skull base
     7) may have laryngeal or tracheal calcifications

II. **Dysplasia Epiphysealis Hemimelica (synonyms: Trevor's disease, tarsoepiphyseal aclasis)**

   a) **General features**
   - not genetically transmitted
   - three general forms: monostotic; classical form (more than one area in an

extremity); polyostotic (involving an entire lower extremity)

b) Clinical features

- male predominance (3:1)
- presents in first decade
- asymmetrical epiphyseal overgrowth (usually medial)
- usually monomelic
- most often affects distal femur, distal tibia, talus
- hard, bony swellings; usually painless
- occasionally affects upper limb

c) Radiologic features

- asymmetrical focal overgrowth of epiphysis
- medial side more often (2:1)

III. Epiphyseal Dysplasia Multiplex (synonyms: dysplasia epiphysealis multiplex, multiple epiphyseal dysplasia, Fairbank-Ribbing disease, dysplasia polyepiphysaire)

a) General features

- autosomal dominant transmission
- possibly a tarda form of chondrodysplasia punctata

b) Clinical features

- waddling gait, difficulty running
- premature, often severe, DJD
- shortened extremities; short, thick hands
- genu vara or valgum; coxa vara; flexion deformities
- tibiotalar slant in 50% of cases
- usually lower limbs: bilateral and symmetrical

c) Radiologic features

- delayed, irregular epiphyseal development
- hypoplastic tarsals, carpals
- short, thick tubular hand (and sometimes foot) bones
- mature to irregular joint surfaces: flat femoral heads, condyles
- slipped femoral capital epiphysis (SFCE) with coxa vara
- Scheuermann's-like spinal changes
- vertebral wedging, scoliosis
- occasionally: platyspondyly, dens agenesis

IV. Spondyloepiphyseal Dysplasia: two forms: congenita and tarda

- **Spondyloepiphyseal dysplasia congenita**

a) General features

- autosomal dominant
- **DDX** consideration: Morquio's syndrome, which shows central beaking of vertebrae and normal disc height; congenital

Spondyloepiphyseal Dysplasia has bulbous vertebrae and thin discs

b) Clinical features

- apparent at birth
- short limbs, flat faces, widely spaced eyes
- cleft palate, hearing loss, myopia, retinal detachment
- short neck and spine (grow to less than 52 inches), very short trunk
- hyperlordosis, hyperkyphosis, scoliosis
- pectus carinatum
- genu varum or valgum; hip contractures
- hands and feet are normal

c) Radiologic features

- delayed ossification at pubis, distal femur, proximal tibia, calcaneus, talus, femoral head
- horizontal acetabular roofs, short iliac wings
- vertebrae: bulbous (*pear-shaped*), develop platyspondyly, hypoplastic in thoracolumbar region, odontoid malformations
- thin discs
- abnormal curvatures (see above)
- proximal long bones shortened (rhizomelia), flared metaphyses

- **Spondyloepiphyseal Dysplasia Tarda**

a) General features

- usually X-linked, recessive transmission
- expressed in males

b) Clinical features

- males, usually diagnosed at 5–10 years old
- mildly shortened height (grow to 52–62 inches)
- reports of back pain
- premature osteoarthritis (beginning shortly after puberty)

c) Radiologic features

- vertebrae: hump-shaped, pear-shaped, or "*heaped-up*" (Fig. 3.2); platyspondyly in thoracics; non-ossified ring epiphysis; early DJD
- thin disc spaces
- mild curvature abnormalities
- early, severe hip arthritis; deformed femoral head and neck
- small pelvis; broad thorax; prominent sternum

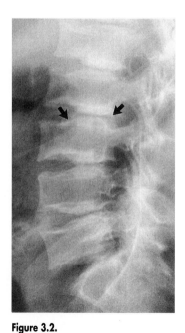

Figure 3.2.

"Heaped-up" vertebrae. Reprinted with permission from Yochum TR, Rowe LJ. Essentials of Skeletal Radiology, 2nd ed. Baltimore: Williams & Wilkins, 1996:1519.

REVIEW—STUDY QUESTIONS

1. What complications occur with achondroplasia, and why do they happen?

2. Which entities must be differentially diagnosed from spondyloepiphyseal dysplasia, and what features help in the differentiation?

3. The following vertebral appearances are characteristic of which dysplasias? Biconvex vertebra; non-ossified ring epiphyses; bullet-nosed vertebra; vertebral wedging; pear-shaped (or bulbous) vertebra; heaped-up vertebra

4. Name and describe the two forms of chondrodysplasia punctata (clinical presentation, roentgen signs, progression and prognosis).

5. Of the foregoing dysplasias, which is not genetically transmitted?

6. Would manipulation be contraindicated for any of the foregoing dysplasias? Should it be approached with special caution for any of them? Which, and why?

7. Which of the above dysplasias show a gender predilection, and for which gender?

8. What pathologic process produces cleidocranial dysplasia?

9. Name and give general descriptions of four epiphyseal dysplasias.

10. List ten roentgen signs present in achondroplasia.

---

4. **Fibrodysplasia Ossificans Progressiva (synonyms: Munchmeyer's disease; fibrogenesis ossificans progressiva; myositis ossificans progressiva; fibrositis ossificans progressiva)**

   a) **General features**
- idiopathic etiology
- soft tissue ossification
- autosomal dominant transmission; may be random spontaneous occurrence
- affects striated muscles only
- manipulation is contraindicated
- drug therapy leads to osteomalacia: pathologic fractures common
- death from cardiopulmonary failure usually results

   b) **Clinical features**
- torticollis
- SCM masses: hot, painful, edematous
- sometimes post-traumatic onset
- possibly accompanied by fever
- may entail respiratory difficulty with intercostal involvement
- phalangeal synostosis
- 75% of patients have microdactyly of great toe
- thumb anomalies

☞   **c) Radiologic features**
- anomalous digits: great toe and thumb especially affected
- short metacarpals (usually first and fifth)
- hallux valgus
- broad femoral neck
- hypoplastic discs calcify
- ectopic ossifications: muscles, tendons, ligaments, fascia

☞   **5. Holt-Oram Syndrome (synonyms: heart-hand syndrome; cardio-limb syndrome; cardiomelic syndrome)**

a) General features
- familial transmission, autosomal dominant
- spares the lower extremities

b) Clinical features
- cardiovascular abnormalities: patent atrial septum most common; also see ventricular septal defects, great vessel anomalies
- limited elbow range of motion; elbow dislocation
- shoulder anomalies
- chest wall anomalies, pectoral muscle deficiencies
- may have aplastic anemia

☞   **c) Radiologic features**
- thumb anomalies very common: triphalangeal thumb (extra phalanx), agenesis of thumb
- carpal abnormalities very common: scaphoid abnormalities, extra carpals, carpal fusions
- fifth finger middle phalanges short, usually with clinodactyly
- hypoplasia or agenesis of radial head
- radio-ulnar and/or humero-ulnar synostosis
- radial ray deficiency (or dysplasia), agenesis of radius
- hypoplastic humeri, clavicles, scapulae
- Sprengel's deformity
- pectus excavatum, pectus carinatum

☞   **6. Infantile Cortical Hyperostosis (synonyms: Caffey's disease; Caffey's syndrome)**

a) General features
- no gender predilection; no population prevalence
- often familial presence over several generations
- probably inherited
- incidence is decreasing
- presents within first 5 months of life

b) Clinical features
- hyperirritability
- soft tissue swellings

- usually symmetrical involvement
- hard masses over affected bones
- fever
- elevated ESR and alkaline phosphatase, anemia
- pseudoparalysis
- pleuritis
- marked swelling over mandible

☞   c) **Radiologic features**
- periosteal new bone formation at sites of swelling: may appear laminated during healing phase
- commonly seen at mandible, clavicle, ribs, ulna (without radial involvement)
- usually not affected: vertebrae, carpals, tarsals, phalanges
- spares epiphyses

☞ 7. **Marfan's Syndrome (synonyms: arachnodactyly; dolichostenomelia)**

a) **General features**
- incidence 4 to 6 per 100,000 (cannot be considered ''rare'')
- familial transmission, autosomal dominant
- normal mentation
- no gender or population predilection
- involves skeletal, ocular, and cardiovascular systems
- connective tissue disorder; inferior quality collagen
- atlantoaxial instability may be present, contraindicates upper cervical manipulation
- radiologically similar to homocystinuria: DDX by vertebral body flattening, osteoporosis, and mental retardation in homocystinuria

b) **Clinical features**
- tall, thin individuals (usually taller than 6 feet)
- elongate extremities (especially distally, and more marked in lower extremities)
- hypoplastic, hypotonic muscles, with scant subcutaneous fat
- joint laxity and dislocations (hips and patellae; bilateral perilunate dislocations)
- genu recurvatum, pes planus
- thoracic scoliosis
- dolichocephaly: elongate face, arched palate, prominent jaw
- normal mentation
- anomalous dentition (may have two rows or irregularly placed teeth)
- ocular abnormalities: dislocated lens (ectopia lentis), iridodonesis (trembling iris), retinal detachment, cataracts, myopia, absent dilator muscles

(permanently contracted pupils), strabismus

- congenital heart disease: atrial septal defect, abnormal tunica media, cystic medial necrosis (aortic or pulmonary artery dissection/ rupture), dilatation of ascending aorta, valve abnormalities ("floppy valve syndrome": valvular incompetence and left- heart insufficiency)
- "thumb sign": flexed thumb protrudes beyond closed fist
- chest wall deformities: pectus excavatum, pectus carinatum

   c) Radiologic features
- arachnodactyly (spider-like fingers); long, thin extremities
- thin cortices and delicate trabeculation but NO osteoporosis
- protrusio acetabulae
- vertebrae: tall, with posterior scalloping
- scoliosis or kyphoscoliosis
- widened spinal canal (usually lumbosacral)
- thin lamina and pedicles (caused by dural ectasia)
- pectus carinatum, or pectus excavatum with elongated ribs
- may be meningocele with nerve root compression
- slipped capital femoral epiphysis
- may see atlantoaxial hypermobility and/or dislocation

8. **Metaphyseal Dysplasia (synonyms: Pyle's disease, familial metaphyseal dysplasia)**

   a) General features
- autosomal recessive transmission
- craniometaphyseal dysplasia (as distinct from metaphyseal dysplasia) involves mental, motor retardation; craniofacial abnormalities; cranial nerve involvement; hemi- or quadriplegia
- manifests in late childhood
- subperiosteal remodeling fails in metaphyses
- possibly caused by chronic hyperemia in perichondral ring of osteoblasts; hyperplasia of perichondral ring arteries (congenitally)

   b) Clinical features
- tall patient
- lower extremity involvement: genu valgum, bulbous joints
- patient occasionally has joint pain or contractures, weakness

   c) Radiologic features
- as newborn, skeleton looks osteoporotic

- Erlenmeyer flask deformity (splayed metaphyses) with thin cortices
- predisposed to fracture at affected metaphyses (usually lower extremities)
- most commonly affected: distal femur, tibia (proximal and distal) proximal fibula
- upper extremity involvement may include: distal radius, ulna, proximal humerus
- small tubular bones of hands and feet occasionally involved
- sternal end of clavicle; ribs; ischial and pubic rami
- sinus hypoplasia
- hyperostosis at calvarium and mandible
- ocular hypertelorism (widened interocular space)
- vertebrae: platyspondyly or vertebra plana with dense vertebral body centra

9. **Nail-Patella Syndrome (synonyms: HOOD [hereditary osteo-onychodysplasia], osteo-onychodysostosis, Fong's syndrome)**

   a) **General features**
   - autosomal dominant transmission
   - early death because of kidney dysplasia with renal osteodystrophy
   - paired posterior iliac horns are present from infancy; occasionally these are absent; a single posterior iliac horn is not associated with this syndrome

   b) **Clinical features**
   - dysplastic fingernails: hypoplastic, splitting (first and second digits usually)
   - may see clinodactyly, short fifth metacarpals
   - absent patellae (palpably evident)
   - asymmetric femoral condyles cause deformity, gait abnormalities, genu valgum
   - increased elbow carrying angle; radial head subluxation or dislocation
   - soft tissue abnormalities: joint contractures, webbing fingers and toes, muscle hypoplasia
   - abnormal iris pigmentation

   c) **Radiologic features**
   - paired posterior iliac "horns" (pathognomonic)
   - flared or shortened iliac wings
   - small or absent patellae
   - asymmetric femoral condyles
   - hypoplastic medial humeral condyle, hypoplastic capitellum

REVIEW—STUDY QUESTIONS

1. Describe the clinical presentation of a patient with Marfan's syndrome.
2. For which of the above might spinal manipulation be contraindicated or might caution be advised when manipulating?
3. Which of the above dysplasias specifically affects the thumbs? Describe the effect in each case.
4. What roentgen feature is pathognomonic for Fong's syndrome?
5. What body systems are affected by Marfan's syndrome?
6. Describe the pathologic process that causes metaphyseal dysplasia.
7. Give two synonyms for Holt-Oram syndrome, and describe it clinically and radiologically.
8. Describe fibrodysplasia ossificans progressiva. What is the common cause of death for these patients?
9. Describe the Erlenmeyer flask deformity. What dysplasias feature it? Why does it develop?
10. Which of the nine dysplasias that we have covered so far entails defective mentation?

10. **Osteopenic Dysplasias**

I. **Ehlers-Danlos Syndrome (synonyms: arthrochalasis multiplex congenita, cutis hyperelastica, dermatorrhexis)**

a) **General features**
- ten types identified (I–X): most autosomal dominant, some autosomal recessive, and some X-linked recessive
- connective tissue disorder (mesenchymal tissue)
- systems affected: bronchopulmonary, genitourinary, cardiovascular, alimentary, CNS, eyes, integument
- normal mentation
- predilection for white, European males
- billed as *"Elastic Lady, Pretzel Man, Rubber Man"*

b) **Clinical features**
- joint hyperextensibility, hypermobility (ligament and capsule laxity)
- vascular fragility, easy bruising
- skin hyperelasticity, fragility; feels velvety, chamois-like
- subcutaneous nodules: spherules (necrotic fat), hematomas, molluscoid fibrous tumors
- *"cigarette-paper skin"* caused by many large scars covered by thin skin
- type IV most serious: very fragile vessels and thin, fragile skin, but no skin elasticity and little joint involvement

- patients often tall, with characteristic gait
- hip hyperextension and genu recurvatum
- pes planus
- hyperextensible wrists, thumbs, knees and elbows
- lop ears
- drooped skin folds around eyes
- blue sclerae
- poor dentition
- high arched palate
- cardiovascular abnormalities: tetralogy of Fallot, aortic dissection, aneurysms, arteriovenous fistulas, varicosities, valve abnormalities
- bronchopulmonary abnormalities: spontaneous pneumothorax, bronchiectasis, pulmonary hypertension
- genitourinary abnormalities: bladder diverticula, hydronephrosis, medullary sponge kidney
- GI abnormalities: dilatation or spontaneous perforation and hemorrhage of the large bowel

c) **Radiologic features**
- calcified subcutaneous spherules (2–15 mm) in pretibial soft tissue and along the forearms (ringlike, non-laminated)
- heterotopic ossifications (e.g., around the hip)
- platyspondyly
- posterior vertebral body scalloping (CSF pulsates in ectatic thecal sac)
- diminished (even lordotic) thoracic kyphosis, thoracic scoliosis
- spondylolysis and spondylolisthesis
- thoracic cage asymmetry, pectus excavatum or pectus carinatum
- acroosteolysis (terminal finger tufts resorbed) when Raynaud's phenomenon is associated
- may see delayed cranial vault ossification, micrognathia, hypertelorism, fifth digit clinodactyly, ulnar styloid elongation, radioulnar synostosis, arachnodactyly, club foot, pes planus

II. **Massive Osteolysis of Gorham (synonyms: hemangiomatosis, massive osteolysis, disappearing bone disease, vanishing bone disease)**

a) **General features**
- no gender predilection
- usually evidenced before age 40
- idiopathic: may or may not follow significant trauma; no familial links
- any bone, but more often in long bone, pelvis, thorax, and spine
- spreads to adjacent bones
- unpredictable progression, prognosis

- spinal involvement may lead to cord transection, paraplegia
- pulmonary complications with thoracic involvement
- soft, spongy bone with eroded cortices
- hemangiomas replace bone; these are replaced by vascular fibrous tissue
- hypervascular marrow spaces (hypervascularity appears to cause the bone resorption)

b) Clinical features
- acute pain onset or insidious onset, progressing from dull pain and soft tissue atrophy
- may present with pathologic fracture and deformity
- lab findings unremarkable

c) Radiologic features
- subcortical, intramedullary patchy osteoporosis
- numerous fractures, bony fragmentation, total disappearance of bone
- remaining ends of bone tapered
- atrophied soft tissues with calcified thrombi (phleboliths)

III. Mucopolysaccharidoses (MPS)
- inherited metabolic disorders
- skeletal, visceral, and mental abnormalities
- aberrant storage of mucopolysaccharide macromolecules in body tissues
- excessive urinary excretion of mucopolysaccharides
- six distinct syndromes classified:
    1) MPS-I: three varieties; Hurler, Scheie, and Hurler-Scheie
    2) MPS-II: Hunter
    3) MPS-III: Sanfilippo (subtypes A, B, C, D)
    4) MPS-IV: Morquio (subtypes A, B)
    5) MPS-V: Maroteaux-Lamy
    6) MPS-VI: Sly
- most commonly encountered: MPS-I-H (Hurler's) and MPS-IV (Morquio's)

1) MPS-I-H: Hurler's Syndrome (synonyms: lipochondrodystrophy, gargoylism, osteochondrodystrophy, dysostosis multiplex)

a) General features
- autosomal recessive
- excessive lipid accumulation in CNS and viscera
- about 1 in 100,000 births
- dermatan sulfate and heparin sulfate in urine

b) Clinical features
- normal at birth
- gradual development of large head,

hypertelorism, sunken nose, large lips, protruding tongue, coarsened features
- hydrocephalus
- short, malformed teeth
- corneal opacities
- deteriorating mentation
- gradually increasing deafness
- cardiomegaly, heart murmurs (heart failure is a concern)
- protruding abdomen (hepatosplenomegaly)
- umbilical and inguinal hernias
- early cessation of growth: dwarfism
- severe thoracolumbar kyphosis, flexion contractures
- *trident* hands, may be clawed
- short life span (usually under 20 years)

☞   **c) Radiologic features**
- skull: macrocephaly, frontal bossing, calvarial thickening, premature closure of sagittal and lambdoid sutures, enlarged sella turcica ("J"-shaped), small facial bones, wide mandibular angle
- spine: vertebral body hypoplasia (leading to dorsolumbar kyphosis); *inferiorly beaked* vertebrae in thoracolumbar area; other vertebra with ovoid bodies (convex curvature of endplates); long, slender pedicles; odontoid hypoplasia may cause atlantoaxial subluxation and instability
- appendicular skeleton: *paddle ribs* (spatulated); flared ilia; acetabular roofs are angled obliquely; coxa valga or vara; humerus varus deformity; widened diaphyses in tubular bones (upper more than lower extremities); *trident* hand (short, wide metacarpals and phalanges)
- General osteoporosis

☞   2) MPS-IV: Morquio's Syndrome (synonyms: chondrodystrophy, familial osteodystrophy, eccentro-osteochondrodysplasia, Morquio-Ulrich syndrome, Morquio-Brailsford syndrome)

a) General features
- autosomal recessive transmission
- about 1 in 100,000 births
- keratosulfaturia (detected at birth)
- two types, based on severity: A more severe than B

b) Clinical features
- skeletal changes appear with weight-bearing
- dwarfism (less than 4 feet tall)
- weak, hypotonic muscles
- dorsal kyphoscoliosis
- pectus carinatum (protuberant, horizontally oriented sternum)
- very short neck ("no-neck" appearance)

- wide-set eyes, short nose with depressed bridge
- wide maxillae, teeth deformed, poorly spaced
- corneal opacities, deafness
- normal mentation
- genu valgum, flexion contractures
- enlarged wrists, deformed hands
- respiratory paralysis and paraplegia may result from cord injury caused by atlantoaxial dislocations
- aortic valve abnormalities lead to cardiomegaly
- life-span is usually 30 to 40 years

☞ 　　c) **Radiologic features**
- platyspondyly with *central beaking* (in infants, vertebrae are still rounded, but by age 2 or 3 they flatten)
- first or second lumbar may be hypoplastic, and displaced posteriorly
- normal or widened disc spaces
- hypoplastic or absent odontoid (atlantoaxial instability)
- unstable acetabular joints: hypoplastic acetabuli, femoral heads; wide femoral necks; often coxa valga or vara
- short, thick tubular bones in extremities (upper more than lower)
- carpal, tarsal, phalangeal abnormalities

☞ **IV. Osteogenesis Imperfecta (synonyms: osteopsathyrosis idiopathica, mollities ossium, fragilitas ossium, Lobstein's disease)**

　　a) **General features**
- affects skeleton, ligaments, skin, sclera, inner ear and teeth
- autosomal dominant transmission
- abnormal maturation of collagen in all types of bone; possibly caused by deficiency of ATPase
- may have slight predilection for females
- has traditionally been classified in two major forms: congenita and tarda
- congenita has high rate of stillbirths and infant mortality
- tarda can have normal life expectancy; has two classes: one acquires bowed long bones, the other (less severe) without bowing
- new classification gives five major forms:
  1) Type I: autosomal dominant, variable penetrance (most common, comprises most tarda cases)
  2) Type II: autosomal recessive; congenita cases, very severe
  3) Type III: may be autosomal dominant or recessive, or sporadic; severe progressive skeletal deformities; fractures present at birth; dramatic dwarfism

4) Type IV: autosomal dominant; no blue sclera (present in Types I–III), variable skeletal findings
5) Type V: minimal skeletal fragility, but other criteria for diagnosis are met (see clinical features below)

☞ **b) Clinical features**
- diagnosed when two of four major criteria are present
    1) osteoporosis with abnormal skeletal fragility
    2) blue sclera
    3) abnormal dentition (*dentinogenesis imperfecta*)
    4) premature otosclerosis
- general ligament laxity
- episodic diaphoresis, and abnormal temperature regulation
- easy bruising, premature vascular calcification
- hyperplastic scars
- *Saturn's ring*: ring of normal, white sclera around cornea
- teeth may be blue-gray or yellow-brown opalescent teeth because of malformed, defective dentin, though enamel is normal; teeth often are chipped, with many cavities (dental caries)
- otosclerosis resembles idiopathic conduction deafness
- bleeding tendencies because of platelet aggregation defect
- may have growth retardation; also fractures contribute to short height, as do kyphoscolioses and limb bowing
- bones less fragile with maturity, females seem to remiss after puberty, and estrogen therapy may be helpful

☞ **c) Radiologic features**
- numerous fractures which heal with exuberant callus and a poor cellular matrix
- callus presents as *pseudotumors*
- bowing deformities and pseudarthroses may follow fracture healing
- diffuse osteopenia; pencil-thin cortices
- bones may appear thin and gracile (most commonly); short and thick (seen usually with the congenita form); or cystic (with flared metaphysis)
- persistent, multiple Wormian bones; enlarged sinuses; thin, lucent calvarium; platybasia, often with basilar impression
- kyphoscoliosis
- vertebrae may be flattened, anteriorly wedged, or biconcave (*biconcave lens vertebra*)

- protrusio acetabuli; shepherd's crook deformity of proximal femur
- premature DJD (because of lax ligaments and articular fractures)

REVIEW—STUDY QUESTIONS

1. What systems are affected in Ehlers-Danlos syndrome? Describe the effects on each.

2. What is the underlying pathology in Ehlers-Danlos syndrome?

3. What four criteria define osteogenesis imperfecta? What is its underlying cause?

4. Compare and contrast achondroplasia and Morquio's syndrome in terms of pathologic process, clinical presentation, prognosis, and radiographic findings.

5. Compare Morquio's syndrome and Hurler's syndrome in the same way.

6. In which of the osteopenic dysplasias above is manipulation contraindicated, and why?

7. What is MPS, what is its underlying pathology, and how are its syndromes classified?

8. Describe massive osteolysis of Gorham and explain its process and prognosis.

9. Which two dysplasias (among those we have reviewed thus far) feature the *trident hand*?

10. Among the dysplasias we have reviewed, which offer a normal life-span expectancy?

---

11. Sclerosing Dysplasias

☞ The first three—melorheostosis, osteopathia striata, and osteopoikilosis—appear to be closely related, and cases of signs of all three in a single patient have been recorded. This phenomenon is termed *overlap syndrome.*

☞ **I. Melorheostosis (synonyms: Leri type of osteopetrosis, osteosi eberneizzante monomelica, flowing hyperostosis)**

a) General features
- in addition to the *overlap syndrome* mentioned above, this may be associated with linear scleroderma, neurofibromatosis, tuberous sclerosis, hemangiomas
- melorheostosis means "*limb,*" "*flow,*" and "*bone*" in Greek
- no sex predilection
- etiology unknown; appears to be congenital
- becomes symptomatic in late childhood/ early adolescence
- slow progression, periods of arrest and exacerbation
- usually monomelic, more commonly lower limb

- ipsilateral innominate or scapula often affected
- progression is proximal to distal
- vertebrae, ribs, skull and face have been involved
- lesions appear to follow sclerotomes and myotomes supplied by a single spinal sensory nerve
- laboratory findings normal
- thermography may indicate early soft tissue changes, before osseous findings are demonstrable
- bone scintigraphy will show increased uptake in affected areas

b) Clinical features

- pain, joint swelling, limited motion
- joint contractures and deformities
- genu varum and valgum, valgus foot deformities, patellar dislocations
- in severe cases: premature epiphyseal closure, shortened limbs
- soft tissue: anomalous pigmentation, scleroderma-like skin atrophy; muscle wasting
- lymphedema caused by pressure on adjacent vessels; arteriovenous malformations

c) Radiologic features

- classic: streaked, wavy cortical thickening (endosteal in children, primarily periosteal in adults); *candle drip* or *flowing candle wax* appearance
- hyperostosis under periosteum along one side of a long bone (classic)
- endosteal hyperostosis encroaches upon medullary space
- osteochondroma-like masses extend into joint area
- carpal and tarsal bone reactions resemble osteopoikilosis
- flat bones (ilia and scapula) dense radiations extend from the joint
- soft tissue calcification, heterotopic bone formation may ankylose joint

II. Osteopathia Striata (synonym: Voorhoeve's disease)

a) General features

- genetic transmission suspected; etiology still unknown
- may be a variant of osteopoikilosis
- may also show signs of osteopetrosis, focal dermal hypoplasia (Goltz syndrome), or cranial sclerosis
- no gender predilection
- usually bilateral involvement of long bones

- seems to reflect old remodeling of bone; no scintigraphic uptake
- laboratory results normal

b) Clinical features

- usually an incidental finding; asymptomatic
- sometimes vague joint pain

☞ **c) Radiologic features**

- vertical linear opacities from metaphysis into diaphysis
- occasionally, striations cross into epiphysis
- longest striations are in femur
- ilium: from acetabulum to iliac crest—fanlike *sunburst effect*
- may have densities in small tubular bones of hands and feet, or in spine
- may be thickening and sclerosis of skull base

☞ **III. Osteopoikilosis (synonyms: osteopathia condensans disseminata; spotted bones)**

a) General features

- autosomal dominant transmission
- may be more prominent in succeeding generations
- seems to be remodeling of spongy bone; caused by mechanical stress
- no microfractures involved
- lesions may be small foci that fail to become cancellous; they are compact lamellar bone with haversian systems, like bone islands, but usually not metabolically active
- suspected link with metabolic connective tissue disorder
- associated with cutaneous abnormalities; one with osteosarcoma
- laboratory findings normal

b) Clinical features

- usually asymptomatic, incidental findings
- rarely found before third year of life
- male predilection
- about 25% have cutaneous abnormalities: dermatofibrosis lenticularis disseminata, keloid formation, scleroderma-like lesions
- about 20% report mild joint pain, may have joint effusion

☞ **c) Radiologic features**

- juxtaarticular small round or ovoid radiopacities (pathognomonic)
- epiphyseal and metaphyseal regions affected
- symmetric involvement: predilection for long bones, carpals and tarsals
- may occur in ilium adjacent to acetabulum, in scapula adjacent to

glenoid; rarely in skull, spine, ribs, clavicles

- occasionally disappear, reappear, or change size
- usually 1–10 mm diameter; rarely larger
- usually uniform density, but may have lucent centers
- rarely become more dense with age
- **DDX**: blastic metastasis, tuberous sclerosis, mastocytosis

☞ IV. **Osteopetrosis (synonyms: Albers-Schönberg's disease, osteosclerosis, osteopetrosis generalisata, osteosclerosis generalisata, marble bones, chalk bones)**

   a) **General features**
   - hereditary, familial
   - no resorption of normal primitive osteochondroid tissue: osteoclasts may not respond to parathyroid hormone; primitive calcified cartilage persists
   - results in inhibition of medullary canal formation; absence of marrow; anemia and extra-medullary hematopoiesis (therefore, hepatosplenomegaly)
   - may be intermittent: often vertical or horizontal striations of normal bone are interspersed with the predominant primitive tissue (see *endobones* or *bone within a bone* in radiologic features)
   - four general forms
      1) benign, autosomal dominant heterogeneous form
      2) severe malignant autosomal recessive form
      3) intermediate recessive form
      4) recessive form with tubular acidosis (carbonic anhydrase II deficiency syndrome)
   - severe malignant form associated with consanguinity
   - severe forms fatal within about 2 years; massive hemorrhage or recurrent infections
   - florid cases inevitably stillborn
   - laboratory results: invariably show anemia (myelophthisic, aplastic, or hypoplastic); thrombocytopenia may be severe; may have elevated serum calcium
   - **DDX**: idiopathic hypercalcemia; heavy metal poisoning

   b) **Clinical features**
   - severe anemia, hepatosplenomegaly, lymphadenopathy, thrombocytopenia, failure to thrive
   - brittle, dense bones which fracture easily with transverse fractures; heal quickly

with callus of defective, osteopetrotic bone

- skull involvement: optic nerve atrophy with blindness, acoustic nerve compression with deafness, other cranial nerve defects
- leukemia and sarcoma often associated
- benign cases: 50% completely asymptomatic; others may show anemia, facial palsies, deafness, hepatosplenomegaly
- with persistent hip pain, evaluate for ischemic necrosis of the femoral head
- defective dentition: severe caries, may provide route for osteomyelitis

c) **Radiologic features**

- generalized skeletal sclerosis
- homogeneous increased density, absence of trabeculation, absence of medullary canal
- *bone within a bone* appearance or *endobones*
- flared, elongated metaphyses (*Erlenmeyer flask deformity*) on long bones; may have widened shafts
- hands and feet show similar changes, may have tuftal erosion
- ilium: multiple, dense lines parallel the crest
- spine: uniformly dense vertebrae, or *sandwich vertebrae* with dense bone adjacent to endplates and normal centra, or *bone within a bone*
- lumbar spondylolysis; cervical spinal stenosis with myelopathy
- skull: macrocephaly, hydrocephalus
- prognathism

V. **Progressive Diaphyseal Dysplasia (synonyms: PDD, Engelmann-Camurati, Engelmann's disease)**

a) **General features**

- congenital, familial, hereditary disorder
- predilection for diaphyses
- autosomal dominant with extremely variable expression
- new bone formation due to increased osteoblastic activity
- endosteal involvement most prominent
- possible cause: insufficient vascular supply
- complications with skull involvement: increased intracranial pressure and cranial nerve encroachment

b) **Clinical features**

- manifests < 10 years of age
- male gender predilection
- waddling gait

- weak, poorly developed muscles, especially in lower extremities
- malnutrition
- tenderness over involved long bones
- slow, unpredictable progression
- always symmetric involvement
- weakness, malnutrition resolve in adulthood; radiographic findings persist
- laboratory findings: elevated serum alkaline phosphatase, ESR, and CPK (sporadic findings, not always present)

☞
    c) Radiologic features
- symmetrically distributed long bone fusiform diaphyseal widening
- diameter of diaphyses expanded, medullary cavity encroached
- bone may also be elongated
- process begins midshaft, progresses proximally and distally
- metaphyses spared
- usually involves femur, tibia, radius, ulna, humerus
- usually spares pelvis, carpals and tarsals
- skull: may have basilar sclerosis, calvarial hyperostosis
- exophthalmos occurs with severe skull involvement
- occasional involvement of ribs, clavicles and spine
- posterior vertebral body and posterior arches affected, but no stenosis

☞
VI. Pyknodysostosis

    a) General features
- autosomal recessive transmission
- male gender predilection (2:1)
- dense, fragile bones and dwarfism
- laboratory findings normal
- maxillary or mandibular osteomyelitis due to untreated dental carries (feature of faulty dentition)
- sleep apnea (hypoventilation) due to long uvula and small facial bones
- may have cerebellar or brain stem encroachment due to skull base thickening and platybasia
- Toulouse-Lautrec may have suffered pyknodysostosis
- manipulation contraindicated because of fragility of bones
- **DDX**: osteopetrosis, cleidocranial dysplasia

☞
    b) Clinical features
- usually less than 5 feet tall
- fracture easily
- beaked nose, small face, prominent forehead, enlarged head

- prognathic jaw
- anomalous dentition; high, arched palate
- stubby hands and feet; finger clubbing; spoon-shaped nails (koilonychia)
- mentation usually normal—lowered in about 10%

    c) Radiologic features

- general increase in bone density, preserving medullary canal
- long bones most affected
- transverse pathologic fractures; stress fractures of weight-bearing bones
- may see fractures of clavicles, mandible
- skull abnormalities: patent sutures, wide anterior fontanelle, numerous Wormian bones, platybasia, thickened skull base
- hypoplastic facial bones and sinuses
- hypoplastic mandible with obtuse angle
- retained deciduous teeth; unerupted or malformed permanent teeth
- hypoplastic or absent lateral clavicles
- acroosteolysis (hypoplastic/absent terminal tufts of fingers and toes)
- pelvis: shallow, obliquely roofed acetabulae; coxa valga
- radius: Madelung's deformity (bowed, overgrown radius); abnormal radioulnar articulations
- spine: hyperlordosis, scoliosis, kyphosis, block vertebrae (usually at craniocervical and lumbosacral junctions)
- vertebrae: *spool-shaped*, with persistent anterior infantile notching
- primary C2 spondylolysis
- lower lumbar spondylolisthesis

VII. Tuberous Sclerosis (synonyms: epiloia, Bourneville's disease)

    a) General features

- epiloia means: "*mindless epileptic*"
- autosomal dominant transmission
- neuroectodermal origin; multisystem effects
- classed as a phakomatosis (most common example: neurofibromatosis)
- laboratory: may see high serum alkaline phosphatase; abnormal GTT

    b) Clinical features

- classic clinical triad: mental retardation, epilepsy, skin lesions
- usually diagnosed in adolescence or early adulthood
- seizures manifest in first decade of life because of CNS lesions
- hamartomas: skin, eyes, lungs, kidneys, liver, spleen, brain, heart, bone
- skin lesions: hypopigmented macules (irregularly marginated ovals or leaf-

shapes on legs and trunk); café au lait spots; peau-chagrin patches (shagreen); gingival and periungual fibromas; skin tags
- most common skin change: adenoma sebaceum (a hamartoma)
- eyes: 52% of cases have retinal phakomas (white patches) at birth
- cranial: early detection of lesions via ultrasonography
- visceral hamartomas: myolipomas, angiomyomas, angiofibromas, adenomas, rhabdomyomas (rarely present at birth, slow growing)
- kidneys: angiomyolipomas (renal hamartomas) in up to 80% of cases; cause flank pain and hematuria; usually bilateral; may undergo malignant degeneration; chronic hypertension, renal insufficiency
- renal artery tortuosity and aneurysms often associated
- heart: rarely involved; multiple rhabdomyomas; cor pulmonale
- colon: rare adenomas
- lungs: very rarely affected, almost always females with late involvement in disease process; uniform diffuse or basilar interstitial pattern; may have progressive volume loss; rare *honeycomb lung* (poor prognosis); lead to pneumothorax, hemoptysis, dyspnea, aspiration pneumonia
- insidious onset of acute dyspnea and chest pain: spontaneous pneumothorax
- dysfunction of pituitary, adrenal, or thyroid glands

☞   **c)   Radiologic features**
- skull: intracranial calcifications (basal ganglia, paraventricular cortical tubers and subependymal nodules, cerebellar calcifications); thickened, hyperostotic cranial vault
- tubular hand and foot bones: irregular subperiosteal nodules; small cysts (especially in distal phalanges); coarsened trabeculae
- diffuse or discrete islands of density in vertebral bodies and pedicles and along pelvic brim
- *periosteal warts*: tibial cortical excrescences
- rib enlargement and sclerosis
- scoliosis
- renal hamartomas visible on plain films due to fatty component, associated kidney enlargement and contour irregularity
- lung interstitial changes also visible on plain film
- cranial lesions best found with MRI or ultrasound

REVIEW—STUDY QUESTIONS

1. In which of the sclerosing dysplasias, if any, is manipulation contraindicated? Why?
2. Explain the *overlap syndrome.*
3. Which sclerosing dysplasias are not clearly known to be genetically transmitted?
4. Define *epiloia* and *melorheostosis.*
5. In which dysplasia do you see spool-shaped vertebrae: bone within a bone or sandwich vertebrae?
6. Describe the pathologic process of tuberous sclerosis. What body systems are affected, and how?
7. Sleep apnea may complicate pyknodysostosis. Why?
8. Compare and contrast the effects on long bones of pyknodysostosis and osteopetrosis.
9. What dysplasia features café au lait spots and is related to neurofibromatosis?
10. Which, if any, of the sclerosing dysplasias adversely affect mentation?

anomaly: a marked deviation from the normal standard, especially as a result of congenital or hereditary defects. Dorland's Illustrated Medical Dictionary; twenty-sixth edition. Philadelphia: WB Saunders, 1981.

B. CONGENITAL ANOMALIES

1. Craniovertebral Anomalies

I. Atlas Occipitalization

a) General features

- assimilation of C1; atlas fused to base of occiput
- failure of segmentation of caudal occipital sclerotome
- may cause compression of medulla and cord by odontoid process at foramen magnum, or by transverse ligament laxity
- may be asymptomatic, or cause headaches, restricted range of motion, visual and auditory abnormalities, upper extremity neurologic signs, nuchal pain, vertigo
- early DJD at subadjacent segments
- may be associated with platybasia, basilar impression, Arnold-Chiari malformation (Type I), atlantoaxial dislocation or instability, Sturge-Weber syndrome, Klippel-Feil syndrome

b) Radiologic features

- lateral skull film: decreased or absent space C1 posterior arch-occipital base
- flexion-extension views: bony ankylosis at the occiput to C1

☞ **II. Occipital Vertebrae**

    a) General features

- third condyle, epitransverse and paracondylar processes
- caused by failure of normal fusion of terminal basiocciput
- anterior defective fusion = *third condyle*
- lateral anomalies are *paracondyloid, paramastoid, epitransverse*
- may be other accessory ossicles around foramen magnum
- *third condyle*: *condylus tertius*; usually no clinical significance
- *epitransverse*: unilateral or bilateral, from C1 TP to unite or articulate with skull near jugular process
- *paracondylar processes* or *paramastoid process:* from jugular process toward C1 TP
- these lateral ossicles may limit lateral flexion in upper cervical area
- paracondylar processes may cause cervical contracture and pain, may "shim" the occiput, tilting the head to one side
- Occiput-C1 articulations cannot be manipulated due to fusion
- epitransverse increases risk of posttraumatic basal subarachnoid hemorrhage

    b) Radiologic features

- third condyles, if large enough, show on lateral film as oval/round densities about same size as atlas anterior arch; may articulate with C1 anterior arch
- CT or tomography will visualize this anomaly
- laterally placed ossicles: usually not visible on APOM, but rotating the head slightly may permit viewing an occipital/TP bony connection
- accessory joint may be seen between ossicle and C1 TP, or bony ankylosis may exist
- optimal imaging is via CT or MRI

III. Accessory Ossicles

    a) General features

- possible etiologies: types of occipital vertebrae; secondary ossifications within ligaments around foramen magnum

    b) Radiologic features

- small, round or oval sesamoid-like bones above the C1 anterior arch

☞ **IV. Platybasia/Basilar Impression**

    a) General features

- platybasia means "*broad base*"
    1) caused by congenital sphenoid and/ or occipital maldevelopment

2) determined by a Martin's basilar angle > 152°, measured on lateral skull film

3) clinically insignificant alone; often found with occipitalization of C1 and Klippel-Feil syndrome, syringomyelia

- basilar impression synonymous with basilar invagination

    1) odontoid encroachment into foramen magnum

    2) elevation of posterior fossa floor

    3) *primary*: caused by congenital defects: may be associated with C1 occipitalization; C1 SBO; agenetic or hypoplastic C1; anomalous odontoid; Arnold-Chiari malformation

    4) *secondary*: caused by diseases that soften bone; associated with Paget's disease, osteomalacia, fibrous dysplasia

    5) causes headache and nystagmus; pyramidal tract signs, posterior column signs, wasting of upper limbs; neuroelectrodiagnostic signs, sudden hearing loss

    6) cervical hyperextension can be lethal

☞   **b) Radiologic features**

- lateral skull film

- angle formed by plane of clivus and plane of floor of the anterior fossa is unusually flat and wide (> 152°)

- with no evidence of bone-softening pathology: platybasia

- with bone-softening: posterior fossa floor elevation; upward convexity of posterior foramen magnum; dens apex above foramen magnum; this is basilar invagination or basilar impression

☞   **V. Arnold-Chiari Malformation**

    a) General features

- downward displacement of brainstem and cerebellar tonsils through the foramen magnum

- may have hydrocephalus in varying degrees

☞ - Types I and II most common

☞ - Type I = tonsilar herniation or tonsilar ectopia; female predilection (3:2); headache, cervical pain, vague symptoms; adult presentation with mild brain changes, mild hydrocephalus, variable syringomyelia

☞ - Type II: childhood or infancy presentation with stridor, apnea, feeding problems; nystagmus, cranial nerve palsies; severe hydrocephalus; medulla dorsally kinked at cervicomedullary junction; upward displacement of upper cervical nerves;

associated spina bifida and
meningomyelocele
- treatment (type II) - posterior fossa and
upper cervical decompression
(suboccipital craniectomy and cervical
laminectomy); may insert shunt within
syrinx for spinal cord decompression
(spinal myelotomy)
- condition can involve autonomic
dysfunction: impotence, dyspnea,
anhidrosis, hyperhidrosis, constipation

b) Radiologic features
- MRI is modality of choice to establish
diagnosis
- shows: triangular-shaped, prolapsed
cerebellar tonsils; elongation or kinking of
fourth ventricle with a sharp clivoaxial
angle
- syringomyelia shows as a spinal cord
cavitation: may be cervical, cervicodorsal,
or holocord
- skeletal abnormalities will be visualized
on plain film: C1 occipitalization,
platybasia and basilar impression, cervical
block vertebrae, cervical ribs, fused
thoracic ribs

2. Cervical Spine Anomalies

I. C1 Posterior Arch Agenesis

a) General features
- lacks cartilage template for ossification
- normally begins in lateral masses at about
seventh fetal week, proceeds posteriorly;
at 2 years, secondary growth center for
posterior tubercle develops; fusion
completed by age 5
- complete or partial agenesis is rare; arch
defects alone clinically insignificant, but
may be associated with other anomalies
- cervical flexion/extension films screen for
instability due to possible compromise of
transverse ligament

b) Radiologic features
- lateral cervical projection
- associated enlargement of C2 SP (*mega-
spinous process*), actually a fusion of
rudimentary C1 posterior tubercle and C2
SP
- enlarged, sclerotic C1 anterior
arch—stress related

**II. Posterior Ponticle (synonyms: Kimmerly anomaly;
foramen arcuale; pons posticus; posticus ponticus)**

a) General features
- arcuate foramen formed when oblique
portion of atlanto-occipital ligament
calcifies or ossifies
- transmits vertebral artery and first cervical
nerve

- most often unilateral
- may cause vertebral artery traction and compression during flexion and extension; especially significant with small caliber foramen
- may increase risk of posttraumatic basal subarachnoid hemorrhage
- requires caution with upper cervical manipulation because of increased risk of post-manipulative vasospasm or vertebral artery dissection

b) **Radiologic features**
- lateral cervical projection
- at anterosuperior surface of C1 posterior tubercle

III. **C1 Anterior Arch Agenesis**

a) **General features**
- rarely seen
- may be associated with median cleft face syndrome and Pierre-Robin syndrome (micrognathia with cleft palate, glossoptosis and absent gag reflex)

b) **Radiologic features**
- lateral cervical projection
- absence of "D"-shaped anterior C1 arch
- flexion/extension studies to screen for C1-C2 hypermobility (C1 may retrosubluxate on C2)

IV. **Down's Syndrome (synonyms: Mongolism, Trisomy 21)**

a) **General features**
- most common autosomal syndrome; 1 in 600 births
- trisomy of the 21st chromosome
- identified at birth: small skull A-P; small nose with flat bridge, slanting eyes (epicanthal folds), simian creases, protruding tongue
- mental retardation
- ligamentous laxity: hip and patellar dislocations
- predisposed to leukemia
- 20% born without transverse ligament at C1; atlantoaxial instability
- prone to cervical spondylosis, cervical myelopathy

b) **Radiologic features**
- flexion lateral projection
- most clinically significant sign: increased ADI, indicates atlantoaxial instability resulting from agenesis of transverse ligament of the atlas
- C1 A-P diameter reduced
- decreased iliac index

- hypoplastic middle phalanx of fifth finger; clinodactyly
- manubrium: multiple ossification centers
- small (underpneumatized) paranasal sinuses
- small A-P diameter of lumbar vertebrae
- 11 or 13 rib pairs
- clavicles may have prominent conoid processes

V. Ossiculum Terminale Persistens of Bergman

a) General features

- normal secondary growth center appearing at about 2 years of age at cephalic tip of odontoid process
- normally this should unite with the dens at about 10–12 years of age
- occasionally it remains a separate ossicle
- no clinical significance
- **DDX**: os odontoideum or fracture

b) Radiologic features

- APOM or lateral cervical projection
- discrete, round, oval or diamond-shaped bone at cephalic tip of dens

VI. Os Odontoideum

a) General features

- potential for significant neurologic damage (death, paralysis) from relatively trivial trauma or even manipulation
- normally developed cephalic part of dens is not fused with C2 body
- neurocentral synchondrosis (growth plate) is below this lesion, so this may be a fracture nonunion of the base of the dens, or may be congenital nonunion (should be fused by age 7)
- sometimes occurs familially, or in identical twins
- transverse ligament is usually intact
- associated sometimes with: absent or hypoplastic posterior C1 arch, Down's syndrome, Klippel-Feil syndrome, Morquio's syndrome, spondyloepiphyseal dysplasia
- atlantoaxial instability with cord compression; vertebral artery compression

b) Radiologic features

- adult: smooth, wide, lucent defect between dens and C2 body at level of articular processes
- associated stress hypertrophy C1 anterior tubercle
- may find "molding" of C1 anterior arch into ventral aspect of dens
- child: before age 5, diagnosis depends on finding hypermobility of dens on the C2 body during flexion/extension

- MRI used to evaluate cord (angulation, compression, contusion)

VII. Hypoplastic/Aplastic (Agenetic) Odontoid Process

a) General features
- agenesis extremely rare
- flexion/extension views to rule out instability
- with instability, upper cervical spinal manipulation contraindicated
- may get surgical opinion on arthrodesis

b) Radiologic features
- APOM shows abbreviated stump
- may be complete lack of osseous shadow where dens should be

☞ VIII. Congenital Block Vertebra

a) General features
- adjacent vertebrae osseously fused from birth
- caused by failure of segmentation of somites in fetus
- may predispose to early DJD above or below, but especially below the level of fusion
- discogenic spondylosis and arthrosis may ensue
- a unilateral bar conduces to scoliosis
- most common at: C5–6, C2–3, T12–L1, L4–5
- possible association with lax atlantooccipital ligaments, excessive motion at that level, and brainstem or cord compression

☞ b) Radiologic features
- diminished AP body diameter
- hypoplastic or rudimentary disc space (may have faint calcification)
- 50% have fused apophyseal joints
- spinous processes may be malformed or fused
- anterior margin of fused bodies is concave (*wasp waist*)
- osseous fusion of the neural arches

☞ IX. Klippel-Feil Syndrome

a) General features
- short, webbed neck (*pterygium coli*)
- low hairline
- decreased cervical range of motion
- this "classic triad" is seen in about 52% of cases
- facial asymmetry, torticollis, neck webbing
- deformation of thorax caused by scoliosis or Sprengel's deformity

- systems affected: musculoskeletal, genitourinary, cardiopulmonary, nervous
- possibly caused by developmental disturbance in fourth or fifth embryonic week
- MRI to image spinal cord effects: compression, hydromyelia, diplomyelia

   b) **Radiologic features**
- multiple block vertebrae (cervical and upper thoracic areas)
- anomalous ribs
- scoliosis
- possible platybasia
- Sprengel's deformity (elevation of scapula) in 25% of cases

☞   **X.   Sprengel's Deformity**

   a) **General features**
- probably a failure of scapular descent in second month of gestation
- 2:1 female predilection
- usually unilateral; can be bilateral
- limited humeral abduction
- may be associated with torticollis, omovertebral bone, Klippel-Feil syndrome, scoliosis, hemivertebrae, block vertebrae, spina bifida occulta, cervical ribs

   b) **Radiologic features**
- elevation of the scapula
- scapula is hypoplastic, vertically shortened and broad
- rotated so glenoid process is directed inferiorly
- inferior angle rests above the T7 level (normal level)

☞   **XI.   Omovertebral Bone**

   a) **General features**
- cartilage, fibrous tissue, or bone
- from SP, lamina, or TP of C5 or C6, to superior scapular angle
- present in 30–40% of Sprengel's deformity cases

   b) **Radiologic features**
- bony density projecting inferolaterally toward superior angle of scapula from C5 or C6
- seen on AP lower cervical and lateral cervical views

XII.   Cervical Spondylolisthesis

   a) **General features**
- congenital form: caused by bilateral agenesis of pedicles, dysplasia of articular processes
- most commonly involves C6, next most

common is C2, may be seen at other levels

- male predilection
- may be asymptomatic, or may involve occipital headache, nuchal rigidity, torticollis, dysphagia, depression of DTRs, radicular arm pain

b) Radiologic features

- cervical AP, lateral, or oblique views display anomalies
- absent pedicle shadows bilaterally
- hypoplastic or dysplastic articular processes
- neural arch dysplasia
- involved vertebra may show slight anterolisthesis
- AP projection images spina bifida occulta (at C6 this is a rare finding as an isolated anomaly, usually suggests spondylolisthesis)
- bilaterally enlarged neural foramina (absent pedicles)
- may be intersegmental instability (flexion/ extension films)
- smooth cortical margins of pedicle defects shown on CT
- may be an incidental finding after trauma: use MRI to rule out acute injury to discs or spinal cord (edema should be absent)

XIII. Cervical Rib

a) General features

- articulates with TP of cervical vertebrae
- most common at C7; next most common, C6, then C5
- **DDX** from elongate TP (apophysomegaly, transverse mega-apophysis): rib articulates, elongate TP has no articulation
- cervical TP is caudally oriented, thoracic TP is cephalically oriented
- 2:1 female predilection
- present in about 0.5% of population, 6% of them bilateral
- may cause neurovascular compression later in life
- usually brachial plexus and subclavian vessels are superior to rib
- rib may "split" brachial plexus
- fibrous band may extend from rib tip, causing neurovascular compression- thoracic outlet syndrome, diagnosed by contrast study

b) Radiologic features

- rib forming a joint with caudally oriented TP
- variable length, from stub to full rib articulating with sternum

3. Cervical/Thoracic/Lumbar Anomalies

☞ **I. Pedicle Agenesis**

    a) General features

- failure of development of cartilage anlage for pedicles
- cervical spine affected (in descending order of frequency) at: C6, C5, C4, C7

☞
- invariably unilateral; may be either side
- may be associated with paresthesia or pain (head, neck, arms)
- **DDX:** pathologic destruction of pedicle

☞   **b) Radiologic features**

- oblique projection, pillar projection are optimal images
- enlarged IVF
- may have dysplastic TPs (bilaterally) and superior articular process
- malformed articular process is displaced posterior
- hallmark: contralateral pedicle hypertrophy, sclerosis
- sclerosis of remaining pedicle more pronounced in lumbar spine
- vertebral body unaffected
- **DDX:** neurofibroma (dumbbell tumor)—these scallop posterior body

II. Butterfly Vertebra (Coronal Cleft Vertebra)

    a) General features

- etiologic theories: failure of regression of chorda dorsalis; persistent ventrodorsal extension of perichordal sheath; failure of union of lateral ossification centers; placement of intraosseous blood vessels
- most commonly in thoracic and lumbar spine
- as isolated anomaly, clinically insignificant
- multiple butterfly vertebrae with meningocele, myelomeningocele, diastematomyelia

    b) Radiologic features

- demonstrated on AP projection
- indentation of endplate cortices toward central vertebral body
- hourglass central lucency (disc material)
- slightly enlarged pedicles, increased interpediculate distance are sometimes associated

III. Hemivertebrae

    a) General features

- failure of development of a lateral ossification center
- lateral hemivertebra is most common presentation, dorsal hemivertebra is rare, and ventral hemivertebra extremely rare
- rarely an isolated anomaly

- lateral hemivertebrae usually associated with block vertebrae, diastematomyelia, Klippel-Feil syndrome, meningocele, multiple enchondromatosis, spondylothoracic dysplasia
- dorsal hemivertebrae may be associated with achondroplasia, cretinism, chondrodystrophy, Morquio's disease, gargoylism
- remember other systems are often involved when there are spinal anomalies: e.g., VATER syndrome: vertebral (and vascular) anomalies, anal atresia, tracheo-esophageal fistula with esophageal atresia, renal and radial dysplasia

b) Radiologic features
- laterally wedged: seen on AP projection
- laterally wedged: triangular vertebral body, endplates taper to a point
- adjacent discs normal
- adjacent vertebral endplates slightly deformed: trapezoid vertebral bodies
- isolated wedge causes a scoliosis
- multiple hemivertebrae with block vertebrae cause *scrambled spine*
- lateral projection shows dorsal hemivertebra pointed anterior: causes gibbus deformity

IV. Schmorl's Nodes (synonyms: cartilaginous nodes, intraspongy nuclear herniations)

a) General features
- nucleus pulposus herniation through fractured vertebral endplate
- may be developmentally weak endplate (e.g., with penetrating blood vessels or chorda dorsalis regression)
- traumatic or pathological acquisition (osteoporosis, osteomalacia)
- usually asymptomatic; occasionally causes pain
- **DDX:** nuclear impression (persistent notochord)—smooth, undulating cortical surface involving most of the endplate; lateral view shows indentation of inferior endplate; AP view shows *Cupid's bow contour* or *double hump*; on CT this yields *owl's eyes* appearance in either inferior or superior endplate
- most commonly thoracic or lumbar

b) Radiologic features
- best seen on lateral projection
- squared-off, sharp, rectangular sclerotic margin protruding into vertebral body from disc space
- may be central or peripheral
- Schmorl's node phenomenon: giant, enlarged, squared-off indentations,

anterosuperior placement; reduced supra-adjacent disc space; increased AP body diameter

☞ **V. Spina Bifida**

    a) General features

- may be occult or manifest: *spina bifida occulta* or *spina bifida manifesta (spina bifida vara)*
- in occult form (SBO): failure of lamina to fuse posteriorly, usually with a cleft spinous process
- SBO is clinically insignificant
- SBO has a 9:1 male predilection; occurs at L5 and S1
- when at C1, termed a *spondyloschisis*, because there is no SP there
- spina bifida vara has larger defect, may allow the meninges and/or spinal cord to protrude
- about 60% of cases appear to be genetic
- elevated alpha fetoprotein in amniotic fluid allows in utero diagnosis
- often has "cutaneous signature" in the form of a hair patch, lipoma, or dimple
- spina bifida manifesta (vara) may involve local cord and nerve root deficits, increased risk of hydrocephalus and cord infection

☞   **b) Radiologic features**

- SBO: AP projections give optimal view; lucent cleft between laminae, small or absent SP at that level
- lateral projection may display absence of spinolaminar junction line
- *Spina Bifida Vera*: AP and lateral projections: wide defect in posterior neural arch at multiple levels; possible soft tissue mass posterior to the spine (see VI, below)

☞ **VI. Meningocele; Myelomeningocele**

    a) General features

- spina bifida vara occurs due to failure of neural arch posterior fusion
- late in first month of gestation (21st to 29th day)
- early diagnoses via alpha fetoprotein in amniotic fluid, by 18th week
- leptomeninges or meninges plus cord may protrude through defect
- upper thoracic herniations occur laterally, through IVF (e.g., in neurofibromatosis)
- herniations may occur anteriorly through the sacrum
- severe cases: visible protruding sac, bilateral clubbed feet, paralysis
- mild cases: gait disturbances begin to manifest around 5 or 6 years

    b) **Radiologic features**
- increased interpediculate distance
- absent lamina, spinous process; usually at multiple levels
- when anterior sacrum is involved, curvilinear erosion on anterior sacral canal: *scimitar sacrum* (resembles shape of a curved Turkish sword)
- water-density mass posterior to spine
- myelography, MRI, or US to define cord involvement

VII. **Diastematomyelia**

    a) **General features**
- spinal dysraphism
- osseous, cartilaginous, or fibrous bar partitions spinal cord or cauda equina
- tethers the cord in the midline
- most common in thoracolumbar area
- may be diagnosed any time: prenatal to adulthood
- clinically may show anal dimple, hairy lumbar patch, asymmetrical lower extremity size, lipoma

    b) **Radiologic features**
- wider interpediculate distance
- osseous bar is visible; 50% accompany other osseous defects

VIII. **Transitional Vertebrae**

    a) **General features**
- found at cervicothoracic, thoracolumbar, and lumbosacral junctions
- most common is lumbosacral where we see:
  1) sacralization: fifth lumbar appears to be a sacral segment
  2) lumbarization: first sacral segment appears to be a lumbar vertebra
- debate of clinical significance still pending: disc above the transitional segment may be prone to herniation because of abnormal stresses
- accessory joints between large lumbar TPs and sacral alae may degenerate, produce low back pain
- *Bertolotti's syndrome:* scoliosis and sciatica caused by transitional vertebrae

    b) **Radiologic features**
- L5: TP (one or both) vertically > 19 mm; TP (one or both) fused with the sacrum or forming a joint with the sacrum
- accessory joint (if unilateral) may show DJD: subchondral sclerosis, marginal osteophytes
- L5 body normal
- interposed disc hypoplastic or vestigial; short vertically

4. **Lumbar or Lumbosacral Anomalies**

  I. **Facet Tropism**

  a) **General features**
  - lumbar facets are curved rather than planar
  - asymmetric articular planes at a single level are called *tropism*
  - so far clinical significance is unknown
  - most common at L5-S1, but seen at any lumbar level
  - scoliosis or intersegmental rotation may simulate tropism
  - CT can define true plane of the facets
  - has been associated with sclerotic pedicle

  b) **Radiologic features**
  - AP projection gives optimal view
  - unilateral linear radiolucent joint space, not visible contralaterally

  ☞ II. **Clasp Knife Syndrome**

  a) **General features**
  - spina bifida of S1 with associated L5 SP caudal enlargement
  - creates pain upon lumbosacral extension
  - elongated SP may be caused by fusion of first sacral tubercle with L5 SP ossification center
  - L5 may have increased ROM in extension, causing pain by pressure over sacral defect, or pressure on laminar stumps at S1

  ☞ b) **Radiologic features**
  - visible on AP: spina bifida occulta at S1 and elongate L5 SP
  - tilt-up view (30° cephalad angulation) through L/S disc may help
  - lateral projection shows SP enlargement
  - myelography with patient in extension will demonstrate block
  - CT can image SP intrusion through the SBO

REVIEW—STUDY QUESTIONS

1. What radiographic findings are typical of Down's syndrome, and which are particularly clinically significant?
2. How may os odontoideum be differentiated from fracture?
3. What clinical signs suggest the possible presence of SBO?
4. What is Sprengel's deformity and with what other anomalies and/or syndromes is it associated?
5. What is a "wasp-waist" and with what anomaly is it associated?
6. What causes the development of a "butterfly vertebra"?

7. What is the clinical significance of the "clasp knife syndrome"?

8. Describe the Klippel-Feil syndrome, both the clinical presentation and radiographic findings.

9. Discuss the distinctions between platybasia and basilar invagination or basilar impression.

10. What and where are third condyles? Epitransverse processes? Paracondylar processes?

11. Discuss the potential clinical significance of a posterior ponticle.

12. How can one differentiate congenital absence of a pedicle from pathologic pedicle destruction?

13. What is the triad that is comprised by the Giant Schmorl's node?

14. Where are transitional vertebrae found, and can they be clinically significant?

15. Explain tropism and its significance.

5. **Thoracic Cage Anomalies**

I. **Congenital first rib pseudoarthrosis**

a) **General features**
- midportion of first rib shows incomplete ossification
- usually painless
- **DDX:** stress fracture from heavily loaded shoulder strap

b) **Radiologic features**
- first rib slightly enlarged
- smooth, sclerotic cortical margins at lesion site

II. **Srb's anomaly**

a) **General features**
- involution of one or both first ribs
- incomplete fusion of first and second ribs

b) **Radiologic features**
- chest or rib projections demonstrate this
- broad, solid bony plate at fusion site
- lack of normal interspace between first and second ribs
- may have pseudoarthrosis in midportion of fused rib

III. **Luschka's Bifurcated Rib**

a) **General features**
- anterior upper rib may split
- clinically insignificant
- **DDX:** cavity within lung

b) **Radiologic features**
- anterior rib "branches" into two clearly marginated osseous structures

IV. Rib Foramen

    a) General features
- clinically insignificant

    b) Radiologic features
- radiolucent foramen within rib

V. Intrathoracic Rib

    a) General features
- anomalous rib protruding through thoracic cavity

    b) Radiologic features
- clear osseous rib shadow at incongruous angle across lung field

☞ **VI. Pectus Excavatum (synonym: funnel chest)**

    a) General features
- most common chest wall anomaly
- clinically: see midline depression of sternum

    b) Radiologic features
- lateral projection is optimal
- posteriorly displaced sternum
- diminished retrosternal clear space

☞ **VII. Pectus Carinatum (synonym: pigeon breast)**

    a) General features
- prominent sternum
- associated with Morquio's syndrome

    b) Radiologic features
- lateral projection is optimal
- anteriorly displaced sternum
- increased retrosternal clear space

☞ **VIII. Straight Back Syndrome (synonym: cobbler's chest)**

    a) General features
- diminished thoracic kyphosis
- heart and mediastinal structures compressed: "pancake heart"
- altered hemodynamics cause ejection systolic murmur which abates when patient sits up or inspires (functional murmur)
- significant increase in mitral valve prolapse with this syndrome
- possibly autosomal dominant transmission; chromosome 6 implicated

☞   **b) Radiologic features**
- PA projection shows unusually vertical orientation of anterior ribs
- heart shadow displaced left
- no heart shadow on right side of lower thoracic spine
- prominent upper left heart border
- lateral projection shows loss of kyphosis; possibly pectus excavatum

- less than 1.2 cm from mid-anterior T8 to a vertical line from T4 to T12 is considered a positive sign of straight back syndrome

6. **Anomalies of the Hip and Pelvis**

☞   I. **Congenital Hip Displasia**

      a) **General features**

- malformed acetabulum; possible hip dislocation
☞ - Ortolani's or Barlow's tests aid diagnosis of dislocation
- dislocation caused by inversion of fibrocartilage limbus and capsular contraction
- reduction of the dislocation is difficult or impossible

☞   b) **Radiologic features**

- *Putti's triad:* absent or small proximal femoral epiphysis; lateral displacement of femur; increased inclination of acetabular roof
- femoral head luxated proximally and posteriorly
- after attempts at weight bearing: shallow pseudoacetabulum formed superior to primary site

II. **Sacral Agenesis (synonym: caudal regression syndrome)**

      a) **General features**

- agenesis may extend as high as T10
- association with maternal diabetes
- clinically apparent at birth
- associated with spinopelvic instability, scoliosis, myelomeningocele, hip dislocation or contracture, knee contracture, foot deformity
- may be teratogenically induced, or spontaneous genetic mutation
- linked with sixth chromosome, histocompatibility system coded there
- link with diabetes and histocompatibility system

      b) **Radiologic features**

- absence of sacrum
- possibly absent lumbar segments

☞   III. **Coxa Vara**

      a) **General features**

- vara means distal angulation toward the midline
- coxa refers to the hip
- normal angle of incidence of proximal femur: 120–130° (Mikulicz's angle) (Fig. 3.3)
- coxa vara is an angle < 120° (Fig. 3.4)
- results from eccentric growth arrest at

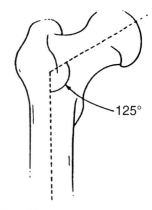

Figure 3.3.

Mikulicz's angle (normal). Reprinted with permission from Magee JA. Orthopedic Physical Assessment. Philadelphia: WB Saunders, 1987:246.

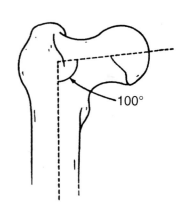

Figure 3.4.

Mikulicz's angle (coxa vara). Reprinted with permission from Magee JA. Orthopedic Physical Assessment. Philadelphia: WB Saunders, 1987:246.

medial aspect of growth plate between femoral epiphysis and femoral neck
- may be associated with: femoral focal deficiency, osteogenesis imperfecta, rickets, fibrous dysplasia, cleidocranial dysplasia
- 75% of cases unilateral
- no gender predilection

☞   **b)   Radiologic features**
- decreased femoral angle
- radiolucent inverted "V" in proximal femoral metaphysis
- enlarged greater trochanter
- may have some deformation of the acetabulum and DJD

☞   **IV.   Coxa Valga**

a)   General features
- valgus means distal angulation away from the midline
- angle greater than 130° (Fig. 3.5)
- caused by muscle imbalance involving hip abductors; reduces traction on the physis at the greater trochanter base, effecting angulation of femoral neck and shaft

b)   Radiologic features
- increased femoral angle
- often tends to laterally dislocate femoral head from acetabulum
- seen with chronic lower limb injuries as acquired condition

7.   Lower Extremity Anomalies

☞   **I.   Multipartite Patellae**

a)   General features
- normal patellar development: from single ossification center by about 6 years of age
- fragmented ossification center may not unite osseously
- usually does have a unifying fibrous bridge

☞
- most common is bipartite, 80% of these are unilateral
- three-piece is "tripartite"
- more than three is "multipartite" or "segmented"
- no gender predilection
- **DDX:** fracture
- usually clinically insignificant; some report associated pain, possibly caused by loosening of fibrous connection; exacerbated by activity; treated best by excision of accessory portion of the patella

☞   **b)   Radiologic features**
- for clear DDX, AP, lateral and axial views should be taken

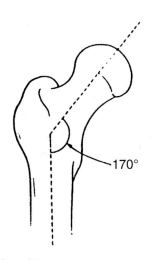

Figure 3.5

Mikulicz's angle (coxa valga). Reprinted with permission from Magee JA. Orthopedic Physical Assessment. Philadelphia: WB Saunders, 1987:246.

- most commonly see non-united segment in superolateral patella
- smooth, rounded, and well corticated margins

II. Fong's Syndrome (synonym: iliac horn syndrome)

a) General features

- may be associated with nail-patella syndrome, hereditary onycho-osteo dysplasia
- autosomal dominant transmission
- associated abnormalities of nails in hands and feet, renal dysplasia, bone deformities

b) Radiologic features

- hypoplastic and laterally placed patellae
- iliac horns (exostoses on posterior ilia)
- malformations of elbow articulations

III. Tarsal coalition (synonym: tarsal bars)

a) General features

- fibrous union or bony bar between two or more tarsals
- majority are congenital, but condition may be acquired post-traumatically or from inflammatory arthritis
- symptomatic usually after age 10
- symptoms secondary to osteoarthritis from biomechanical stress
- 1–2% of population affected
- clinically: tarsal pain, limited motion in subtalar or midtarsal joint, rigid or semirigid pes planus, prominent peroneal tendons
- associated with chronic inversion injuries
- surgical correction effective
- associated with phocomelia, hemimelica, other limb anomalies
- bar may fuse by syndesmoses, synchondroses, or synostoses

b) Radiologic features

- to diagnose, take dorsiplantar, lateral and medial oblique foot views and axial calcaneus projection
- bony bar will be continuous with normal bones and will obstruct view of a normally seen joint
- most commonly seen at talocalcaneal and calcaneonavicular joints
- talar beak is often present

IV. Vertical Talus

a) General features

- congenital talonavicular dislocation
- seems to be caused by short Achilles tendon
- "rocker bottom" foot: rounded prominence of medial plantar surface

- associated with spina bifida manifesta, myelomeningocele, Down's syndrome
- equal gender incidence

   b) Radiologic features
- dorsiplantar projection shows calcaneus valgus, metatarsus adductus
- lateral view shows plantar flexion of calcaneus; talus shows increased plantar inclination
- navicular articulates with dorsal talus

V. Morton's Syndrome (synonyms: Morton's foot; first ray insufficiency syndrome)

   a) General features
- activity causes pain at plantar surface near second cuneiform-metatarsal joint
- callus develops under second and third metatarsal heads
- may be complicated by stress fractures of second and third metatarsals

   b) Radiologic features
- dorsiplantar projection shows short first metatarsal as compared to second metatarsal; unusually broad based second metatarsal
- varus deformity of first metatarsal
- sesamoids at first metatarsal head are both proximally displaced

8. Upper Extremity Anomalies

I. Humeral Supracondylar Process (synonyms: supracondyloid process;supraepitrochlear process; epicondylic process)

   a) General features
- rudimentary exostosis that occurs in humans and other animals
- on anteromedial distal humeral metaphysis
- **DDX:** osteochondroma (which points away from joint, while supracondylar process points toward the elbow joint)
- clinical significance: may compress median nerve and/or median, brachial or radial arteries; subject to fracture; rarely causes a median nerve neuralgia or nerve palsy
- Struther's ligament: fibrous or fibro-osseous ligament from tip of process to medial humeral epicondyle
- also a feature of rare condition "Cornelia de Lange syndrome"

   b) Radiologic features
- beaklike bony spur with cortical and trabecular bone, at anteromedial distal humeral metaphysis
- angled toward elbow
- usually less than 1 cm long
- lateral or oblique projections show it best
- may not be visible on frontal projection

II. Radioulnar Synostosis

a) **General features**

- caused by failure of longitudinal segmentation of the proximal radius and ulna
- autosomal dominant transmission
- no gender predilection
- 80% are bilateral
- 3 to 6 cm of osseous or fibrous fusion
- limited or completely absent pronation/ supination range of motion
- detectable at birth, but most often diagnosed in childhood
- may be associated with dislocated hip, clubfoot, Madelung's deformity (see below), syndactyly or polydactyly, Holt-Oram syndrome
- surgery permits functional hand position

b) **Radiologic features**

- AP and lateral elbow projections demonstrate deformity
- show bone between proximal radius and ulna (up to 6 cm)

☞ **III. Madelung's Deformity**

a) **General features**

- may be isolated anomaly, or part of dyschondrosteosis
- autosomal dominant transmission
- female predilection
- two-thirds of cases are bilateral
- usually diagnosed in early adolescence
- wrist pain during growth period; may subside after growth period
- distal medial radial epiphysis growth is retarded
- asymmetric prominence of ulnar styloid, posterior subluxation of distal ulna
- *bayonette* appearance

☞ b) **Radiologic features**

- PA projection (Fig. 3.6) shows triangular distal radial epiphysis, retarded medial growth causes an ulnar slant of distal radial articular surface
- shortened radius; lucent defect along medial metaphysis
- widened distal radioulnar joint
- decreased carpal angle ($< 117°$)
- lateral projection (Fig. 3.7) shows volar tilt of distal radial articular surface $> 5°$
- dorsal subluxation of ulna
- altered carpal alignment: lunate at proximal apex of carpal arc

---

Madelung's Deformity is seen with:

"RED HOT"

Radial ray dysplasias

Epiphyseal dysplasias

Dyschondrosteosis

Hereditary multiple exostosis

Ollier's disease

Thalidomide

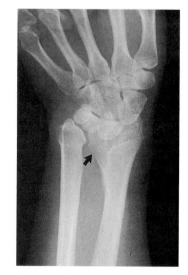

Figure 3.6. Madelung's Deformity.

Features seen in PA projection. Reprinted with permission from Yochum TR, Rowe LJ. Essentials of Skeletal Radiology, 2nd ed. Baltimore: Williams & Wilkins, 1996:250.

IV. Negative Ulnar Variance (synonym: ulnar minus variant)

  a) General features

  - thickened triangular fibrocartilage complex at distal ulna
  - ulna unusually shorter than radius
  - measurement of variance: ulna appears more foreshortened with supination, less so with pronation (than in neutral position)
  - may increase likelihood of Kienböck's disease (questionable)
  - treatment attempts to encourage revascularization of the lunate by "unloading" it through osteotomy to shorten the radius; reduces compressive force on the lunate
  - appears effective if there is no carpal DJD

  b) Radiologic features

  - distal ulnar articular surface more proximal than radial articular surface
  - may be seen with posttraumatic scapholunate dissociation
  - may be seen in patients with Kienböck's disease

V. Carpal coalition

  a) General features

  - fusion of two or more carpal bones
  - isolated anomaly, or often occurs with other skeletal anomalies
  - lack of segmentation and cavitation in cartilage template for these bones
  - female predilection: 2:1
  - most common bridge connects lunate and triquetrum
  - may be associated with: Madelung's deformity, Holt-Oram syndrome, Turner's syndrome, Ellis-van Creveld syndrome
  - when it is an isolated anomaly, usually only one row of carpals is involved
  - with congenital syndromes, fusions may exist between the rows
  - clinical significance lies in risk of fracture of bony bar

  b) Radiologic features

  - multiple views needed to demonstrate bridge
  - see continuous cortical and trabecular bone between carpals
  - cannot be diagnosed radiographically until ossification is complete
  - **DDX:** arthritic, infectious processes via history and clinical behavior

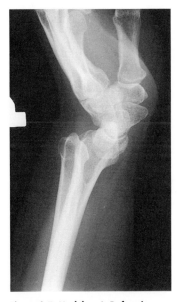

Figure 3.7. Madelung's Deformity.
Features seen in lateral projection. Reprinted with permission from Yochum TR, Rowe LJ. Essentials of Skeletal Radiology, 2nd ed. Baltimore: Williams & Wilkins, 1996:250.

VI. Polydactyly

a) General features

- increased number of fingers or toes
- more prevalent among black patients
- significance depends on which side of hand is affected
- preaxial (radial) side: associated with Apert's syndrome, Fanconi's syndrome, Holt-Oram syndrome
- postaxial (ulnar) side: associated with Ellis-van Creveld syndrome and Laurence-Moon-Biedl syndrome

b) Radiologic features

- x-ray identifies osseous development in digits, associated osseous anomalies in the extremities

VII. Syndactyly

a) General features

- most common developmental anomaly of the hand, also affects feet
- syndactyly (skin, soft tissue fusion) or synostosis (osseous fusion)
- predilections: white:black = 10:1; clear male predominance
- partial (proximal phalanges only) or complete (distal phalanges too)
- acrosyndactyly: distal phalanges only
- mesenchymal organization defect in fifth week of gestation
- classified into five types:
    1) zygodactyly: third and fourth fingers and/or second and third toes (most common)
    2) synpolydactyly of third and fourth fingers with partial or complete duplication of fingers three and four in the web (or may affect fourth and fifth toes)
    3) fourth and fifth finger syndactyly: middle phalanx of fifth finger rudimentary or absent
    4) complete syndactyly: involves all fingers
    5) syndactyly with metacarpal and/or metatarsal synostosis; usually affecting medial side of the hand
- associations include: Poland's syndrome, Apert's syndrome, Saethre syndrome, Pfeiffer's syndrome

b) Radiologic features

- plain films show osseous and soft tissue fusions
- may show interphalangeal fusion of a single digit or interdigital fusions

VIII. Kirner's Deformity (synonym: dystelephalangy)

  a) General features

   • fifth finger palmar curvature of distal phalanx
   • autosomal dominant transmission; may occur sporadically
   • usually bilateral
   • usually not diagnosed before fifth year of life
   • may be preceded by soft tissue swelling
   • clinically insignificant

  b) Radiologic features

   • volar curvature of fifth digits
   • separation (widening)of growth plate
   • deformity of epiphysis

REVIEW—STUDY QUESTIONS

1. Discuss the development and significance of bipartite, tripartite, and multipartite patellae.
2. What is Morton's syndrome?
3. Which anomalies of the extremities have clear male predilection? Female predilection?
4. Describe straight back syndrome and its clinical significance.
5. What is Srb's anomaly?
6. Describe coxa vara and coxa valga and explain what conditions they may accompany and why.
7. What is the possible clinical significance of a supracondylar process?
8. Describe Madelung's deformity.
9. What is the distinction between syndactyly, acrosyndactyly, and synostosis?
10. What is a carpal coalition and what is its clinical significance?

variant: differing in some characteristic from the class in which it belongs

C. NORMAL SKELETAL VARIANTS

 1. Skull and Face

  a) choroid plexus calcification

  b) falx cerebri calcification

  c) pineal gland calcification

  d) basal ganglia calcification
   • may be associated with pseudohypoparathyroidism or pseudopseudohypoparathyroidism

  e) calcification of petroclinoid ligament

  f) osseous bridging of sella turcica

        g) hyperostosis frontalis interna; **DDX:** meningioma

        h) persistent metopic suture
- may be associated with cleidocranial dysplasia
- **DDX:** fracture

        i) parietal foramina (conduct veins of Santorini)

☞   **j)** Wormian bones
- may be associated with cleidocranial dysplasia; osteogenesis imperfecta, or other anomalies

        k) prominent external occipital protuberance (EOP)

☞   **l)** Mach effect: lucent pseudofracture at base of dens (atlas posterior arch overlying dens)

2. Cervical Spine

☞   **a)** pseudo-Jefferson's fracture (APOM shows overhanging C1 lateral masses), normal in a child

        b) Viking helmet sign: osseous "horns" protrude laterally from dens

        c) calcified cervical lymph nodes (lateral to cervical spine)

        d) calcified stylohyoid ligament

☞   **e)** thyroid cartilage calcification (may appear ectopically beneath base of tongue)
- often bilateral
- oblique orientation aids **DDX** from calcified vertebral artery

☞   **f)** laryngeal shadow: **DDX** from SBO or vertical fracture of C6 body

        g) trapped air shadows: in esophagus or in vallecula of the larynx

☞   **h)** sclerotic C1 anterior tubercle
- normal variant = sclerosis without enlargement
- sclerosis with enlargement is usually compensatory stress hypertrophy

☞   **i)** short C1 posterior arch
- mimics anterolisthesis of C1 with RA or ankylosing spondylitis (AS); but this variant has no increased ADI
- may cause canal stenosis, even without instability

        j) small C1 anterior tubercle

        k) enlarged C1 posterior tubercle

☞   **l)** central incisor gap: simulates vertical Type I dens fracture

        m) C1 anterior spondyloschisis

        n) atlantoaxial "ball and socket" articulation

o) C1–2 accessory joint
- posterior arch of C1 with superior C2 lamina
- limits C1–2 flexion/extension

p) posterior tubercle notches (Yochum's notch)
- notched superior C1 tubercle

q) persistent infantile odontoid process
- base of odontoid is asymmetric
- lateral mass of C1 and superior facet of C2 articulate at anomalous angle

☞ **r)** "V"-shaped ADI: normal in children

☞ **s)** pseudohypermobility of C2: normal in children, "V"-shaped ADI, wide posterior gap

t) trapezoidal cervical vertebrae: normal in children

u) apparent C2–3 ankylosis of facet joints (on lateral projection: appearance due to orientation of joints)

v) facet notch—facet surface of C3 appears "notched" by C2 inferior process
- do not mistake this for joint erosion or fracture

w) bifid C2 spinous: bifurcation may be transverse or sagittal

x) C2 SP nonunion (ununited tip is not caudally displaced)

☞ **y)** supraspinous ligament or ligamentum nuchae ossifications (nuchal bones)

☞ **z)** non-union of SP secondary growth center
- especially at C7, T1 or T2
- **DDX:** clay shoveler's avulsion fracture

aa) congenital bifid SP (C7)
- **DDX:** fractured SP

bb) elongated cervical TP (superimpose upon IVD in lateral projection)

cc) pseudotumor (normal TP superimposed upon vertebral bodies in lateral projection)

dd) pseudofracture:
- slight rotation projects normal facet joint lucency over vertebral body
- hypertrophied uncovertebral joints create vertebral body lucency in lateral view

ee) enlarged cervical TP anterior tubercles: may create anomalous articulation

☞ **ff)** notochordal persistence (nuclear impression)

3. Chest, Thorax, and Thoracic Spine

a) bent SP: caudally angulated (most common in mid-thoracic spine)

b) tracheal cartilage calcification

☞   **c)** calcified axillary lymph nodes (**DDX:** blastic bone lesions; pulmonary nodules)

     d) normal thymus gland in infant (paraspinal density above the heart)

☞   **e)** calcified mediastinal lymph node
- may constrict trachea, bronchus
- can erode through bronchial wall, become a broncholith

     f) azygos fissure; azygos vein; azygos lobe

☞   **g)** aortic arch "thumbnail sign"—atherosclerosis within aortic arch

     h) prominent aortic knob (may indicate systemic hypertension)

     i) hiatal hernia (fundus of stomach in retrocardiac space, above diaphragm)

     j) tortuous descending thoracic aorta (with hypertension or advancing age)

     k) costochondral joint irregularities (irregular and prominent calcifications)

     l) costochondral cartilage calcification (seen in infants and senior citizens and is of no pathological significance)

     m) manubrium secondary growth center nonunion (lateral margins of manubrium)

☞   **n)** rhomboid fossae (inferomedial clavicles)

     o) supraclavicular foramen
- small, circular radiolucency at superior surface of medial third of clavicle
- may transmit supraclavicular nerve

     p) clavicular conoid tubercle prominence
- **DDX:** ossification of coracoclavicular ligament

     q) venous clefts of Hahn (usually in lower thoracic vertebral bodies)

     r) nipple shadows: **DDX:** pulmonary nodules

     s) conoid tubercle: exostosis from clavicle, may articulate with coracoid process

     t) T1 TP secondary growth center nonunion: double articulation at costotransverse

☞   **u)** ununited secondary ossification centers may occur anywhere in the spine: SPs, TPs, superior or inferior articulating processes

☞   **v)** limbus bone
- ossicles at anterior corners of vertebral bodies
- nonunion of secondary ossification center due to migration of nuclear material from disc herniation

  4. Abdomen, Pelvis and Lumbar Spine

☞   **a)** pseudotumor: fluid in stomach fundus, under left hemidiaphragm

b) calcified mesenteric lymph nodes

c) residual contrast media (angiogram, lymphangiogram, KUB, barium studies, myelogram)

d) ossified iliolumbar ligament (unilateral or bilateral)

e) calcified Cooper's ligament (parallel to superior line of pubic bones)

f) calcification of sacrotuberous ligaments
  - may be a variant or may occur with DISH or fluorosis

g) phleboliths

h) calcified scrotal lymph nodes

i) lumbar Harris' growth arrest lines (parallel endplates)

j) "step defect" in juvenile lumbar vertebra: will disappear with full ossification

k) lumbar rib

l) trapezoid lumbar vertebral body (commonly at L5)

☞ **m)** pig snout vertebra
  - transverse process malformation (seen on "Scotty Dog" in oblique view)

☞ **n)** L5 thin pars interarticularis (may predispose to spondylolysis)

o) widened SI joints—normal in youth

p) accessory sacral foramina

q) iliac fossa (**DDX:** SI joint erosion)

r) sacral ossification defect (lateral margin of distal sacral foramina does not ossify)

☞ **s)** paraglenoid sulci (lateral to inferior margin of SI joint)
  - female predilection, usually bilateral but asymmetrical
  - also called "preauricular" sulcus

t) sacrococcygeal angulation
  - may be an anatomic variation or post-traumatic
  - may present a problem in labor and delivery

u) iliac vascular groove: nutrient artery passageways; "V" or "Y" shapes

☞ **v)** triradiate cartilage: medial acetabulum of immature hip shows this lucency

w) ischiopubic synchondrosis variants
  - bulbous ossification with lucencies within it
  - callus-like bony expansion at ischiopubic synchondrosis
  - originally erroneously thought to be osteonecrosis (Van Neck's)

- separate growth center, ununited with rami
- may be unilateral or bilateral

    x) ischial agenesis (failure of ossification of ischium)

☞   **y)** pubic ears (protuberances project toward obturator foramen from medial pubis)

    z) agenetic lumbar transverse processes

5. Hip and Lower Extremities

☞   **a)** os acetabulum (at lateral margin of acetabulum)

    b) third leg syndrome (accessory acetabulum)
- rudimentary femoral head and neck
- articulates with inferior pubic ramus
- ischium is incomplete

☞   **c)** femoral herniation pits (synonym: Pitt's pits)
- geographic radiolucency within femoral neck
- bone reaction to an irregular capsular surface

☞   **d)** Harris' growth arrest line
- radiopaque transverse bands in metaphyses of long bones
- **DDX:** heavy metal poisoning, bone-sclerosing dysplasias; metabolic abnormalities

    e) bone bars (confluent trabeculae create narrow, linear densities)

☞   **f)** fabella: sesamoid bone within lateral gastrocnemius tendon

☞   **g)** talar beak (isolated variant, or associated with tarsal coalition)

☞   **h)** os trigonum: accessory ossicle posterior to talus
- **DDX:** fracture of talar posterior process

☞   **i)** calcaneal apophysis
- sclerotic appearance is normal in pediatric patient
- erroneously called "Sever's disease" (osteonecrosis)

    j) os tibiale externum: accessory ossicle medial to tarsal navicular

    k) os supranaviculare (synonym: Pirie's bone)
- accessory ossicle at proximal superior margin of tarsal navicular

    l) os peroneum: accessory ossicle at inferior margin of cuboid

    m) sesamoid bones
- commonly found at many articulations in hands and feet
- may be bipartite, tripartite (**DDX:** fractures)

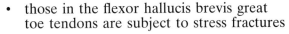

• those in the flexor hallucis brevis great
toe tendons are subject to stress fractures

6. **Shoulder and Upper Extremities**

   a) humeral pseudotumor
   • visual presentation of articular surface of
     humeral head superimposed with the
     tuberosities

   b) radial pseudotumor
   • proximal metaphysis of radius may appear
     radiolucent if radial tuberosity is
     unusually large

   c) os centrale
   • accessory ossicle at carpal dorsum,
     between scaphoid, trapezoid and capitate

   d) ununited secondary ossification center at
     distal ulna
   • ulnar styloid fails to fuse osseously with
     ulna
   • **DDX:** styloid fracture

REVIEW—STUDY QUESTIONS

1. What are the most common sites for sesamoid bones?
2. What is the largest sesamoid bone in the body, and what
    are its normal variants?
3. What is the cause of femoral herniation pits?
4. Name four intracranial structures that are commonly
    calcified.
5. What is the Mach effect?
6. What is the clinical significance of sacrococcygeal
    variations?
7. What is a "pig snout vertebra"?
8. Name four common accessory ossicles not found in the
    hands or feet.
9. Describe the location and reasons for three different
    "pseudotumors" seen on plain film.
10. Describe five normal variants that might be mistaken for
    fractures.

1. Encroachment into the foramen magnum by the odontoid is called:

   a) primary platybasia.
   b) basilar impression.
   c) tonsilar ectopia.
   d) Arnold-Chiari syndrome.

2. A helpful radiologic sign in distinguishing congenital from acquired vertebral fusion is:

   a) the "wasp waist" of the acquired fusion.
   b) the fused apophyses of the acquired fusion.
   c) the "wasp waist" of the congenital block vertebrae.
   d) the lack of rudimentary disc space in a congenital fusion.

3. Congenital hemivertebrae are apparently caused by:

   a) exaggerated lateral bending of the fetus during the second and third months of gestation.
   b) failure of development of the anterior ossification center.
   c) failure of development of the apophysis.
   d) failure of development of a lateral ossification center.

4. Clinical indications of Morton's syndrome may include:

   a) a shortened Achilles tendon.
   b) severe pain at the first metatarsal-phalangeal joint.
   c) a callus under the second and third metatarsal heads.
   d) excessive pronation.

5. Differential considerations with pseudoarthrosis of the first rib must include:

   a) elongated transverse process.
   b) stress fracture.
   c) cervical rib.
   d) bifurcated rib.

6. The most commonly encountered forms of mucopolysaccharidoses are:

   a) MPS-I-H (Hurler) and MPS-II (Hunter).
   b) MPS-II (Hunter) and MPS IV (Morquio).
   c) MPS-I-H (Hurler) and MPS IV (Morquio).
   d) MPS-II (Hunter) and MPS VI (Sly).

7. Linear opacities in a fanlike sunburst from the acetabulum to the iliac crest may be a sign of:

   a) Paget's disease.
   b) osteopoikilosis.
   c) melorheostosis.
   d) osteopathia striata.

8. Holt-Oram syndrome features all of the following radiologic abnormalities except:

   a) periosteal new bone formation on the ulna.
   b) Sprengel's deformity.
   c) thumb agenesis.
   d) triphalangeal thumb.

9. All of the following diseases are considered phakomatoses except:

   a) multiple sclerosis.
   b) cerebroretinal angiomatosis.
   c) tuberous sclerosis.
   d) neurofibromatosis.

10. Chondrodystrophia calcificans congenita is also known as:

    a) spondyloepiphyseal dysplasia congenita.
    b) Munchmeyer's disease.
    c) stippled epiphyses.
    d) cardio-limb syndrome.

11. Platybasia is determined by:

    a) Martin's basilar angle less than 140°.
    b) Martin's basilar angle less than 120°.
    c) Martin's basilar angle greater than 152°.
    d) Martin's basilar angle greater than 125°.

12. The radiologic finding of a dense and hypertrophied C1 anterior tubercle:

    a) helps in differentiation of odontoid fracture and os odontoideum.
    b) indicates the presence of an odontoid fracture.
    c) indicates cervical osteopetrosis.
    d) is of no diagnostic significance.

13. Multiple butterfly vertebrae are associated with:

    a) myelomeningocele.
    b) aberrant intraosseous blood vessels.
    c) Arnold-Chiari syndrome.
    d) persistent notochord.

14. Tarsal coalition may result from any of the following except:

    a) congenital malformation.
    b) trauma.
    c) neoplastic overgrowth.
    d) inflammatory arthritis.

15. The radiologic appearance of tropism may be simulated by:

    a) spondylolysis.
    b) intersegmental lateral flexion.
    c) intersegmental rotation.
    d) spondylolisthesis.

16. A young or middle-aged adult with extensive pathologic fractures, normal laboratory studies, and no familial history of similar conditions may be suspected to have:

    a) massive osteolysis of Gorham.
    b) Pyle's disease.
    c) HOOD.
    d) Holt-Oram syndrome.

17. Osteopathia striata is thought by some to be a variant of:

    a) osteopoikilosis.
    b) osteopetrosis.
    c) melorheostosis.
    d) tuberous sclerosis.

18. Chiropractic spinal manipulation is contraindicated for patients with:

    a) Holt-Oram syndrome.
    b) Munchmeyer's disease.
    c) hereditary osteo-onychodysplasia (HOOD).
    d) Conradi-Hunermann syndrome.

19. Epiloia is a Greek word meaning:

    a) "flowing bone."
    b) "vanishing bone."
    c) "mindless epileptic."
    d) "above (or over) bone."

20. The "hot cross bun" look refers to the widely separated cranial sutures seen in:

    a) Conradi-Hunermann syndrome.
    b) Trevor's disease.
    c) cleidocranial dysplasia.
    d) infantile cortical hyperostosis.

21. Third condyles (condylus tertius) may articulate with:

    a) the paracondyloid process.
    b) the C1 lateral mass.
    c) the C1 posterior arch.
    d) the C1 anterior arch.

22. The anomaly known as "os odontoideum":

    a) is also called "os terminale."
    b) is of little or no clinical significance.
    c) represents a potentially significant risk of cord compression from trivial trauma.
    d) requires CT or MRI imaging for definitive diagnosis.

23. Congenital agenesis of the pedicle is:

    a) invariably unilateral.
    b) most frequently seen at C4.
    c) always associated with neck pain and upper limb paresthesia.
    d) frequently associated with "butterfly vertebra."

24. The radiologic features of hypoplastic patellae, elbow malformations, and iliac horns are seen in:

    a) Putti's triad.
    b) Morton's syndrome.
    c) Fong's syndrome.
    d) Klippel-Feil syndrome.

25. Bertolotti's syndrome is associated with all of the following except:

    a) scoliosis.
    b) transitional vertebrae.
    c) sciatic pain.
    d) autonomic dysfunction.

26. Spontaneous bowel perforation, spontaneous pneumothorax, aortic aneurysms, genu recurvatum, and molluscoid fibrous subcutaneous tumors might be expected in a patient with:

    a) Marfan's syndrome.
    b) Fong's syndrome.
    c) Holt-Oram syndrome.
    d) Ehlers-Danlos syndrome.

27. When melorheostosis is manifested in carpal or tarsal bones, it may resemble:

    a) endosteal hyperostosis.
    b) osteopoikilosis.
    c) osteopetrosis.
    d) fibrous dysplasia.

28. Calcified, hypoplastic intervertebral discs, and ectopic ossification in soft tissues are indicative of:

    a) metaphyseal dysplasia.
    b) Morquio's syndrome.
    c) fibrodysplasia ossificans progressiva.
    d) osteopoikilosis.

29. Faulty dentition with dental carries is a feature of:

    a) melorheostosis.
    b) osteopoikilosis.
    c) pyknodysostosis.
    d) tuberous sclerosis.

30. Chondrodysplasia punctata is characterized by:

    a) stippling of the epiphyses.
    b) accessory epiphyses on the second metacarpals.
    c) hypoplastic epiphyses.
    d) asymmetrical focal overgrowth of the epiphyses.

31. Paracondyloid and epitransverse processes are examples of:

    a) atlas occipitalization.
    b) block vertebrae.
    c) occipital vertebrae.
    d) supernumerary zygapophyses.

32. The clinician working with a patient who has clinical signs of trisomy 21 should be especially aware of the possibility of:

    a) underdeveloped paranasal sinuses.
    b) cervical ribs.
    c) atlanto-axial instability.
    d) lumbar stenosis.

33. Cervical ribs most commonly:

    a) lie above the brachial plexus.
    b) divide the brachial plexus from the subclavian vessels.
    c) lie inferior to the brachial plexus and subclavian vessels.
    d) "split" the brachial plexus.

34. The most commonly seen form of multipartite patella is:

    a) unilateral tripartite patella.
    b) bilateral bipartite patellae.
    c) bilateral tripartite patellae.
    d) unilateral bipartite patella.

35. Clinical manifestations of diastematomyelia include all of the following except:

    a) intermittent low-grade fever.
    b) asymmetrical lower extremity size.
    c) lipoma.
    d) hairy lumbar patch.

36. Defective mentation is a feature of all of the following dysplasias except:

    a) familial metaphyseal dysplasia.
    b) rhizomelic chondrodysplasia punctata.
    c) MPS-I-Hurler syndrome.
    d) tuberous sclerosis.

37. Flowing hyperostosis is a term applied to:

    a) melorheostosis.
    b) osteopoikilosis.
    c) osteopetrosis.
    d) osteogenesis imperfecta.

38. All of the following are synonyms for Fibrodysplasia ossificans progressiva except:

    a) Munchmeyer's disease.
    b) fibrositis ossificans progressiva.
    c) epiphyseal dysplasia multiplex.
    d) myositis ossificans progressiva.

39. Progressive diaphyseal dysplasia (PDD):

    a) manifests around puberty, with symmetrical bilateral involvement.
    b) manifests before age 10, with bilateral symmetrical involvement.
    c) manifests before age 10, with asymmetrical involvement.
    d) manifests around puberty, with asymmetrical involvement.

40. "Trident hand" is characteristic of:

    a) achondroplasia.
    b) Caffey's syndrome.
    c) Morquio's syndrome.
    d) Holt-Oram syndrome.

41. The clinical signs of atlas occipitalization:

    a) are usually negligible.
    b) may include mental retardation.
    c) may include vertigo, visual difficulties, and auditory abnormalities.
    d) are usually caused by atlantoaxial instability.

42. The arcuate foramen transmits:

    a) the basilar artery.
    b) the first cervical nerve.
    c) the external carotid artery.
    d) the recurrent nerve of Luschka.

43. Bilaterally enlarged cervical neural foramina may suggest the presence of:

    a) neurofibroma.
    b) vertebral artery aneurysm.
    c) congenital spondylolisthesis caused by agenesis of pedicles.
    d) hyperplastic articular processes.

44. The normal angle of incidence of the proximal femur is:

    a) 115–120°.
    b) 105–115°.
    c) 120–130°.
    d) 130–145°.

45. Spinal dysraphism is most commonly seen in:

    a) the cervical spine.
    b) the thoracolumbar spine.
    c) the lumbar spine.
    d) the thoracic spine.

46. Synonyms for HOOD include all of the following except:

    a) osteo-onychodysostosis.
    b) nail-patella syndrome.
    c) Fong's syndrome.
    d) Holt-Oram syndrome.

47. "Overlap syndrome" refers to cases in which a single patient has signs of:

    a) Marfan's syndrome, osteogenesis imperfecta, and mucopolysaccharidosis.
    b) osteopoikilosis, osteogenesis imperfecta, and osteopathia striata.
    c) mucopolysaccharidosis, osteogenesis imperfecta, and osteopoikilosis.
    d) melorheostosis, osteopoikilosis, and osteopathia striata.

48. In spinal films of a patient with spondyloepiphyseal dysplasia tarda, one might expect to see:

    a) normal disc heights, but "beaked" vertebrae with posterior scalloping.
    b) thin disc spaces, with "heaped-up" vertebrae and non-ossified ring epiphyses.
    c) tall vertebrae with posterior scalloping and normal disc heights.
    d) widened disc spaces with centrally beaked, flattened vertebrae.

49. Progressive diaphyseal dysplasia most prominently involves:

    a) the endosteum.
    b) the periosteum.
    c) the medullary cavity.
    d) the articular surface.

50. The spine of an achondroplastic dwarf may typically have:

    a) anteriorly scalloped vertebral bodies.
    b) "heaped-up" vertebra.
    c) "bullet-nosed" vertebra.
    d) "rugger jersey" vertebra.

51. *Putti's triad* is a group of radiologic features associated with:

    a) congenital hip dislocation.
    b) malum coxae senilis.
    c) protrusio acetabulum.
    d) coxa valga.

52. The cervical vertebra most commonly involved in congenital spondylolisthesis is:

    a) C5.
    b) C2.
    c) C4.
    d) C6.

53. The Kimmerly anomaly is commonly known as:

    a) posterior ponticle.
    b) agenesis of the C1 posterior arch.
    c) atlanto-occipital fusion.
    d) a nuchal bone.

54. Acroosteolysis is a feature of:

    a) pyknodysostosis.
    b) massive osteolysis of Gorham.
    c) osteogenesis imperfecta.
    d) rheumatoid arthritis.

55. Engelmann's disease is commonly called:

    a) nail-patella syndrome.
    b) metaphyseal dysplasia.
    c) progressive diaphyseal dysplasia.
    d) osteopathia striata.

56. Diagnosis of osteogenesis imperfecta requires:

    a) osteoporosis with abnormal dentition.
    b) osteoporosis with blue sclera.
    c) premature otosclerosis with skeletal fragility.
    d) at least two of the four major criteria to be present.

57. Paired posterior iliac "horns" are pathognomonic for:

    a) Gaucher's disease.
    b) metaphyseal dysplasia.
    c) nail-patella syndrome.
    d) Ehlers-Danlos syndrome.

58. Agenesis of the anterior sacrum may be seen on x-ray as:

    a) the scimitar sacrum sign.
    b) the inverted Napoleon hat sign.
    c) the domed sacrum sign.
    d) the clasp knife appearance.

59. The clinical picture of a young boy (younger than 10 years) with unilateral hard, painless swelling in the distal tibia, and distal femur suggests a diagnosis of:

    a) epiphyseal dysplasia multiplex.
    b) dysplasia epiphysealis hemimelica.
    c) Morquio's syndrome.
    d) spondyloepiphyseal dysplasia tarda.

60. The rhomboid fossae are anomalies that may be seen:

    a) along the superomedial border of the scapulae.
    b) along the inferomedial border of the scapulae.
    c) along the inferomedial border of the clavicles.
    d) along the transverse processes of T3 and T4.

61. Ortolani's test and Barlow's test are used to help diagnosis:

    a) protrusio acetabulae.
    b) hip dislocation.
    c) Legg-Calvé-Perthes disease.
    d) slipped femoral capital epiphysis.

62. An omovertebral bone:

    a) projects from the hyoid bone to the thyroid cartilage.
    b) is always present in Klippel-Feil syndrome.
    c) consists of cartilage, fibrous tissue, or bone attached to the superior angle of the scapula.
    d) descends from the transverse process of C2, C3, or C4 to the superior scapular angle.

63. The modality of choice for diagnosis of Arnold-Chiari malformation is:

    a) CT.
    b) CT myelography.
    c) MRI.
    d) tomography.

64. Bone density is generally increased, but the medullary canal is preserved in:

    a) osteoporosis.
    b) osteopetrosis.
    c) pyknodysostosis.
    d) Ehlers-Danlos syndrome.

65. All of the following are true of patients with osteopetrosis except:

    a) they have fragile, brittle bones and suffer multiple pathologic fractures.
    b) they may be completely asymptomatic.
    c) they are subject to blindness or deafness when the skull is involved.
    d) their condition is always diagnosed at birth.

66. All of the following are true of osteogenesis imperfecta except:

    a) it may be detectable at birth.
    b) the tarda form has a life expectancy of two to three decades.
    c) it affects skin, ligaments, the sclera, the inner ear, and the skeleton.
    d) may be caused by an ATPase deficiency.

67. Platyspondyly, hyperostotic calvarium and mandible, ocular hypertelorism, and Erlenmeyer flask deformities (especially in the femur, tibia and fibula) are radiologic features common to:

    a) Marfan's syndrome.
    b) Fong's syndrome.

c) metaphyseal dysplasia.

d) Holt-Oram syndrome.

68. By the 18th week of gestation, alpha fetoprotein in the amniotic fluid may indicate:

a) the presence of spina bifida occulta.

b) the presence of a meningocele.

c) the presence of Down's syndrome.

d) the presence of a neurofibroma.

69. All of the following are correct about Trevor's disease (dysplasia epiphysealis hemimelica) except:

a) it is monostotic.

b) it is polyostotic.

c) in its classical form, it is present in more than one area in an extremity.

d) is known to be a genetic disorder.

70. Syndactyly has a clear predilection for:

a) white females.

b) black females.

c) white males.

d) black males.

71. A chest wall anomaly commonly associated with Morquio's syndrome is:

a) pectus carinatum.

b) pectus excavatum.

c) straight back syndrome.

d) Srb's anomaly.

72. The normal scapula usually is positioned with its inferior angle:

a) at the T7 level.

b) below the T7 level.

c) above the T7 level.

d) above the T6 level.

73. The clinical picture of a patient with a Type I Arnold-Chiari malformation may involve:

a) autonomic dysfunctions, such as anhidrosis and hyperhidrosis.

b) impotence.

c) headaches and neck pain.

d) dyspnea.

74. A patient with tuberous sclerosis has a poor prognosis if there:

a) is epilepsy.

b) is peau-chagrin.

c) is honeycomb lung.

d) are renal hamartomas.

75. Because of the pathological process involved in osteopetrosis, these patients will develop:

a) irritable bowel syndrome.

b) hepatosplenomegaly.

c) adult respiratory distress syndrome.

d) bleeding disorders.

76. A "no-neck" appearance, wide-set eyes set beside a depressed nose bridge, deformed teeth, and deafness but normal mentation characterize:

a) an achondroplastic dwarf.

b) Hurler's syndrome.

c) Morquio's syndrome.

d) Klippel-Feil syndrome.

77. Pyle's disease (metaphyseal dysplasia):

a) is familial and involves autosomal recessive transmission.

b) primarily involves the upper extremities and spares the lower extremities.

c) is manifested at birth.

d) is a form of dwarfism.

78. Spina bifida occulta:

a) is most common at C1..

b) is most common at T1.

c) is most common at L5 and S1.

d) is most common at T12 and L1.

79. Premature DJD, short thick hands, and bilaterally, symmetrically shortened legs characterize:

a) epiphyseal dysplasia multiplex.

b) dysplasia epiphysealis hemimelica.

c) spondyloepiphyseal dysplasia.

d) metaphyseal dysplasia.

80. The most common carpal coalition connects the:

a) scaphoid and trapezoid.

b) lunate and triquetrum.

c) trapezium and trapezoid.

d) hamate and pisiform.

81. "Pancake heart" is a common complication of:

a) Srb's anomaly.

b) pectus carinatum.

c) cobbler's chest.

d) intrathoracic rib.

82. Sprengle's deformity is:

a) an omo-hyoid bone.

b) congenital elevation of the scapula.

c) congenital cervical block vertebra.

d) scoliosis with an elevated shoulder.

83. Downward displacement of the brainstem and cerebellar tonsils through the foramen magnum is known as:

a) platybasia.

b) Arnold-Chiari malformation.

c) basilar impression.

d) basilar invagination.

84. Café au lait spots are characteristic of neurofibromatosis,

a) fibrous dysplasia, and tuberous sclerosis.

b) fibrous dysplasia, and epilepsy.

c) tuberous sclerosis, and osteopoikilosis.

d) fibrous dysplasia, and pyknodysostosis.

85. Juxtaarticular small, round, or ovoid opacities are pathognomonic for:

a) bone islands.

b) osteoid osteoma.

c) osteopathia striata.

d) osteopoikilosis.

86. Morquio's syndrome is also known as:

   a) MPS-IV.
   b) gargoylism.
   c) dysostosis multiplex.
   d) Sly syndrome.

87. A patient with protrusio acetabulae, tall vertebrae, pectus excavatum, and atlantoaxial hypermobility may be suspected of having:

   a) metaphyseal dysplasia.
   b) Fong's syndrome.
   c) Holt-Oram syndrome.
   d) Marfan's syndrome.

88. The "Cupid's bow" contour seen on an AP lumbar or thoracic film indicates the presence of:

   a) persistent notochord.
   b) Schmorl's node.
   c) butterfly vertebra.
   d) congenital hemivertebra.

89. Trevor's disease and tarsoepiphyseal aclasis are both synonyms for:

   a) dysplasia epiphysealis punctata.
   b) dysplasia epiphysealis hemimelica.
   c) multiple epiphyseal dysplasia.
   d) spondyloepiphyseal dysplasia congenita.

90. A beaklike bony spur at the anteromedial distal humeral metaphysis that angles toward the elbow is most likely:

   a) an osteosarcoma.
   b) a chondrosarcoma.
   c) an osteochondroma.
   d) a supracondylar process.

91. Srb's anomaly involves:

   a) lumbar ribs.
   b) involuted ribs.
   c) cervical ribs.
   d) agenesis of the first ribs.

92. The *pterygium coli* is the:

   a) low hairline seen in Klippel-Feil syndrome.
   b) short, webbed neck seen in Klippel-Feil syndrome.
   c) omovertebral bone.
   d) triad of features seen in Klippel-Feil syndrome.

93. Primary basilar impression is generally caused by:

   a) Paget's disease.
   b) osteomalacia.
   c) fibrous dysplasia.
   d) congenital malformations.

94. The classic clinical triad of tuberous sclerosis is:

   a) mental retardation, visual abnormalities, and hepatosplenomegaly.
   b) mental retardation, skin lesions, and kidney failure.
   c) mental retardation, epilepsy, and skin lesions.
   d) epilepsy, lung hamartomas, and visual abnormalities.

95. Osteopoikilosis involves:

   a) microfractures.
   b) abnormally low serum calcium levels.
   c) abnormally high serum calcium levels.
   d) autosomal dominant transmission.

96. Frontal bossing, an enlarged "J" shaped sella turcica, inferiorly beaked thoracolumbar vertebrae, "paddle ribs," and a "trident hand" are all characteristic of the radiologic features of:

   a) Morquio's syndrome.
   b) achondroplasia.
   c) Hurler's syndrome.
   d) Holt-Oram syndrome.

97. Marfan's syndrome:

   a) seldom involves the spine.
   b) has a 3:1 male predilection.
   c) is essentially a connective tissue disorder.
   d) may involve significant mental retardation.

98. The VATER syndrome may involve all of the following except:

   a) vascular anomalies.
   b) retinal dysplasia.
   c) anal atresia.
   d) vertebral anomalies.

99. Conradi-Hunermann syndrome is a form of:

   a) chondrodysplasia punctata.
   b) metaphyseal dysplasia.
   c) Ehlers-Danlos syndrome.
   d) mucopolysaccharidoses.

100. Although probably genetic in etiology, Caffey's disease may not be detectable until:

   a) puberty.
   b) a child begins weight-bearing (i.e., standing and walking).
   c) the third decade of life.
   d) a child is 2 or 3 months old.

PRACTICE TEST CHAPTER 3—ANSWER KEY

1.	b	11.	c	21.	d	31.	c	41.	c	51.	a	61.	b	71.	a	81.	c	91.	b
2.	c	12.	a	22.	c	32.	c	42.	b	52.	d	62.	c	72.	a	82.	b	92.	b
3.	d	13.	a	23.	c	33.	c	43.	c	53.	a	63.	c	73.	c	83.	b	93.	d
4.	c	14.	c	24.	c	34.	d	44.	c	54.	a	64.	c	74.	c	84.	a	94.	c
5.	b	15.	c	25.	d	35.	a	45.	b	55.	c	65.	d	75.	b	85.	d	95.	d
6.	c	16.	a	26.	d	36.	a	46.	d	56.	d	66.	b	76.	c	86.	a	96.	c
7.	d	17.	a	27.	b	37.	a	47.	d	57.	c	67.	c	77.	a	87.	d	97.	c
8.	a	18.	b	28.	c	38.	c	48.	b	58.	a	68.	b	78.	c	88.	a	98.	b
9.	a	19.	c	29.	c	39.	b	49.	a	59.	b	69.	d	79.	a	89.	b	99.	a
10.	c	20.	c	30.	a	40.	a	50.	c	60.	c	70.	c	80.	b	90.	d	100.	d

Chapter 4

TRAUMA
Terminology for Traumatic Lesions, Fracture Repair, Most Common Fractures

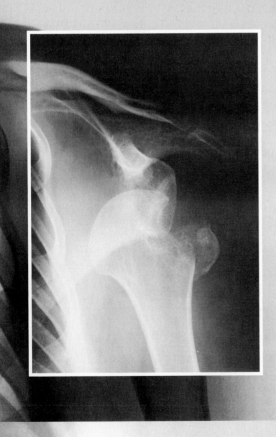

A. FRACTURE TERMINOLOGY

   1. Types of Fractures

a) Closed fracture: skin intact; older term—"simple fracture"

b) Open fracture: skin ruptured and bone exposed; older term—"compound fracture"

c) Comminuted fracture: more than two fragments

- butterfly fragment: triangular cortical fragment; usually on concave side of injury

d) Noncomminuted fracture: bone separated into two fragments

e) Avulsion fracture: portion of bone torn away by muscle or ligament tractional force

f) Impaction fracture: bone fragments driven into one another

- plain film shows radiopaque white line of impaction
- two sub-types: depressed and compression
    1) depressed fracture: inward bulging of outer cortical surface
        - often seen at tibial plateau and in frontal bone
    2) compression fracture: trabecular telescoping
        - typically in vertebrae with hyperflexion injuries
- term *compression fracture* used for spinal injury; in appendicular skeleton (e.g., femoral neck), term *impaction fracture* is used

g) Incomplete fracture: one side of cortex broken; bone buckled or bent

- may see angular deformity, but no displacement

- two sub-types: greenstick fracture and torus fracture
    1) Greenstick (Hickory stick) fracture: bent bone fractures on convex side, concave side intact (Fig. 4.1)
        - usually in infants and young children
    2) Torus (Buckling) fracture: compression bulges cortex outward (Fig. 4.2)
        - usually in metaphysis
        - especially painful

h) Infraction fracture: moderately severe impaction fracture; minor, localized cortical break

i) Chip fracture (also called "corner fracture"): form of avulsion fracture, term is used to

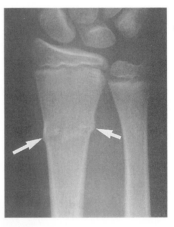

Figure 4.1.

Greenstick fracture. Reprinted with permission from Yochum TR, Rowe LJ. Essentials of Skeletal Radiology, 2nd ed. Baltimore: Williams & Wilkins, 1996:656.

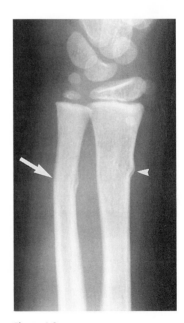

Figure 4.2.

Torus fracture. Reprinted with permission from Yochum TR, Rowe LJ. Essentials of Skeletal Radiology, 2nd ed. Baltimore: Williams & Wilkins, 1996:656.

describe small chip avulsed from phalangeal corner or from another tubular bone

j) Pathologic fracture: fracture through bone weakened by a pathological process
- usually smooth, straight transverse breaks

k) Stress fracture (also called fatigue fracture): repetitive stress causes microfractures and eventually a true fracture
- actual fatigue failure of bone
- insufficiency fracture: stress fracture through diseased bone

l) Occult fracture: clinically evident but not visible radiologically
- may become visible a week or 10 days later due to bone resorption at the site, callus formation, or frank displacement
- commonly occur at carpal scaphoid (navicular), and in ribs

m) Bone bruise: hemorrhage and edema occur with microfractures; imaged only by MRI
- most common at articulating surfaces of the knee

☞ **n)** Stable fracture: one that is unlikely to move during healing
- especially critical in spine: stable fracture poses no threat to cord or exiting nerve root

☞ **o)** Unstable fracture: one that may shift position during healing
- especially in spine, an unstable fracture may cause neurologic lesions

2. **Fracture Orientation**

a) Oblique fracture: common in long bone shaft; fracture line at an angle (often about 45°) to the long axis of the bone; blunt fracture ends

b) Spiral fracture: pointed ends of fracture, fracture line curves in spiral along shaft

c) Transverse fracture: at right angle to long axis of bone; almost always in diseased bone
- *"banana fracture"*: transverse pathologic fracture seen with Paget's disease

☞ 3. **Descriptors for Spatial Relationship of Fragments**

a) Alignment: angulation (or lack thereof) of distal fragment in relation to proximal fragment
- angulation must be assessed in at least two views at 90° to one another

b) Apposition: distance between fragments
- good apposition means almost complete surface contact of fractured fragments
- partial apposition means partial bony contact

- poor apposition is complete lack of bony contact
- distraction refers to separation of fractured ends by muscles or traction devices

c) Rotation: twisting forces causing rotation around long axis
- proximal and distal joints must be seen on film to assess rotational malposition

B. TRAUMATIC ARTICULAR LESION DESCRIPTORS

1. Growth Plate Fractures

 a) Salter-Harris classification of physeal/epiphyseal fractures (Fig. 4.3 A–E)
- Type I: a horizontal fracture through the growth plate
    1) plain film may appear normal if there is no misalignment or significant distraction
    2) diagnosis by clinical evidence of pain, swelling
    3) may occur with rickets, scurvy, osteomyelitis, hormone imbalance
    4) classic example: slipped capital femoral epiphysis
- Type II: displaced growth plate and fractured metaphyseal corner
    1) *Thurston-Holland sign*: metaphyseal fracture fragment
    2) about 75% of epiphyseal fractures are this type
    3) 50% of Type II fractures are at the distal radius
    4) other common sites: tibia, fibula, femur, ulna
- Type III displaces the physis and fractures the epiphysis
    1) intraarticular lesion; may need open reduction
    2) most often at distal tibia
- Type IV is obliquely vertical, through metaphysis, physis, and epiphysis
    1) most common at distal humeral lateral condyle (pediatric patients)

Figure 4.3.

Salter-Harris Types I–V. **A**. *Type I.* **B**. *Type II.* **C**. *Type III.* **D**. *Type IV.* **E**. *Type V. Reprinted with permission from Yochum TR, Rowe LJ. Essentials of Skeletal Radiology, 2nd ed. Baltimore: Williams & Wilkins, 1996:659.*

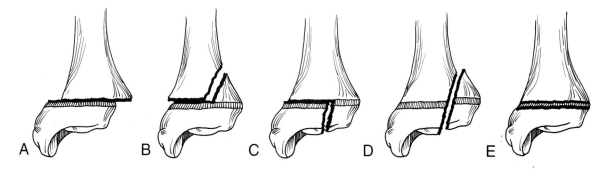

A   B   C   D   E

and distal tibia in patients > 10
years old

    2) ·open reduction needed; permanent
deformity may result

- Type V is an impaction fracture of the
physis

    1) initial plain films appear normal;
monitor child for 2 years

    2) growth of bone inhibited; abnormal
shortening or angulation results

    3) distal femur and distal tibia most
frequently affected

    4) this is the least common type

2. Chondral and Osteochondral Fractures

a) Joint surface fractured by shearing, rotary, or
tangential impaction force

b) Cartilage fracture only (chondral)

c) Cartilage and underlying bone fractured
(osteochondral)

d) Common osteochondral fracture:
osteochondritis dissecans

- at femoral condyles, talar dome,
capitellum

3. Diastasis

a) Separation or displacement of a syndesmosis
(slightly movable joint)

b) Most commonly at pubic symphysis, skull
sutures, distal tibiofibular syndesmosis

c) Called a *diastatic fracture*

4. Dislocation (Luxation)

a) Luxated joint has complete loss of contact
between normal articular surfaces

b) A fracture dislocation involves both
fractured structure and dislocated joint

c) Extremity dislocation described in relation to
proximal bone

d) Spinal dislocation described in relation to
subadjacent segment

5. Subluxation

a) Partial loss of normal articular contact or
orientation

C. FRACTURE REPAIR

1. Circulatory (Inflammatory) Phase

a) First of three phases, itself has three sub-
phases, each about 10 days long; comprises
necrosis, hematoma, vascular spindle
formation and primary callus development

b) Cellular phase: hematoma and clot formation

- hematoma is central to callus formation;
the less it is disturbed the better

- cellular inflammatory response: granulation tissue creates a mesenchymal blastema, which matures into callus over time
- granulation tissue replaces hematoma

   c) Vascular phase: auxiliary circulatory network develops around fracture

- forms a vascular spindle
- active hyperemia around injury
- passive hyperemia or congestion within injured area's vascular "swamp"
- prompts mesenchymal blastema cells to secrete osteoid matrix
- peripheral osteoclastic activity promoted; subchondral and submetaphyseal resorption
- may note temporary hypertrichosis and tanning skin due to regional hyperemia
- periosteum stripped by fracture, elevated by newly formed matrix; new periosteum formed between normal muscle and callus in injured muscle adjacent to bone, results in *Codman's triangle* periosteal response visible on x-ray

   d) Primary callus phase: plastic exudate develops around fragmented surfaces, eventually unites them

- undifferentiated mesenchymal cells from injured bone and soft tissue elements form about 70% of callus (in femur fractures, specifically)
- within callus coarsely woven bone (osteoid) deposited, then mineralized
- cartilage formed within callus simultaneously
- developing repair visible on x-ray at about 14 days

2. Reparative (Metabolic) Phase

   a) More orderly callus secretion

   b) Coarsely woven osteoid removed; replaced by more mature bone

   c) Remodeling process

   d) Callus functions: sealing, buttressing, bridging and uniting

- sealing callus fills medullary cavity, "seals" marrow from fracture site
- buttressing callus is adjacent to outer cortex; formed by periosteum and muscle
- bridging callus fills gap between buttress ends
- uniting callus connects cortical ends of fractured bone

3. Remodeling (Mechanical) Phase

   a) Realignment and remodeling of bone and callus along stress lines

b) Wolff's law applies here: bone deposited in stress (or highest stress) areas, removed from non-stress (or lower stress) areas

c) Final stage is restoration of medullary cavity and bone marrow

4. **General Features**

a) Hematoma should not be disturbed, as it stimulates granulation tissue production and ultimately, callus formation: injured soft tissue should be left to heal

b) Phagocytosis removes bone fragments, but may impede callus formation

c) Sequestered fragments may have to be surgically removed

d) Correlation between fractures in bone with little or no adjacent musculature damage: healing will be poor in these sites

e) Bone is clinically healed before it is anatomically reconstituted: remodeling proceeds over years

f) Usually, anatomic reconstitution realigns and reforms bone to normal contours

5. **Radiologic Features**

a) First 5 days: osteoclastic activity visibly increases width of fracture line

b) Next 10–30 days: callus appears as a "veil" of new bone adjacent to fracture site

c) Next 4 to 12 weeks: gradual remodeling, repair of cortical integrity
- 4 to 6 weeks in pediatric patients
- 6 to 12 weeks in geriatric patients

D. FRACTURE COMPLICATIONS

1. **Immediate Complications**

a) Vascular injury
- especially likely with open or comminuted fractures
- most common arterial rupture with fracture: popliteal
- next: superficial femoral artery at the adductor canal

 b) Compartment syndromes
- unrelenting pressure increase due to edema and hemorrhage in closed compartments
- may cause permanent necrosis of compromised muscles
- e.g., anterior tibial compartment; anterior forearm (Volkmann's contracture)

c) Gas gangrene
- skin or intestine penetrated; blood supply compromised

- these conditions can precipitate clostridium perfringens infection
- infection occurs within 1 to 3 days
- buttocks and thighs most frequently affected
- x-ray indication: thin, linear, parallel streaks within muscle planes

☞ **d)** Fat embolism syndrome
- pulmonary fat embolism up to five days after fracture
- emboli mobilized by vasoactivity and fat hydrolysis
- femur fracture most frequently involved
- other fractures often involved: tibia, pelvis
- more than 50% are associated with multiple fractures

☞ **e)** Thromboembolism
- deep vein thrombosis facilitated by immobilization and bed rest after fracture
- potential for pulmonary emboli; may be fatal
- especially associated with fracture of hip, pelvis, lower extremity

2. **Intermediate Complications**

☞ **a)** Osteomyelitis
- *Staphylococcus aureus* causes 60–70% of these infections
- rarely seen with closed fractures; a complication of open fracture or surgical reduction
- most frequently seen with femoral and tibial fractures
- usually manifest within one month of trauma or reparative surgery
- plain films show "moth-eaten" lytic lesions, sequestra formation, periosteal response at painful area

b) Hardware failure
- screws and plates used to stabilize the healing bone may fail
- loosening, bending, breaking, or migration
- metal-bone interface may widen visibly (plain film)
- pins may be transported via blood vessels; rarely have migrated to heart or great vessels

☞ **c)** Reflex sympathetic dystrophy syndrome (synonym: Sudeck's atrophy)
- painful, severe regional osteoporosis
- may also follow trivial trauma

☞ **d)** Posttraumatic osteolysis
- common at pubic bones and distal clavicle
- posttraumatic osteolysis of the clavicle (PTOC) is most frequent
- PTOC may follow clavicular fracture;

acromioclavicular trauma; shoulder overuse syndromes

e) Refracture
- usually secondary to bone pathology, noncompliance by patient, inadequate immobilization, or bone weakened at pin site

f) Myositis ossificans
- heterotopic bone formation at trauma site
- occurs with or without fracture
- usually at thigh or anterior arm
- plain film shows confluent ossification in muscle tissue

g) Synostosis
- between closely apposed bones
- most commonly: radius-ulna, tibia-fibula, small bones of hands or feet
- clinical significance: loss of functional motion

h) Delayed union
- may be caused by inadequate immobilization, poor vascularity, disease, or age
- especially vulnerable sites: scaphoid (navicular), proximal femur, tibia

3. Delayed Complications

a) osteonecrosis (synonyms: avascular necrosis, ischemic necrosis, aseptic necrosis)
- loss of blood supply to bone
- factors: fracture site, normal bone vascularity, appropriate early treatment
- common sites: femoral head, humeral head, scaphoid, talus

b) Degenerative joint disease
- intraarticular fracture damages articular cartilage
- most frequent at hip, knee, ankle
- posttraumatic DJD most likely if weight-bearing axis is altered

c) Lead arthropathy and toxicity
- gunshot wounds
- especially near joints where more acidic fluid and mechanical friction hasten breakdown of lead pellets

d) Osteoporosis
- if functional weight-bearing is delayed, bone is lost
- factors: pain, nerve palsy, altered function, failure to mobilize

e) Aneurysmal bone cyst
- rare sequela of fracture
- proposed mechanism: subperiosteal hematoma converts to expansile tumor

f) Malunion

- union occurs but not in correct anatomic position
- altered joint mechanics and loss of function result
- limb may be shortened: alters gait, causes unleveled pelvis, scoliosis

 g) Nonunion

- failure of full osseous fusion at fracture site
- factors include: inadequate immobilization, impaired circulation, infection, distraction
- most commonly seen at midclavicle, ulna, and tibia
- x-ray signs become apparent months after trauma: fracture margin rounding, sclerotic fracture margins, pseudoarthrosis, lack of callus formation

REVIEW—STUDY QUESTIONS

1. What factors affect the probability of osteonecrosis developing after a fracture and what are the most frequently affected sites?

2. Describe diastasis. Where is it most often seen?

3. What are the three general, overall stages of bone healing?

4. Describe in detail the three sub-phases of the circulatory (inflammatory) phase of fracture repair.

5. Explain apposition, alignment, distraction, and rotation of fracture fragments. What is the orientation or point of reference for these terms in appendicular fractures? In spinal fractures?

6. Define and differentiate the two terms commonly used for partial fractures.

7. Differentiate stress fracture and insufficiency fracture.

8. Describe five complications of fracture that are "delayed" or late in manifesting themselves.

9. Describe five intermediate (neither early nor delayed) complications of fracture.

10. What is Sudeck's atrophy?

11. What are the functions of callus in the healing process of fractures?

12. Describe the subtypes of impaction fractures. When is the term *compression fracture* used, and when is *impaction fracture* preferred?

13. List and describe Salter-Harris classifications of epiphyseal fractures. Which is most common? Where?

14. Explain the distinction between stable and unstable fractures.

15. What are the radiologic signs of fracture nonunion?

E. SKULL AND FACIAL BONE FRACTURES

1. Introduction

a) Plain films demonstrate less than 10% of skull fractures: CT is optimal modality

b) MRI may not show early hematoma or fracture, takes too long for acutely injured patient to endure, and presents technical difficulties in working around life support systems

c) Films done for medicolegal reasons: minimum set is left and right lateral, AP Towne's and PA Caldwell

d) Head injuries often include hematomas and other intracranial lesions, and many of these do not involve fracture

e) Neurologic indications of intracranial trauma: loss of consciousness, abnormal reflexes, sensory or motor changes, ear discharge, discolored ear drum, vomiting, amnesia

f) Complications of skull fractures
   • leptomeningeal cyst
     1) "pocket" forms where torn dura adheres to bone fragment
     2) CSF fills this "pocket"
     3) pulsations of CSF in the cyst erode adjacent bone, increasing size of fracture (*growing fracture*)
     4) clinical significance: focal neurological deficit due to pressure on subadjacent cerebral cortex
   • subdural and extradural hematoma
     1) these more often occur without fracture, but may be associated with fracture
     2) contrecoup injury creates hematoma on contralateral side of brain
     3) CT is imaging modality of choice
     4) appearance: bright crescent (concave medially) adjacent to internal skull table
   • pneumocephalus
     1) possible with fracture of paranasal sinus or mastoid air cell
     2) air admitted to subarachnoid space, thence into ventricular system

g) Facial fractures demonstrated in four projections: PA Water's, PA Caldwell, lateral (side of trauma), submentovertex

h) X-ray exam for facial fracture must visualize entire mandible

i) CT preferred to assess complex facial structures, such as sinuses

2. **Linear Skull Fracture**

    a) Most common type of skull fracture (up to 80%)

    b) Usually several centimeters long

    c) Varied orientation: straight, angular, curvilinear

    d) Radiologic signs: sharp, irregular radiolucent lines with no sclerotic rim

    e) Most common sites: temporal and parietal bones

     f) **DDX**
- suture lines: sutures often serrated
- vascular grooves: fracture more lucent (involves inner and outer skull tables), may cross sutures

3. **Depressed Skull Fracture**

    a) About 15% of skull fractures; usually within cranial vault

    b) Usually several bone fragments are angulated inward at the site

    c) Must image them in profile to determine depth of fragment displacement

    d) May cause dural tears, which require surgical repair (about ⅓ of depressed fractures)
- high probability of dural tear with depression > 5 mm beyond inner table

    e) Radiologic signs: radiopaque in *en face* view, may be stellate

4. *Ping Pong* **Fracture**

    a) Type of depressed fracture

    b) Seen in pediatric patients: pliable skull

    c) Deep, broad depression in skull

    d) Most often occur on lateral skull, seen on frontal views

5. **Basal Skull Fracture**

    a) Difficult to demonstrate

    b) Look for air/fluid level or opacification of sphenoid sinus on upright patient
- this is hemorrhage in sinus
- seen in 75% of basal skull fracture cases

    c) Compression can (rarely) cause occipital condyle fractures
- often in conjunction with other fractures
- demonstrated on CT (coronal reconstruction of axial images)

6. **Diastatic Fracture**

    a) Sutural separation

    b) Usually in children, usually unilateral

    c) Most commonly in lambdoidal or sagittal sutures

    d) Radiologic sign: suture more than 2 mm wide

☞   **7. Tripod Fracture**

    a) Most common facial bone fracture

    b) Blow to malar eminence and zygoma

    c) Results in restriction of jaw movement: coronoid process of mandible entrapped by zygoma

    d) Three limbs of zygoma broken: zygomatic arch, orbital process and maxillary process

8. Nasal Bone Fracture

    a) Most are transverse

    b) Usually depress distal bone

    c) Occasionally, fracture may be longitudinal

    d) *Underexposed* lateral projection is optimal

☞   **9. Orbital Blowout Fracture**

    a) Infraorbital plate of maxillary bone fractured

    b) May leave orbital rim intact

    c) Impact is directly on the orbit or just caudal to it

    d) Globe of eye often damaged too, diplopia a frequent result

    e) Optimal projection: Water's projection

    f) Radiologic signs: maxillary sinus opacification; inverted dome or polypoid mass hangs from maxillary sinus roof (inferior rectus muscle); possibly intraorbital emphysema; inferior orbital rim usually intact, but may be displaced; thin spicule of bone caudal to orbit (depressed orbital floor)

10. Mandibular Fracture

    a) Most commonly at mandibular body; may also fracture mandibular angle, condyle, symphysis, ramus, coronoid process or alveolar process

    b) Majority are multiple fractures

    c) Optimal projection is *overpenetrated* Towne's projection

    d) Slowest healing bone in body; clinical union long precedes radiographic union

11. LeFort Fractures

    a) Classification of consistent fracture patterns depending on vector and strength of impact to face

    b) Best definitively demonstrated by tomography or CT

    c) More commonly seen in combination than as single specific type

- *LeFort 1:* fracture through mid-maxilla and pterygoid plates
- *LeFort II:* nasofrontal blow obliquely fractures ethmoid bone, medial maxillary surface of orbital and lateral maxilla (between inferior orbital fissure and lateral maxillary wall)
- *LeFort III:* fracture line from nasofrontal area across ethmoid, posteriorly to inferior orbital fissures and pterygoid process, then laterally through lateral wall of orbit and zygomatic arches
  1) separates facial bones from skull
  2) optimal projections: Caldwell or Water's (not well shown on lateral)

REVIEW—STUDY QUESTIONS

1. What are the optimal views for detection of basilar skull fractures?
2. What are the radiographic signs of a blowout fracture?
3. What diastatic fractures are most common in the skull, and what are their radiographic signs?
4. Describe a tripod fracture.
5. What is the optimal projection for detection of a nasal bone fracture?
6. Describe three common complications of skull fractures, and when they are most likely to occur.
7. What are the clinical signs of neurologic involvement with skull trauma?
8. Describe the locales of mandibular fracture, and the optimal view for demonstrating them.
9. What is the most common skull fracture, and from what must it be differentiated?
10. Describe the depressed fracture and its radiologic signs.

F.   SPINAL FRACTURES AND DISLOCATIONS

1.   General Features

a) Most commonly affected segments: C1, C2, C5-C7, T12-L2

b) 10–14% of spinal fractures or dislocations involve cord injuries
- about 40% of cervical spine injuries involve neurologic damage
- about 10% of thoracic spine injuries involve neurologic damage
- about 4% of thoracolumbar injuries involve neurologic damage

c) Vectors of fracture force in descending order of frequency: flexion, extension, rotation, shearing, compression, distraction

    d) Significant paraspinal injury occurs without fracture (see *whiplash* below)

    e) Minimum study for cervical trauma: APOM, APLC, right and left obliques, lateral

    f) Clinical indications or initial findings may indicate need for flexion/extension, or pillar views

    g) All seven cervical vertebrae must be visualized as completely as possible: may require additional projections, e.g., swimmer's lateral

    h) With neurologic deficits, MR or CT with myelography should be considered

2. Cervical Spine Fractures

    a) Atlas posterior arch fracture
- most common atlas fracture (at least 50% of all atlas fractures)
- usually bilateral
- fractures vertically through neural arch, close to junction with lateral masses
- severe hyperextension injury: atlas arch is compressed between occiput and posterior arch of the axis
- most (about 80%) involve additional spinal fractures
- optimal projection is lateral, but this fracture is easily missed
- complications: seldom neurologic deficit; potential for vertebral artery injury

    b) Jefferson's fracture (synonym: "bursting" fracture of the atlas)
- anterior and posterior arches of ring of atlas fractures, usually bilaterally
- up to one-third of atlas fractures are this type
- caused by compression due to blow on vertex of head: diving injuries, auto accidents
- clinical signs: pain, stiffness, occipital dysesthesia; seldom cause significant neurologic deficit, seldom fatal
- optimal visualization: APOM, supplemented with CT
- radiologic signs: increased lateral paraodontoid space bilaterally, offset lateral edge of atlas lateral masses above axis superior articular processes (usually more than 3 mm); often prevertebral swelling is present
- sign of transverse ligament rupture: total offset > 8 mm
- may be simulated by: pediatric patient, for whom overhanging lateral mass is normal; atlas developmental anomalies (combined AP spina bifida of atlas; lateral mass malformation); rotary atlantoaxial

subluxation; torticollis (these usually overhang 2 mm or less)

c) Atlas anterior arch fracture
- usually horizontal segmental avulsions at anterior longitudinal ligament and longus colli insertions
- essentially these are hyperextension injuries
- often in conjunction with odontoid fractures
- best displayed on lateral projection; CT for definitive diagnosis
- radiologic signs: avulsed fragment displaced inferiorly from anterior arch

d) Atlas lateral mass fracture
- rare
- requires CT for visualization
- TP may be fractured
- transverse ligament ruptured from medial surface of lateral mass may create an avulsion fracture (see below)

e) Transverse ligament rupture
- rare to see this as an isolated injury, usually dens will fracture first
- may occur with Jefferson's fracture, RA, psoriasis, AS, or Reiter's syndrome
- agenesis of ligament (or laxity) found in about 20% of Down's syndrome
- radiologic signs: increased ADI (> 3 mm in adults, > 5 mm in children); disrupted posterior cervical line
- clinical evidence may not occur until up to 10 mm of atlas anterior displacement, due to anatomical composition at that level
- *Steele's Rule of Thirds*: Atlas ring divided into approximate thirds: (Fig. 4.4) one third cord, one third space, one third odontoid
- with intact dens, transverse ligament rupture can produce "guillotine" or "pincers" effect on cord

f) Hangman's fracture (traumatic spondylolisthesis)
- very common: up to 40% of C2 fractures
- hyperextension fracture

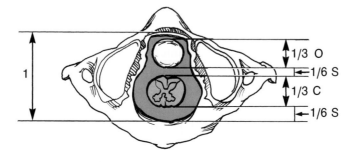

Figure 4.4.

Steele's rule of thirds. Reprinted with permission from Yochum TR, Rowe LJ. Essentials of Skeletal Radiology, 2nd ed. Baltimore: Williams & Wilkins, 1996:672.

- bilateral axis pedicle fracture
- clinical findings: usually no neurologic findings; airway compromise due to prevertebral swelling; potential for vertebral artery injury
- lateral projection optimal; CT for definitive identification
- radiologic signs: fracture lines anterior to inferior facet; C2 anterior on C3; C2 may be in flexion and superior distraction; increased retropharyngeal space; often with teardrop fracture (see below)
- 25% have other fractures, most often atlas

g) Vertebral body wedge fracture
- a compression fracture, usually due to forced hyperflexion
- stable fracture (ligaments intact anteriorly and posteriorly)
- most frequently affected: C5, 6, 7 (⅔ of wedge fractures)

h) Odontoid process fractures
- 40–50% of axis fractures
- categorized by location of lesion (Anderson and Dalonzo)
  1) Type I: uncommon, avulsion of tip of dens caused by apical or alar ligament stress; may be complicated by nonunion

  2) Type 2: most common; fractures at dens/body junction; most frequent dens fracture to result in nonunion (lack of vascularity in dens); also, hypertrophic callus may induce myelopathy during healing; also can result in post-fracture osteolysis of the dens
  3) Type 3: below base of dens/body junction; also very common but heals more easily as it does not compromise blood supply to the dens
- radiologic signs: fracture line, dens displacement, disruption of axis "ring," apparent enlargement of C2 body, retropharyngeal swelling
- optimal projection is APOM, but CT or MRI may be necessary for identification of the lesion; type 3 fracture line may show on lateral film
- anterior or posterior dens displacement, usually less than 3 mm
- atlas posterior cervical line will be offset
- lateral tilt of dens greater than 5° indicates dens fracture
- axis body enlargement ("fat C2" sign): sagittal dimension increases with significant comminution into axis body
- nonunion signs: smooth sclerotic margins,

widened fracture line, progressive dens osteolysis, mobility at fracture site with flexion-extension; "vacuum" within fracture

- treatment for nonunion: posterior fusion (Gallie fusion) or screw fixation

- **DDX:** Mach band, dentocentral synchondrosis (usually fused by age 7, but may persist), congenital odontoid tilt (these are < 3°), paraodontoid notch, os odontoideum (has wide, smooth, sclerotic cleft; atlas anterior arch may be enlarged and sclerotic with posterior surface protruding into odontoid cleft)

- space between frontal incisors may resemble vertical fracture: these do not occur

- bone scan may be used to show active healing site, help DDX from os odontoideum

i) Vertebral body burst fracture

- caused by vertical compression

- nucleus pulposus driven through endplate into vertebral body

- comminution of vertebral body; fragments migrate centrifugally

- unstable fracture; threatens cord; neural arch may also fracture

- best evaluated by CT; optimal plain film views are AP and lateral

- radiologic signs: lateral shows comminuted body, flattened centrally; AP shows vertical fracture line through body

j) Teardrop fracture

- triangular fragment avulsed from anteroinferior vertebral body (often axis)

- acute hyperextension fracture; also caused by acute hyperflexion

- frequently associated with hangman's fracture

- unstable fracture; ligaments are disrupted, instability and misalignment; rupture of anterior longitudinal ligament, disc torn, partially avulsed from endplates

- posterior longitudinal ligament disruption may involve unilateral or bilateral facet dislocation

- associated with acute anterior cervical cord syndrome: immediate, complete paralysis; loss of pain and temperature (anterior column sensations)

- upper extremities more severely affected

- radiologic signs: lateral view shows avulsed, inferiorly displaced fragment; may show local kyphosis, widened interlaminar and interspinous spaces; disc may be narrowed or widened

☞   **k)** Articular pillar fracture
- frequently missed: requires pillar view or CT bone window to demonstrate it
- commonly at C4-C7
- usually compression injury (compressive hyperextension with lateral flexion)
- may involve anterolisthesis, altered shape, shortening
- on AP this fracture may resemble a joint space ("horizontal facet" sign)

☞   **l)** Clay shoveler's fracture (synonyms: coal miner's fracture, root-puller's fracture)
- avulsion of spinous process tip due to abrupt flexion or repeated stress pulls on trapezius, latissimus dorsi, and rhomboid muscles
- most common site: C7; frequent sites: C6, T1
- stable fracture, no neurologic deficits
- optimal view: lateral projection; may be seen on AP
- radiologic signs: lateral view shows inferiorly displaced SP tip; frontal view shows "double spinous process" sign (two SPs on a single vertebra)

☞   - **DDX:** nonunion of secondary growth center or nuchal bone—fracture will be displaced caudally, with jagged edges

m) Lamina and transverse process fractures
- C5 and C6 most vulnerable to laminar fracture; best displayed by CT
- C7 most exposed for TP fracture, but these are very rare in cervical spine
- brachial plexus lesions, other cervical fractures usually associated with these
- TP fractures near junction with pedicle; may injure vertebral artery

3. **Cervical Spine Dislocations**

a) Atlanto-occipital dislocation
- caused by hyperextension and distraction of the head
- rare; usually fatal
- pediatric patients more likely to survive

b) Atlantoaxial dislocation
- anterior atlantoaxial dislocation with ruptured transverse ligament (see above)
- four types of rotary atlantoaxial fixation (subluxation)
    1) most common: no anterior displacement; within normal range of motion
    2) with 3–5 mm anterior atlas displacement
    3) > 5 mm anterior atlas displacement

4) with posterior atlas displacement (occurs only with deficient dens)

- occurs with trauma (even minor trauma), upper respiratory infection, oral surgery, inflammatory arthritis

- possible causes: joint effusion, damaged joint capsule, entrapment of joint inclusions (meniscoids, fat pads, synovium, capsular rim)

- clinical signs: torticollis; head cocked in lateral flexion, slight flexion, and contralateral rotation; pain; possible subjective upper limb weakness

- radiologic signs: anteriorly rotated side, lateral mass widened, closer to dens; posteriorly rotated side, narrowed lateral mass, farther from dens; atlantoaxial joint space obscured; rotation of C2 spinous process (lateral bending or cervical rotation views do not alter these findings)

- lateral film may show entire posterior C1 arch as a ring; possibly an increased ADI (> 3 mm); cervical spine lateral flexion-rotation (caused by torticollis)

c) Bilateral interfacetal dislocation (BID)

- caused by severe hyperflexion

- most often at C4-C7

- torn posterior soft tissues: PLL, posterior ligamentous complex, annulus fibrosus; occasionally ALL may also be torn, disc may be herniated

- unstable lesion; cord is very much at risk

- segment above a congenital or surgical fusion is most vulnerable

- superior facets lie anterior to inferior facets, within IVF

- radiologic signs: dislocated body displaced anteriorly, "naked facet" sign (axial CT: absent articular surface), lateral films show divergent SPs, displaced prevertebral fat stripe, altered posterior cervical line

- treatment: surgical arthrodesis

d) Unilateral interfacetal dislocation (UID)

- caused by flexion/rotation force

- single inferior facet dislocates into IVF ("*jumped facet*")

- visible on lateral projection: forward displacement of vertebral body; articular pillars are not superimposed; "bow tie sign"

- AP projection shows SP rotated and elevated, body rotated

- oblique projections are optimal for diagnosis

- "*naked facet*" sign will be seen on CT

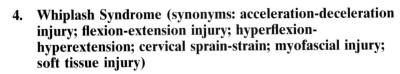

4. Whiplash Syndrome (synonyms: acceleration-deceleration injury; flexion-extension injury; hyperflexion-hyperextension; cervical sprain-strain; myofascial injury; soft tissue injury)

a) **General features**
- clinical manifestations varied: minor complaints of pain to severe incapacitation
- posterior neck pain most common; radiation of pain to head, shoulder, arm, or interscapular region
- stiffness, loss of range of motion, painful facet joints, headache, visual disturbances, memory impairment, dizziness
- soft tissue damage is usually present; imaging must rule out fractures and dislocations, look for evidence of soft tissue injury
- plain film: minimal study APOM, APLC, lateral, obliques
- lateral film is usually optimal (positive in 70–90% of cases)
- if there are no contraindications, "Davis series" should be considered to assess flexion/extension for hypermobility or hypomobility
- special attention should be paid to assessment of soft tissues, vertebral alignment, and joint spaces

b) **Soft tissue abnormalities**
- widened retropharyngeal space
   1) soft tissue anterior to anteroinferior C2 body should be < 7 mm wide
   2) longus colli hematoma or edema; torn ALL, torn discovertebral junction will widen this
- widened retrotracheal space
   1) soft tissue anterior to anteroinferior C6 body should be < 14 mm in children, < 22 mm in adults
   2) hematoma or edema in esophagus, longus colli, ALL; or discovertebral junction tear will widen this
- displaced prevertebral fat stripe
   1) normal thin vertical lucency anterior to C6–7 vertebral bodies
   2) displaced by hematoma, edema, or fractures in this region
- tracheal deviation, laryngeal dislocation
   1) lateral or anterior tracheal displacement
   2) hematoma, edema, or torticollis may do this
   3) tracheal transection will elevate the hyoid above C3 superior endplate
- soft tissue emphysema
   1) tracheal laceration or transection,

pneumomediastinum or pneumothorax will permit gas to accumulate in the cervical soft tissues

2) may also see pneumorrhachis (air in spinal canal)

c) Vertebral alignment abnormalities

- cervical lordosis diminution or loss
  1) the most common radiologic finding following whiplash injury
  2) significance is controversial: does not prove underlying soft tissue injury
  3) frequently secondary to muscle spasm
  4) **DDX:** hypolordosis caused by positioning or DJD

- acute kyphotic angulation
  1) "acute kyphosis sign" with "divergent spinous process sign"
  2) strongly suggests ruptured posterior ligamentous complex
  3) most common at C5-C6
  4) flexion view exaggerates it; may cause facet subluxation almost to the point of dislocation
  5) demonstrated on lateral and AP projections

- widened interspinous spaces
  1) multisegmental, uniform interspinous widening ("fanning")
  2) coexists with reversed cervical curve: "arcual kyphosis"

- altered flexion patterns
  1) loss of flexion movement can occur at a single motion segment or in multiple segments, up to and including all cervical segments
  2) motion at three or more levels suggests normal pattern
  3) total loss of motion, or only single segment motion is correlated with significant soft tissue injury

- vertebral body rotation
  1) subtle, but may be significant
  2) can accompany serious facet subluxation or dislocation
  3) sagittal rotations (flexion-extension): >11.5° intersegmental angular incongruence may signify ligament injury
  4) coronal rotations (lateral flexion): facet instability, joint capsule disruption or facet dislocation permits this deviation
  5) axial rotation (rotatory): spinous processes displaced from midline (mid and lower segments) on AP projections; lateral projection show

articular pillars superimposed over vertebral bodies and posterior pillar borders duplicated

    6) rotation caused by torticollis; head position; facet subluxation or dislocation

- sagittal translation
  1) lateral film gives appropriate view
  2) four "cervical arc lines": connect anterior body margins, connect posterior body margins, connect spinolaminar junctions, connect spinous tips
  3) functional displacements demonstrated on flexion/extension studies
  4) intersegmental excursion > 3.5 mm denotes significant intersegmental instability
- torticollis
  1) AP projection shows unleveling of inferior mandible, scoliosis with intersegmental coupled motions (lateral flexion and rotation)

d) Joint abnormalities

- widened medial atlantoaxial joint
  1) ADI > 3 mm in adults, or > 5 mm in children
  2) disruption of transverse ligament
- widened or narrowed intervertebral disc
  1) height or symmetry may be altered
  2) severe ligamentous disruption signaled by widened space
  3) sometimes clearly demonstrated by axial distraction
  4) ALL disruption may show as anterior "gaping" during extension
  5) ruptured disc may manifest in loss of disc height
- vacuum phenomenon
  1) smooth lucent cleft adjacent to anterior vertebral endplate
  2) may require extension lateral to demonstrate it
  3) etiology may be degenerative rather than traumatic
- displaced ring epiphysis
  1) young patient may have a dislodged ring epiphysis
  2) signifies significant discovertebral damage
  3) flexion injury displaces superior epiphysis, extension injury avulses inferior epiphysis
  4) prevertebral hematoma usually accompanies this finding

- widened zygapophyseal joint
    1) joint space > 2 mm may denote torn joint capsule
    2) tetrad: wide facet joint, wide interspinous space, loss of cervical lordosis with compression fracture (denotes significant instability with torn posterior ligament complex

e) Imaging in whiplash

- plain film
    1) basic Davis series; use caution and do flexion/extension studies only if other films show no contraindications
    2) first priority: exclude fracture, dislocation, significant instability
- computed tomography (CT)
    1) detection, assessment of fractures; relationships between bone fragments and cord
    2) evaluation of disc herniations, hematomas, cord lesions and other paravertebral soft tissue lesions
- magnetic resonance imaging (MRI)
    1) useful in both acute and chronic cases
    2) soft tissue lesions well imaged
    3) healing process demonstrated
    4) detection of bone contusion
- nuclear bone scan
    1) high sensitivity for occult fracture
    2) does not image non-fracture articular damage

5. Thoracic Spine Fractures

a) Most common thoracic fracture site: T11–12

b) Compression fracture due to axial compression with flexion

c) At T4–8: convulsions or electric shock trigger violent muscle contractions, cause compression fractures

d) Results usually are wedge-shaped vertebrae, few have neurologic consequences

e) X-ray signs: wedge-shaped vertebra; sometimes paraspinal mass (edema)

f) Pathologic fractures: reduced posterior vertebral body height, pedicular damage, paraspinal mass (edematous swelling); MR shows marrow abnormalities

g) May require swimmer's lateral, tomography, CT, or MRI, especially in upper T-spine

6. Thoracic Spine Dislocation (or fracture dislocation)

a) Fracture dislocation most frequent T4–7

b) Associated with fractured lamina, facets, or vertebral body

c) Often accompanied by paralysis due to small diameter canal and sparse vascularization

d) Optimal projection is an *overpenetrated* frontal view

e) Radiologic signs: reduced vertebral height, displacement, widened interpediculate distance, paraspinal widening; on lateral view look for "step sign" and paraspinal line displacement

f) Associated injuries: aortic arch tears, sternal fracture, disc herniation, instability

g) May involve *Kummel's disease*: delayed posttraumatic vertebral collapse due to avascular necrosis

7. Lumbar Spine Fractures

☞ **a)** Compression fractures
- general characteristics
  1) most common lumbar spine fracture
  2) caused by axial compression/flexion force
  3) in children, these are often torus fractures
  4) elderly may have spontaneous compression fracture (pathologic, insufficiency fracture) sometimes called "grandma fracture"
  5) pathologic fractures caused by: early menopause, corticosteroid therapy, hyperthyroidism, or malignancy
  6) symptomatic for about 2 weeks; without dislocation these are stable fractures
- evaluation for stability
  1) Denis classification:
     - anterior column: ALL to mid-vertebral body
     - middle column: mid-vertebral body to PLL
     - posterior column: PLL to supraspinous ligament
  2) if two or more "columns" are disrupted, fracture is unstable, with high likelihood of neurologic damage; surgical stabilization required
☞ - radiologic signs
  1) lateral projection is optimal view
  2) step defect: buckled anterior cortex shows sharp step off anterosuperior vertebral margin (anteriorly displaced superior corner overhangs the anterior cortical line)
  3) wedge deformity: anterior vertebral body compression makes triangular wedged vertebra; may cause angular kyphosis; 30% loss of height is

significant (normal variant is usually 10–15%)

4) linear white band of condensation (zone of impaction): occasional sign—radiopacified band below fractured superior endplate, site of bone impaction and later callus formation; denotes recent fracture

5) endplate disruption: best seen on CT; jagged, irregular edges; most commonly superior endplate fracture

6) paraspinal edema: unilateral or bilateral paraspinal masses indicate hemorrhage or edema; usually on AP thoracic, but may displace psoas margins on lumbar AP film

7) abdominal ileus: high likelihood of fracture if excessive large or small bowel gas distends the lumen; indicates visceral autonomic reaction to injury, pain, edema or hematoma

☞ • differentiation of old versus recent compression fracture

1) hemorrhage, hematoma (best demonstrated by MRI), step defect, and zone of impaction indicate fracture less than 2 months old

2) old fractures often show contiguous disc degeneration

3) bone scan may show "hot spots" for up to 24 months

☞ **b)** Burst fractures

• form of compression fracture

• posterosuperior fragment is displaced into the spinal canal

• high impact axial compression/flexion force

• up to 50% cause cord injury (or conus medullaris or cauda equina injury)

• differentiated from simple compression:

1) AP film shows vertical fracture line often

2) interpediculate distance widened

3) may cause "acquired coronal cleft vertebra"

4) lateral film shows central depression of both endplates

5) may see disruption of posterior vertebral body line

• CT is definitive imaging modality: depicts degree of fragmentation and position of fragments

• MRI used to assess neurologic lesions

c) Fractures of posterior apophyseal ring

• posterior limbus bone

1) posterior vertebral body ring apophysis separation

    2) uncommon; seen before apophyseal fusion

    3) stiffness and pain; neurological indications include spasm, numbness, weakness, neurogenic claudication, cauda equina syndrome

    4) usually L4 and L5; may happen at T12-L3 also

    5) 50% caused by auto accident, weight lifting, or gymnastics

    6) various configurations occur, some with disc herniation

- imaging

    1) only 15–20% are identifiable via plain film

    2) lateral projection has best chance of demonstrating lesion

    3) thin, linear arc of calcification crossing disc space near posteroinferior vertebral body

    4) may show a posterior focal Schmorl's node

    5) may have slightly diminished disc height

    6) definitive imaging via CT

d) Kummel's disease

- delayed posttraumatic vertebral collapse
- possibly caused by avascular necrosis
- rarefaction with progressive compression
- plain film may show vacuum phenomenon
- controversial entity: only a few recorded cases

e) Neural arch fractures

- transverse process fractures

    1) second most common lumbar spinal fractures

    2) hyperextension/lateral flexion force causes avulsion

    3) most often at L2 and L3

    4) imaged on AP projection: jagged vertical lucency across TP

    5) fragment may displace inferiorly

    6) horizontal fracture line may indicate a Chance fracture (look for it)

    7) TP fractures frequently occur at multiple levels

    8) L5 TP fractures often occur with pelvic fractures

    9) may see hemorrhage: blurring or loss of psoas shadow

    10) LOBS = lumbar ossified bridging syndrome: due to myositis ossificans within the hemorrhage from the fracture

    11) associated renal damage suspected if hematuria occurs, or with subsequent persistent hypertension

☞   12)   **DDX:** simulated by overlying fat lines, intestinal gas, developmental nonunion (especially at L1)—rule these out via oblique or tilt views

- pars interarticularis fractures
  1) traumatic pars fractures rare: caused by violent hyperextension
  2) occur at L4 or L5
  3) vertically oriented jagged lucency seen best on oblique projections
  4) *"Scotty dog's collar"* sign
  5) differentiate acute pars interarticularis fracture from spondylolysis, (usually a stress fracture): acute fracture is almost always unilateral, while spondylolysis (stress fracture) is usually bilateral (see below)
  6) healing is usually uncomplicated and without anterolisthesis

☞   - Chance fracture (synonyms: lap seat belt fracture, fulcrum fracture)
  1) horizontal splitting of neural arch and vertebral body
  2) auto accidents with lap belted passengers increased the incidence
  3) severe abrasions on lower anterior abdominal wall; internal visceral damage (splenic, pancreatic rupture; intestinal, mesenteric tears)
  4) 15% involve neurologic deficit
  5) most common at L1-L3
  6) classified by location of fracture line:
     - horizontal splitting SP, pedicle, and posterior body to superior endplate (Chance fracture)
     - horizontal splitting SP, pedicle, posterior body without extension to the endplate
     - Smith injuries:
       a. Type A: ruptured interspinous ligaments and partial rupture of IVD
       b. Type B: avulsed posteroinferior body corner
       c. Type C: fractured superior articular process
  7) AP view: transverse fracture line through posterior elements; wide gap between upper and lower fragments (*empty vertebra sign*)
  8) lateral view: lucent split through posterior elements, posterior body

☞   **8. Spondylolysis**

     a) Etiologies

       - repetitive microtrauma causing stress fracture of pars

- acute stress fracture: e.g., severe overlifting
- no recorded incidents of spondylolysis in newborns
- higher incidence in Native American people: question cradleboard as source of spinal stress in infancy
- congenitally slender pars may predispose to stress fracture (familial incidence)

b) Stress fracture factors
- fatigue fracture caused by mechanical stress at lumbosacral lordosis
- hyperextension loading (e.g., carrying heavy backpack)
- onset in patients is most commonly after 5 years of age; implicating upright posture and ambulation stresses
- premature walking may increase incidence
- high incidence among divers and gymnasts, pole-vaulters, weight lifters
- nonunion because of lack of immobilization at the time of lysis
- Boston overlap brace (antilordotic) will permit healing of fresh pars defect

 9. Spondylolisthesis

a) General features
- "slippage" of the vertebral body to the anterior or posterior
- anterolisthesis; posterolisthesis
- five types identified: dysplastic, isthmic, degenerative, traumatic, pathologic
  1) Type I: dysplastic
     - congenital malformation of L5 neural arch and/or upper sacrum
     - anterolisthesis of L5 on sacral promontory
     - often with SBO
     - often progressive slippage but without pars defects
  2) Type II: isthmic
     - four times more common than dysplastic type
     - three subtypes:
       a. fatigue fracture caused by biomechanical stress (see above)
          - most common type in patients < 50 years; not found in newborns
       b. pars elongated but without defect
          - looks like Type I, but etiology is thought to be repetitive stress and healing with gradual

              elongation, displacing vertebral body anteriorly

- may eventually develop pars defect, essentially becoming Type IIa

    c. rare: caused by acute pars fractures; seldom displaced

    3) Type III: degenerative (synonym: pseudospondylolisthesis)

- neural arch is intact
- most common at L4 (10 times greater incidence than at L3 or L5)
- anterior displacement of L4 body is not > 25%; usually 10–15%
- female predilection (6:1)
- rare in patients < 50 years old
- more common in blacks than whites (3:1)
- predisposition with sacralized L5 (4 times more common)
- altered stresses caused by facet arthrosis, disc degeneration lead to remodeling of articular processes and pars
- angle of long axis of pedicle with long axis of articular pillar is increased because of more horizontal orientation of facets
- overriding articular surfaces

    4) Type IV: traumatic

- caused by acute, severe injury with fracture of neural arch (not at pars)
- most often seen at C2 ("hangman's fracture")
- heals well with proper immobilization

    5) Type V: pathologic

- Paget's disease, osteopetrosis, metastatic carcinoma will weaken bone, predispose to spondylolysis
- iatrogenic spondylolisthesis: postsurgical development due to added stress on isthmus when segments below or above are fused
- too much bone removed during posterior decompression laminectomy, added stress on neural arch opposite the surgical defect

- Hyland's alternate classification: based on history and clinical presentation

    1) RSS: Recent Spondylolytic Spondylolisthesis

- acute, painful traumatic or stress fracture of pars

- usually in young athletes
- linked with inherited weakness or biomechanical factors: e.g., high sacral base angle, increased disc angle

2) PSS-S: Preexisting Spondylolytic Spondylolisthesis—Stable
- nonunion old pars fracture
- permanent fibrous defect
- no progression nor increased low back pain expected
- most common type: look past the defect for the pain source

3) PSS-U: Preexisting Spondylolytic Spondylolisthesis—Unstable
- incomplete fibrous union
- hypermobility and biomechanical instability at level of defect
- rare
- may cause recurrent episodes of back pain; prolonged disability in adults
- may cause progressive slipping in adolescent

4) DS: Degenerative Spondylolisthesis (pseudospondylolisthesis)
- in late middle age and older
- about 25% of all spondys; female predilection
- no pars defect
- usually at L4
- secondary to disc degeneration, facet joint arthrosis
- may be predisposed by a straight, stable L/S joint, seated high between the ilia (may include sacralization of L5)
- seldom slips > 25% (usually 10–15%)
- may see lateral nerve root entrapment, with intermittent neurogenic claudication

b) **Clinical features**
- presence or level of pain does not correlate with amount of displacement
- pain is more likely to be present during development of the lysis defect
- posture is often affected: hyperlordotic
- spinal crepitation may be heard with active flexion/extension
- gait changes, especially in children, because of tight hamstrings: pelvic waddle—stiff legged short steps with pelvic rotation; walk on toes with knees bent
- no neurologic signs; may have sclerotomal pattern pain into lower extremities

- palpation: prominent SP with lytic spondy; "step off" non-palpable SP with non-lytic spondylolisthesis

☞ **c) Progressive displacement**
- controversial: only 2–3% tend to displace progressively, usually from 5–15 years of age; female predilection (2:1)
- displacement risk increased with associated SBO
- in adults, displacement is usually < 15%, and is associated with DJD
- trapezoidal L5 with "domed" sacral promontory predispose to slippage
- anterior S1 may develop "buttressing" to resist slippage by L5
- with no demonstrable instability; no limitation of activities is needed

☞ **d) Radiologic features**
- assessment includes upright AP, tilt-up AP, lateral, bilateral obliques
- CT is most definitive diagnostic modality for pars defects
- upright (weightbearing) AP projection:
  1) may show lucency roughly parallel to inferior cortex of pedicle
  ☞ 2) with significant anterolisthesis: *inverted Napoleon's hat* or *gendarme's cap* sign, or *bowline of Brailsford* (Fig. 4.5)
  3) may see single lumbar SP deviated in rotation (without scoliosis)
- upright (weightbearing) AP angulated projection (tilt-up view)
  1) may be called Ferguson's view or Hibbs' projection
  2) clearer visualization of L5 pars
  3) 25–30° cephalad tube angulation
  4) defect shows as focal lucency below pedicle margin
- weightbearing lateral projection
  1) clearly demonstrates degree of listhesis
  ☞ 2) mensurations: George's line (posterior vertebral body margin; Ulmann's line (perpendicular to sacral base at sacral promontory); Meyerding classifications (grading displacement by 25% increments) (see Chapter 1, Mensurations)
  3) may see trapezoidal L5 or domed S1, which indicate instability
  4) buttressing at sacral promontory denotes stabilization
  5) defect is an oblique linear lucency below the pedicle
  6) flexion/extension lateral views improve visualization

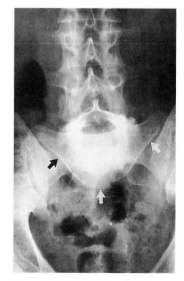

Figure 4.5. Grade IV Spondylolis-thesis.

Bowline of Brailsford. Reprinted with permission from Yochum TR, Rowe LJ. Essentials of Skeletal Radiology, 2nd ed. Baltimore: Williams & Wilkins, 1996:1515.

☞

- oblique projections (done bilaterally, not necessarily weight-bearing)
    1) optimal for visualizing pars defects above L5
    2) if done upright, use anterior obliques
    3) 30° cephalic tube tilt elongates pars, shows subtle defects
    4) oblique shows "*Scotty dog*" margins, and pars defect appears as a "*broken neck*" or "*collar*"—lucency across the neck of the dog
    5) "*stepladder*" sign: facet joints are misaligned at level of defect

e) Assessment of stability
- instability of the spondylolisthetic segment itself is assessed
- erect flexion and extension lateral lumbar films
- > 4 mm additional displacement is considered unstable
- angular motion > 11° more than that of adjacent segments indicates instability; conservative treatment has a poor prognosis
- lateral spot films with axial traction and compression show translatory movement in unstable segments (significant movement is > 4 mm)

f) Single-photon emission computed tomography (SPECT)
- sectional, multiplanar imaging: good for complex spinal areas
- early identification of "active" or developing lesions
- gives more specific localization than planar bone scintigraphy
    1) may be used to assess postsurgical spine for pseudoarthrosis

g) Unilateral spondylolysis
- may cause Wilkinson's syndrome: stress hypertrophy of contralateral pedicle
- sclerotic contralateral pedicle due to stress: **DDX** osteoid osteoma, osteoblastoma

☞

h) Management
- conservative means should be used first
- sports activities or manual labor are not contraindicated by the presence of an asymptomatic spondylolysis or spondylolisthesis
- pain in presence of spondy may be from another source—look further

10. **Lumbar Fracture Dislocation**

a) Most are thoracolumbar

b) Force is a violent flexion mechanism

c) Frequently associated with teardrop avulsions

d) Severe dislocation often involves cord or cauda equina paralysis

e) Most dislocate anteriorly, no lateral displacement

f) Shearing force disrupts disc, ligaments, and posterior arch elements

g) *"Naked facet"* sign indicates dislocation (seen on axial CT)

REVIEW—STUDY QUESTIONS

1. Name and describe five types of spondylolisthesis.

2. How do old compression fractures differ radiographically from new compression fractures?

3. Describe and explain the reasons for the clinical indicators of spondylolisthesis in children.

4. List and describe five JOINT abnormalities that may be seen radiographically with a whiplash patient.

5. Name three cervical dislocation patterns and describe their radiologic signs.

6. What spinal segments are most often involved in compression fracture, and what forces are responsible?

7. Name and describe four common "named" cervical spine fractures.

8. Describe Steele's "rule of thirds" and explain its significance.

9. What projection(s) are optimal for clearest presentation of spondylolisthesis of L5 on S1?

10. What areas of the thoracic spine most often fracture, and what forces cause these fractures?

11. Describe atlanto-axial subluxations: categories, causes, signs, and symptoms.

12. Give the categories of spondylolistheses and their probable etiologies.

13. What is the difference between a crush fracture and a burst fracture?

14. When is a fracture considered "unstable"?

15. Name as many stable spinal fractures as you can. List as many unstable fractures as you can.

G. PELVIC FRACTURES AND DISLOCATIONS

1. Sacral Fracture

a) General features

- usually caused by falling on buttocks, or direct blow to the sacrum

- often occur with fractures of the ilia, ischia, or pubic arches

- may see horizontal (transverse) or vertical sacral fracture

☞   **b)**   Horizontal (transverse) sacral fracture
- most common sacral fracture, usually at third or fourth sacral tubercle
- AP projection: check for disruption of foraminal lines
- lateral projection: may show disrupted anterior cortex, with forward angulation of inferior segment
- *suicide jumper's fracture*: horizontal upper sacral fracture caused by fall from great height

         c)   Vertical sacral fracture
- caused by indirect trauma
- > 50% have associated pelvic organ damage
- visible on frontal projections; tilt-up view is optimal; foraminal line disruption
- may require tomography or CT to demonstrate

2. Coccygeal Fracture

         a)   General features
- usually transverse
- lateral projection is optimal

         b)   Radiologic features
- oblique fracture line
- slight anterior displacement of distal coccyx
- **DDX:** congenital variants

3. Iliac Fracture

☞   **a)**   Iliac wing fracture (synonym: Duverney fracture)
- force is from lateral direction
- oblique projection displays fracture optimally
- may be a lucent line, or may be a stellate pattern of lucent lines
- stable fracture

☞   **b)**   Malgaigne fracture
- ipsilateral double vertical fractures: superior pubic and ischiopubic rami fracture and sacroiliac joint fractures or dislocates
- often, L5 TP fractures and hemipelvis displaces anteriorly or posteriorly
- most common pelvic fracture (about 33% of all pelvic fractures)
- caused by vertical shearing force
- pelvic organ damage commonly associated: high morbidity and mortality
- unstable fracture

☞   **c)**   Bucket-handle fracture
- fracture is contralateral to impact site
- superior pubic ramus and ischiopubic junction fracture

- sacroiliac joint dislocates on side of impact
- pubis displaces inward and superiorly
- caused by force with an oblique vector
- abdominal and thoracic viscera (heart, lungs) also injured often

d) Iliac avulsion fracture (synonym: tug lesion)
- may be acute traumatic lesion or caused by repetitive stress
- young athletes suffer these; have acute, severe muscle contracture–spasm
- common in sprinters, long jumpers, gymnasts, hurdlers, cheerleaders
- anterosuperior iliac spine (ASIS) avulsion by sartorius muscle
- **DDX:** healed displaced ASIS avulsion from osteochondroma
- anteroinferior iliac spine (AIIS) avulsion by rectus femoris muscle (seen often in soccer, rugby, football players)

4. Acetabular Fracture

a) General features
- about 20% of all adult pelvic fractures
- majority are caused by indirect injury, where femur is driven into the acetabulum
- capsular distention may displace obturator internus muscle, distort psoas and gluteus medius fascial planes
- in children, the teardrop space may be widened (unusual in adults)
- medial displacement or asymmetry of the obturator internus fat pad (*obturator internus sign*)

b) Posterior rim fracture (synonym: dashboard fracture)
- knee impacted with leg in flexion and adduction
- may involve posterior dislocation of the femoral head
- comprises about one-third of all acetabular fractures

c) Simple posterior column fracture
- rare; separates ilioischial line from teardrop, displaces it medially
- optimal projection: oblique; may also be visible on frontal projection

d) Central acetabular fracture (synonym: explosion fracture)
- most common acetabular fracture
- splits ilium into superior and inferior halves
- may be oriented transversely or obliquely
- transverse: fracture line bisects ischial spine

- oblique: fracture line goes posterosuperior to sacrosciatic notch
- if not severe: obturator internus sign may be only evidence radiographically
- if severe: femoral head may protrude through acetabulum

   e) Simple anterior column fracture
- iliopubic line interrupted
- teardrop medially displaced
- terminates along pubis or ischiopubic junction
- anterior oblique view is optimal

5. Ischial and Pubic Fractures

   a) Straddle fracture
- comminuted fracture of pubic arches
- most common *unstable* pelvic fracture
- bilateral double vertical fractures: superior pubic rami and ischiopubic junctions fractured
- central fragment displaces posterosuperiorly
- 20% result in bladder/urethra damage

   b) Symphysis pubis avulsion
- adductor muscles avulse bone from superior or inferior pubic rami
- common injury for soccer players
- see irregular symphysis joint surface with roughened pubic bone cortex; may have both sclerotic and lucent areas
- **DDX:** osteitis pubis

   c) Ischial tuberosity avulsion
- ischial tuberosity apophysis avulsed by hamstring contractions
- often bilateral
- healing leaves overgrowth of apophysis with radiolucent gap between ischium and avulsed fragment
- **DDX:** osteochondroma (avulsion has history of hamstring injury and the lesion will be asymptomatic by the time overgrowth is apparent)
- common injury in cheerleaders, hurdlers, horseback riders
- residual fragment called *"rider's bone"*

6. Sprung Pelvis (synonym: open book pelvis)

   a) General features
- complete separation of symphysis pubis and one or both SI joints
- pelvis "opened like a book": one or both ilia displaced laterally
- pelvic viscera often damaged

   b) Radiologic features
- pubic articulation widely opened (> 8 mm in adults, > 10 mm in children)
- one or both SI joints significantly widened

7. **Pubic Diastasis**

a) **General features**
- shearing separation of pubic articulation (> 8 mm adult; > 10 mm child)
- unilateral SI dislocation may easily be missed
- almost always associated with soft tissue damage

b) **Soft tissue damage**
- vascular: intrapelvic hemorrhage—look for scrotal, labial, inguinal, or buttock ecchymosis
- urethra, bladder, ureter rupture (often at the trigone)—look for bruised perineum, urine retention, blood at tip of urethra
- bowel laceration, or rectal obstruction
- ruptured diaphragm (usually on left)

H. FEMORAL FRACTURES AND DISLOCATIONS

 1. **Proximal Femur Fractures**

a) **General features**
- most commonly occur in elderly patients
- predisposed by osteoporosis, Paget's disease, fibrous dysplasia, malignancies, osteomalacia, osteonecrosis (radiation-induced)
- females more frequently affected (2:1)
- death secondary to pulmonary or cardiac complications is common
- nonunion and avascular necrosis risk greatest with intracapsular lesions
- nonunion in about 25% of intracapsular fractures
- avascular necrosis caused by disruption of medial and lateral femoral circumflex arteries
- avascular necrosis detectable on plain film at 3 months, or not for 3 years: average appearance at about 1 year (visible much earlier with MRI)

b) **Imaging**
- standard plain film views: AP full pelvis, AP hip spot, frog-leg, or oblique

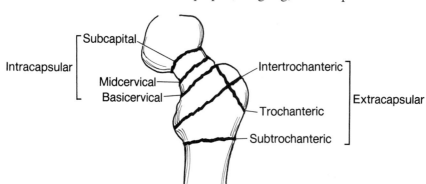

Figure 4.6.

Proximal femur fracture classification. Reprinted with permission from Yochum TR, Rowe LJ. Essentials of Skeletal Radiology, 2nd ed. Baltimore: Williams & Wilkins, 1996:714.

- may need a groin lateral (horizontal beam, grid cassette)
- CT good for occult fracture, fragment location, soft tissue injury identification
- MRI excellent for occult fracture, stress fracture
- bone scan used for occult and stress fracture detection

c) Classification by location of fracture (Fig. 4.6)

- intracapsular: subcapital, midcervical, basicervical
- extracapsular: intertrochanteric, trochanteric, subtrochanteric

d) Intracapsular fractures

- fractured proximal to trochanters
- subcapital: junction of head and neck (most common)
- midcervical: through femoral neck
- basicervical: through base of femoral neck, at junction with trochanters
- midcervical and basicervical lesions usually involve both lateral and medial cortices
- basicervical fractures are frequently pathologic

e) Subcapital fractures

- may be impacted or displaced
- Garden classification:
  1) Stage 1: lateral cortex impacted without angulation
  2) Stage 2: entire neck impacted with no displacement
  3) Stage 3: entire neck fractured, with partial displacement
  4) Stage 4: entire neck fractured and fully displaced
- subcapital fractures at stage 1 or 2 frequently missed

f) Extracapsular fractures

- often intertrochanteric fractures are comminuted (greater and/or lesser trochanter form separated fragments)
- intertrochanteric fracture line oblique, separates head and neck from shaft
- subtrochanteric (rare) is about 2" below lesser trochanter: usually pathologic
- avulsions of greater trochanter in elderly when they fall
- lesser trochanters avulsed in young athletes; in adult, usually pathologic
- severe trauma produces very unstable mid-diaphyseal fracture, prone to malalignment

☞ **2. Slipped Femoral Capital Epiphysis (synonyms: SFCE, adolescent coxa vara, epiphyseal coxa vara, epiphyseolisthesis)**

    a) General features

- patient usually around 10–15 years of age
- during rapid adolescent growth, femoral neck slips up off femoral head
- actually a stress fracture (Salter-Harris Type 1), 20–30% bilateral
- only about 50% have trauma history
- femoral neck displaces upward, externally rotates, and adducts on the head
- femur suffers varus deformity, with external rotation and adduction
- more common in males, but bilateral involvement more common in females
- usually one side slips, and if it is to be bilateral, the second slips within a year
- associated with: renal osteodystrophy, rickets, radiotherapy, Fròlich's syndrome (adiposogenital dystrophy—marked obesity with gonadal hypodevelopment)
- complications: DJD (by far most common), avascular necrosis, chondrolysis
- pinned in situ; or conservatively: tractioned and held with a spica cast

☞   **b) Clinical features**

- typical presentation: obese young teen with pain referred to knee, limps
- pain is more often in thigh and knee than in the hip itself
- usually limitation of abduction and internal rotation
- when advanced, Trendelenburg test will be positive; gluteus medius inadequate
- *"waddling gait"* with bilateral SFCE—bilateral gluteus medius weakness

☞   **c) Radiologic features**

- bilateral AP and "frog-leg" hip views essential
- posteromedial slippage (more marked posterior slip seen best on oblique; more marked medial slip seen best on AP)
- shortened epiphysis (vertically); slight metaphyseal osteopenia
- widened physis with irregular margins
- roughened, or frayed metaphyseal/growth-plate margin
- beaking of inferomedial epiphysis
- teardrop distance increased
- medial buttressing or lateral buttressing ("Herndon's hump") on femoral neck
- "Capener's sign": metaphysis is lateral to the posterior acetabular margin
- abnormal Klein's line: line does not intersect femoral head

- "pistol-grip deformity": curved, deformed proximal femur

3. Distal Femur Fractures

    a) Supracondylar fractures
- just proximal to condyles
- usually transverse or oblique
- may be comminuted, may be intraarticular
- caused by severe impaction force to femur
- associated fractures frequent at the hip or tibia
- "floating knee": supracondylar fracture with tibial shaft fracture

    b) Femoral condyle fractures
- intraarticular fractures: frequently deform the joint
- may affect one or both condyles
- often "T" or "Y" shaped
- single condyle fracture usually oblique
- if articular surface is affected, may result in an intraarticular loose body

4. Hip Dislocations

    a) Posterior hip dislocation
- 85% of hip dislocations are posterior
- knee is impacted when hip is in flexion, driving the femoral head posterior
- especially with thigh abduction, posterior acetabular lip may fracture (90%)
- small anterior femoral head fracture occurs in about 13%
- CT required to image these small fractured fragments

    b) Anterior hip dislocation
- caused by forceful abduction and extension of the femur
- femoral head lodges near obturator foramen (migrates caudally and medially)

    c) Complications of hip dislocation
- sciatic nerve paralysis (10–15% of posterior dislocations)
- myositis ossificans (10%)
- avascular necrosis of the femoral head (10%)
- hip DJD

I. PROXIMAL TIBIAL, FIBULAR, AND PATELLAR FRACTURES AND DISLOCATIONS

1. Proximal Tibial Fractures

    a) Tibial plateau fracture (synonyms: bumper fracture, fender fracture)
- femoral condyles impacting tibial plateau
- 80% affect lateral plateau, 5–10% medial plateau, 10–15% both

- lateral plateau fracture commonly seen in elderly, osteoporotic patients
- 10–12% involve injury to ligaments; severe valgus stress; collateral ligaments and cruciate ligaments are at risk
- DJD ensues in about 20% of plateau fracture cases
- radiographic signs: oblique fracture line or actual displacement
- CT visualizes fragments: number, size, location

b) Anterior tibial spine avulsion

- knee hyperextension with tibial internal rotation
- anterior cruciate ligament avulses anterior tibial spine
- most often affects children: e.g., falls from bicycles
- radiographic signs: undisplaced, horizontal fracture at anterior base of tibial spine; displaced may show inverted fracture fragment

c) Trampoline fracture

- through proximal tibial metaphysis
- often with young child jumping on trampoline with much heavier person

d) Tibial tuberosity avulsion

- proximal displacement of fragment by infrapatellar tendon
- may be predisposed by Osgood-Schlatter's disease
- most commonly in adolescent athletes
- associated with infrapatellar tendon rupture, subcondylar or comminuted proximal tibial fractures

e) Segond's fracture

- lateral tibial condyle avulsion by TFL (iliotibial band) at its insertion
- radiographic sign: small flake of bone near lateral tibial condyle margin
- MRI good for confirmation of soft tissue and bone lesions
- almost always associated with anterior cruciate tears
- disruption of lateral capsule, meniscal tears commonly associated

2. Proximal Fibular Fractures

a) General features

- rarely isolated proximal fibular fracture
- usually associated with fractures of lateral tibial plateau, ankle
- impacted, comminuted fracture of fibular head
- avulsion of fibular styloid or proximal pole (biceps femoris insertion)

- associated injuries: lateral compartment syndrome of the knee or ligamentous peroneal nerve syndrome (ruptured lateral capsule and ligaments with peroneal nerve damage)

☞ **3. Patellar Fractures**

  a) **General features**
  - fractured by both direct and indirect trauma
  - 60% are transverse or slightly oblique
  - 25% are comminuted (stellate), 15% are vertical
  - **DDX:** developmental bipartite or tripartite patella (superolateral fragments)

  b) **Radiologic features**
  - AP and lateral views display most fractures
  - vertical fracture best displayed on skyline (tangential) projection

4. Knee Dislocations

  a) Patellar dislocation
  - usually superolateral dislocation: may also move horizontally or vertically
  - often associated with "flake" fractures (osteochondral): patellar medial facet impacts lateral femoral condyle
  - fragment discernible on tangential projection, or with CT
  - fragment removal may preclude development of DJD

  b) Femorotibial dislocation
  - dislocates anteriorly or posteriorly
  - associated collateral ligament, cruciate ligament, popliteal artery, and peroneal nerve lesions

  c) Proximal tibiofibular dislocation
  - may be anterior, posterior, or superiorly displaced, with fibular head as point of reference
  - infrequent injury, but anterolateral is most often seen
  - seen in parachutists
  - lateral projection shows anterior fibular head displacement
  - AP shows almost full fibular head, very little overlap with tibial condyle

5. Associated Soft Tissue Injuries of the Knee

☞ a) Lipohemarthrosis
  - with intraarticular fractures: marrow fat extruded into joint fluid
  - hemarthrosis due to bleeding into joint
  - fat floats on blood and synovial fluid
☞ - in suprapatella bursa you see: FBI (**f**at, **b**lood **i**nterface) sign

- lateral projection done horizontally will demonstrate this
- indicates presence of occult intraarticular fracture (often lateral tibial plateau)
- absence of FBI sign DOES NOT rule out fracture
- seen also in other synovial joints, second most common is shoulder

b) Ligament lesions
- varus-valgus stress views assess for collateral ligament damage
- Pelligrini-Stieda disease: calcifications in medial collateral ligament at distal femur due to previous avulsions
- ACL tears often involve bone contusion on anterior lateral femoral condyle and posterolateral tibia
- MRI is definitive modality for ligament damage
- signs: distention, discontinuity, edema
- optimal images: sagittal; cruciates also delineated on coronal images

c) Meniscal lesions
- MRI is optimal modality showing tears and cysts (usually in lateral joint)
- degenerative tears usually horizontal; traumatic tears more often vertical

J. ANKLE FRACTURES AND DISLOCATIONS

1. Ankle Fractures

a) General features
- standard evaluation requires AP, lateral, and medial oblique projections
- occult fractures may require stress views or CT
- CT is optimal for subtalar joint visualization
- MRI is necessary for demonstrating associated soft tissue lesions
- ankle fractures classified by two methods:
  1) Laug-Hansen: according to forces producing the fracture
  2) Danis-Weber: according to fibular fracture position
     - Type A: fibula fractured below tibiotalar joint
     - Type B: oblique fibular fracture at tibiotalar joint level
     - Type C1: oblique fibular fracture above distal tibiofibular ligaments
     - Type C2: high fibular fracture with ruptured syndesmosis
- Type A simply cast; Types B and C often require internal fixation

b) Complications
- nonunion: most often with medial malleolar fracture without internal fixation

- nonunion more symptomatic at plafond level than below
- traumatic degenerative arthritis due to inexact mortise reduction, plafond comminution, and aging
- ligamentous instability: lateral collateral, medial collateral (deltoid), tibiofibular ligament (or syndesmosis)
- lateral ligaments most often ruptured
- stress studies advisable to rule out ligament ruptures, especially with significant swelling, even in the absence of fracture
- compare left and right: > 10° difference in tilt or > 3 mm difference in joint space is significant; as is > 6° tilt in neutral position
- lateral view: anteroposterior (drawer) stress tests for anterior talofibular ligament lesion: > 2 mm difference between left and right is significant
- arthrography is optimum diagnostic modality

c) Medial malleolus fracture
- usually transverse or oblique
- talar pressure against distal tibia fractures malleolus
- fracture proximal to plafond (tibiotalar joint line) is unstable; distal is stable
- AP is optimal projection

d) Lateral malleolus fracture
- oblique or spiral fracture due to external foot rotation, pressure on distal fibula
- optimally imaged by medial oblique projection
- McKenzie's sign: soft tissue swelling adjacent to oblique radiolucency
- may be associated with flake fractures at tip of lateral malleolus and the talar dome

e) Bimalleolar fracture
- one side fractures transversely because of tensile force
- opposite fracture is oblique or spiral

f) Trimalleolar fracture (synonym: Cotton's fracture)
- third malleolus is the posterior lip of the tibia
- seen with tibiotalar dislocations
- caused by foot external rotation: posterolateral displacement
- optimal projection is lateral
- third malleolus fragment displaced posteriorly and/or superiorly

g) Pott's fracture (Fig. 4.7)
- partial dislocation: fibular fracture 6–7 cm above lateral malleolus
- distal tibiofibular ligaments ruptured
- does NOT involve any malleolar fracture

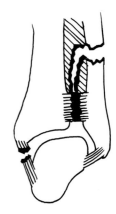

Figure 4.7.

Pott's fracture. Reprinted with permission from Yochum TR, Rowe LJ. Essentials of Skeletal Radiology, 2nd ed. Baltimore: Williams & Wilkins, 1996:731.

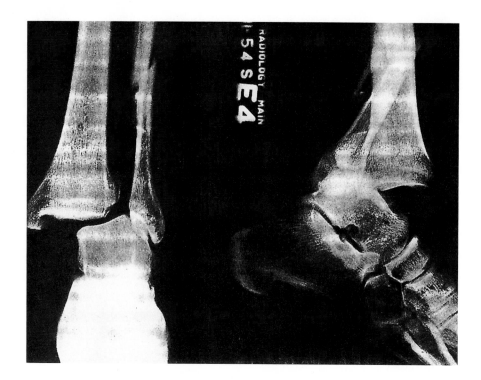

Figure 4.8.
Dupuytren's fracture. Reprinted with permission from Traumatic disorders of the ankle and foot. CIBA: Clinical sumposia reprint 1965;17(1):22.

h) Dupuytren's fracture (Fig. 4.8)
- lateral malleolus (distal fibula) fractures, ruptured distal tibiofibular ligaments with diastasis of the syndesmosis, lateral dislocation of talus
- foot is displaced upward and outward, tibia is displaced medially

i) Maisonneuve's fracture (Fig. 4.9)
- proximal fibular shaft fracture with ruptured inferior tibiofibular syndesmosis
- fibula fractures within its proximal third, levered out from its distal end
- caused by forceful inversion and external ankle rotation
- proximal fracture missed due to extreme ankle pain

j) Tillaux's fracture
- medial malleolus fracture with distal tibiofibular syndesmosis diastasis; tibial anterior tubercle avulsion; fibula fracture 6–7 cm from distal end
- AP is optimal projection

k) Toddler's fracture
- tibial spiral fracture; undisplaced
- children 3 years and younger
- do AP and lateral projections: one of these will display the fracture
- occasionally fibula is also fractured
- occasionally an adult has this, as a *boot-top* fracture
- when both tib and fib are fractured: *BB* or *both bones* fracture

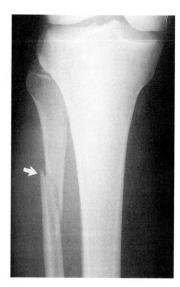

Figure 4.9.
Maisonneuve's fracture. Reprinted with permission from Yochum TR, Rowe LJ. Essentials of Skeletal Radiology, 2nd ed. Baltimore: Williams & Wilkins, 1996:732.

2. Ankle Dislocations

    a) General features
- talus may be dislocated with or without fracture to the talar neck
- talar dislocation may represent extrusion of the talus from the mortise joint
- medial or lateral dislocations almost always occur with fracture (see above)
- anterior or posterior dislocations do fracture the adjacent tibial margins

    b) Anterior dislocation
- when tibia is displaced posteriorly on fixed foot, talus dislocates anteriorly
- all tibiotalar and fibulotalar ligaments and capsular elements rupture
- clinical appearance: foot in slight dorsiflexion, looks anteriorly elongated
- disappearance of the depressions normally flanking Achilles tendon
- talus anteriorly prominent
- sometimes dorsalis pedis pulse is absent
- occasionally the posterior talofibular ligament is spared

    c) Posterior dislocation
- more common than anterior (both are rare)
- caused by blow to posterior tibia: tibia driven forward, talus displaces posteriorly
- clinical appearance: plantar flexion with "shortened" foot
- reduced by long axis traction combined with anterior lift of the heel
- may require operative repair of ligaments

K. FOOT FRACTURES AND DISLOCATIONS

1. General Features

    a) Routine views include: dorsoplantar, 35° medial oblique, lateral

    b) calcaneal fracture requires axial projection

    c) direct trauma, ligament/tendon avulsions, diabetic neurotrophic arthropathy, repeated stress all may cause fractures in feet

☞ **2. Calcaneal Compression Fracture**

    a) General features
- calcaneus is the most frequently fractured tarsal bone, talus is second
- 75% involve subtalar joint and calcaneal body

    b) Compression fracture of calcaneus
- 10% are bilateral
- 10% associated with thoracolumbar spinal fractures
- fracture is usually comminuted, involving subtalar joint

- posterior facet often depressed
- fracture lines often cannot be visualized; Boehler's angle crucial for diagnosis
- Boehler's angle norm: 28° to 40°; < 28° shows depression, probable fracture

3. **Calcaneal Avulsion Fracture**

   a) Spare subtalar joint

   b) Most commonly affect anterior process of calcaneus

   c) Talar beak (posterior margin of tuberosity) may be avulsed by Achilles tendon

4. **Talar Body Fracture**

   a) Usually obliquely or transversely oriented

   b) Talar dome prone to osteochondral chip fractures

5. **Talar Neck Fracture**

   a) Most frequent are anterior surface avulsions; second: vertical fractures

   b) Tibia is forced down into talar neck

   c) Sometimes vertical fracture is called *"aviator's fracture"*

   d) Vertical fracture prone to avascular necrosis of the talus
   - the more anterior the fracture, the greater likelihood of avascular necrosis
   - *Hawkin's sign:* subcortical lucency in talar dome, good prognosis for revascularization, less probability of avascular necrosis

6. **Talar Head Fracture**

   a) Rare fracture well forward of talar neck

7. **Navicular Fracture**

   a) Most often: avulsion of dorsal cortical surface

   b) Medial tuberosity may be avulsed by tibialis posterior in acute eversion

   c) **DDX:** os tibiale externum (accessory ossicle)

8. **Lisfranc's Injury**

   a) Distal fractures of cuneiforms, with tarsometatarsal dislocation

9. **Metatarsal Fracture**

   a) Usually in shaft or neck

   b) Fracture is oblique, spiral or transverse, may be difficult to visualize

   c) Stress fractures: most frequent at second and third metatarsal necks

   d) Jones' fracture (synonym: Dancer's fracture)
   - transverse fracture at proximal fifth metatarsal

- plantar flexion and inversion exert traction upon peroneus brevis tendon and plantar aponeurosis
- the more distal the fracture, the more prone to nonunion, slow to heal
- often missed because pain may indicate mortise lesion
- radiologic sign: transversely oriented lucency about 15–20 mm from base
- **DDX:** juvenile apophysis (longitudinally oriented lucency)

10. **Phalangeal Fracture**

    a) Crush fracture: comminuted phalanx, frequently distal phalanx is affected

    b) Bedroom fracture: "stubbing the toe," first and fifth digits especially vulnerable

    c) Chip fracture: articular margins, usually hyperextension injury

11. **Sesamoid Fracture**

    a) Jumping, running, dancing—especially barefoot

    b) Acute or stress fractures occur

    c) May result in avascular necrosis

    d) Medial hallux sesamoid more vulnerable

    e) May be comminuted, or show single fracture line

    f) Optimal view: axial submetatarsal

    g) **DDX: bipartite sesamoid variant (85% bilateral)**

12. **Hallux Rigidus**

    a) Sequela of phalangeal fracture of great toe

    b) Painful, stiffened first metatarsophalangeal joint

    c) May be followed by DJD at that site

13. **Talar Dislocation**

    a) Most commonly dislocated foot bone

    b) Single or multiple dislocations at talotibial, talocalcaneal (subtalar) and talonavicular joints

    c) Talar avascular necrosis may ensue

14. **Midtarsal Dislocation (synonym: Chopart's dislocation)**

    a) Rare

    b) Foot separated at talonavicular and calcaneocuboid joints

15. **Tarsometatarsal Fracture Dislocation (synonym: Lisfranc's dislocation)**

    a) Dorsal dislocation of metatarsal bases from their contiguous tarsals, with fractures at the dislocation sites (usually base of second metatarsal and lateral cuboid)

b) Metatarsals may be laterally displaced too

c) Longitudinal compression, or twisting of forefoot; most commonly in motor vehicle, industrial, and equestrian accidents

d) Lisfranc amputated injured feet at this site, hence the eponym

e) CT is optimal imaging modality

REVIEW—STUDY QUESTIONS

1. What is the most common dislocation of the hip, and where does it leave the femoral head?

2. Describe the locations of intracapsular fractures of the proximal femur. With what complications are these commonly associated ?

3. What three joints are involved in tarsal dislocations?

4. At which locations in the pelvis, hip, and lower extremity is avascular necrosis most frequently encountered?

5. Describe the Danis-Weber fibular fracture classification. Which of these require surgical fixation?

6. What projections are commonly used to visualize patellar fractures?

7. What is lipohemarthrosis? What is its radiologic sign? Where is it most commonly seen, and on what projections?

8. Describe the injury sustained in a "sprung pelvis." What is a synonym for it?

9. Describe SFCE. What is it? Who does it usually affect? Give its clinical and radiologic signs.

10. What soft tissues of the knee are at risk in dislocation or fracture/dislocation knee injuries?

L. RIB, STERNUM FRACTURES AND COSTAL CARTILAGE LESIONS

1. General Features

a) Require significant force unless they are pathologic (e.g., osteoporotic bone)

b) Rare in childhood

c) Difficult to visualize on plain film: multiple oblique views required

d) May be seen only after callus develops

e) Bone scan is helpful for location of occult rib lesions

f) Multiple rib fractures usually are aligned linearly

g) Associated with pleural fluid in costophrenic recess, pneumothorax, subcutaneous emphysema, diaphragmatic elevation, splenic laceration

h) Lower ribs rarely fracture: check for damage to kidneys; anteriorly check spleen, liver

☞   **2. Radiologic Features**

        a) transverse or oblique radiolucent fracture line (**DDX:** bronchial air shadows)

        b) cortical offset: "step effect"

        c) altered rib orientation distal to fracture site

        d) *"costal hook sign"*: distal end of rib appears hook-like, may indicate flail segment

        e) callus: local bulbous expansion and increased density at fracture site

        f) local hematoma adjacent to fracture may displace or deflect pleura into lung; gives *"extrapleural sign"*: radiopacity convex into lung

3. Upper Rib Fractures

        a) Ribs 1–3 seldom fracture because of inherent strength and firm muscular support

☞   **b)** First three rib fractures associated with: tracheal, brachial plexus, spinal lesions; damage to great vessels (including aorta)

        c) Stress fractures to first rib: throwing injuries

        d) Bench pressing may fracture second rib

☞   **4. Flail Chest**

        a) Single rib with two fractures, isolating a section of the rib from distal and proximal segments

        b) Usually multiple adjacent ribs affected

        c) Isolated portions move opposite to normal respiratory motion: paradoxical motion

        d) Potentially life-threatening interference with respiratory function

        e) Associated radiologic appearance: *"costal hook sign"*

☞   **5. Golfer's Fracture**

        a) Lateral margin of rib fractures

        b) Caused by unexpected impact of golf club with ground in mid-swing

☞   **6. Passion Fracture (synonym: bear-hug fracture)**

        a) Predisposed by osteopenia or other bone pathology

☞   **7. Cough Fracture (synonym: post-tussive fracture)**

        a) Persistent or violent coughing may produce stress fracture

        b) Lower anterior ribs affected: most often sixth and seventh anterior ribs

8. Sternum Fracture

        a) Compressive blunt trauma is most common force

        b) Manubriosternal junction, body of sternum, suffer transverse fractures

  c) Visualized on lateral projection
   • fracture line, hematoma, displacement

  d) May require CT for optimal display of lesions

  e) Search for associated soft tissue, organ, and thoracic spine injury

9. Costal Cartilage Injury

  a) Calcified costal cartilage shows disruption on plain film

  b) Uncalcified cartilage damage may be identified via nuclear bone scan or CT

10. Thoracic Trauma Complications

  a) Traumatic pneumothorax: loss of intrapleural negative pressure causes collapse of lung

  b) Hemothorax: blood in pleural space (blunt costophrenic sulci, widened paraspinal space and apical "capping" are radiologic signs)

  c) Chylothorax: accumulated lymphatic fluid, signs similar to hemothorax

  d) Lung contusion: intrapulmonary hemorrhage, local opacification on film
   • appears within hours of injury, gradually resorbs in 3–10 days

  e) Pneumonia: caused by restricted mobility of chest, hindered lung fluid clearing

  f) Organ damage: ruptured spleen, ruptured diaphragm, lesions of tracheobronchial tree; esophageal tearing, ruptured kidney; heart lesions; lung cyst formation; aortic aneurysm formation

M. SHOULDER GIRDLE FRACTURES AND DISLOCATIONS

 1. Clavicle Fractures

  a) General features
   • clavicle is most frequently fractured bone during birth process
   • in children, this is the most commonly fractured bone
   • in young adulthood, clavicle fracture is frequent, as is shoulder dislocation and acromioclavicular separation
   • in elderly, most common injuries are shoulder dislocation and fracture of the surgical neck of the humerus

  b) Complications
   • neurovascular damage: subclavian artery, vein, brachial plexus and sympathetic chain are vulnerable (most frequently, the artery)
   • rupture during fracture, compression effects from hypertrophic callus
   • nonunion: sclerosis; smooth, rounded margins signal need for surgical fixation
   • malunion: cosmetic deformity due to fragment overlap and massive callus may

require osteotomy, realignment and fixation

- degenerative arthritis: caused by intraarticular clavicle fractures; films show sclerosis, osteophytes, diminished joint space
- posttraumatic osteolysis: 1–3 mm of distal segment resorbs, often after minor injury; may completely regenerate, or may leave permanently tapered distal clavicle

c) Radiologic features

- routinely use "hotlight": parts of shoulder are inherently overpenetrated
- optimal view for clavicle is AP with 15° cephalad tube angle
- evaluation of acromioclavicular separation is with patient holding 10- to 15-pound weights to assess integrity of coracoclavicular ligaments
- for clavicle, use about half the exposure factors as for standard shoulder views
- osteolysis: cystic subarticular cortex; then cortical dissolution; joint widening; clavicular surface is frayed and irregular or cup-shaped

d) Medial clavicle fracture

- least common (5% of clavicle fractures)
- often require CT to depict fracture

 e) Middle clavicle fracture

- most common—about 80% of clavicle fractures
- shearing at middle clavicle for force at distal end
- SCM elevates medial fragment; shoulder weight depresses lateral fragment
- malalignment and overlap are common, with extensive healing callus formed

f) Lateral clavicle fracture

- about 15% of all clavicle fractures
- three types
  1) undisplaced
  2) displaced—distal fragment moved anteroinferior
  3) articular surface extension—prone to future DJD

2. Scapula Fractures

a) Isolated fracture rare: severe trauma fractures scapula

b) Sometimes pushups may result in stress fracture

c) Routine shoulder views usually adequate, but may need specialized views

d) Coracoid view (synonym: scapular "Y" view)

- 25 to 40° tube tilt, AP

    e) Lateral view
- patient rotated 35°; PA
- gives tangential view of scapular body and acromion

    f) Axillary view
- superior-inferior; arm abducted and cassette in axilla
- good image of glenoid, acromion and coracoid process

    g) Fractures usually occur in scapular body or neck (80%)

    h) Coracoid or acromion may fracture at their narrowest point

    i) Bankart lesion: inferior glenoid rim avulsion at insertion of triceps with anterior humeral dislocation

3. Anterior Glenohumeral Joint Dislocation

    a) Glenohumeral dislocations account for 85% of shoulder girdle dislocations (AC joint, 12%; sternoclavicular joint 2%; scapulothoracic joint about 1%)

    b) About 95% of glenohumeral dislocations are anterior

    c) Hill-Sachs defect: impacted humeral head (in 60% of cases)

    d) Humeral head may settle in subcoracoid (most common), subglenoid, subclavicular or intrathoracic position

    e) Radiologic signs: inferior and medial displacement; altered humeral head shape; Hill-Sachs and/or Bankart lesions

    f) MR is optimal for locating Hill-Sachs defect

4. Posterior Glenohumeral Joint Dislocation

    a) Only 2–4% of glenohumeral dislocations

    b) Caused by epileptic convulsions, electric shocks, direct trauma

    c) Radiologic signs: "*rim sign*": joint space > 6 mm; "*trough sign*": double articular surface line; diminished/absent overlap of glenoid fossa and humeral head; "*vacant glenoid sign*": no close anterior joint margin contact; "*tennis racquet appearance*": cystic-looking humeral head; superior displacement

    d) Humeral head looks identical in external and internal rotation, because of fixation in its superiorly displaced position

5. Inferior Glenohumeral Joint Dislocation (synonym: luxatio erecta)

    a) Caused by severe hyperabduction trauma

    b) Acromion acts as fulcrum to lever humeral head out and inferior

      c) Humerus locked in hyperabducted position with head in subglenoid position

      d) *"Hanging shoulder"* or *"drooping shoulder"*: partial inferior displacement may occur with stroke, hemarthrosis, joint effusion, or brachial plexus lesions

6. Superior Glenohumeral Joint Dislocation

      a) Rare: occurs with elbow flexed and joint adducted; heavy force required

☞ **7. Rotator Cuff Tears**

      a) May be traumatic or degenerative

      b) Partial superior glenohumeral dislocation with infraspinatus tendon lesion
- caused by imbalance between rotator cuff and deltoid vectors
- may cause eventual pseudoarthrosis between humeral head and both clavicle and acromion

      c) Indicator of rotator cuff tear: acromiohumeral space < 7 mm

      d) May also have inferior acromial erosion and sclerosis

      e) Greater tuberosity may show roughened cortex and cysts

      f) Diagnostic imaging by plain film, arthrography, ultrasound, and MR (optimal)

☞ **8. Glenoid Labral Tears (synonym: SLAP lesions)**

      a) Superior labrum anterior to posterior = SLAP

      b) Associated with shoulder instability

      c) MRI is optimal imaging modality: shows labral avulsion, cleft, or absence

☞ **9. Acromioclavicular Joint Separations**

      a) General features:
- classifications:
    1) Type I: mild sprain—acromioclavicular ligament stretched and coracoclavicular ligament intact
        - weight-bearing does not increase joint space or alter alignment
    2) Type II: moderate sprain—acromioclavicular ligament torn; coracoclavicular ligaments stretched
        - widened joint space, slight elevation of clavicle
    3) Type III: severe sprain—acromioclavicular and coracoclavicular ligaments disrupted
        - widened joint space; clear elevation of distal clavicle above acromion, coracoclavicular space > 5 mm wider than contralateral counterpart

- separation clear on non-weight-bearing internal rotation AP projection
- may need joint repair and open fixation for types II and III
- old injuries of coracoclavicular ligament may ossify

b) Radiologic features

- optimal views: AP projection with 15° cephalad tilt
- take both with and without 10–15 pounds of weight in dependent hands
- bilateral views for comparison
- Type III tears will show without weights because of scapular motion
- three landmarks assessed
    1) acromioclavicular joint space: should be bilaterally symmetrical within 2–3 mm; average normal width is 2–4 mm
    2) acromioclavicular joint alignment
    3) coracoclavicular distance: normally 11–13 mm; should be bilaterally symmetrical within 5 mm

N. FRACTURES AND DISLOCATIONS OF THE PROXIMAL HUMERUS

1. Neer Classification

a) General features

- proximal fractures identified by specific location
    1) anatomic neck
    2) greater tuberosity
    3) lesser tuberosity
    4) surgical neck
- proximal shaft fractures are outside of Neer classification
- in Neer classification the number of fractures is added to give a one part, two part, three part, or four part fracture
- 80% are one part; 10% two part; three part about 3%, four part about 4%
- "head-splitting fracture": comminuted humeral head fracture

b) Radiologic features

- most proximal humeral fractures can be imaged with AP internal and external rotation projections
- CT is valuable for locating fragments, delineating articular involvement

2. Humeral Fracture Proximal to the Anatomic Neck

a) Usually occur with other humeral fractures

b) High risk of avascular necrosis of humeral head

c) Posterolateral humeral head suffers impaction fracture with anterior dislocation (Hill-Sachs defect, or hatchet defect)

d) Best demonstrated with internal rotation projection

3. **Greater Tuberosity Fracture (synonym: flap fracture)**

a) May be fractured by direct trauma or may be avulsed

b) Often fractures with anterior dislocation

c) Displacement > 1 cm = significant rotator cuff rupture: requires open reduction

d) Optimal projection: AP external rotation

4. **Lesser Tuberosity Fracture**

a) Almost always in conjunction with other proximal humeral fractures

 5. **Surgical Neck Fracture**

a) Most common humeral fracture site

b) Usually comminuted, with both tuberosities involved

c) Pectoralis muscle displaces shaft anteromedially

d) Axillary nerve and artery vulnerable to injury

6. **Proximal Humeral Shaft Fracture**

a) Usually caused by direct trauma

b) With fracture proximal to pectoralis major insertion, humeral head rotates and abducts

c) Fracture between deltoid and pectoralis major insertions, head adducts

d) Fracture distal to deltoid insertion: head abducts

e) Complications: malunion, DJD, avascular necrosis, myositis ossificans, neurovascular lesions, residual joint stiffness

O. ELBOW AND FOREARM FRACTURES AND DISLOCATIONS

 1. **General Features**

a) Adults: 50% of elbow fractures involve radial head and neck; 20% olecranon

b) Children: 60% of elbow fractures are supracondylar

c) Occult elbow fractures easily overlooked, produce residual joint dysfunction

d) Minimum radiologic study: AP in full extension; medial oblique, lateral, axial olecranon

e) With children, do comparative bilateral study to rule out growth variations

      f) With forearm fractures, AP and lateral views are adequate

      g) Distal humeral fractures easily detected; 95% disrupt the elbow joint

☞ **2.** **Supracondylar Fractures of the Distal Humerus**

      a) Transverse or oblique fracture above condyles

      b) This is the **most common** "elbow fracture" in children

      c) Distal fragment usually posteriorly displaced

☞ **3.** **Intercondylar Fracture of the Distal Humerus**

      a) Fracture line communicating with supracondylar region, extends between the condyles

      b) May have a "T" or "Y" configuration

      c) This comprises about 50% of adult distal humeral fractures

  4. **Transcondylar Fracture of the Distal Humerus**

      a) Fracture line passes transversely through both humeral condyles

☞ **5.** **"Sideswipe Fracture" (synonym: "baby car fracture")**

      a) Most often comminuted; associated with ulnar and radial fractures

      b) Occurs when the elbow protrudes from a car window .

  6. **Condylar Fracture**

      a) Shearing force may fracture off a single condyle

      b) Articular surfaces of capitellum and trochlea also vulnerable to fracture

      c) Compression fracture of capitellum caused by radial head impact: sometimes both fracture

      d) Osteochondral fragment from convex capitellar surface: "*Kocher's fracture,*" osteochondral fracture, osteochondritis dissecans

  7. **Epicondylar Fracture**

      a) Usually avulsions

      b) Little Leaguer's Elbow: medial epicondyle avulsion caused by stress on immature, ununited apophysis

  8. **Olecranon Fracture**

      a) Comprises about 20% of adult elbow fractures

      b) Direct trauma or avulsion by triceps tendon during acute flexion

      c) Usually fractures adjacent to inferior convex trochlear surface

    d) Best demonstrated on lateral projection

    e) Surgical fixation required: fragments significantly distracted

9. Coronoid Process Fracture

    a) Avulsion by brachialis muscle

    b) Impaction into trochlear fossa

    c) Rarely isolated; usually occurs with posterior elbow dislocation

    d) Usually has small, elusive fragment

    e) Oblique view is the optimal diagnostic projection

10. "Chisel Fracture"

    a) Incomplete radial head fracture, from center of articular surface about 10 mm into bone

    b) May be indicated by a positive fat-pad sign

☞ **11. Radial Head Fracture**

    a) Often occult; watch for positive fat-pad sign

    b) Radiolucent fracture vertically oriented, cortical lesion toward lateral side of radial head

    c) Often a sharp angulation or step-off caused by fragment displacement

    d) *"Double cortical sign"*: depression of fracture fragment

    e) Supinator fat line: on lateral view fat line is obliterated, blurred, or ventrally displaced; and additional 1 to 2 cm (normally it is about 1 cm above anterior radial surface)

    f) Fat pad sign: displaced humeral capsular fat pads
- fat pads between synovial and fibrous layers of joint capsule, fore and aft
- lateral projection normally shows obliquely oriented lucency anteriorly
- edema causes horizontal orientation and elevation of anterior fat pad; and severe edema will obliterate the anterior pad entirely
- posterior pad normally not visible; becomes visible when swelling occurs
- 90% of children's elbow fractures have visible posterior fat pad
- less frequently seen in adults; absence of sign does not preclude fracture

12. Radial Neck Fracture

    a) Impaction at head/neck junction is most common injury at this site

    b) Lateral view may show sharper angle on anterior surface of radial neck

    c) In complete fracture: lucent transverse fracture line

13. **Essex-Lopresti Fracture**

    a) Comminuted radial head fracture with distal radioulnar dislocation

14. **"B-B Fracture" (both bones fracture)**

    a) About 60% of all forearm fractures involve both bones

    b) Most commonly occur mid-shaft

    c) Usually displaced with angulation and rotation, require surgical reduction, fixation

☞ 15. **Distal Ulnar Shaft Fracture (synonyms: nightstick fracture; parry fracture)**

    a) Direct trauma to forearm

16. **Proximal Ulnar Shaft Fracture (synonym: Monteggia fracture) (Fig. 4.10)**

    a) Fractured ulna with radial displacement

    b) In children, ulnar fracture my be incomplete (green-stick fracture)

17. **Distal Radial Shaft Fracture (synonyms: Galeazzi fracture; Piedmont fracture; reversed Monteggia fracture) (Fig. 4.11)**

    a) Rare; results in serious injury

    b) Radial fracture at junction of mid and distal thirds; associated dislocation of distal radioulnar joint

    c) Even with surgical reduction, this is subject to nonunion and redislocation

☞ 18. **Posterior and Posterolateral Elbow Dislocation**

    a) Adults: elbow is third most common site of dislocation (1 = shoulder; 2 = interphalangeal joints of fingers)

    b) Children: elbow is MOST COMMON dislocation site

    c) Dislocations classified according to position of radius and ulna relative to humerus

    d) Posterior and posterolateral are most common (up to 90%)

    e) Both radius and ulna are almost always displaced

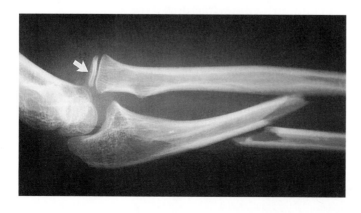

Figure 4.10.

Monteggia fracture. Reprinted with permission from Yochum TR, Rowe LJ. Essentials of Skeletal Radiology, 2nd ed. Baltimore: Williams & Wilkins, 1996:755.

f) More than 50% are associated with fracture: usually medial epicondyle and radial head or neck

g) Children may have avulsed medial epicondyle, which may be entrapped in the joint

h) A few result in myositis ossificans, usually in brachialis muscle

☞ **19. Pulled Elbow (synonyms: toddler elbow, Safeway elbow)**

a) Common in children 2–5 years old

b) Caused by axial traction of forearm

c) Radial head slips from under annular ligament; traps ligament in radiohumeral joint

d) Replace by supinating the hand

e) Recurrence is common

P. WRIST FRACTURES AND DISLOCATIONS

☞ **1. General Features**

a) Wrist is one of the more frequently fractured articulations

b) Complex anatomy makes identification of fracture more difficult

c) Minimum plain film study includes PA neutral, PA with ulnar flexion, oblique, and lateral projections

d) CT is optimal modality for identification of occult fractures and fragment location

☞ **2. Colles' Fracture (Fig. 4.12)**

a) General features
- distal radius fractured about 20–35 mm proximal to joint surface, distal fragment angulated posteriorly
- ulnar styloid is also fractured in about 60% of these
- usually caused by falling on outstretched, extended hand
- clinical appearance: *"dinner fork deformity"*
- incidence increases with age, more in women than in men: at age 65, ratio is 6:1

b) Radiologic features
- fracture line transverse and comminuted with variable degree of impaction on dorsal surface
- PA projection shows sharp cortical overlap (distal fragment migrates proximally)
- decreased overall length of radius due to proximal migration of distal fragment
- lateral view shows dorsal tilt of distal

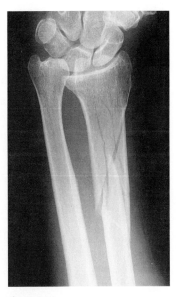

Figure 4.11.
Galeazzi or reversed Monteggia fracture. Reprinted with permission from Yochum TR, Rowe LJ. Essentials of Skeletal Radiology, 2nd ed. Baltimore: Williams & Wilkins, 1996:755.

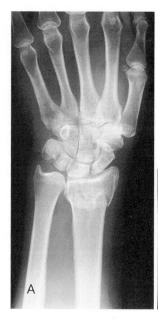

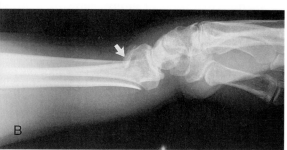

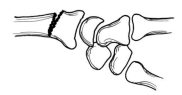

Figure 4.12.

Colles' fracture. Reprinted with permission from Yochum TR, Rowe LJ. Essentials of Skeletal Radiology, 2nd ed. Baltimore: Williams & Wilkins, 1996:756.

fragment (normal articular surface angle is 5 to 15° palmar)

- distorted skin contour and altered plane of pronator quadratus fat pad is evident on lateral projection

 3. **Smith's Fracture (synonym: reversed Colles' fracture) (Fig. 4.13)**

    a) Distal radius fracture with distal fragment angulated anteriorly

    b) Caused by fall with wrist forced into hyperflexion

    c) Radiologic signs same as for Colles' except distal fragment angles anteriorly

4. **Barton's Fracture (synonym: rim fracture) (Fig. 4.14)**

    a) Proximal dislocation of carpus with posterior rim fracture of radius' joint surface

    b) Caused by forced wrist hyperextension

    c) PA projection shows proximal carpal row overlapping radial articulating surface

    d) Lateral view displays posterior rim fracture, posterior and proximal carpal displacement

5. **Reverse Barton's Fracture**

    a) Fracture of anterior rim of radius' joint surface

 6. **Chauffeur's Fracture (synonyms: backfire fracture; Hutchinson's fracture) (Fig. 4.15)**

    a) Caused by sharp blow on dorsal wrist

    b) Radial styloid process avulsed or fractured because of impaction by scaphoid

    c) Transverse or oblique fracture line, usually without displacement

Figure 4.13.

Smith's fracture. Reprinted with permission from Yochum TR, Rowe LJ. Essentials of Skeletal Radiology, 2nd ed. Baltimore: Williams & Wilkins, 1996:757.

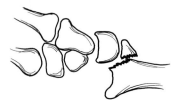

Figure 4.14.

Barton's fracture. Reprinted with permission from Yochum TR, Rowe LJ. Essentials of Skeletal Radiology, 2nd ed. Baltimore: Williams & Wilkins, 1996:757.

7. **Moore's Fracture**

    a) Ulnar styloid process fractured; distal ulna dislocated

    b) This is in conjunction with a Colles' fracture

☞ 8. **Torus Fracture of Wrist**

    a) Most common fracture of wrist in 6- to 10-year-old children

    b) Usually 2–4 cm proximal to distal growth plate

    c) Could occur in any long bone: buckling of cortex

    d) Radiologic sign: small, localized cortical bulge or bump

9. **Slipped Radial Epiphysis**

    a) Childhood version of Colles' fracture: forceful hyperextension injury

    b) Radial epiphysis displaces posteriorly

    c) "*Corner sign*": small, displaced metaphyseal fragment

    d) Salter-Harris Type II: closed reduction treatment; no growth alteration

10. **Ulnar Styloid Process Fracture**

    a) Rare as isolated fracture

    b) May occur as an avulsion when distal radius is fractured

☞ 11. **Scaphoid Fracture**

    a) General features
- most commonly fractured carpal bone
- scaphoid most often fractures in people between 15 and 40 years of age
- most common site for occult fracture
- 70% occur at scaphoid waist; 20% at proximal pole; 10% at distal pole

    b) Complications
- prone to nonunion; avascular necrosis; carpal instability, radiocarpal DJD

    c) Avascular necrosis
- occurs in 15% of cases
- governed by location of fracture line in relation to major arterial supply (fracture proximal to this artery is prone to necrosis)

    d) Nonunion
- 30% of fractures at waist suffer nonunion (again, mediated by relation of fracture to major arterial supply)
- nonunion facilitated by inadequate immobilization, delayed diagnosis
- nonunion promotes DJD

    e) Carpal instability
- manifested by altered carpal alignments

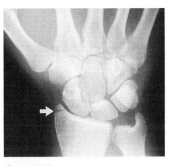

Figure 4.15.
Chauffeur's fracture or Hutchinson's fracture. Reprinted with permission from Yochum TR, Rowe LJ. Essentials of Skeletal Radiology, 2nd ed. Baltimore: Williams & Wilkins, 1996:758.

- associated with DJD and RA; ligament rupture, fractures, dislocations, and repetitive microtrauma (stress injuries)
- dorsal intercalated segment instability (DISI); ventral (or volar) intercalated segment instability (VISI); scapholunate dissociation are most common
- also may see ulnar translocation, dorsal carpal subluxation, palmar carpal subluxation, capitolunate instability, or midcarpal instability

f) Scapholunate dissociation (rotary subluxation of the scaphoid)
- most common carpal instability
- follows acute dorsiflexion injury
- clinically: pain, crepitus, weakened grip
- caused by scapholunate ligament disruption
- radiologically: "Terry Thomas sign," "ring sign"
- scapholunate space > 4 mm (**DDX:** lunotriquetral coalition, with 50% of these there is widened scapholunate space)
- optimal projections: PA ulnar deviation; "clenched fist" views

g) Dorsal intercalated segment instability (DISI)
- lunate tilted dorsally (> 80° angle to radial long axis)
- capitate displaced dorsally, lying posterior to longitudinal radial axis
- optimal view is lateral projection
- this is the second most commonly seen carpal instability

h) Ventral (volar) intercalated segment instability (VISI)
- lunate tilted ventrally
- capitate extended (tilted dorsally)

i) Radiocarpal degenerative arthritis
- sequela of scaphoid fracture, nonunion, avascular necrosis, or radial fracture
- radiologic signs: loss of radiocarpal joint space; subchondral sclerosis, osteophytes, subchondral cysts
- dorsal distal radius hypertrophy (over Lister's tubercle) affects extensor pollicus longus tendon (may lead to tendon atrophy or rupture)
- with no history of trauma, **DDX:** CPPD
- severe radiocarpal joint space loss with scapholunate dissociation and proximal migration of capitate may lead to scapholunate advanced collapse (SLAC)

☞ **j)** Radiologic signs of scaphoid fracture and its complications
- PA ulnar deviation projection is optimal view

- fracture line may not be visualized; fracture will show about 20 days later
- bone scan may be false positive (16%), but not false negative
- fracture line: transverse, occasionally oblique
- soft tissue sign: laterally displaced or obliterated scaphoid fat stripe ("*navicular fat stripe sign*")
- more distal fractures heal faster: no callus forms, fracture line fades out
- necrosis: increased density and fragmentation of segment; fracture line widens, may appear cystic
- nonunion: widened fracture line, cyst formation, sclerotic margins along fracture line
- scapholunate dissociation: wide scapholunate joint space ("*Terry Thomas sign*"), 2 mm wide space is suspicious, > 4 mm is abnormal; foreshortened scaphoid due to rotation ("*ring sign*"); unparallel joint surfaces

☞ **12. Triquetrum Fracture (synonym: Fischer's fracture)**

  a) Second most common carpal fracture

  b) Usually avulsion by radiocarpal ligament (dorsal surface)

  c) Hyperflexion injury

  d) Lateral view shows small, displaced flake fracture

13. Pisiform Fracture

  a) Caused by direct blow

  b) Usually a vertical fracture, divides pisiform into halves

14. Trapezium Fracture

  a) Usually caused by hyperabduction of thumb

  b) Radial portion of trapezium is fractured

15. Trapezoid Fracture

  a) Least often fractured carpal

16. Capitate Fracture

  a) Associated with scaphoid or perilunate dislocation

  b) Most often transverse fracture through capitate waist

17. Hamate Fracture

  a) Various fractures possible: hook fractured by direct blow

  b) Dorsal surface fracture with posterior dislocation; subluxation of fourth or fifth metacarpal; displaced oblong fragment seen

  c) Optimal diagnostic view: tangential projection with wrist in hyperextension

18. **Lunate Fracture**

  a) Rare: usually dislocates instead of fracturing

  b) Fracture likely to precipitate Keinböch's disease (avascular necrosis)

19. **Carpal Dislocations**

  a) **General features**
  - single bone may dislocate relative to other carpals
  - single bone may remain in normal location, while others dislocate

  ☞ b) **Radiologic features**
  - evaluate three carpal arcs
  - arc 1: proximal articular surfaces of the proximal carpal row
  - arc 2: distal articular surfaces of the proximal carpal row
  - arc 3: proximal surfaces of distal carpals (capitate and hamate)
  - disruptions of smooth arcs indicate carpal displacement

☞ 20. **Lunate Dislocation**

  a) Most frequently dislocated carpal

  b) Hyperextension injury

  c) Lunate tilts palmar; articulation with capitate disrupted, articulation with radius intact

  d) Lateral view displays anterior tilt

  e) PA view: lunate looks triangular (apex points distally)—"*pie sign*"

  f) Arcs 2 and 3 disrupted at midcarpal joint

☞ 21. **Scaphoid Dislocation**

  a) Second most frequently dislocated carpal

  b) Usually subluxed rather than fully dislocated

  c) Rotary subluxation: moved laterally with anterior rotation

  d) PA projection shows small, foreshortened scaphoid, somewhat circular: ("*ring sign*," or "*signet ring sign*")

  e) Widened space between scaphoid and lunate (> 4 mm): "*Terry Thomas sign*"

☞ 22. **Perilunate Dislocation**

  a) All carpals except the lunate displace dorsally

  b) Lunate remains in normal apposition to radius

  c) PA view shows capitate overlying the lunate

23. **Trans-scaphoid Perilunate Dislocation**

  a) Similar to perilunate, except there is fracture through the scaphoid waist

  b) Scaphoid proximal fragment retains normal

position with the lunate; distal fragment dislocates dorsally with other carpals

24. deQuervain's Fracture Dislocation

   a) Scaphoid fracture

   b) Anterior displacement of proximal scaphoid fragment, with anterior lunate displacement

Q. HAND AND FINGER FRACTURES AND DISLOCATIONS

1. General Features

   a) Phalanges are most common fracture sites in entire skeleton

   b) Examination requires three projections: PA, oblique, and lateral

   c) For phalanges, single-digit collimated views should be done

   d) **DDX:** nutrient canals, sesamoids (especially with thumb examinations)

   e) Fifth is most commonly fractured metacarpal, most often in distal half

   f) 50% of phalangeal fractures are distal, 15% proximal, 10% middle

2. Boxer's Fracture

   a) Transverse fracture of second or third metacarpal neck

   b) Caused by impact of short, straight jabbing blow

3. Barroom Fracture

   a) Transverse fracture of fourth or fifth metacarpal neck

   b) Caused by "roundhouse" blow

   c) This and boxer's fracture result in anterior angulation of metacarpal head and shortening and rotation of distal fragment

4. Shaft Fracture

   a) Usually third and fourth metacarpals, singly or simultaneously

   b) Dorsal angulation and displacement across fracture site

5. Bennett's Fracture (Fig. 4.16)

   a) First metacarpal fracture/dislocation

   b) Intraarticular fracture through base of first metacarpal

   c) Shaft displaces dorsally and radially

   d) Small proximal/medial fragment retains alignment with trapezium

6. Rolando's Fracture (synonym: comminuted Bennett's fracture)

   a) Intraarticular fracture through base of first metacarpal

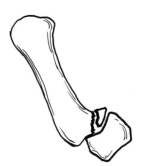

Figure 4.16.

Bennett's fracture. Reprinted with permission from Yochum TR, Rowe LJ. Essentials of Skeletal Radiology, 2nd ed. Baltimore: Williams & Wilkins, 1996:767.

      b) Least common first metacarpal fracture; difficult to treat

7. Transverse Fracture

      a) Most common type of first metacarpal fracture

      b) Fracture line is articular, but may be obliquely oriented

8. Salter-Harris type II Fracture of First Metacarpal

      a) In adolescents

9. Distal Phalangeal Fracture

      a) Most are in middle finger

      b) May be transverse, longitudinal, comminuted, or chip fractures

      c) Transverse are usually near the base

      d) Comminuted are most common, usually at distal tuft

      e) Chip fractures at phalangeal base corners

       f) *"Mallet finger"* or *"baseball finger"*: disabled extension of DIP, flexion deformity caused by chip fracture at posterior corner of base of phalanx

10. Middle Phalangeal Fracture

      a) Distal shaft of middle phalanx most vulnerable

      b) Anterior phalangeal base fracture: "volar plate fracture"

11. Proximal Phalangeal Fracture

      a) Usually in mid- or proximal shaft of the phalanx

      b) Seldom intraarticular

12. Turret Exostosis

      a) Bony prominence on ulnar dorsal base of proximal or middle phalanx

      b) Traumatic subperiosteal hemorrhage; soft tissue mass which has ossified

      c) High rate of recurrence after surgical removal

      d) **DDX:** sessile osteochondroma

13. Metacarpophalangeal Joint dislocation

      a) Most common at digits one and five

      b) Simple dislocation: easily reducible

      c) Complex dislocations: have entrapped, avulsed volar plate in joint; need open reduction: sign is a sesamoid bone within a widened joint space

14. Gamekeeper's Thumb (Fig. 4.17)

      a) First metacarpophalangeal tear or rupture of ulnar collateral ligament

b) Abduction stress view of thumb shows widened ulnar side of MCP joint, indicating instability

c) May have a chip fracture, with small fragment from ulnar margin of proximal phalanx base

d) MR will demonstrate ulnar collateral ligament lesions

15. Interphalangeal Dislocation

a) Usually caused by acute hyperextension

b) Usually phalanx will be dorsally displaced, rarely come to rest anteriorly

c) Most commonly, one joint per digit is dislocated; occasionally two on the same digit

d) May have associated volar plate fracture: this may be entrapped in joint, require open reduction

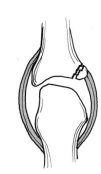

Figure 4.17.
Gamekeeper's thumb. Reprinted with permission from Yochum TR, Rowe LJ. Essentials of Skeletal Radiology, 2nd ed. Baltimore: Williams & Wilkins, 1996:770.

R. STRESS FRACTURES

 1. Etiology and Definitions

a) Repetitive trauma or microtrauma, either tensile (at tendon/ligament insertions) or compressive at point of repeated impact

b) Caused by alterations of balance or of normal stress patterns (e.g., post-surgical)

c) Caused by weakened pathologic bone

d) Fatigue fracture: secondary to stress on normal bone

e) Insufficiency fracture: secondary to normal stress on inadequate or weakened bone, e.g., Paget's disease, osteoporosis, osteomalacia, rickets, osteopetrosis, fibrous dysplasia, osteogenesis imperfecta

2. Clinical Features

a) Pain related to activity and alleviated by rest

b) Soft tissue swelling, local tenderness over site of stress fracture

c) Most common sites:
- metatarsals (middle and distal shafts of second and third metatarsals most frequently); called "*march fracture*," "*Deutchlanders disease*"
- proximal tibia
- calcaneus
- fibular metaphyses (distal more often than proximal)
- pars interarticularis (**most common stress fracture in entire skeleton**)
- hook of the hamate
- outer third of clavicle

3. Radiologic Features

a) Often occult; requires bone scan or delayed plain film images

b) Minimum latent period for plain films: 10 days to 3 weeks

c) Bone scan is sensitive, not specific

d) CT may be able to delineate fracture line through sclerosis

e) Periosteal response: local periosteal and endosteal cortical thickening

f) Viewed *en face*, callus creates linear, transverse, sclerotic band

- characteristic of stress fracture in calcaneus
- seen as vertically oriented, dense radiopaque line in calcaneus
- in other sites, transversely oriented; **DDX:** growth arrest line because the callus margins are hazy and poorly defined

g) **DDX:** growth arrest lines (see above)

- chronic osteomyelitis (Brodie's Abscess): lack of adjacent bone destruction
- osteoid osteoma: use CT to visualize lucent oval nidus
- osteosarcoma: stress fracture gives solid periosteal response; sarcoma renders spiculated pattern and involves bone destruction

S. NON-ACCIDENTAL TRAUMA

1. Synonyms

a) Battered child syndrome

b) Parent-infant traumatic stress syndrome

c) Infant abuse syndrome

d) Shaken infant syndrome

2. General Features

a) Clinical and radiologic evidence of repeated injury

b) Hallmark of physically abusive relationship, whether parent or guardian to child; adult child to elderly or infirm parent; or spouse to spouse (or significant other)

c) Clinically: multiple bruises, burns, localized traumatic alopecia

d) Fractures caused by abuse are most common in children under five; 80% under 18 months

e) Shaken infant syndrome gives whiplash injuries including: retinal hemorrhages, subdural hemorrhages, cerebral edema, and skull fractures

☞   **3. Radiologic Features**

a) Suspected abuse should occasion full skeletal survey:
- PA and lateral chest
- AP bilateral humeri and forearms
- PA hands
- AP pelvis
- AP and lateral lumbar spine
- AP lower extremities
- AP and lateral skull
- repeat imaging on symptomatic sites in 7–10 days; or use bone scan
- cranial CT scan if neurologic abnormalities are observed

T. POSTTRAUMATIC MYOSITIS OSSIFICANS

1. Synonyms

a) Myositis ossificans posttraumatica

b) Ossifying hematoma

c) Traumatic ossifying myositis

d) Heterotopic posttraumatic bone formation

☞   **2. General Features**

a) Bone formation in soft tissues after trauma

b) Happens in muscle, fascia, tendons, joint capsules, ligaments

c) Usually after local injury causing bruising or hemorrhage

d) Most commonly at brachialis anterior, quadriceps femoris, thigh adductors, knee's medial collateral ligament (Pellegrini-Stieda disease), coracoclavicular ligament, or deltoid muscle

e) Prussian's disease (saddle tumor): ossification in adductor magnus found in riders

f) Ischial tuberosities or paravertebral sites may host ossification caused by gravitational stress in invalids

3. Lumbar Ossified Bridge Syndrome (LOBS)

a) Hematoma in psoas muscle may form union between lumbar transverse processes

b) This forms complete bone, with cortex, medullary bone, and marrow

c) Sometimes causes pain; relieved by surgical excision

4. Ossified Achilles Tendon

a) Caused by surgery and sometimes trauma

b) Sometimes occurs with DISH, fluorosis, ochronosis, Wilson's disease, renal failure, Reiter's syndrome, gout, AS

    c) Ossification is within tendon; has mature bone with marrow; is subject to fracture

5. **Cortical Irregularity Syndrome**

    a) Roughened posterior femur in young adults (archaic: periosteal desmoid)

    b) distal linea aspera enthesopathy

    c) **DDX:** osteosarcoma (not likely in this location)

REVIEW—STUDY QUESTIONS

1. Describe a Colles' fracture and compare it with a Smith's fracture.
2. What intrathoracic lesions should be considered when significant trauma with rib fracture is present?
3. What projection is optimal when searching for a clavicle fracture?
4. Describe the soft tissue indicators for a fracture at the elbow.
5. What carpal is most frequently fractured and what complications may arise from this fracture?
6. What is a Galeazzi fracture and what complications accompany it?
7. Describe a Monteggia fracture.
8. What is the most commonly encountered scapulohumeral dislocation and what are its complications?
9. Describe a "mallet finger": the actual lesion, the clinical appearance, and the treatment.
10. Compare the boxer's fracture and the bar room fracture, and explain how they occur.
11. What is a "B-B fracture" and where might it occur?
12. Explain the Neer classification of proximal humeral fractures.
13. What is "game keeper's thumb"? What is the optimal plain film view for its diagnosis?
14. What is Safeway elbow? How is the injury acquired? How is it reduced?
15. What is a Bankart lesion, and with what sort of trauma is it usually associated?

1. A subtrochanteric femoral fracture (about 2 inches distal to the lesser trochanter):

   a) is rare and usually pathologic.
   b) is the most common femoral fracture.
   c) is seen most commonly in young athletes.
   d) is, of all femoral fractures, most prone to subsequent ischemic necrosis.

2. The FBI sign is a radiographic indication of:

   a) hematoma.
   b) lipoma.
   c) lipohemarthrosis.
   d) bilateral fracture to the ilia.

3. Chopart's dislocation is:

   a) a rare midtarsal dislocation.
   b) a proximal fibular dislocation.
   c) a femorotibular dislocation.
   d) a superolateral patellar dislocation.

4. Posterior humeral capsular fat pads:

   a) are normally not visible on lateral elbow projections.
   b) are normally oriented horizontally on lateral elbow projections.
   c) are normally oriented obliquely on lateral elbow projections.
   d) are obliterated completely when there is significant swelling at the elbow.

5. Radiographic evidence of a rotator cuff tear may include:

   a) a hatchet defect.
   b) a decreased acromiohumeral space ($<$ 7 mm).
   c) an increased acromiohumeral space ($>$ 5 mm).
   d) a "hanging shoulder" or "drooping shoulder."

6. A fracture that disrupts the bone between the inferior orbital fissure and the lateral maxillary wall, and also shatters the ethmoid bone, is classified as:

   a) an orbital blowout fracture.
   b) a LeFort I fracture.
   c) a LeFort II fracture.
   d) a LeFort III fracture.

7. The most common lumbar spine fracture is:

   a) a burst fracture.
   b) a fracture of the transverse process of L4 or L5.
   c) a Chance fracture.
   d) a vertebral body compression fracture.

8. Fracture healing involves three major phases, which are:

   a) the circulatory (inflammatory) phase, the reparative (metabolic) phase, and the remodeling (mechanical) phase.

   b) the circulatory (inflammatory) phase, the vascular phase, and the remodeling (mechanical) phase.
   c) the vascular phase, the metabolic phase, and the reparative phase.
   d) the vascular phase, the reparative (metabolic) phase, and the primary callus phase.

9. Ferguson's view, or Hibbs' projection, helpful in detecting L5 pars defects and anterolisthesis, is:

   a) a cross-table lateral projection.
   b) an upright lateral projection.
   c) a "tilt-up" upright AP projection.
   d) a weight-bearing oblique projection.

10. Another term for a stress fracture is:

   a) fatigue fracture.
   b) pseudofracture.
   c) occult fracture.
   d) increment fracture.

11. Risk of nonunion or avascular necrosis is greatest when:

   a) a fracture of the proximal femur occurs in an elderly female.
   b) a proximal femur fracture is subtrochanteric.
   c) a proximal femur fracture is intracapsular.
   d) a proximal femur fracture is intertrochanteric.

12. When an AP radiograph of the knee shows the full fibular head, overlapping very little with the tibial condyle, one may suspect a diagnosis of:

   a) distal tibiofibular diastatic fracture.
   b) anterolateral proximal tibiofibular dislocation.
   c) posteromedial proximal tibiofibular dislocation.
   d) distal fibular malleolar fracture.

13. A dancer's fracture must be differentiated from:

   a) a longitudinally oriented juvenile apophysis.
   b) a horizontally oriented juvenile apophysis.
   c) a transversely oriented juvenile apophysis.
   d) a Jones' fracture.

14. Little Leaguer's Elbow may involve:

   a) lateral epicondyle avulsion.
   b) bilateral epicondylar avulsions.
   c) medial epicondylar avulsion.
   d) triceps tendon rupture.

15. "Luxatio erecta" is a synonym for:

   a) posterior glenohumeral joint dislocation.
   b) inferior glenohumeral joint dislocation.
   c) anterior glenohumeral joint dislocation.
   d) Sprengel's deformity.

16. Mandibular fracture is best demonstrated radiographically by:

a) an overpenetrated Towne's projection.
b) a lateral projection with the injured side adjacent to the film.
c) a lateral projection with the uninjured side adjacent to the film.
d) a Caldwell projection.

17. Adequate radiographic imaging of the upper thoracic vertebrae may require:

a) an apical lordotic projection.
b) a swimmer's lateral projection.
c) filtration of the thoracolumbar region.
d) left and right oblique projections.

18. During the vascular phase of fracture healing:

a) a vascular spindle forms in the area of hyperemia around the injury.
b) a mesenchymal blastema is created by granulation tissue around the injury.
c) the hematoma around the injury is replaced by granulation tissue.
d) cartilage and osteoid are formed or deposited within the healing callus.

19. A "bowline of Brailsford" on a frontal projection is indicative of:

a) advanced degenerative joint disease.
b) spina bifida occulta.
c) spondylolisthesis of L5 on S1.
d) facet imbrication.

20. Pathologic fractures often appear:

a) unusually jagged.
b) smooth, disrupting the bone in a straight, transverse line.
c) in a spiral pattern, with a white line of impaction.
d) comminuted, with excessive fragmentation.

21. An "open book pelvis" or "sprung pelvis" is best described as:

a) a symphysis pubis diastasis.
b) diastasis of the symphysis pubis and one or both sacroiliac joints.
c) fracture/dislocation of one or both ilia.
d) the lateral displacement of one or both ilia, with bilateral fractures of the pubic rami.

22. Transverse (or slightly oblique) patellar fractures:

a) are the most common patellar fractures.
b) are seen less often than stellate patellar fractures.
c) are less common than vertical patellar fractures.
d) are the least common patellar fractures.

23. Lisfranc's injury involves:

a) multiple proximal metatarsal fractures.
b) foot dislocation without fracture.
c) ankle dislocation without fracture.
d) tarsometatarsal fracture dislocation.

24. The position of the humeral head after a proximal humeral shaft fracture may be affected by any of the following muscles except:

a) the rotator cuff muscles.
b) the deltoid muscle.
c) the triceps muscles.
d) the pectoralis major muscle.

25. The most common location for the humeral head after an anterior glenohumeral dislocation is:

a) an intrathoracic position.
b) a subclavicular position.
c) a subglenoid position.
d) a subcoracoid position.

26. Up to 80% of skull fractures are:

a) depressed fractures.
b) in the base of the skull.
c) linear fractures.
d) incomplete fractures.

27. Nuclear bone scan is a useful imaging modality for trauma patients because of its:

a) high specificity for occult fracture.
b) high sensitivity for occult fracture.
c) high specificity for non-fracture articular damage.
d) high sensitivity for non-fracture articular damage.

28. The hematoma at a fracture site:

a) is essential for proper callus formation.
b) should be resorbed within 10 days.
c) may delay healing if it is allowed to remain at the site.
d) is normally resorbed during the cellular phase of healing.

29. Factors that may predispose a patient to the development of a degenerative spondylolisthesis include all of the following except:

a) female gender.
b) hyperlordosis with an unstable lumbosacral joint.
c) sacralization of L5.
d) facet joint arthrosis.

30. When it occurs in the spine, the injury that is called an "impaction fracture" in the appendicular skeleton is called:

a) a torus fracture.
b) a teardrop fracture.
c) a compression fracture.
d) a limbus bone.

31. A "tug lesion" (iliac avulsion fracture):

a) is usually a pathologic avulsion fracture caused by osteochondroma at the ASIS.
b) is usually a pathologic avulsion of the rectus femoris from the AIIS.
c) is often caused by repetitive stress, causing avulsion of the sartorius from the ASIS or avulsion of the rectus femoris from the AIIS.
d) is most commonly an avulsion of osteoporotic bone in a geriatric patient.

32. An avulsion of the lateral tibial condyle by the tensor fascia lata (iliotibial band) tendon is termed:
    a) Segond's fracture.
    b) Cotton's fracture.
    c) Pott's fracture.
    d) Dupuytren's fracture.

33. Ankle fractures include all of the following except:
    a) Tillaux's fracture.
    b) Maisonneuve's fracture.
    c) Jones' fracture.
    d) Dupuytren's fracture.

34. When the surgical neck of the humerus is fractured, the shaft usually is displaced:
    a) posteriorly.
    b) superiorly.
    c) anterolaterally.
    d) anteromedially.

35. A Bankart lesion is:
    a) an avulsion of the inferior glenoid rim at the insertion of the triceps.
    b) an avulsion of the superior glenoid rim at the insertion of the supraspinatus.
    c) a "chip fracture" of the humeral head caused during anterior humeral dislocation.
    d) an impaction fracture of the humeral head acquired during posterior humeral dislocation.

36. On x-ray, a "growing fracture" in the skull may be an indication of:
    a) subdural hematoma.
    b) a leptomeningeal cyst.
    c) arachnoiditis.
    d) cerebral hemorrhage.

37. Nonunion of the secondary growth center for the spinous process must be differentiated from:
    a) a clay shoveler's fracture.
    b) a teardrop fracture.
    c) an articular pillar fracture.
    d) a Chance fracture.

38. The inflammatory (circulatory) phase of fracture repair:
    a) may last as long as 60 days.
    b) has four sub-phases, each of which may last as long as 10 days.
    c) involves necrosis, hematoma formation, vascular spindle formation, and primary callus formation.
    d) is the second phase of repair.

39. Some of the classifications of spondylolisthesis are:
    a) dysplastic, degenerative, or traumatic.
    b) congenital, degenerative, or infectious.
    c) dysplastic, isthmic, or infectious.
    d) infectious, dysplastic, or pathologic.

40. An avulsion fracture is the term used to describe:
    a) the bending of a soft bone, with no cortical disruption.
    b) cortical disruption only on the convex side of the injured bone.
    c) a cortical fragment torn away by tractional force of the ligament or tendon.
    d) a bone fragment driven into another portion of the bone.

41. A bucket-handle pelvic fracture is caused by:
    a) excessive weight-bearing in a geriatric or osteoporotic patient.
    b) an impact contralateral to the actual fracture.
    c) traumatic compressive force, as in a fall from great height.
    d) traumatic impact from behind and above.

42. With traumatic hyperextension of the knee:
    a) the posterior cruciate ligament may avulse the medial tibial plateau.
    b) the posterior cruciate ligament may avulse the lateral tibial plateau.
    c) the anterior cruciate ligament may avulse the anterior tibial spine.
    d) the anterior cruciate ligament may avulse the medial tibial plateau.

43. A distal fibular fracture with rupture of the distal tibiofibular ligament but no malleolar fracture is:
    a) a Colles' fracture.
    b) a Pott's fracture.
    c) a Dupuytren's fracture.
    d) a bumper fracture.

44. Significant displacement (> 1 cm) of the free fragment in a flap fracture indicates:
    a) probable ankle instability.
    b) probable patellar tendon rupture.
    c) probable significant rotator cuff rupture.
    d) probable atlantoaxial instability.

45. The most common fracture of the clavicle is:
    a) a middle clavicle fracture.
    b) a medial clavicle fracture.
    c) a fracture of the distal third of the clavicle.
    d) an avulsion fracture at the insertion of the acromioclavicular ligament.

46. The optimal imaging modality for demonstrating skull fractures is:
    a) CT.
    b) MRI.
    c) plain films.
    d) tomography.

47. Acute anterior cervical cord syndrome (immediate, complete paralysis, loss of pain and temperature) is associated with:
    a) a teardrop fracture.
    b) a burst fracture.
    c) a Jefferson fracture.
    d) a Type 2 odontoid fracture.

48. The Salter-Harris Type V fracture is:

    a) a pathologic fracture seen with rickets.
    b) an oblique fracture requiring open reduction.
    c) the most commonly seen Salter-Harris fracture.
    d) an impaction fracture of the physis.

49. Pars defects in newborns:

    a) are seen more frequently in Native American infants than in other populations.
    b) have never been reported.
    c) are asymptomatic, and are incidental findings on x-rays taken for other purposes.
    d) occur only in approximately 1% of x-rayed infants.

50. A comminuted fracture involves:

    a) a bone separated into two fragments.
    b) a bone separated into more than two fragments.
    c) disruption of the skin over the fracture.
    d) disruption of the bone on the convex surface of the injury only.

51. The posterolateral impaction fracture often occurring with anterior glenohumeral dislocation is best demonstrated radiographically with:

    a) an internal rotation AP shoulder projection.
    b) an external rotation AP shoulder projection.
    c) an axillary view.
    d) a weighted external rotation AP shoulder view.

52. Cotton's fracture is:

    a) a fracture of the medial malleolus distal to the talar plafond.
    b) a fracture of the lateral malleolus distal to the talar plafond.
    c) a bimalleolar fracture.
    d) a trimalleolar fracture.

53. A "bumper fracture" is:

    a) a fracture of the tibial plateau.
    b) a fracture of the proximal fibula.
    c) a "B-B fracture" involving both tibia and fibula.
    d) a fracture of the tibial shaft with distal fibulo-tibial diastasis.

54. A Malgaigne fracture is:

    a) a pelvic fracture.
    b) an elbow fracture.
    c) a fracture/dislocation of the distal radius.
    d) an ankle fracture.

55. Spondylolysis has a higher incidence among:

    a) white North Americans.
    b) Native Americans.
    c) black North Americans.
    d) northern Europeans.

56. The Mach band is:

    a) a shadow on the AP open mouth film caused by nonunion of a Type 3 odontoid fracture.
    b) a shadow on the AP open mouth film caused by the tongue.
    c) a shadow on the AP open mouth film caused by the dentocentral synchondrosis.
    d) a shadow on the AP open mouth film caused by the posterior arch of the atlas.

57. Factors in the development of osteonecrosis after fracture include all of the following except:

    a) vascularity of the bone at the fracture site.
    b) appropriate early treatment of the injury.
    c) extent of soft tissue damage at the fracture site.
    d) site of the fracture itself.

58. Adequate radiologic evaluation for acromioclavicular separation requires:

    a) overpenetrated AP views of the shoulder with external and internal rotation.
    b) bilateral non-weighted and weighted (patient holding 10–15 pound weights) AP views.
    c) bilateral internally and externally rotated AP views.
    d) underpenetrated AP view with 15° cephalad tube tilt.

59. The "Thurston-Holland sign" is:

    a) a humeral head fragment often seen with glenohumeral dislocations.
    b) a glenoid rim lesion seen with posterior glenohumeral dislocation.
    c) an indication of a good prognosis after a talar fracture.
    d) a metaphyseal fragment seen with a Salter-Harris Type II fracture.

60. When the ulnar styloid is fractured as the distal ulna dislocates, the result is called:

    a) a chauffeur's fracture.
    b) a Hutchinson's fracture.
    c) a Barton's fracture.
    d) a Moore's fracture.

61. The Neer classification considers fractures:

    a) of the proximal humeral shaft.
    b) of the femoral head and neck.
    c) of the humeral head and neck.
    d) of the radial head.

62. The ligament most often ruptured in ankle injuries is the:

    a) deltoid ligament.
    b) tibiofibular ligament.
    c) medial collateral ligament.
    d) lateral collateral ligament.

63. The most common hip dislocation leaves the femoral head in:

    a) an anterior superior position.
    b) an anteromedial position.
    c) a superior posterior position.
    d) an inferolateral position.

64. Whenever there is a pelvic or sacral fracture:

    a) there is high probability of nonunion.
    b) there is high probability of subsequent avascular necrosis.
    c) there is high probability of associated injury to pelvic organs.
    d) there is high probability of reflex sympathetic dystrophy syndrome.

65. A Chance fracture:

    a) almost always involves neurologic deficit.
    b) most commonly is seen at L4 or L5.
    c) specifically involves horizontal splitting of the spinous process, pedicle, and posterior body to the superior endplate.
    d) involves the cleaving of an entire lumbar vertebra on a coronal plane.

66. The hangman's fracture is the result of:

    a) traumatic compression.
    b) traumatic hyperflexion.
    c) traumatic hyperextension.
    d) traumatic distraction.

67. Posttraumatic osteolysis is a complication that is likely to be seen after fracture of the:

    a) tarsal navicular.
    b) calcaneus.
    c) distal clavicle.
    d) acromion.

68. Fracture of the distal clavicle may be followed by:

    a) stress hypertrophy of the acromion.
    b) posttraumatic osteolysis of the distal clavicle.
    c) stress hypertrophy of the distal clavicle.
    d) stress hypertrophy of the coracoid process.

69. The most frequently seen type of Salter-Harris fracture is:

    a) Salter-Harris Type I.
    b) Salter-Harris Type II.
    c) Salter-Harris Type IV.
    d) Salter-Harris Type V.

70. In the common childhood injury known as "toddler elbow":

    a) forceful supination of the forearm dislocates the radial head.
    b) pronation coupled with hyperextension of the elbow dislocates the radial head.
    c) the annular ligament becomes entrapped in the radioulnar joint.
    d) the annular ligament becomes entrapped in the radiohumeral joint.

71. A "head-splitting fracture" refers to:

    a) a LeFort Type III fracture.
    b) a cranial diastasis.
    c) a comminution of the humeral head.
    d) an impaction fracture of the radial head.

72. When an ankle fracture exists, ligament ruptures should be ruled out by:

    a) stress studies comparing the ankles bilaterally.
    b) stress studies looking for $> 6°$ combined lateral and medial tilt.
    c) stress studies looking for $> 6°$ tilt in either lateral or medial joint tilt.
    d) stress studies looking for any joint space > 3 mm.

73. A normal Klein's line should:

    a) intersect the superolateral acetabular margin.
    b) intersect the fovea capitus centralis.
    c) intersect the femoral head.
    d) pass tangential to the superolateral margin of the femoral head.

74. The most commonly seen sacral fracture is:

    a) a transverse fracture at the third or fourth sacral tubercle level.
    b) a vertical sacral fracture.
    c) an avulsion of the sacral promontory.
    d) a horizontal fracture at the level of the second sacral tubercle.

75. Traumatic fracture of the lumbar pars interarticularis:

    a) is the third most common occult fracture.
    b) is extremely rare and results only from violent hyperextension.
    c) is the second most common cause of a "pars defect."
    d) is most likely to occur at L1, as opposed to a stress fracture of the pars, which occurs at L4 or L5.

76. A "guillotine" effect may be produced on the cervical spinal cord when there is:

    a) a congenital block vertebra.
    b) a ruptured transverse ligament.
    c) spina bifida occulta of the atlas and axis.
    d) a persistent ossiculum terminale of the axis.

77. The fracture most frequently associated with fat embolism formation is a fracture of:

    a) the pelvis.
    b) the spine.
    c) the femur.
    d) the tibia.

78. The bone most frequently fractured in the birth process is:

    a) the maternal coccyx.
    b) the infant acromion.
    c) the infant clavicle.
    d) the maternal ischial spine.

79. Good apposition of a fracture refers to:

    a) almost complete surface contact of fractured fragments.
    b) lack of angulation between fractured fragments.

c)   optimal alignment of fractured fragments.

d)   little or no rotation of the distal fragment around its long axis.

80. The Galeazzi (or Piedmont) fracture is a serious injury because:

a)   it often results in permanent neurologic damage.

b)   it usually results in rupture of the radial artery.

c)   it is subject to nonunion and redislocation despite surgical reduction.

d)   it usually results in Sudeck's atrophy.

81. All of the following must be assessed in the evaluation of acromioclavicular joint injury except:

a)   coracoclavicular distance.

b)   anterior glenohumeral joint space.

c)   acromioclavicular joint space.

d)   acromioclavicular joint alignment.

82. The optimal imaging modality for demonstration of damage to the knee ligaments or meniscus is:

a)   MRI.

b)   CT.

c)   arthrography.

d)   scintigraphy.

83. An optimal radiologic study for evaluating slipped femoral capital epiphysis should include:

a)   AP and "frog-leg" hip views of the involved side.

b)   bilateral AP and "frog-leg" hip views.

c)   bilateral AP and overpenetrated lateral hip views.

d)   bilateral AP hip views with internal and external rotation of the thigh.

84. Conservative treatment of a patient with spondylolisthesis has a poor prognosis if:

a)   there are bilateral pars defects.

b)   there is a unilateral pars defect.

c)   flexion and extension lateral lumbar films indicate instability at the level of the lesion.

d)   the patient is < 20 years of age.

85. Cauda equina injury is most likely to result from:

a)   a thoracolumbar compression fracture.

b)   a lumbar "burst" fracture.

c)   a Chance fracture.

d)   a lumbar transverse process fracture.

86. Significant trauma to the cervical spine involves neurologic damage in approximately:

a)   10–14% of cases.

b)   40% of cases.

c)   4% of cases.

d)   60–70% of cases.

87. Following a fracture, x-ray indication of clostridium perfringens infection may show as:

a)   thin, linear, parallel lucent streaks within muscle planes.

b)   lucent "bubbles" around the newly formed callus.

c)   lucent "bubbles" just below the skin contour.

d)   lucent streaks between the periosteum and cortical surface.

88. A "golfer's fracture" involves:

a)   the tip of a spinous process, usually between C6 and T2.

b)   a stress fracture of the proximal lateral metatarsals.

c)   fracture of the lateral rib margin.

d)   fracture of the ulnar styloid.

89. A spiral fracture is distinguished by:

a)   sharply pointed ends of the fracture fragments.

b)   an angled fracture line with blunt fracture ends.

c)   a "bulge" in the bone on the concave side of the injury.

d)   a spiral-shaped avulsed bone fragment.

90. A comminuted radial head fracture coupled with distal radioulnar dislocation is called a(n):

a)   "baby car" fracture.

b)   Galeazzi fracture.

c)   Essex-Lopresti fracture.

d)   Monteggia fracture.

91. Glenoid labral tears are called:

a)   Bankart lesions.

b)   rim signs.

c)   SITS lesions.

d)   SLAP lesions.

92. Pelligrini-Stieda disease is defined as:

a)   ununited avulsions at the lateral femoral condyle.

b)   medial collateral ligament calcifications at the distal femur caused by previous avulsions.

c)   ununited avulsions of the medial tibial plateau.

d)   calcifications in the lateral collateral ligament; possibly caused by previous ligament damage.

93. Slipped femoral capital epiphysis (SFCE) is:

a)   now known to be genetically mediated.

b)   now recognized as a pathologic fracture.

c)   actually a Salter-Harris Type 1 stress fracture.

d)   almost always preceded by significant trauma.

94. The Meyerding classification system grades spondylolisthesis displacement:

a)   by 10% increments, based on lateral projections.

b)   by 25% increments, based on lateral projections.

c)   by 10% increments, based on anterior oblique projections.

d) by 25% increments, based on anterior oblique projections.

95. A linear zone of impaction below a vertebral body endplate denotes:

a) an old, healed fracture.
b) a recent fracture.
c) a period of arrested growth.
d) Paget's disease.

96. Spinal fractures are most common in the:

a) lumbar spine.
b) thoracic spine.
c) cervical and thoracolumbar areas.
d) mid-cervical spine.

97. Muscle damage adjacent to a fracture site:

a) must be repaired surgically.
b) has no effect on the healing of the fracture itself.
c) appears to enhance fracture healing.
d) appears to be detrimental to fracture healing.

98. The ''costal hook sign'' may indicate the presence of:

a) costochondral calcifications.
b) atelectasis.
c) bronchogenic carcinoma.
d) a flail segment.

99. MRI is the only imaging modality that is capable of displaying:

a) an occult fracture.
b) a bone bruise.
c) a stress fracture.
d) a torus fracture.

100. Wolff's law, which applies in fracture healing, states that:

a) callus forms only when the hematoma is undisturbed.
b) stress will retard the formation of callus.
c) stress will speed the formation of callus.
d) bone is deposited in stressed areas and removed from non-stressed areas.

PRACTICE TEST CHAPTER 4—ANSWER KEY

1.	a	11.	c	21.	b	31.	c	41.	b	51.	a	61.	c	71.	c	81.	b	91.	d
2.	c	12.	b	22.	a	32.	a	42.	c	52.	d	62.	d	72.	a	82.	a	92.	b
3.	a	13.	a	23.	d	33.	c	43.	b	53.	a	63.	c	73.	c	83.	b	93.	c
4.	a	14.	c	24.	c	34.	d	44.	c	54.	a	64.	c	74.	a	84.	c	94.	b
5.	b	15.	b	25.	d	35.	a	45.	a	55.	b	65.	c	75.	b	85.	b	95.	b
6.	c	16.	a	26.	c	36.	b	46.	a	56.	d	66.	c	76.	b	86.	b	96.	c
7.	d	17.	b	27.	b	37.	a	47.	a	57.	c	67.	c	77.	c	87.	a	97.	c
8.	a	18.	a	28.	a	38.	c	48.	d	58.	b	68.	b	78.	c	88.	c	98.	d
9.	c	19.	c	29.	b	39.	a	49.	b	59.	d	69.	b	79.	a	89.	a	99.	b
10.	a	20.	b	30.	c	40.	c	50.	b	60.	d	70.	d	80.	c	90.	c	100.	d

Chapter 5

ARTHRITIDES

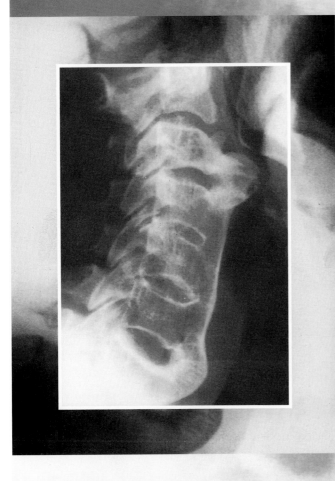

A. JOINT CLASSIFICATION

TABLE 5.1
Joint Classifications

Motion Characteristics	Tissue Type	Examples
Synarthroses essentially immobile	fibrous	cranial sutures, teeth
Amphiarthroses slightly movable	cartilaginous	symphysis pubis, symphysis menti, intervertebral disc
Diarthroses freely movable	synovial	hinge joints, ball and socket, saddle joints, mortise joints

B. TERMINOLOGY

a) *enthesis*—periarticular site of tendon or ligament insertion into bone
b) *enthesopathy*—inflammation at enthesis; seen on plain film as cortical erosion and/or periostitis
c) *monoarticular*—involving a single joint
d) *pauciarticular*—involving two to four (2–4) joints
e) *polyarticular*—involving more than four (>4) joints
f) *uniform loss of joint space*—entire joint space evenly reduced
g) *nonuniform loss of joint space*—most heavily stressed area or compartment of joint space most severely reduced
h) *osteophyte*—extension of cortical bone (often with visible subcortical trabecular bone) at site of periarticular ligament insertion; usually has a cartilaginous cap; indicates degeneration
i) *syndesmophyte*—ossification of a spinal ligament; indicates an inflammatory process
j) *spondylophyte*—spinal osteophyte
k) *hyperostosis*—exuberant ossification of tendons or ligaments
l) *periostitis*—inflammatory elevation of periosteum; leads to formation of periosteal new bone
m) *spondyloarthropathy*—spinal inflammatory arthritis
n) *seronegative arthritis*—inflammatory arthritis without rheumatoid factor
o) *rheumatoid variants*—seronegative arthritides that simulate rheumatoid arthritis clinically, but not radiographically or pathologically

C. CATEGORIES OF ARTHRITIDES

   1. **Inflammatory**

   a) Symmetric, polyarticular

   b) Osteopenic subarticular bone, poorly defined erosions, periostitis

   c) Includes: rheumatoid arthritis, juvenile rheumatoid arthritis, ankylosing spondylitis, enteropathic arthritis, psoriatic arthritis, Reiter's syndrome, systemic lupus erythematosus, Jaccoud's arthritis, idiopathic chondrolysis of the hip, scleroderma, osteitis condensans ilii, osteitis pubis, hypertrophic osteoarthropathy

☞ **2. Degenerative**

  a) Monoarticular or pauciarticular with asymmetric distribution

  b) Sclerotic subarticular bone, osteophytes

  c) Includes: degenerative joint disease, erosive osteoarthritis, diffuse idiopathic skeletal hyperostosis, ossified posterior longitudinal ligament syndrome, neurotrophic arthropathy, synoviochondrometaplasia

☞ **3. Metabolic**

  a) Monoarticular or pauciarticular with asymmetric distribution

  b) Sharply defined erosions

  c) Includes: gout, calcium pyrophosphate dihydrate crystal deposition disease (CPPD), hydroxyapatite deposition disease, ochronosis, tumoral calcinosis, sarcoidosis, pigmented villonodular synovitis (PVNS)

D. JOINT ANATOMY

☞ **1. Synovial Joints**

  a) Fibrous capsule which functions as a ligament

  b) Synovial tissue (*synovium*): lines capsule and intracapsular non-articular bone

  c) Articular cartilage (*hyaline*): chondrocytes in collagen and a ground substance of chondroitin sulfate and water; 1–7 mm thick; lines subchondral bone plate (articular bone)

  d) Synovial fluid: plasma dialysate with mucoid exudate from synovial cells; provides joint nutrition and lubrication

  e) Bare area: at periphery of articular surface, a small area of intracapsular bone is covered by neither synovium nor articular cartilage; vulnerable to inflammatory erosion

  f) Subchondral bone plate: cortical and cancellous bone subadjacent to articular cartilage

  g) N.B., note that there is NO intracapsular periosteum

☞ **2. Intervertebral Discs**

  a) Superior and inferior surfaces: approximately 1 mm of hyaline cartilage, attached to cortical endplates of adjacent vertebrae

  b) Central nucleus pulposus: gelatinous in youth, these desiccate with age to become fibrocartilaginous; slightly post-central within disc

  c) Peripheral annulus fibrosus: medial fibers fibrocartilaginous, lateral fibers collagenous

3. **Fibrous Joint (synarthrosis)**
   a) Fibrous tissue interposed between bones
   b) Radius/ulna
   c) Tibia/fibula
   d) Opposing surfaces roughly parallel
   e) Irregular contour of surfaces is normal

4. **Cartilaginous Joint (amphiarthrosis)**
   a) Fibrocartilage is main interposed tissue
   b) Some hyaline cartilage may be present
   c) Symphysis pubis
   d) Sternoclavicular joint
   e) Intervertebral disc (IVD)

E. COMMONLY ENCOUNTERED ARTHRITIDES

TABLE 5.2
Common Arthritides

Incidence	Entity	Age/Gender Predilections
Very common	Osteoarthritis (DJD)	< 45: female, > 45: male
Common	rheumatoid arthritis (RA) diffuse idiopathic skeletal hyperostosis (DISH) ankylosing spondylitis (AS) pseudogout (CPPD) osteitis condensans ilii psoriatic Arthritis synoviochondrometaplasia	< 40: female, > 40: equal > 40: male < 40: male > 30: equal < 40: female < 40: equal < 30: male
Less Common	gout systemic lupus erythematosus (SLE) scleroderma Reiter's syndrome juvenile rheumatoid arthritis (JRA) (Still's)	> 40: male < 40: female < 40: female < 40: male 2–16: female

REVIEW—STUDY QUESTIONS

1. List three joint types as classified by tissue type; by motion characteristics. Give examples of each.
2. Describe the anatomy of a synovial joint.
3. Describe the anatomy of an intervertebral disc.
4. What is the most commonly occurring arthritis?
5. Name four arthritides with predilection for females. Specify their age predilections.
6. Name four arthritides with predilection for males. Specify their age predilections.
7. List five characteristics of inflammatory arthritides.
8. Contrast these characteristics with the characteristics of degenerative arthritis and with those of metabolic arthritides.

F. DEGENERATIVE JOINT DISEASE (DJD)

1. General Considerations

a) The most commonly seen arthritis

b) Noninflammatory, progressive process

c) Most commonly involves finger joints, weight-bearing joints

d) a.k.a. osteoarthritis (or . . .arthrosis); degenerative arthritis (or arthrosis); arthritis deformans; Kellgren's arthritis; hypertrophic arthritis

e) result of cartilage degeneration caused by insult (trauma, wear and tear, unidentified)

☞ **f)** classified as *primary* (idiopathic), *secondary* (caused by identified stress or trauma), or *erosive* (variant occurring in the hands, involving inflammation)

☞ **2. Clinical Features**

a) General features
- < 45 more common in males
- > 45 more common in females
- most common sites: proximal interphalangeal (PIP) joints; distal interphalangeal (DIP) joints; first metacarpal-trapezium joint; first metatarsal phalangeal joint; spine, hips, knees, and acromioclavicular (AC) joint
- onset is gradual; intermittent signs and symptoms
- usually stiffens with rest and improves with activity
- decreased articular or intersegmental motion
- complications: spinal stenosis; nerve entrapments; vertebral artery impingement

b) Features at specific sites
- most common spinal sites: C5–7; L4-S1; T6-L1
- cervical spine:
  1) C1 and C2 less commonly involved
  2) apophyseal joints: may develop degenerative spondylolisthesis
  3) most common cervical degenerative spondylolisthesis: C7 anterolisthesis
  4) neurocentral (uncovertebral, von Luschka) joint involvement (uncinate hypertrophy) may lead to foraminal encroachment; yields "pseudofracture" line seen on lateral cervical projection (most commonly at C5, 6, 7); can impinge on vertebral artery
  5) IVD narrowing, endplate sclerosis, osteophytes; sometimes vacuum cleft

6) reduced cervical lordosis; early hypermobility (instability); later reduced intersegmental mobility

7) osteophytes rarely produce dysphagia; more often cause spinal stenosis, reducing sagittal canal dimensions to < 12 mm

8) intercalary bone: calcification of anterior annulus

- thoracic spine:

1) affected at IVD, apophyseal joints (facet arthrosis), costovertebral and costotransverse joints

2) apophyseal involvement in lower thoracic spine

☞ 3) apophyseal pain from lower thoracic segments may refer to lower lumbar segments (*Maigne's syndrome*)

4) costal joint involvement in lower thoracic segments can simulate gastrointestinal disease (*Robert's syndrome*)

5) senile kyphosis (usually > 70 years old); infrequent, anterior IVD ankylosis

☞ - lumbar spine:

1) apophyseal (facet) joint involvement most common at L4 and L5

- leads to anterolisthesis (as in cervical segments), most common in females > 40 years old; most common at L4; occasionally retrolisthesis

- most diagnostic plain film for facet visualization is *oblique*

- specific roentgen signs: interruption of Hadley's "S" curve; pars sclerosis

2) IVD degeneration most common at L4 and L5

3) lumbar DJD roentgen signs:

- early: retrolisthesis, anterior lipping, vacuum cleft (of Knuttson), mild loss of disc height

- late: body displacement, severe disc space diminution, loss of intersegmental motion, large claw osteophytes

4) synovial (juxtaarticular, ganglion) cysts: usually at L4 and L5 facets

5) hemispheric spondylosclerosis (HSS): most common at L4 and L5 bodies; simulates appearance of neoplasm, infection

6) kissing spinous (*Baastrup's syndrome*)

7) anterolisthesis

- caused by reduced disc height and facet remodeling from a more

vertical to a more horizontal plane

- gives a broadened pedicle/facet angle
- may lead to lateral and/or central canal stenosis

- Sacroiliac joint
    1) visible changes in synovial portion (lower two-thirds) of joint
    2) joint space diminution (normal = 2–5 mm)
    3) iliac surface of joint may show 1–2 mm of sclerosis
    4) osteophytes form at superior or inferior margin of synovial joint area
    5) occasionally iliolumbar ligaments ossify
    6) occasional *senile ankylosis*
        - ossified interosseous ligaments
    7) vacuum cleft here is a **normal** physiologic finding, not a DJD sign

- Hip
    1) advanced cases termed *malum coxae senilis*; coxarthrosis
    2) may entail any of the eight universal DJD signs (see radiologic features, below); plus cortical buttressing
    3) correlation between hip arthrosis and decreased risk of osteoporosis
    4) decreased joint space
        - most common: decreased superiorly, widened medially (*Waldenstrom's sign*); femoral head migrates anterosuperiorly
        - occasionally, femoral head migrates posteromedially with medial joint space loss; may be associated with mild *protrusio acetabulae*
        - rarely, femoral head migrates superomedially; shows uniform loss of joint space, which is more common with inflammatory or infectious arthritides
    5) osteophytes usually form at superolateral acetabular rim or at the lateral and inferomedial surfaces of the femoral head
    6) commonly, large subchondral cysts appear in superior femoral head or at the supraacetabular margin; DDX neoplasm, avascular necrosis
    7) sclerosis appears in the same regions
    8) buttressing: stress reaction; thickens inferomedial femoral head and neck
    9) remodeling: deformities may include flattened superior femoral head, acetabular roof, "tilt" deformity

(resembles a "slipped" femoral head in appearance)

- Knee
    1) three compartments: lateral or medial femorotibial; patellofemoral
    2) usually single compartment affected—most often the medial
    3) femorotibial
        - best diagnosed (early) via MR
        - decreased medial joint space
        - little or no sclerosis
        - seldom cysts (if present, most likely in tibial plateau)
        - minimal osteophyte formation
        - early sign: "sharpened" tibial eminences   *spiking*
        - "joint mice" loose bodies; often calcified in concentric laminations (if not calcified, may need contrast arthrogram for detection)
        - varus deformity is a late sign
        - may see chondrocalcinosis in the decreased joint space
    4) patellofemoral changes: usually an adjunct to medial compartment degeneration
        - anterior femoral erosion (2–3 cm above patella)
        - sclerosis (usually on patellar surface)
        - osteophytes develop from the four patellar poles
        - irregular anterior patellar surface (spiculated: "tooth sign")
    5) chondromalacia patellae
        - most common in adolescents
        - idiopathic pain, crepitus, buckling, locking, stiffness, swelling
        - best visualization via MR; no radiologic features
        - provoked by stair climbing, long sitting ("movie sign")
        - "Q" angle > 20° may indicate chondromalacia risk (Fig. 5.1)
        - test for pain with patellofemoral compression, knee slightly flexed
        - patella alta may be contributing factor
- Foot and ankle
    1) ankle, tarsals rarely involved
    2) most common site in foot: first metatarsophalangeal (MTP) joint
    3) **DDX:** gout
    4) osteophytes, remodeling, valgus deformity (lateral displacement of phalanx)
    5) produces characteristic bunion

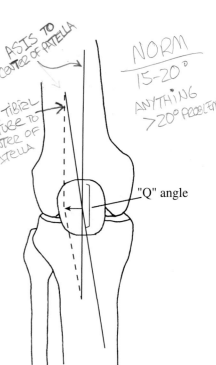

ASIS TO CENTER OF PATELLA

TIBIAL TUBE TO CENTER OF PATELLA

NORM 15-20° ANYTHING >20° PROBLEM

"Q" angle

Figure 5.1.

Reprinted with permission from Kessler AW. Management of Common Musculoskeletal Disorders. New York: Harper & Rowe, 1983:440.

- Shoulder
    1) most common in AC joint
    2) glenohumeral involvement usually post-traumatic
        - **DDX:** CPPD, ochronosis, acromegaly
        - rotator cuff degeneration (humeral head migrates superiorly)
        - erosion of inferior acromial surface
    3) calcific tendinitis, bursitis
        - often bilateral
        - most common at supraspinatus insertion into greater tuberosity
        - optimal view: external rotation
        - subacromial bursa calcifications also frequent
- Elbow
    1) secondary to trauma, repetitive microtrauma
    2) olecranon spur, loose bodies
- Wrist and hand
    1) most commonly secondary EXCEPT: primary in PIP, DIP, and first metacarpal-trapezial joints
    2) first metacarpal/trapezium
        - universal signs (see radiologic features, below) plus radial subluxation at the first metacarpal base
    3) radiocarpal joint
        - usually after fracture of scaphoid or radius
        - sequela: ischemic necrosis (lunate or scaphoid); CPPD
        - **DDX:** CPPD (where radioulnar triangular cartilage calcifies)
    4) hand
        - clinically visible phalangeal joint osseous nodules
            a) DIP joints: Heberden's nodes
            b) PIP joints: Bouchard's nodes
        - DIP malalignment common

☞   **3. Erosive Osteoarthritis (EOA)**
    a) DJD variant occurring in DIP, PIP joints
    b) Most common in middle-aged females (age 30–50 years)
    c) Episodic acute inflammation
    d) Symmetric involvement
    e) Swelling, pain, redness, decreased mobility, nodules
    f) May slightly elevate ESR; otherwise, lab results are normal
    g) Residual deformities

h) About 15% go on to develop RA

i) May involve radial carpals; invariably spares ulnar carpals

j) Radiographically resembles DJD, *except* it features:
- periostitis
- "gull wings" pattern (Fig. 5.2)
- sometimes bony ankylosis results

k) DDX: RA, DJD, psoriatic arthritis

Figure 5.2.
"Gull wings" sign. Reprinted with permission from Yochum TR, Rowe LJ. Essentials of Skeletal Radiology, 2nd ed. Baltimore: Williams & Wilkins, 1996:863.

4. **Pathologic Process and Laboratory Findings**

a) Mechanical (or chemical) disruption of chondrocyte function

b) Loss of chondroitin sulfate; collagen fibers exposed

c) Cartilage develops fissures, crevices

d) Vessels infiltrate, ulceration occurs

e) Cartilage is shed, exposing subchondral bone

f) Subchondral cysts develop (geodes)

g) Debris irritates synovium causing hypertrophy of synovial tissue

h) Altered joint space leads to altered function, causing joint capsule stress

i) Osteophytes form (cortical bone with cartilage cap)

j) Process can progress to osseous fusion of joint

k) IVD degeneration theories: mechanical stressors, autoimmune function, vascular insufficiency

l) In *erosive osteoarthritis*, the ESR may be slightly elevated, otherwise laboratory findings are unremarkable

5. **Radiologic Features**

a) Eight "universal" radiologic features characteristic of DJD:
- asymmetric distribution
- nonuniform loss of joint space
- osteophytes
- subchondral sclerosis (eburnation): trabecular thickening in areas of mechanical stress
- subchondral cysts (geodes): synovial fluid intrudes into subchondral bone
- intra-articular loose bodies (joint mice): cartilage fragmentation and subchondral bone flaking or synovial metaplasia with debris (synoviochondrometaplasia)
- articular deformity: remodeling of articular surfaces
- joint subluxation: instability

b) N.B., vacuum cleft: denotes degeneration in *spinal DJD*, but not in other joints

REVIEW—STUDY QUESTIONS

1. Name three classifications (subtypes) of DJD.
2. What are the most common sites of each subtype?
3. What are their age/gender predilections?
4. Trace the pathologic development of DJD.
5. List the (eight) universal features of DJD that might appear in various sites.
6. What are the most common spinal sites for DJD?
7. What potential complications can result from cervical DJD?
8. Define Maigne's syndrome and Robert's syndrome.
9. How does degenerative spondylolisthesis develop?
10. What is the significance of the vacuum cleft in an IVD? In a peripheral joint?
11. Define HSS. Where is it most commonly seen, and what DDX must be considered?
12. Describe the characteristics of SI joint DJD.
13. How does hip DJD correlate with osteoporosis?
14. Describe the various patterns of joint space loss in the hip.
15. Which of these patterns is most common with DJD, and what radiographic sign is associated with it?
16. What DDX must be considered for femoral head geodes?
17. Describe and explain "buttressing" in hip DJD.
18. Describe early and late radiographic signs of knee DJD and the involvement of the various knee joint compartments.
19. Describe the clinical presentation of chondromalacia patellae and its clinical and radiographic signs.
20. How is the "Q" angle measured? What is its significance in the context of DJD?
21. What wrist and hand joints are most commonly involved in DJD?
22. Give the location and explain the significance of triangular cartilage calcification.
23. What are the eponyms of the characteristic nodes of DJD at the DIP and PIP joints?
24. Describe the clinical presentation (including age and gender predilections) of erosive osteoarthritis.
25. What are the radiologic hallmarks of erosive osteoarthritis?

G. DISH (DIFFUSE IDIOPATHIC SKELETAL HYPEROSTOSIS)
(synonyms: spondylosis hyperostotica; spondylitis ossificans ligamentosa, senile ankylosing hyperostosis, Forestier's disease)

1. **General Considerations**

   a) Estimated incidence (in the United States): about 12% of middle-aged and elderly population

b) Frequent correlation with diabetes mellitus

c) Pathogenesis
- provocation is idiopathic
- ossifying diathesis: predisposition to form bone in ligamentous and tendinous attachments
- anterior longitudinal ligament (ALL) calcification and, eventually, ossification
- discal extensions may prevent ossification at disc level

2. Clinical Features

a) Often asymptomatic, even while radiographically evident

b) Male predominance; > 40 years old

c) 20–50% have diabetes mellitus

d) Morning stiffness, pain

e) Increased kyphosis; decreased cervical and lumbar lordoses

f) Extraspinal sites: pelvis, knee, foot, elbow

g) Most common spinal sites: thoracolumbar first, then cervical and lumbar

h) Synovitis; tendon pain

i) Dysphagia caused by esophageal obstruction

j) Apophyseal joints spared: spinal motion may be maintained

k) "Carrot stick" fractures may lead to neurologic sequela (90% at C5–7)

l) Spinal stenosis rare; occurs with posterior longitudinal ligament (PLL) ossification, hypertrophic ligamentum flavum, or posterior osteophytes

3. Radiologic Features

a) Diagnostic criteria require:
- flowing calcification/ossification of anterior portions of at least four contiguous vertebral segments
- preservation of IVD height, lack of disc degeneration
- no ankylosis of facet joints
- no degeneration of SI joints (absence of joint erosion, sclerosis, osseous fusion)

b) Flowing calcification/ossification described as:
- "dripping candle wax"
- "flame-shaped" osteophytes
- flowing hyperostosis
- undulating (bumpy) contour ossifications

c) Cervical spine:
- cervical involvement most often C4-C7
- hyperostosis from anteroinferior body margin tapering downward

- eventually bridges disc space; may be > 1 cm thick
- linear radiolucent clefts due to disc extrusions: **DDX** fracture or pseudoarthrosis
- lateral film may show displaced pharyngeal air shadow; clinically, dysphagia
- may see posterior involvement: osteophytes, hyperostosis of posterior body, and PLL ossification (OPLL); these can lead to myelopathy

d) Thoracic spine
- most common area of spinal involvement (T7–11 especially)
- right-sided involvement (aortic pulsations inhibit left-sided hyperostosis)
- ossification can be 2 cm thick; can obstruct esophagus to T9 or T10 level
- vertical radiolucency may separate ossified ligament from vertebral body
- up to 20% have costovertebral and costotransverse hyperostotic bridging
- apophyseal joints **not** affected

e) Lumbar spine
- usually L1–3
- hyperostosis starts in mid- and upper anterior body, tapering upward (resembling a candle flame)
- similar to cervical appearance: discal extrusion clefts
- may displace aorta
- less posterior involvement; but may involve interspinous ligaments

f) Sacroiliac joints
- later development (spine involved earlier)
- ossification may occur in superior and extreme inferior ligaments
- synovial joint remains unaffected

g) Extraspinal involvement
- any ligament or tendon insertion may calcify/ossify
- most common sites: pelvis, patella, calcaneus, foot, elbow
- about 30% of cases show extraspinal involvement
- "whiskering" at insertion points; ligament/tendon ossification
- adjacent joint spaces remain normal

 4. Differential Considerations

a) DJD, AS, psoriasis, Reiter's syndrome, acromegaly, fluorosis, axial neuropathic arthropathy

b) AS: usually involves the synovial portion of the SI joint; will not ossify pelvic ligaments, as commonly seen with DISH

H. OSSIFIED POSTERIOR LONGITUDINAL LIGAMENT SYNDROME (OPLL)

1. **General Considerations**

   a) Associated with DISH

   b) Japanese people are predisposed, although it does occur in other populations

   c) most common site: cervical spine

   d) with progressive myelopathy, decompressive laminectomy may be necessary

2. **Clinical Features**

   a) Often asymptomatic

   b) Most symptomatic in cervical spine; least often symptomatic in thoracic spine

   c) Insidious onset of lower limb motor and sensory effects

   d) Associated cord myelopathy leads to progressive problems with walking

   e) Paresthesias, diminished tactile sensations; areas of involvement gradually enlarge

   f) Possible pain similar to musculoskeletal back pain

   g) Symptomatic when PLL ossifications occupy > 60% of cervical canal sagittal diameter

   h) No laboratory correlations

   i) Pathologic process
   - thicker, broader PLL than normal
   - hard, nondeforming ossified band over three or four segments; across disc spaces
   - ossifications form cortical, lamellar bone with Haversian canals and rudimentary marrow cavities in superficial ligament layers
   - deeper layers of ligament unaffected
   - adjacent body may have hyperostosis
   - rarely occurs with posterior disc protrusion
   - spinal cord flattened; gray matter infarcted; posterior and lateral white columns demyelinated

3. **Radiologic Features**

   a) Optimal view: lateral (for any affected region)

   b) Dense, linear opaque strip parallel to posterior body margins

   c) Calcific density about 1–5 mm thick

   d) Radiolucent zone between ossification and vertebral body

   e) May be single body length or may traverse several contiguous segments

f) IVD and facet joints usually unaffected, but may show some degeneration

g) May see evidence of concurrent DISH (with about 85% of OPLL cases)

h) Tomography, CT, or MRI needed to determine extent of encroachment

i) MR optimal for detecting myelopathy

I. NEUROTROPHIC ARTHROPATHY
(synonyms: neurogenic arthropathy; neuroarthropathy; neurogenic osteoarthropathy; Charcot's joints)

☞   **1. General Considerations**

a) Secondary to impaired (or absent) sensory or proprioceptive function in joints

b) Excessive traumatic DJD

c) Results in severe instability; joint destruction

d) Specifically associated with tabes dorsalis; affects ankle, subtalar joints, feet

e) 5% of diabetics develop peripheral neuropathy; usually in the ankle, subtalar joints, feet

f) Syphilis patients (in about 20% of cases) may show arthropathic changes in lumbar spine, knee, ankle

g) Traumatic spinal paraplegia may result in neurotrophic arthropathy below the lesion

h) 25% of syringomyelia patients have upper extremity arthropathy: shoulder, elbow, wrist

  2. Clinical Features

a) Altered gait patterns

b) Reduced/absent DTRs

c) Local pain insensitivity

d) Relatively painless instability of affected joint

e) Joint enlargement (recurrent, painless joint effusion) and crepitus

☞   **f)** Pathologic process
- French theory (Charcot): lack of nutrition from CNS trophic centers
- German theory (Volkmann and Virchow): unprotected mechanical microtraumas
- neurotraumatic theory: ineffective protective neurologic mechanism
- weight-bearing leads to osteophytes, sclerosis, loose bodies (hypertrophic phase)
- neurovascular hyperemia stimulates bone resorption (atrophic phase)
- fractures and joint damage ensue; bone fragmentation

- articular cortex undergoes cartilaginous fibrillation, flaking, denudation
- extensive osseous and cartilaginous intraarticular debris
- laboratory findings do not indicate arthropathy, but reflect underlying diseases

3. **Radiologic Features**

    a) General features
- early: chronic, painless effusion; DJD; spontaneous fractures
- later signs reflect phase of process: hypertrophic and atrophic stages
- ☞ **"six Ds"** of hypertrophic stage: (most common in weight-bearing joints)
  1) **d**istention of joint
  2) **d**ensity of subchondral sclerosis
  3) **d**ebris within joint
  4) **d**islocation due to chronic and severe instability
  5) **d**isorganization of all joint elements
  6) **d**estruction of bone
- ☞ atrophic pattern: may succeed hypertrophic stage, or develop from normal joint
  1) usually in non-weight-bearing joints, but also seen in hip and foot
  2) tapered bone; may end in "licked candy stick" at joint space
  3) amputated bone appearance without tapering

    b) Spinal sites
- most commonly lumbar
- hypertrophic pattern
- IVD height loss, sclerosis, osteophytes, vacuum phenomena
- vertebral fragmentation: "jigsaw vertebra"
- vertebral malalignment: "tumbling building-block spine"
- most frequent with syphilitic neuroarthropathy; may be only affected site at earlier stages

    c) Knee
- hypertrophic pattern
- early stage: joint effusion, DJD
- may fracture early; especially medial tibial plateau
- changes in medial compartment of joint occur first
- later, extensive subchondral sclerosis, as far as adjacent metaphyses
- prominent feature: joint debris
- articular surface destruction (especially tibial plateau)

- severe malalignment: tibia and fibula laterally displaced
- lateral dislocation of patella

d) Foot
- subtalar joint shows early hypertrophic changes
- talocalcaneal joint: collapse of inferior talar cortex
- talar destruction, involvement of entire tarsus
- malleolar fractures; tibiotalar destruction with sclerosis, fragmentation and malalignment
- forefoot: atrophic changes
- metatarsal shaft and neck fractures; occasional fracture near metatarsal bases
- atrophic changes in metatarsals and adjacent phalanges
- metatarsals spread apart as soft tissue support is destroyed

J. SYNOVIOCHONDROMETAPLASIA
(synonyms: synovial chondromatosis, osteochondromatosis, osteochondral loose bodies, "joint mice")

1. General Considerations

a) Distinctly separate entity from osteochondritis dissecans

b) Benign arthropathy, with metaplastic transformation of synovial tissue into cartilaginous foci

c) Results in multiple loose bodies in joint

2. Clinical Features

a) Range from asymptomatic to total joint locking with pain

b) Most common in ages 20–50 years

c) Male predilection: (3:1)

d) 70% of cases affect knee

e) Second most common site: elbow; then hip, ankle, shoulder, wrist

f) Rarely impacts spine or extraarticular synovial tissue (bursae or tendon sheaths)

g) May form in popliteal cysts and move around: "migrating mouse sign"

h) Insidious onset without history of trauma

i) Mild, chronic pain, intermittent swelling, crepitus, loss of motion

j) With fragment entrapment in joint: acute pain, swelling, and joint locking

k) Joints function surprisingly well despite large masses

l) Gradual progression of symptoms over years

    m) Tend to promote DJD

    n) May regress with time or may require surgical removal and may recur

    o) Pathologic process
- primary form: spontaneous origin (may involve recurrent microtrauma)
- secondary form: follows DJD, neuropathic arthropathy, osteochondritis dissecans, osteochondral fractures, dislocations
- may be a benign neoplasia
- synovial cells transform to foci of cartilage cells and cartilage matrix
- minimum of 2 cm of synovium involved
- neocartilage enlarges, protrudes beyond synovial surface, may break free
- even free fragments may grow, with nutrition from synovial fluid
- may calcify, ossify; rarely undergo malignant transformation
- lead to premature DJD

3. Radiologic Features

    a) Laminated or stippled masses within an opaque matrix

    b) Some are homogeneously sclerotic, structureless; some have trabecular patterns

    c) Uncalcified or unossified masses may be invisible on film, or may appear as indistinct soft tissue masses

    d) Loose body size: usually 1–20 mm in diameter

    e) Giant synovial chondromatosis: concretions up to 20 cm in diameter

    f) Mostly round/ovoid; occasionally a flat facet contacting adjacent bone

    g) Sharp, well-defined margins

    h) Extrinsic intraarticular pressure erosions: concave cortical indentations with sclerotic margin and no periosteal new bone formation

    i) "*Apple core deformity*": concentric erosion of femoral neck

    j) Erosions resolve within a year of removal of loose bodies

4. Differential Considerations

    a) Pseudogout

    b) Synovioma

    c) Chondrosarcoma

    d) Pigmented villonodular synovitis

    e) Tuberculous arthritis

    f) Sesamoid bones (e.g., fabella)

REVIEW—STUDY QUESTIONS

1. Explain the pathologic process that produces synoviochondrometaplasia.
2. What is Forestier's disease?
3. What conditions predispose to neuropathic arthropathy?
4. Explain the French theory and German theory of neurotrophic arthropathy.
5. What is the most common radiographic presentation of synoviochondrometaplasia?
6. What population is most predisposed to OPLL?
7. What clinical features are associated with DISH?
8. What other disease processes frequently occur in conjunction with DISH?
9. What are the "six Ds" associated with the hypertrophic presentation of neurotrophic arthropathy?
10. Describe the radiographic appearance of atrophic neurotrophic arthropathy.

K. RHEUMATOID ARTHRITIS

1. **General Considerations**
    a) Generalized connective tissue disorder; targets synovial tissue selectively
    b) Bilateral symmetry
    c) Progresses to deformity
    d) May affect heart, lungs, small blood vessels, nervous system, eyes, reticuloendothelial system
    e) Spares cartilaginous joints (except: cervical IVDs)
    f) May (rarely) cause enthesopathy

2. **Clinical Features**
    a) General features
        • onset between 20 and 60 years of age (most commonly in the 40s)
        • age 20–40 years, female predilection is 3:1
        • > 40 years old, no gender preference
        • usually periodic remission/exacerbation with progressive deformity and disability
        • poor prognosis indicated by:
            1) symmetric polyarthritis, subcutaneous nodules, high rheumatoid factor levels
            2) sustained episode of active disease (> 1 year)
            3) early onset: < 30 years old
            4) extraarticular rheumatoid arthritis manifestations

b) Constitutional (nonarticular) symptoms

- fatigue, malaise
- general muscle weakness
- fever
- Raynaud's phenomenon
- generalized osteopenia
- 3–5 cm diameter, firm, nontender rheumatoid nodules (20% of cases) on forearms, knees, ankles, hands, sacrum (most often just distal to olecranon); their presence indicates more severe prognosis
- neurologic effects: exacerbation of compression syndromes; e.g., carpal tunnel
- scleromalacia perforans: perforation of sclera (leads to other ocular problems)
- Sjogren's syndrome: lacrimal gland atrophy causes dry eyes (keratoconjunctivitis sicca), generalized drying of mucus membranes
- skin ulcerations, gangrene: caused by vasculitis
- "Caplan's syndrome": pneumoconiosis with rheumatoid arthritis
- "Felty's syndrome": leukopenia, splenomegaly, and rheumatoid arthritis

c) Articular involvement

- insidious onset of pain, tenderness, swelling, and stiffness of joints
- "jelling phenomenon" : symptoms worse in the morning
- bilateral, symmetric peripheral joint involvement is a hallmark
- does **not** affect paralyzed limbs
- interphalangeal and metacarpophalangeal joints initially affected, with disease progressing proximally
- 80% of cases eventually involve the cervical spine
- rheumatoid soft tissue nodules at MCP joints: "Haygarth's nodes"
- cervical subluxations, eventually dislocations
- arthritis mutilans: severe polyarticular destruction and joint deformities
- Baker's cyst: fluid-filled gastrocnemius-semimembranosus bursa
- "button hole" rupture: rupture of extensor digitorum tendon at PIP
- boutonniere deformity: (Fig. 5.3) PIP flexes, DIP extends as extensor digitorum tendon ruptures at PIP joint
- swan-neck deformity: (Fig. 5.4) PIP extends, DIP flexes
- mallet finger: DIP fixed in flexion; when extensor digitorum communis tendon ruptures at base of distal phalanx

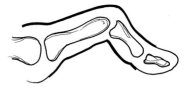

Figure 5.3.

Boutonniere deformity. Reprinted with permission from Yochum TR, Rowe LJ. Essentials of Skeletal Radiology, 2nd ed. Baltimore: Williams & Wilkins, 1996:863.

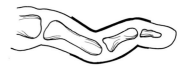

Figure 5.4.

Swan-neck deformity. Reprinted with permission from Yochum TR, Rowe LJ. Essentials of Skeletal Radiology, 2nd ed. Baltimore: Williams & Wilkins, 1996:863.

- hitchhiker's thumb: thumb's interphalangeal joint flexed, with extended first MCP joint
- spindle digit: fusiform digits because of PIP swelling
- fibular deviation: toes dislocate, pointing to the lateral side of the foot
- Lanois deformity: MTP dorsal subluxation, with digits in fibular deviation
- ulnar deviation: ("ulnar drift") fingers deviated toward ulnar side (starts at MCP joints)

d) Pathologic process
- general features
  1) initially:
     - acute synovitis; edema, congestion in synovial membrane
     - joint effusion, periarticular edema, juxtaarticular hyperemia
  2) subsequently:
     - formation of *pannus*: vascular granulation tissue
     - spreads over intraarticular bone and cartilage
  3) resulting bone destruction:
     - *pannus* erodes cortex in "bare area": marginal bone erosions
     - *pannus* intrudes into marrow of subchondral bone, producing subchondral cysts
  4) cartilage destruction:
     - hyaline cartilage eroded by *pannus'* chondrolytic collagenase enzymes
  5) progression:
     - cartilage is replaced and joint space filled with proliferating *pannus*
     - *pannus* undergoes fibrosis
     - joint suffers fibrous ankylosis, and sometimes bony ankylosis
- atlantoaxial features (common to all inflammatory spondyloarthropathies)
  1) synovium affected between anterior tubercle and anterior odontoid, between transverse ligament and posterior odontoid
  2) synovium adjacent to odontoid apex may become involved
  3) pannus at these sites leads to odontoid erosion, or complete dissolution
  4) transverse ligament stretched; its attachments loosened by decalcification

     5) results in severe atlantoaxial instability, subluxation, or dislocation

     6) may create cord compression or vertebrobasilar insufficiency

- intervertebral disc consequences
  1) mechanisms poorly understood
  2) cervical endplate erosion and reduced disc height
  3) may be invasion of pannus from neurocentral (von Luschka) joints
  4) may be due to Schmorl's nodes caused by facet joint instability

- consequences at entheses
  1) enthesopathy is less common with RA than with seronegative arthropathies
  2) cervical SP tips may be eroded and sclerotic, appearing tapered
  3) may be caused by pannus within interspinous bursae

- pathologic features of rheumatoid nodules
  1) central focus of necrotic tissue
  2) middle layer: pallisaded histiocytes
  3) outer fibrous layer with plasma cell and lymphocytic infiltrate
  4) usually subcutaneous, but may occur in viscera (often lungs), in serous linings, and within bone

- laboratory findings
  1) 70% have positive RA latex (sheep agglutination test)
  2) may have anemia
  3) elevated ESR unless disease is in a period of remission
  4) synovial fluid has poor mucin precipitate
  5) biopsy of synovium may show:
     - villous hypertrophy
     - superficial synovial cell proliferation
     - inflammatory cell infiltrate fibrin deposition
     - foci of cell necrosis

☞ **3. Radiologic Features**

   a) General considerations

- bilateral symmetry
- periarticular soft tissue swelling: fat lines displaced, soft tissue density increased, peripheral skin contours displaced
- juxtaarticular osteoporosis: inflammatory hyperemia causes epiphyseal and metaphyseal osteopenia; steroid therapy and disuse cause further osteopenia, predispose to fracture

- uniform loss of joint space
- marginal erosions ("rat bite" erosions): loss of cortex at bare areas, no sclerotic border
- juxtaarticular periostitis: (occasional sign) solid or single lamination adjacent to involved joint
- pseudocysts: frequently 4–6 cm in diameter; intraosseous pannus and synovial fluid; simulate subarticular neoplasm or infection
- articular deformity: joint destruction, ligament laxity, altered muscle function; leads to subluxations, dislocations, osseous misalignments
- early x-ray signs may be visible within 3–6 months of onset

b) RA x-ray signs in hands
  - PIP and MCP joints involved; DIP spared
  - spindle digit: fascial planes, skin contours displaced; increased tissue density
  - first articular sign: marginal erosion
    1) first appears at radial margins of second and third metacarpal heads, distal and proximal ends of proximal phalanges
    2) **Norgaard view** ("*ball-catcher's*") displays these lucent defects
    3) irregular, poorly defined defects with no sclerotic borders
  - early bone sign: juxtaarticular osteoporosis
    1) epiphyseal and metaphyseal osteopenia
    2) "dot-dash" interruptions of articular cortex caused by bone mass loss
    3) later, osteopenia extends into diaphysis
  - periosteal new bone forms solid or single lamination at metaphysis and proximal diaphysis
  - ivory phalanx: homogenous sclerosis of terminal phalanx (not specific to RA)
  - characteristic digital deformities
    1) boutonniere (button hole) deformity
    2) hitchhiker's thumb
    3) swan neck deformity
    4) ulnar deviation (ulnar drift)
    5) zig-zag deformity (digital ulnar drift with carpal radial deviation)
  - arthritis mutilans: complete disorganization of anatomic relationships

c) RA x-ray findings at the wrist
  - may be site of first x-ray findings
  - 60% of cases: wrist findings more severe than those in hands

---

Demineralizing Arthritides

"HORSE"

Hemophilia

Osteomyelitis

Rheumatoid arthritis, Reiter's syndrome

Scleroderma

Erythematosus (lupus)

- distal ulna periarticular swelling
- ulnar styloid erosions
    1) pannus causes subperiosteal resorption: radioulnar joint, prestyloid recess, extensor carpi ulnaris tendon sheath
- distal radius
    1) marginal erosions of radial styloid and adjacent scaphoid
    2) uniform radiocarpal joint space loss without subchondral sclerosis
- carpus
    1) multiple carpals show erosions: especially triquetrum, pisiform; called "*spotty carpal sign*," not specific to RA
    2) uniform loss of midcarpal joint space (with radiocarpal narrowing)
    3) may progress to midcarpal ankylosis (rarely to radiocarpal fusion)
    4) radial rotation of proximal carpal row (in "*zig-zag deformity*")
    5) "*Terry Thomas sign*": scapholunate separation; may accompany palmar scaphoid and lunate subluxation
    6) radioulnar diastasis: dorsal ulnar displacement leads to extensor tendon rupture (caput ulnae syndrome)

Carpal Erosions
"GS RAT"
Gout
Sudeck's atrophy
Rheumatoid Arthritis
Trauma

d) RA x-ray findings at the foot
- feet show initial involvement in 15% of cases
- great toe interphalangeal joint and all MTP joints characteristically involved
- fifth MTP joint is most commonly involved, then fourth, third, second, and first
- marginal erosions most prominent on medial joint surfaces
- hallux sesamoids may show erosions
- plantar and posterior calcaneal surfaces may show poorly defined erosions
- digital MTP joint fibular deviation (but **not** at fifth digit)
- Lanois deformity: toe flexion deformities with fibular deviation
- prominent hallux valgus
- flattened longitudinal arch; metatarsal spread
- MTP plantar callus and bunion at great toe
- may have rheumatoid nodules adjacent to Achilles tendon

e) x-ray findings of spinal RA
- general considerations
    1) cervical spine involvement up to 80% of cases

2) only 5% show thoracic spine involvement: DJD-like changes

3) intravertebral vacuum cleft sign: gas in vertebral body with osteopenic fracture or with avascular necrosis caused by corticosteroids

4) cervical involvement usually post-dates extremity involvement

5) include APOM and flexion lateral with standard views to demonstrate instability and RA effects at C1/C2; CT and MRI are valuable here

6) summation effect: neck length loss caused by invagination, osteolysis, disc space loss (neck can lose 50% of length)

- atlanto-occipital involvement
  1) pseudobasilar invagination may prove fatal (Chamberlain's or McGregor's line evaluations useful)
  2) erosions, sclerosis, joint space loss are common here

- atlantoaxial involvement
  1) 30–50% show atlanto-odontoid involvement
  2) **atlantoaxial instability**: transverse ligament disruption leads to atlas displacement (most commonly anterior)
  3) flexion lateral will show ADI > 3 mm
  4) posterior arch of C1 may encroach on spinal cord: spinolaminar junction line will be disrupted
  5) instability is a late development, usually after 10–20 years of disease
  6) **erosions**: pannus from adjacent synovium
  7) affects odontoid base circumferentially; most prominently anterior and posterior surfaces
  8) affects C1 anterior tubercle, posterior surface
  9) alters shape of dens: base narrowed
  10) may erode apex of dens
  11) severe erosion may leave only an osseous stump
  12) dens is increasingly vulnerable to fracture with RA

- subaxial involvement (C3-C7)
  1) **subluxation**: C2–4 most commonly affected
  2) invariably anterolisthesis (most frequent at C3 and C4)
  3) "stepladder" or "doorstep" look with multiple anterolistheses
  4) **apophyseal joint** erosions, joint space diminution, instability

5) occasionally progresses to bony ankylosis

6) instability demonstrated in flexion lateral views: widened joint

7) **IVD and discovertebral effects**: loss of disc height

8) endplate erosions, cortical contour disruption, especially at posterior margin (rheumatoid discitis)

9) frequently multisegmental

10) **DDX** from DJD: with RA there *usually* is no sclerosis or osteophytic development at involved level

11) **bone changes:** generalized osteopenia (especially with steroid therapy), which may predispose to vertebral compression fractures

12) "sharpened pencil" lower cervical SPs (tapered)

f) X-ray findings of RA at the hip

- hip manifestations occur in about 35% of patients with long-term RA
- axial migration of femoral head
- in about 15% of patients, this results in protrusio acetabulae (arthrokatadysis, or Otto's pelvis)
- bilateral protrusio acetabulae, often accompanied by small, eroded femoral heads (steroid therapy implicated)
- bilateral protrusio acetabuli is most often secondary to RA, DJD and traumatic fractures
- secondary degeneration:
    1) subchondral sclerosis
    2) osteophytes
    3) femoral head erosions, cysts, osteonecrosis
- prominent generalized osteoporosis
- "steplike" defect in weight-bearing surface of femoral head indicates cortical collapse
- after hip replacement: insufficiency fractures in the sacral ala or the pubis

g) X-ray findings of RA at the sacroiliac joint

- SI involvement in less than 35% of RA patients, regardless of duration
- iliac erosions; slightly reduced joint space
- little or no sclerosis; ankylosis is rare
- SI involvement will be unilateral or asymmetric; when it occurs, it usually is a counterpart of pelvic osteoporosis

h) X-ray findings of RA at the shoulder

- bilateral, symmetric glenohumeral and acromioclavicular involvement
- prominent bursa involvement with extensive swelling

Protrusio Acetabulae May Be Caused By

"PORT"

Paget's disease

Osteomalacia, Osteoarthritis

Rheumatoid arthritis

Trauma

- rotator cuff rupture is common, with humeral head elevation
- humeral head/acromial proximity leads to sclerosis, cysts on their articulating surfaces, and a concavity on the inferior acromion
- inflammatory synovial erosions near greater tubercle (**DDX:** Hill-Sachs lesion)
- entire humeral head may eventually be resorbed (**DDX:** atrophic arthropathy)
- distal clavicular erosions, eventually resorption of distal clavicle (**DDX:** hyperparathyroidism)
- inferior distal clavicle may develop a concave defect; adjacent coracoid process surface develops irregularities

i) X-ray findings of RA at the elbow
- rheumatoid nodules protrude on forearm's extensor surface
- olecranon bursa enlargement
- lateral view shows displaced anterior and posterior fat-pads (90% of cases involving elbows show the *"fat-pad sign"*)
- supinator notch sign: erosion (visible on AP and oblique films) on proximal ulna opposite radial neck
- eventually joint components undergo osteolysis (similar to neuroarthropathy)
- extrinsic pressure erosions from rheumatoid nodules are rare

j) X-ray findings of RA at the knee
- frequently involved joint
- prominent suprapatellar and popliteal synovial effusion
- large Baker's cysts
- uniform, bicompartmental joint space loss **(hallmark of RA)**
- tibial and femoral peripheral erosions are early sign
- frequently see large subchondral cysts

k) X-ray findings of RA at the ankle
- mortise and tarsal joints frequently involved, difficult to demonstrate on film
- swelling, osteoporosis, erosions
- at mortise: uniform joint loss, linear periostitis (occasionally)
- eventually, ankle may ankylose

l) X-ray findings of RA in the rib cage
- in long-term disease: superior margin erosions in third, fourth, fifth posterior ribs
- may be broad, shallow concave defect: up to 6 cm long
- may be short (< 1 cm long), discrete excavations
- **DDX:** lytic malignancies

m) X-ray findings of visceral effects of RA
- heart: cardiomegaly; sometimes valvular insufficiency and pericarditis
- lungs:
  1) pulmonary rheumatoid nodules
     - necrobiotic nodules: cavitate (**DDX:** pulmonary metastases)
  2) *"honeycomb lung"*: diffuse interstitial fibrosis
     - both patterns may occur simultaneously
     - Caplan's syndrome: rheumatoid arthritis in lung; pneumoconiosis
- pleura: pleural effusions, often chronic
  1) blunt lateral and posterior costophrenic sulci
  2) *"meniscus sign"*: sweeping concave fluid interface on upright chest film
  3) localized pleural adhesions

REVIEW—STUDY QUESTIONS

1. List the classic, general radiographic signs of rheumatoid arthritis.
2. What sites does RA affect most commonly?
3. Describe the pathologic process that occurs with RA.
4. What are Baker's cysts and where are they found?
5. Where do "rat bite" erosions appear, and why?
6. Why might upper cervical manipulation be contraindicated in a patient with RA?
7. What films would be taken to evaluate the advisability of upper cervical manipulation?
8. Describe the visceral effects of RA that can be discerned radiographically.
9. Describe the changes brought about by RA in the hip.
10. Explain the pathomechanics behind the "swan neck," "boutonniere," and "hitchhiker's thumb" deformities.

L. JUVENILE RHEUMATOID ARTHRITIS (JRA)
(synonyms: Still's disease, juvenile chronic polyarthritis)

    1. General Considerations

a) Not one, but a group of related diseases

b) Most common is Still's disease: a seronegative arthritis with three distinct forms: classic systemic; polyarticular; and monoarticular or pauciarticular

c) onset is < 16 years of age; disease course and prognosis differ from adult RA

d) prognosis usually good: < 20% have progressive destruction

2. **Clinical Features**

    a) Seropositive JRA
- adult type, but with juvenile onset
- poorest prognosis of any form of JRA
- affects about 10% of JRA patients

☞   **b)** Still's disease
- classic systemic form: seen in about 20% of juvenile patients
  1) equal gender occurrence
  2) onset with high, acute, intermittent fever
  3) lymphadenopathy
  4) hepatosplenomegaly
  5) polyserositis
  6) carditis
  7) leukocytosis and anemia
  8) fleeting, migratory, pale erythematous rash late in the day
  9) mild to absent joint manifestations
- polyarticular form: affects about 50%
  1) female predilection (2:1)
  2) bilateral, symmetric joint involvement
  3) pain and swelling: metacarpophalangeal joints, wrist, foot, ankle, knee, cervical spine
  4) may occur spontaneously or as sequel to classic systemic form
  5) may include milder systemic manifestations: fever, lymphadenopathy, rash
  6) chronic course leads to "birdlike" frail features and limbs, small, receded jaw
- pauciarticular-monoarticular form: affects about 30%
  1) female predilection (3:1)
  2) involves four or less joints
  3) most commonly seen at: knee, ankle, hip, elbow, wrist
  4) rarely occurs in hands or feet
  5) monoarticular form most often found in knee; commonly occurs with iridocyclitis which can progress to blindness if untreated
  6) insidious onset of mild swelling, stiffness, pain
  7) rarely has systemic manifestations

    c) Pathologic process and laboratory findings
- pathology:
  1) less inflammation, less fibrinous exudate, and less cellular proliferation in the synovium than seen in adult RA
  2) pannus is present, but less extensive

3) bony ankylosis of carpal, tarsal and cervical facet joints is frequent

4) frequent growth disturbances: premature fusion or accelerated activity at physis

5) periostitis is a prominent response

- laboratory findings:
    1) rheumatoid factor in < 10% of cases; poor prognosis when it exists
    2) erythrocyte sedimentation rate (ESR) elevated in active phase
    3) positive C-reactive protein (CRP) in active phase
    4) anemia and leukocytosis commonly seen
    5) with spinal involvement: HLA-B27 and other histocompatibility antigens occur

3. Radiologic Features

a) Early radiologic features

- intraarticular and periarticular soft tissue swelling
- juxtaarticular or diffuse osteoporosis
- "growth arrest lines": transverse linear densities
- metaphyseal linear periostitis, especially common in hands and feet

b) Later radiologic manifestations

- uniform loss of joint space
- marginal and central articular erosions
- growth disturbances:
    1) in length or diameter of long bones
    2) lengthened or shortened enchondral bones
    3) ballooned epiphyses with constricted metaphyses and diaphyses
- intraarticular bony ankylosis: most common in hands, feet, and cervical spine
- joint subluxations: secondary to effusion and soft tissue fibrosis
- epiphyseal compression fractures: especially in lower extremities
- radiolucent submetaphyseal bands
- ectopic calcifications: in arteries and soft tissue

c) X-ray signs of JRA in hands and feet

- distal joints spared
- brachydactyly common; single or multiple digit lengths altered
- tibiotalar slant deformity
- usually carpals and tarsals are involved
- carpal, tarsal, and interphalangeal ankylosis commonly occur
- N.B., carpal and tarsal ankylosis in one patient strongly suggests JRA

- residual effect in adult is small ossific carpal mass, *"squashed carpi"*

d) X-ray signs of JRA in the spine
- C1-C4 most often (and earliest) affected; about 20% JRA patients
- atlantoaxial instability in 30% of these; caused by transverse ligament lesions
- check ADI in flexion lateral films (should be < 5 mm in a child)
- may see erosions on dens; *increased* dens length
- may have facet ankylosis C2–4, with hypoplastic IVD, vertebral bodies and SPs
- possibly caused by lack of mechanical stimulation for bone growth (**DDX:** congenital block vertebrae)
- spinal canal and IVF are normal
- steroid therapy may lead to general osteopenia: compression fractures in thoracic and lumbar spine

e) X-ray signs of JRA in the pelvis, hip, and sacroiliac joint
- SI joint seldom involved, but unilateral SI erosions can lead to eventual ankylosis
- enlargement of femoral head and trochanters; flattening of femoral head
- obturator foramen appears enlarged

f) X-ray signs of JRA in the mandible
- vertical rami and body of mandible shortened
- antegonal notching (concave notch anterior to angle of mandible) because condylar growth plate is inhibited

M. ANKYLOSING SPONDYLITIS (AS)
(synonym: Marie-Strümpell's disease)

☞ **1. General Considerations**

  a) Chronic inflammatory condition

  b) Predilection for males 15–35 years of age

  c) Predilection for axial skeleton

  d) Greek roots for the name: *ankylos* = stiffening of a joint; *spondylos* = vertebra

  e) Recently, a higher incidence in females is noted, but a clear male preponderance exists

  f) Ratio of whites affected to blacks affected is reported as 4:1

☞ **2. Clinical Features**

  a) Early findings
  - classic presentation is a young man with chronic low back pain, progressively worsening
  - age of onset 15–35 years, although earlier and later onsets are reported

- usually starts with stiff, aching sacrum, buttocks and thighs; occasionally cervical, thoracic, hip, or shoulder pain
- diminished chest expansion because of costovertebral ankylosis
- pain pattern shifts: unilateral, bilateral, contralateral
- sciatic pattern pain may extend to the knee
- pain worse in morning, evening, and during the night
- early in course of disease: periods of complete remission

b) Later findings
- may include cauda equina syndrome
- paraspinal muscle spasm, atrophy
- straightening of normal spinal curves
- reduced mobility

c) Axial skeletal findings
- pain, stiffness, rigidity in thoracolumbar, lumbosacral areas
- SI pain, stiffness, restricted motion
- restricted chest expansion
- anterior chest pain (with costochondral and manubriosternal involvement)

d) Peripheral skeletal findings
- 50% of patients have manifestations in large peripheral joints
- about 30% have small peripheral joints involved
- hips, shoulders, knees and heels are most commonly involved peripheral joints
- pain, tenderness (enthesopathy) over bony protuberances (commonly at calcaneus, pubic symphysis, iliac crests, trochanters, ischial tuberosities, costal cartilages)

e) Extraskeletal manifestations
- ocular, pulmonary, gastrointestinal, genitourinary, and cardiovascular effects
- recurrent, unilateral iritis (may precede spinal effects) in 25% of patients
- tachycardia conduction defects, aortitis, aortic aneurysms
- upper lung cavitating fibrosis (**DDX:** tuberculosis)
- ulcerative colitis, Crohn's disease; inflammatory gastroenteritis
- 80% of male AS patients develop chronic prostatitis
- renal failure secondary to amyloidosis

f) Pathologic process
- synovial effects
  1) pannus forms with synovial proliferation and inflammatory cell infiltrate
  2) pannus layers over articular

cartilage, destroys it, erodes subchondral bone

3) pannus undergoes fibrosis, transforms to cartilage/bone-producing tissue

4) eventual osseous ankylosis

- cartilage effects
    1) subchondral osteitis; inflammatory cells and granulation tissue invade bone
    2) fibrous tissue replaces the bone and fibrocartilage (erosions seen on film)
    3) this fibrous tissue ossifies: osseous trabeculae traverse joint space

- effects at entheses
    1) normal enthesis: gradual transition from fibrous tissue to cartilage, to calcified cartilage, and finally to bone
    2) this area is predilected to connective tissue disease; possibly caused by high metabolic activity, blood flow, and mechanical stresses
    3) first: inflammatory cell infiltrate replaces chondrified and calcified parts of ligament at the bone-ligament junction
    4) this causes bone erosion, which repairs with deposition of woven bone, projecting out in spurlike spicules
    5) this remodels and is replaced by lamellar bone

g) Laboratory findings
- ESR elevated only in active, inflammatory stage of disease
- HLA-B27 present in up to 90% of cases
- absence of rheumatoid factor aids in differential diagnosis

☞ **3. Radiologic Features**

a) General findings
- bilateral, symmetrical osteoporosis, erosions, and reactive sclerosis
- eventual bony ankylosis
- characteristic sites: SI joints, facet joints, costovertebral joints, pubic symphysis, discovertebral junctions, manubriosternal joints
- distinctive sequence of involvement:
    1) early bilateral SI involvement
    2) spinal effects ascending from thoracolumbar junction; less commonly, ascending from lumbosacral junction
    3) earliest cervical changes at C2–3 and C6–7

- with equivocal early films, re-take in 3–6 months: clear changes should be visible
- women more frequently show peripheral effects and SI changes with little or no spinal involvement

b) X-ray findings of AS at the SI joint
- SI involvement is the hallmark of AS
- optimal projection: angulated spot views (AP or PA)
- earliest sign may be a subtle widening of the SI joint space
- diagnosis is most commonly made at Stage 2 of SI involvement: erosive and sclerotic changes in the SI joint (see below)
- CT scan gives excellent delineation of erosive osteoarthritic lesions
- characteristic involvement is bilateral/symmetrical
- iliac side demonstrates earliest signs: protective cartilage is three times thicker on sacral side helps explain why
- synovial portions suffer predominant pathology (lower ⅔ of joint)
- stages reflect sequence: inflammation, bone destruction, ossification
- Forestier classification of sequential changes:
    1) Stage 1: pseudowidening of joint space—loss of cortical bone margin via subchondral osteoporosis; hazy joint margins
    2) Stage 2: erosive and sclerotic changes—discrete erosions in subarticular bone; irregular joint margin ("*rosary bead*" appearance); reactive sclerosis in adjacent ilium
    3) Stage 3: ankylosis—eventual (over 7–23 years) bony bridging of joint
- after ankylosis, sclerosis dissipates, generalized osteoporosis ensues
- *ghost joint*: anterior SI joint cortical margin is visible through the ankylosis
- ligamentous upper SI joint may ossify: appears on AP film as triangular opacity ("*star sign*")
- about 50% of patients progress to complete SI fusion
- about 40% progress to stage 2 and then resolve
- symphysis pubis often undergoes a parallel sequence of stages

c) X-ray findings of AS in the spine
- discovertebral junction, apophyseal joints, costovertebral joints, atlantoaxial articulation, and spinous process entheses are the affected spinal sites

- earliest visible changes: thoracolumbar junction; then at lumbosacral junction
- process ascends from first sites, may eventually ankylose vertebral column
- discovertebral junction
    1) syndesmophyte formation: inflammation, destruction, and ossification of ligaments
    2) starts at outer annulus enthesis as a lytic vertebral body rim lesion: *Romanus lesion*—lucent corner erosion
    3) this creates "squared contour"—decreased anterior concavity of vertebral body margin
    4) repair may actually create a convex margin: *"barrel-shaped vertebra"*
    5) erosions heal with transient sclerosis: *shiny corner sign*
    6) later, outer annulus and tissue **beneath the ALL** ossify
    7) only innermost ALL fibers ossify, and only very late in the disease
    8) *marginal syndesmophytes* are fine, vertical bridging ossifications at outer disc, originating at adjacent vertebral body margins
    9) multiple ankylosed segments create undulating contour: *bamboo spine* or *poker spine*
- vertebral body
    1) prominent osteoporosis, throughout course of disease, caused by inflammation, immobility after ankylosis, steroid therapy
    2) higher incidence of compression fractures than in average population
    3) pathologic Schmorl's nodes through osteoporotic bone
    4) *Andersson lesion*: irregular, poorly defined endplate because of pseudoarthrosis, due to *carrot stick fracture* through a previously ankylosed motion segment (**DDX:** IVD infection, neuropathic arthropathy)
    5) mid and lower cervical vertebrae appear narrower (sagittally) due to chronic disuse atrophy
- intervertebral disc
    1) entire disc may ossify late in process, with trabeculae and marrow
    2) with osteoporosis, vertebral endplates acquire increased concavity: result is a "ballooning" appearance of the disc
- apophyseal joints
    1) erosions, sclerosis, loss of joint space are early signs

2) optimal views: oblique lumbar; lateral cervical

3) difficult to visualize in thoracic spine

- costovertebral joints

    1) erosions, blurring of joint margins

    2) initially visible on AP projection of upper thoracic region

    3) with ankylosis, trabeculae are continuous across previous joint space

- joint capsules, ligaments, other soft tissues

    1) lumbar spine undergoes joint capsule ossification, with ossified ligamentum flavum and interspinous ligaments: on AP films, this shows as three parallel, vertical linear densities: *trolley track sign*

    2) when only interspinous and supraspinous ligaments ossify, AP films show a single, central vertical density connecting SPs: *dagger sign*

    3) especially in cervical spine: SP erosions (due to enthesopathy) cause reactive bone formation, resulting in tapered SPs

    4) periostitis associated with these SP erosions

    5) especially in cervical spine: arachnoid dilation may enlarge IVFs

- temporomandibular joint (TMJ): changes here parallel involvement of the cervical spine

- atlantoaxial joint

    1) less often and less severely affected than with RA

    2) involvement often asymptomatic, but potentially serious, may be life-threatening

    3) flexion lateral view shows increased ADI (> 3 mm), indicates transverse ligament instability

    4) dens erosions, dens sclerosis (*shiny odontoid sign*)

    5) joint may undergo ankylosis in position of rotary subluxation

- spinal alignment changes

    1) loss of both lumbar and cervical lordoses, seen on lateral films

    2) flexion/extension studies show complete loss of intersegmental motion

    3) cervical lateral film shows marked anterior carriage of the head

d) X-ray findings of AS in peripheral joints

- most frequently involved: hips, shoulders, heel
- bilateral, symmetric involvement is most common
- peripheral joint involvement in about 50% of patients
- hip
    1) uniform loss of joint space
    2) axial migration of femoral head
    3) may result in protrusio acetabulae
    4) subchondral cysts; small osteophytes
    5) eventual ankylosis sometimes occurs
    6) hip prosthesis can become ankylosed within about 6 months; happens in > 30% of cases
    7) erosion, periostitis at trochanters and adjacent ischial tuberosity caused by enthesopathy
- shoulder
    1) lateral humeral head erosions
    2) elevated humeral head due to rotator cuff tears
    3) distal clavicle erosions; eventual resorption
    4) enthesopathic erosions at coracoclavicular ligaments, humeral tuberosities
- calcaneus
    1) erosions, local osteoporosis and periostitis at insertions of Achilles tendon and plantar aponeurosis

e) X-ray findings of enthesopathy with AS

- bone-ligament entheses most prominently affected at iliac crest, ischial tuberosity, femoral trochanters, spinous processes, calcaneal plantar surface
- cortical erosion, sclerosis, periosteal "*whiskering*" extending from bone into ligament or tendon

f) X-ray findings of dural ectasia with AS

- most often in lumbar spine; sometimes thoracic; rarely cervical
- linked with cauda equina syndrome
- arachnoid diverticula may erode pedicles, lamina, and SP or cause posterior vertebral body scalloping
- CT is best imaging modality
- N.B., myelography is contraindicated: exacerbates patient's condition
- **DDX:** cauda equina caused by postirradiation ischemia; demyelination, arachnoiditis

TERMINOLOGY ASSOCIATED WITH ANKYLOSING SPONDYLITIS

a) *Andersson lesion*: pseudoarthrosis due to pathologic fracture through ankylosed motion segment (see "pseudoarthrosis")

b) *ballooning discs*: biconcavity of vertebral endplates; due to osteoporotic vertebral bodies

c) *bamboo spine*: undulating segmented appearance of spine with multiple contiguous bilateral syndesmophytes

d) *barrel vertebra*: exaggerated convexity of anterior body margin

e) *carrot stick fracture*: transverse pathologic fracture (see "Andersson lesion")

f) *dagger sign*: midline vertical linear opacity on AP lumbar film; caused by ossified supraspinous and interspinous ligaments

g) *enthesopathy*: inflammatory infiltration at bone junction with tendon or ligament

h) *ghost joint*: articular cortex visible through the ossific mass of an ankylosed joint

i) *poker spine*: undulating segmented appearance of spine with multiple contiguous bilateral syndesmophytes (see "bamboo spine")

j) *pseudoarthrosis*: instability caused by nonunion of a fracture; e.g., Andersson lesion

k) *Romanus lesion*: anterior vertebral body marginal erosion; caused by enthesopathy at annular fibers' insertion site

l) *rosary bead*: appearance of multiple erosions along sacroiliac articular margins

m) *seronegative*: negative for rheumatoid factor in the blood

n) *shiny corner sign*: transient reactive sclerosis at anterior vertebral body margin

o) *shiny odontoid sign*: increased opacity of the dens caused by reactive sclerosis

p) *star sign*: triangular opacity caused by ossification of superior sacroiliac ligaments

q) *squared vertebra*: loss of anterior vertebral body concavity; caused by periostitis and Romanus lesions

r) *syndesmophyte*: ossification of spinal ligament; due to inflammatory process

s) *trolley track spine*: three parallel vertical opacities over spine; seen on AP lumbar film; caused by ossification of apophyseal joints and interspinous and supraspinous ligaments

t) *whiskering*: ossified spicules extending from bone into ligaments or tendons at entheses

N. ENTEROPATHIC ARTHRITIS

(synonyms: colitic arthritis, enteropathic arthropathy, entero-pathic spondylitis)

 1. General Considerations

    a) Many gastrointestinal disorders produce arthropathies

    b) Most common causes: ulcerative colitis, regional enteritis (Crohn's disease)

    c) Some familial predilection for these two diseases

    d) May also result from various intestinal infections: *Salmonella, Shigella, Yersinia*

    e) Young adults most prone to ulcerative colitis, regional enteritis

    f) About 15% of these patients develop musculoskeletal symptoms

    g) Barium studies, laboratory studies required for definitive diagnosis

    h) Musculoskeletal manifestations parallel GI episodes; self-resolving in 1–3 months

☞   **2. Clinical Features**

    a) Systemic
- malaise, anorexia, weight loss
- abdominal pain
- altered stool characteristics

    b) Appendicular skeleton
- intensifies with chronicity of bowel disorder
- arthralgia, joint effusion, erythema
- most commonly affected: knees, ankles, elbows, wrists
- usually no permanent peripheral joint damage

    c) Axial skeleton
- sites identical to those affected by ankylosing spondylitis
- bilateral sacroiliac effects
- spondylitis: most commonly at thoracolumbar and lumbosacral regions
- 5–10% of ulcerative colitis patients develop full-fledged ankylosing spondylitis
- isolated SI involvement is more common than combined SI/spondylitis (4:1)

    d) Pathologic process
- etiology still in question
- current theory: antigen/antibody complexes create inflammation when antigens are released from the bowel
- spinal changes are identical to those of AS

☞   **e)** Laboratory findings
- HLA-B27 present in 10–12% of cases
- negative for rheumatoid factor (a seronegative spondyloarthropathy)

☞   **3. Radiologic Features**

    a) Sacroiliac manifestations
- bilateral, symmetric erosions, sclerosis and altered joint space
- leads to bony ankylosis
- especially with regional enteritis, SI may be affected with no spinal involvement
- appears identical to AS

    b) Spinal manifestations
- identical to AS
- discovertebral erosions and sclerosis
- vertebral body squaring
- thin, bilateral, marginal syndesmophytes
- apophyseal ankylosis

- tends to progress upward; results in *"bamboo spine"*

 c) Peripheral joint manifestations
- soft-tissue swelling at peripheral joints
- periarticular osteoporosis
- less often: hypertrophic osteoarthropathy; periosteal new bone formation, especially along the long bone metaphyses and diaphyses
- most often seen at radius, ulna, tibia, fibula

O. PSORIATIC ARTHRITIS

  1. General Considerations

 a) About 15% of patients with psoriasis have the associated arthritis

 b) Distribution usually is in hands and feet

 c) Occasionally affects spine, SI joints, hips, knees, shoulders

 d) Wide variety of presentations; may appear to be RA, but lacks rheumatoid factor

 e) Seronegative spondyloarthropathy

 f) **DDX:** RA, Reiter's syndrome (sometimes almost impossible to differentiate), DJD, erosive osteoarthritis

  2. Clinical Features

 a) Patient has psoriatic lesions (extensor forearm, knee, back, scalp, pubic area)

 b) Onset between 20–50 years of age

 c) No gender predilection

 d) One notable relationship: if psoriasis affects nails, patient is more likely to have arthritis
- 80% of psoriasis patients with nail lesions get psoriatic arthritis
- nail lesions: pitting, ridging, discoloration, nail loss, subungual hyperkeratosis (thickened skin under nail tip)

 e) Early manifestations
- distal interphalangeal joint (DIP) redness, swelling, pain
- *cocktail sausage digit* or *sausage digit*: tenosynovitis swells entire digit

 f) Late manifestations:
- arthritis mutilans: disrupted intraarticular relationships, especially in the fingers

 g) Chronic, low-grade back pain: spondyloarthropathy usually at thoracolumbar area

 h) Pathologic process
- pathology in synovial joints:
  1) resembles RA: proliferative synovitis produces pannus

2) pannus undergoes fibrosis
3) erosions of cartilage and cortical margins
4) narrowing of joint space
5) periostitis, with new-bone formation adjacent to inflammatory erosions
6) joint may be widened by fibrous tissue, which eventually ossifies, ankylosing the joint
7) **no** synovial hyperemia, **no** periarticular osteoporosis

- atlantoaxial and SI joints affected, similar process to that in peripheral joints
- enthesopathy also results in erosions and proliferative changes: e.g., at calcaneus, hand, and foot
- in spine:
    1) woven bone, remodeling to lamellar bone, ossifies loose areolar tissue adjacent to vertebral bodies
    2) produces non-marginal syndesmophytes
    3) may progress to ossify annulus and longitudinal ligament

i) Laboratory findings
- ESR elevated in acute phase
- negative rheumatoid factor
- occasionally, hyperuricemia
- in patients with SI involvement: 75% have HLA-B27 antigen
- patients with only peripheral joint effects: 30% have HLA-B27 antigen

☞ **3. Radiologic Features**

a) General features
- asymmetric distribution
- prominent soft tissue swelling:
    1) very early sign; may be only visible manifestation
    2) periarticular, fusiform soft tissue displacement (*spindle digit*)
    3) entire digit swelling (*cocktail sausage digit*)
- lack of osteoporosis: normal bone mineralization is characteristic
- cortical erosions
    1) early erosions are marginal
    2) over time, result is an increasingly tapered bony end
- fluffy periostitis
    1) adjacent to marginal erosions
    2) at ligament and tendon insertions
    3) fluffy, spiculated new bone; external surface is frayed, hazy
- farther from joint, linear periosteal new bone may be formed

- endosteal periostitis: results in sclerotic bone
    1) most prominent at terminal phalanges (*ivory phalanx*)
- joint space alterations: may be narrowed or widened
- ankylosis more common than with RA, especially in interphalangeal joints
- deformity: *pencil-in-cup* telescoping of joint; *opera glass* hand; arthritis mutilans; ulnar and fibular digital deviation; boutonniere and swan-neck deformities (far less common than with RA)

b) X-ray signs of psoriatic arthritis in the hand
- distribution
    1) usually DIP and PIP joints
    2) rarely MCP joints, wrists
    3) *ray pattern* (occasional, but *specific to psoriatic arthritis*, all three joints of single ray): DIP, PIP, and MCP joints
    4) asymmetric distribution (both side to side and digit to digit)
- erosions and deformity
    1) at joint margins, flanked by fluffy periosteal new-bone formation (*mouse ears sign*) (Fig. 5.5)
    2) progresses to form a whittled distal articular end on phalanx
    3) whittled end erodes into adjacent articular surface, forming *pencil-in-cup* deformity (synonyms: *pestle and mortar, mushroom and stem, balancing pagoda, cup and saucer*) (Fig. 5.6)
    4) subsequent shortening of digit creates *opera glass hand*
    5) arthritis mutilans
    6) rarely: acro-osteolysis (resorption of distal phalangeal tuft)

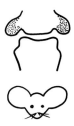

Figure 5.5.

Mouse ears sign. Reprinted with permission from Yochum TR, Rowe LJ. Essentials of Skeletal Radiology, 2nd ed. Baltimore: Williams & Wilkins, 1996:898.

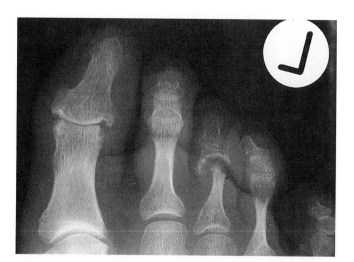

Figure 5.6.

Pencil-in-cup deformity. Reprinted with permission from Yochum TR, Rowe LJ. Essentials of Skeletal Radiology, 2nd ed. Baltimore: Williams & Wilkins, 1996:899.

- joint space alterations
    1) initial widening caused by bone erosion, intraarticular fibrous tissue
    2) 15% of patients progress to osseous ankylosis

c) X-ray signs of psoriatic arthritis in the foot
- characteristic early changes occur at great toe interphalangeal joint
- soft tissue swelling, erosions, fluffy periostitis
- widened joint space, normal bone density
- lysis at metatarsal heads and distal tufts
- sometimes *ivory phalanx* at distal tuft of great toe
- calcaneus: erosions, periostitis at Achilles and plantar ligament insertions
- rarely intertarsal ankylosis

d) X-ray signs of psoriatic arthritis at SI joints
- 30–50% of psoriatic arthritis patients have SI involvement
- involvement is bilateral but asymmetric; may initially be unilateral
- iliac surface of joint shows:
    1) erosions
    2) sclerosis
    3) hazy joint margins
- enthesopathy creates erosive changes and periostitis at iliac crests, ischial tuberosities, femoral trochanters
- infrequently, femoral head erosion with protrusio acetabuli may mimic RA

e) X-ray signs of psoriatic arthritis in the spine
- cervical spine (affected in up to 75% of psoriatic arthritis patients)
    1) apophyseal joint narrowing or fusion
    2) marginal and nonmarginal syndesmophytes
    3) subluxations
- atlantoaxial joint
    1) atlantoaxial instability (in up to 45% of psoriatic arthritis patients)
    2) flexion lateral film to evaluate ADI (should be < 3 mm)
    3) anterior, posterior or lateral dens surfaces may show erosions, sclerosis
- thoracic, lumbar spine (affected in about 60% of patients with psoriasis)
    1) coarse, asymmetric nonmarginal syndesmophytes (paravertebral ossifications)
    2) apophyseal joints are spared in this area of the spine
- nonmarginal syndesmophytes (parasyndesmophytes or paravertebral ossifications)
    1) unilateral or asymmetric

2) usually best visualized on AP projection
3) most common T11-L3
4) early: ossifications lateral to and separate from vertebral body
5) may be thick and fluffy, or thin and well-defined curvilinear opacity
6) later: extends to vertebral body, and includes annular fibers
7) forms thick excrescence from mid-body area
8) four commonly seen variations (Fig. 5.7A-D)
   - *complete*: (Fig. 5.7A) attached to mid-body of two contiguous vertebrae, thick at bases, thinner mid-portion crossing disc
   - *incomplete, comma shaped; inverted comma; teardrop*: (Fig. 5.7B) contiguous with mid-vertebral body, tapering distally

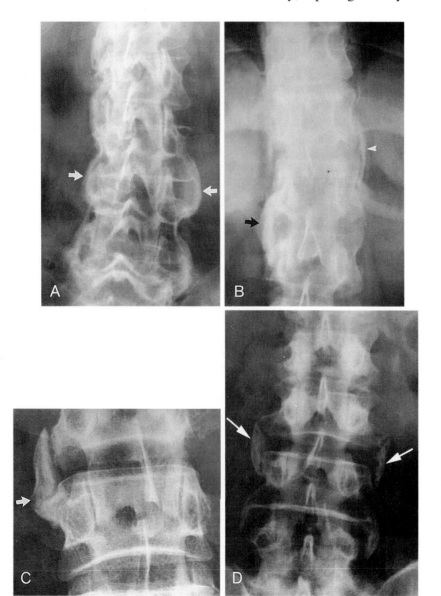

Figure 5.7.

*Psoriatic arthritis: manifestations of syndesmophytes. **A**. Complete. **B**. Incomplete. **C**. Bagpipe. **D**. Floating. Reprinted with permission from Yochum TR, Rowe LJ. Essentials of Skeletal Radiology, 2nd ed. Baltimore: Williams & Wilkins, 1996:903.*

- *bagpipe*: (Fig. 5.7C) bulkier base ("bag") attached to mid-body
- *floating; Bywater's-Dixon*: (Fig. 5.7D) unattached ossification bridging disc space
- marginal syndesmophyte (Fig. 5.8)
    1) rarely seen in psoriatic arthritis
    2) thin, vertical ossification of outer annulus fibers
    3) originate from peripheral body-endplate junctions
    4) usually bilateral; may be complete or incomplete
    5) characteristically seen in AS

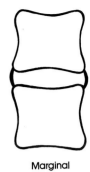

Marginal

Figure 5.8.
Marginal syndesmophyte. Reprinted with permission from Yochum TR, Rowe LJ. Essentials of Skeletal Radiology, 2nd ed. Baltimore: Williams & Wilkins, 1996:903.

P.   REITER'S SYNDROME

1.   General Considerations

a) Definitive triad: urethritis, conjunctivitis, polyarthritis (not necessarily simultaneously)

b) Male predilection (50:1)

c) Most common with venereal etiology, but may also be linked to bowel disorders

d) Self-limiting joint involvement; primarily peripheral (lower extremity, usually)

2.   Clinical Features

a) Venereal origin
- dysuria, discharge, prostatitis
- nonspecific inflammation: no causative organism has been identified
- later, arthritis, iritis, and sometimes skin lesions

b) Enteric origin
- first: dysentery caused by *Shigella flexneri, Yersinia enterocolitica, Salmonella*
- arthritis symptoms appear 1–3 weeks later

c) Lesions of eyes, skin, mucosa
- conjunctivitis (often bilateral), sometimes iritis
- about 30% of patients develop skin lesion very like pustular psoriasis (*keratoderma blenorrhagica*) on palms and soles of feet
- *balanitis circinata*: mucocutaneous lesions on penis
- lesions on oral mucosa, tongue and hard palate

d) Arthritis symptoms
- asymmetric painful effusion
- common sites: knee, ankle, forefoot, calcaneus, low back, shoulder, wrist
- typical: young male with pain at plantar or Achilles calcaneal insertions ("*lover's heels*")
- self-limiting within 2–3 months; prone to recurrence

- residual joint damage with multiple episodes, usually in feet, SI, spine

e) Complications
- urinary tract obstructions
- iritis, retrobulbar neuritis, corneal ulceration
- aortitis, AV blocks
- cranial nerve palsy

f) Pathologic process
- etiology:
    1) no single agent identified, but various enteric organisms, viruses, and *Mycoplasma,* and *Bedsonia* may be implicated
    2) dissemination to SI joints and spine via Batson's venous plexus
    3) immunologic basis also possible (presence of HLA-B27 may indicate this)
- process:
    1) synovitis, fibrous proliferation, periostitis
    2) erosions and periostitis at entheses: especially noted at calcaneal insertions of Achilles tendon and plantar fascia, at malleoli, and metatarsals
    3) spine: nonmarginal syndesmophytes form with paravertebral ossification in loose areolar tissue beside vertebral body; these later attach to vertebral bodies (process appears identical to that occurring in psoriatic arthritis)

g) Laboratory findings
- negative for rheumatoid factor (a seronegative spondyloarthropathy)
- in acute phase, ESR is elevated
- anemia and leukocytosis
- 75% or more show HLA-B27 antigen

☞ **3. Radiologic Features**

a) General signs
- articular and periarticular soft tissue swelling
- osteoporosis
- uniform loss of joint space
- marginal erosions
- periostitis

b) Distribution
- metatarsophalangeal and interphalangeal foot joints
- calcaneus
- ankle
- knee
- sacroiliac joints

- less common at thoracolumbar and cervical spine, shoulder, elbow

c) X-ray signs of Reiter's syndrome in foot and ankle

- toes
  1) prominent soft tissue swelling, especially in toes
  2) metatarsophalangeal and interphalangeal erosions (especially great toe interphalangeal joint)
  3) associated osteoporosis and linear or fluffy periostitis
  4) *Lanois deformity*: proximal phalanges dorsally subluxated, fibular deviation of digits
- calcaneus (*lover's heels*)
  1) erosions
  2) signs at Achilles and plantar insertions
  3) fluffy periostitis
  4) soft tissue swelling
- ankle
  1) prominent swelling
  2) periostitis at malleoli

d) X-ray signs of Reiter's syndrome in the knee

- usually, only visible change is effusion
- occasionally, periostitis at distal femoral metaphysis
- with long-standing disease, Pelligrini-Stieda type of calcification may develop in medial collateral ligament

e) X-ray signs of Reiter's syndrome in the sacroiliac joint

- involved in up to 70% of Reiter's syndrome patients
- no visible changes in some cases, but bone scan indicates involvement
- variable patterns: bilateral and unilateral, symmetric and asymmetric; most common is bilateral and asymmetric
- erosions, hazy joint margin, variable sclerosis, especially on iliac margin
- altered joint space
- can progress to bony ankylosis, but not as likely as with AS

f) X-ray signs of Reiter's syndrome in the spine

- occasionally may result in atlantoaxial instability, atlas dislocation
- thoracolumbar manifestations:
  1) coarse nonmarginal syndesmophytes: early, they are fluffy, poorly defined, though thick; later becoming more clearly defined
  2) may be complete or incomplete
  3) may be *floating* type: vertical, but unattached to vertebral bodies, or

may be attached, forming *teardrop*,
comma, or *bagpipe* shapes

4) distributed unilaterally and
asymmetrically in vertebral column

REVIEW—STUDY QUESTIONS

1. Name four seronegative spondyloarthropathies.
2. Describe the pathologic progression of psoriatic arthritis.
3. How would you screen a patient with psoriasis for upper cervical manipulation? Why?
4. What classic triad indicates a diagnosis of Reiter's syndrome?
5. What histocompatibility antigen is commonly associated with the seronegative arthropathies?
6. How does the prognosis for JRA differ from the prognosis for RA?
7. What radiographic signs would make you suspect a diagnosis of enteropathic arthritis?
8. What enteric disorders are most commonly associated with enteropathic arthritis?
9. Describe the most common presenting symptoms of AS and its usual progression.
10. Describe the definitive radiographic signs of psoriatic arthritis.
11. Give a detailed description of five varieties of syndesmophytes.
12. What spondyloarthropathy (or arthropathies) would most likely have marginal syndesmophytes?
13. Which arthropathies tend to involve the SI joints bilaterally and symmetrically? Bilaterally but asymmetrically? Unilaterally?
14. Describe the progression of the radiologic appearance of the SI joints from early AS to late AS.
15. What are the clinical variations of Still's disease?

Q. SYSTEMIC LUPUS ERYTHEMATOSUS (SLE)

 1. General Considerations

    a) *Lupus* is Latin for "*wolf*": malar erythema resembles facial markings of a wolf

    b) significant immunologic abnormalities

    c) multiple system involvement: urinary system, cardiopulmonary system, nervous system, integument, musculoskeletal system

    d) female predilection; onset between 10–40 years of age

 2. Clinical Features

    a) Initial signs are constitutional: malaise, fever, anorexia, weight loss, polyarthralgia, skin rash

b) Sunlight precipitates the skin rash: symmetric, erythematous rash on face, neck, elbows, and dorsal hands

- classic *butterfly rash* over bridge of the nose and malar eminences is present in a minority of patients

c) Alopecia often accompanies rash; Raynaud's phenomenon may be associated

d) Kidney involvement often leading to renal failure

e) Spontaneous tendon rupture: sometimes presenting symptom

f) Joint involvement

- up to 90% of SLE patients have associated arthritis
- most common presenting complaint
- bilateral, symmetric joint pain in hands, knees, wrists and shoulders
- swelling, pain and stiffness (distribution simulates RA)
- spinal effects often absent or minimal and nonspecific

g) Pathologic process

- etiology: autoimmune connective tissue disorder
- process:
  1) deposition of immune complexes and fibrinoid material in body tissues
  2) prevalent depositions in blood vessels, synovium, serous membranes
  3) result
     - skin edema and necrosis
     - vasculitis (especially smaller vessels)
     - synovitis
     - pleuritis
     - pericarditis
     - myocarditis
     - glomerulitis: leads to diffuse membranous glomerulonephritis, and to eventual renal failure

h) Laboratory findings

- bone marrow biopsy may show characteristic "LE" cells
- "LE" cell: a mature neutrophil with a vacuole filled with nuclear chromatin that is breaking down
- normochromic, normocytic anemia
- thrombocytopenia
- leukopenia
- elevated ESR
- abnormal plasma proteins: antinuclear factor (ANF) (antinuclear antibodies)

☞   **3.** **Radiologic Features**

    a) General features
- bilateral, symmetric, reversible hand/finger deformities
- osteoporosis
- soft tissue atrophy and calcification
- minimal arthropathy
- increased osteonecrosis
- hands are most prominently affected
- proximal long bones may be involved in up to 10% of adults, 40% of youths
- spinal involvement rare

    b) X-ray signs of SLE in the hands
- flexible deformities caused by lax ligaments and tendons
  1) digital ulnar deviation
  2) boutonniere deformity
  3) swan-neck deformity
- arthropathy
  1) joint space usually is normal
  2) **no** subchondral bone changes
  3) generalized osteopenia may be prominent
  4) when Raynaud's phenomenon is present: may be some tuftal resorption (identical to this effect in scleroderma)
- soft tissue effects
  1) muscle atrophy
  2) sometimes punctate or sheetlike calcification in myofascial planes and subcutaneous tissue
  3) peripheral vascular calcifications

    c) X-ray signs of SLE in the spine
- unusual to have spinal manifestations
- may develop atlantoaxial instability ($<$ 5% of cases): ADI $>$ 3 mm in flexion lateral projection
- with corticosteroid therapy, compression fractures

    d) X-ray signs of SLE in long bones
- osteonecrosis, most commonly in femoral and humeral heads
- seen in about 10% of adults, 40% of youth
- effects are likely to be simultaneously bilateral
- other affected sites: femoral condyles, talus, wrist, tarsus, metacarpal heads, metatarsal heads
- severe osteoporosis, conducive to fracture

    e) X-ray signs of SLE in the chest
- small, bilateral pleural effusions, and pleural thickening
- cardiomegaly (mild to moderate)
- pericardial effusion

R. JACCOUD'S ARTHRITIS
(synonyms: Jaccoud's syndrome, Jaccoud's arthropathy, chronic postrheumatic fever arthropathy)

1. **General Considerations**

    a) A consequence of rheumatic fever; infrequently seen

    b) Predominantly affects hands; may affect feet

    c) Hallmarks: ulnar deviation and flexion of MCP joints

2. **Clinical Features**

    a) History of rheumatic fever
    - antecedent streptococcal pharyngitis
    - transitory migratory peripheral myalgias, arthralgias, and skin rash
    - fever, sweating, pallor
    - fatigue and weight loss

    b) If there have been several recurrences, Jaccoud's arthritis may develop

    c) Obvious deformities in hands: ulnar drift, boutonniere and swan-neck deformities

    d) Palmar subluxation at MCP joints: most likely at fourth and fifth digits
    - these are flexible deformities, as in SLE

    e) Less frequently, parallel changes in feet: fibular deviation and MTP subluxations

    f) Pathologic process
    - acute phase:
        1) mild synovitis
        2) some superficial synovial edema and cellular infiltrate
        3) fibrinous change of collagen in deeper synovium and joint capsule
    - changes may regress with no residual effects
    - chronic recurrence:
        1) progressive fibrosis in capsular and periarticular tendons and fascia
        2) rarely: uniform loss of MCP joint space

3. **Radiologic Features**

    a) Acute
    - joint swelling with normal joint space and contour

    b) Chronic
    - ulnar deviation and MCP palmar subluxations, especially fourth and fifth digits
    - interphalangeal deformities: boutonniere and swan-neck configurations
    - usually joint space is normal; occasionally there is uniform diminution

- lack of erosions (clear sign differentiating this from RA)
- occasionally: hook protuberance off radial side of metacarpal head surrounds a lucent cyst
- feet show parallel changes

S. IDIOPATHIC CHONDROLYSIS OF THE HIP

1. **General Considerations**

    a) Primary chondrolysis is rare; idiopathic

    b) Secondary chondrolysis is a sequel to:
    - slipped femoral capital epiphysis (most common)
    - extended immobilization
    - paraplegia
    - septic arthritis
    - rheumatoid arthritis
    - trauma

    c) Strong female predilection (6:1)

2. **Clinical Features**

    a) Typical patient: adolescent girl with hip pain, stiffness, restricted range of motion
    - age of onset usually 11–20 years of age

    b) Prognosis variable
    - spontaneous resolution (about 30% of patients)
    - progression to crippling flexion contracture and inability to stand, increased lumbar lordosis
    - total ankylosis of hip (about 20% of patients)
    - avascular necrosis and hip deformities

    c) Therapies
    - non-weightbearing
    - physical therapy
    - analgesia
    - regular swimming advocated

    d) Pathologic process
    - loss and thinning of superficial cartilage
    - synovium: no inflammatory changes, some villous formation
    - subsynovium: nodular lymphoid hyperplasia
    - perivascular infiltrates: lymphocytes, plasma cells, monocytes
    - joint capsule becomes thickened
    - adjacent bone is osteoporotic, with synovium-filled cysts
    - late in process: cysts, osteophytes, obliteration of joint cavity, deformity
    - possibly find underlying osteonecrosis

3. **Radiologic Features**

    a) Diminished joint space

    b) Protrusio acetabuli

    c) Local periarticular osteopenia, subchondral cysts, erosion, blurred articular cortex

    d) Premature epiphyseal closure

    e) Femoral head shows lateral overgrowth, with broadened femoral neck

    f) Hallmark: young female with narrowed hip joint space, no osteophytes, but periarticular osteopenia

    g) Delayed isotopic bone scan shows increased uptake at femoral head and acetabulum

    h) Arthrography shows "dappled" contrast over femoral head (patchy cartilage loss)

    i) MR shows patchy cartilage loss

4. **Differential Considerations**

    a) Strongly suspect when protrusio acetabuli is seen in asymptomatic patient

    b) Patients may be asymptomatic through adolescence: develop secondary DJD in their 40s

    c) With acute presentation, **DDX** may include: idiopathic protrusio acetabuli, slipped femoral capital epiphysis, trauma, septic arthritis, tuberculosis, migratory or transitory osteoporosis, reflex sympathetic dystrophy, Perthe's disease, pigmented villonodular synovitis, synovioma, rheumatoid arthritis

T. SCLERODERMA
(synonyms: CREST syndrome (Calcinosis, Raynaud's Phenomenon, Esophageal, Scleroderma and Telangiectasia), progressive systemic sclerosis (PSS), acrosclerosis)

1. **General Considerations**

    a) Systemic inflammatory connective tissue disease

    b) Idiopathic etiology

    c) Affects: skin, lungs, gastrointestinal tract, heart, kidneys, musculoskeletal system

    d) Thibierge-Weissenbach syndrome: combined scleroderma, soft tissue calcinosis, Raynaud's phenomenon, and generalized telangiectasia

2. **Clinical Features**

    a) Female predilection (3:1)

    b) Onset 30–50 years of age

    c) Skin progresses through three stages
- edema
- induration
- atrophy

d) Early presentation
- puffy, painful extremity swelling
- Raynaud's phenomenon in > 90% of cases (may precede skin changes)
    1) due to exposure to cold or to emotional stress
    2) peripheral vasoconstriction: pallor or white fingers, then blue
    3) peripheral vasodilation follows: painful swelling, redness

e) Later presentation
- skin thickening, induration, adherence to underlying structures (hidebound)
- in face: *mauskopff*: "mouselike" facies
- fingers and dorsum of hands and feet have most notable skin changes
- telangiectasia, vitiligo, hyperpigmentation may be present
- nodular subcutaneous calcific masses may ulcerate through skin: especially in pressure areas such as fingers, ulnar forearm, ischial tuberosities
- prominent muscle weakness and atrophy

f) Systemic effects
- GI tract effects most prominent
    1) esophageal dilation and loss of motility cause early, severe dysphagia and heartburn (90% of cases)
    2) sluggish, dilated bowel: causes distention, constipation, reduced absorption
- lung and heart involvement leads to dyspnea and heart failure

g) Pathologic process
- low-grade inflammation in perivascular tissue
- atrophy and fibrosis of adjacent collagen
- small arterioles undergo progressive intimal thickening, medial fibrosis, eventual thrombosis
- previously perfused tissues suffer inflammation, decreased vascularity, fibrous tissue deposition and induration
- inflammatory myositis and muscle degeneration
- synovial inflammatory cellular infiltration: external and internal fibrin deposits

3. Radiologic Features

a) Spine, pelvis, large peripheral joints spared

b) X-ray signs of scleroderma in the hand and wrist
- soft tissue
    1) overlying skin contour of distal fingertips altered

2) tapered, conical fingertip, tip retracted proximally (mensuration to determine this: vertical thickness of soft tissue < 20% of width at base of distal phalanx)

3) periarticular skin folds obliterated

4) 20% of cases show soft tissue calcifications: 75% of these in hands

5) calcifications may be punctate or sheetlike

6) calcification appears at stress areas: radial surface of second digit, ulnar forearm (more pronounced in dominant hand)

7) tissue sites:
   - subcutaneous: *calcinosis cutis*
   - along myofascial planes (sheetlike calcification)
   - joint capsules
   - sometimes intraarticular

- bones
  1) distal phalanges, especially terminal tufts affected
  2) resorbing osteolysis starts at tip and lateral palmar tuft
  3) becomes a sharpened, tapered distal phalanx (in 80% of cases)
  4) may progress to complete osteolysis of phalanx
  5) local osteolysis adjacent to soft tissue calcifications
  6) disuse, immobilization lead to general osteopenia

- joints
  1) variable signs: bilateral resorption of first metacarpal base and trapezium
  2) occasional intraarticular calcification
  3) may see changes resembling RA, erosive osteoarthritis, psoriatic arthritis

c) X-ray signs of scleroderma at other sites
- bone
  1) rare: femoral head avascular necrosis due to vasculitis
  2) osteolysis adjacent to overlying skin at distal clavicles, mandible, posterior ribs
- soft tissue
  1) calcifications in stress areas: wrist, elbow, ischial tuberosities, hip, knee
  2) radiolucent periodontal membrane 3–4 times thicker than normal
  3) pulmonary interstitial fibrosis, especially at lung base
  4) barium studies show bowel dilation, decreased peristalsis (especially in

esophagus and small bowel); colon shows broad-based, wide-mouthed pseudodiverticula on antimesenteric surface

U. OSTEITIS CONDENSANS ILII (OCI)

☞ **1. General Considerations**

    a) Isolated sacroiliac arthropathy predominantly in childbearing women

    b) Usually a multiparous woman
- 20–40 years old

    c) Female predominance > 9:1

    d) Same process occurs at medial clavicle: osteitis condensans of the clavicle
- history of localized sternoclavicular stress with swelling and pain
- adjacent joint space remains normal

2. Clinical Features

    a) Chronic low back pain and stiffness

    b) SI motion may be excessive or may be restricted

    c) Orthopedic tests for SI involvement are positive

    d) Pain and tenderness with palpation over SI joint

    e) Lumbar paraspinal muscle spasm

    f) **DDX:** intervertebral disc lesion, facet syndrome, AS, psoriatic spondylitis, DJD

☞   **g)** Pathologic process
- etiology unknown: may involve hormonal, mechanical, infectious, inflammatory or degenerative factors
- predominant theory: combined hormonal and mechanical stress factors
- postulated process
  1) ligamentous laxity of pregnancy (sometimes within menstrual cycle) may predispose to ligament damage
  2) this increases physical stress through the subchondral bone of the ilium
  3) supporting trabeculae thicken in response to this increased stress
- at involved SI joint: increased osseous vascularity, thickened trabeculae, mild inflammatory cellular infiltrate, marrow changes
- joint cartilage may be normal, or may show mild degenerative changes
- all signs and symptoms may completely resolve over several years

☞ **3. Radiologic Features**

    a) Optimal view: tilt-up view (AP pelvis with 30° cephalad tube tilt)

    b) Bilateral, symmetric, triangular sclerotic areas on lower half of ilium (hyperostosis triangularis ilii)

    c) Joint margins and joint space usually normal

V. OSTEITIS PUBIS

1. General Considerations

    a) Painful pubic symphysis articulation

    b) Commonly a sequel to prostate or bladder surgery

2. Clinical Features

    a) Recent history of lower pelvic surgery
- within 3 months
- surgeries might involve bladder, prostate, urethra, uterus, cervix
- other implicated events: pregnancy, trauma; often no identified provocation

    b) Localized pain at symphysis pubis
- exacerbated by palpation, thigh adduction, trunk flexion

    c) May have an audible click when joint is moved

    d) Antalgic gait: waddling gait with antalgic flexion posture

    e) Pain gradually subsiding over time (up to 2 years)

    f) Therapies (varying degrees of effectiveness)
- mobilization
- vitamin B supplementation
- antibiotics
- radiation
- diathermy
- injected cortisone, local anesthetics, and other anti-inflammatory drugs
- arthrodesis may be required

    g) Pathologic process and laboratory findings (correlated with etiologic theories)
- theory of vascular etiology
  1) local venous stasis
  2) intraosseous venous engorgement
  3) localized osteoporosis
- theory that this is a variant of Sudeck's atrophy: no laboratory findings
- theory of low-grade infection
  1) biopsy may show acute and chronic inflammatory changes, cultured bacteria
  2) most commonly cultured agents: gram negative bacilli
     - *Pseudomonas aeruginosa* and *Escherichia coli*

3. Radiologic Features

a) 1–3 weeks latent period after onset of symptoms

b) Some cases never have radiologic manifestations

c) Characteristic: bilateral symmetric pubic bone and rami changes
- irregular joint margins
- subchondral sclerosis
- moth-eaten osteopenia
- widened joint space

d) With resolution: normal bone density but residual irregularity of joint margin

e) May progress to ankylosis

f) May resolve with residual instability and offset of opposing pubic bones

W. HYPERTROPHIC OSTEOARTHROPATHY (HOA)

 ### 1. General Considerations

a) Skeletal signs occur as a sequel to visceral disorder (usually intrathoracic)
- most commonly, bronchogenic carcinoma
- about 10% of bronchogenic carcinomas result in classic triad of HOA

b) May relate to abnormal neurovascular reflexes; especially vagus nerve

c) Classic triad may manifest before primary causative disease becomes symptomatic

d) Surgical excision of primary lesion and vagal resection causes rapid regression of HOA symptoms

2. Clinical Features

a) May simulate RA or other rheumatologic processes

b) Classic triad
- digital clubbing
- symmetric arthritis
- periostitis

c) Thickened soft tissue causes digital clubbing
- bulbous enlargement of fingertips
- increased curvature of nail contour
- **DDX:** digital clubbing caused by thoracic and abdominal disease or heroin addiction

d) Arthritis manifests as:
- synovitis with effusion, warmth, redness
- common at knees, ankles, elbows, wrists, proximal fingers

e) Periostitis manifests as:
- vague, diffuse pain along long bone diaphyses
- commonly in legs and forearms

f) Pathologic process
- periostitis sites
    1) round cell infiltration in outer fibrous layer
    2) cambium new-bone proliferation
    3) fibrous tissue adjacent to cortex
- clubbed digits
    1) hypervascularity
    2) leads to hypertrophy and hyperplasia
- two theories of pathogenesis
    1) humoral: less well accepted; visceral lesion produces a substance that increases peripheral blood flow
    2) neurogenic: considered most likely; vagal efferent reflex vasodilation of peripheral vessels

g) Laboratory findings: elevated ESR

 3. Radiologic Features

a) Periostitis
- most consistent and apparent sign
- solid or single lamination
- outer surface may be undulating
- early: separated from cortex by lucent stripe
- later: no separation from cortical bone
- bilateral, symmetric distribution in metaphyses and diaphyses of long bones

b) Commonly at (in descending order of frequency): tibia, fibula, radius, ulna, metacarpals, metatarsals, femur, humerus

c) Radionuclide studies: periosteal uptake appears as a *double stripe sign*, highlighting the two apposed cortices

d) Joint effusion, but no other signs of arthritis

e) Digital clubbing: bulbous enlargement at fingertips

f) Chest films may demonstrate pulmonary mass or abnormality

REVIEW—STUDY QUESTIONS

1. What disease precedes the onset of Jaccoud's arthritis?
2. Describe the clinical manifestations of SLE.
3. What arthritides are manifested in reversible, or flexible, deformities of the hands?
4. What is the probable etiology of osteitis condensans ilii?
5. What population is most prone to scleroderma?
6. What are the radiologic features of SLE?
7. What are the theories explaining the development of HOA?

8. What is the classic triad of HOA, and what are its most common sites?

9. What are the radiologic features of scleroderma?

10. What is the most common pathologic antecedent of HOA?

X.   GOUT

 1.   General Considerations

    a) Gout is from Latin *gutta*: a drop (Hippocrates believed poison fell "drop by drop" into the joint)

    b) Hyperuricemia with acute inflammatory arthritis

    c) Recurrent episodes

    d) A metabolic arthritis: intraarticular deposits of sodium monourate

    e) *Podagra*: descriptive of predilection for the foot

    f) *Tophus*: Greek term for chalk stone, describes chalky deposits of urate in joints and periarticular tissues

2.   Clinical Features

    a) General characteristics
- characteristically appears in 40–60-year-old males
- 20:1 male predominance
- postmenopausal women on diuretics are susceptible, especially with familial incidence
- Polynesian and New Zealand natives are particularly susceptible
- primary: hyperuricemia due to overproduction (or underexcretion) of uric acid; inborn enzymatic defect (this is most common form)
- secondary: hyperuricemia with another disease or resulting from drug actions
- four clinical stages recognized: asymptomatic, acute, polyarticular, chronic

    b) Asymptomatic hyperuricemia
- predisposed to renal calculi
- later may develop gouty arthritis

    c) Acute gouty arthritis
- acute inflammatory monoarticular (or oligoarticular) arthritis
- attacks usually occur in early morning hours
- lower extremity is the site, 60% at metatarsophalangeal joint of great toe; also hits intertarsal joints and knees

- joint is swollen, hot, and dry
- attack usually lasts a few days, but may be expected to recur
- renal calculi occur more frequently after articular manifestations

d) Polyarticular gouty arthritis
- with multiple attacks, simultaneous polyarticular involvement develops
- lower extremity is still prime site, shows first radiographic changes
- small joints of hand and wrist may be involved, also the elbow
- over time, hip, spine and SI joints are affected

e) Chronic tophaceous gout
- drug therapy has minimized this sequel
- local tophi (sodium monourate deposits) were deposited with numerous attacks over 10 to 12 years
- predilection for more avascular tissues: tendons; subcutaneous layers at elbows, forearms, hands, knees, feet, helix of ear; synovium; periarticular soft tissues; subchondral bone
- destructive, deforming effects on bone and joints; ulcerate through skin
- rarely: tophi in spinal canal lead to neurologic effects
- cause renal damage, kidney stones, hypertension, atherosclerosis, thrombophlebitis

f) Lesch-Nyhan syndrome
- hereditary clinical syndrome (rare)
- hyperuricemia, mental retardation, abnormal self-destructive/aggressive behavior

g) Pathologic process
- precursor: hyperuricemia
- inflammatory agent: sodium monourate crystals
- process: purine nucleic acids (adenine and guanine) break down to produce uric acid
- crucial enzyme: xanthine oxidase
- exacerbators: dietary purine; chronic lead poisoning (impairs uric acid clearance); aspirin; diuretics; alcohol; nicotinic acid (reduce uric acid excretion)
- uric acid crystals are deposited and cause acute inflammation in synovium, cartilage, joint capsules, periarticular tissues and subchondral bone
- mechanisms involved in deposition:
  1) lower temperature in peripheral joints may enhance deposition there
  2) microtrauma
  3) serum globulin abnormalities
  4) tissue levels of proteoglycan

- with chronicity: synovial hyperplasia, pannus formation; degradation of articular cartilage, marginal erosions
- within bone: intraosseous tophi form; subchondral trabeculae are resorbed
- histopathology of tophi:
    1) layers of urate crystals in mineralized crystalline matrix
    2) around tophi: low-grade granulomatous reaction
    3) tophi may develop peripheral calcification or ossification

☞ **3. Radiologic Features**

a) Clinical manifestations may precede visible signs by 5–10 years

b) Soft tissue
- joint effusion
- tophi: soft tissue density 5 mm to 5 cm in diameter, eccentric, usually periarticular in forearm, elbow, dorsum of hand, knee, ankle, forefoot; may show peripheral calcification

c) Joint space
- normal space usually preserved through early stages
- late: uniform loss of joint space
- very rare to progress to ankylosis
- secondary joint changes mimic DJD: subchondral sclerosis, osteophytes, misalignments

d) Bone erosions
- marginal: pannus reaction on "*bare area*"; 2–3 mm cortical loss at bare area; may spread to central intraarticular cortex
- periarticular: extrinsic pressure erosions, especially with tophi; eccentric locations in metaphysis or diaphysis; dense, sclerotic margin; "*overhanging margin sign*" (Fig. 5.9); lip of bone protrudes into soft tissues (this may also occur at edge of marginal erosions)
- intraosseous: well-circumscribed, oval or round "*punched out*" lucent tophi in medullary cavity; usually in subchondral bone adjacent to joint

e) Bone density
- in acute attack, mild subchondral osteopenia
- bone density is usually normal

f) Periosteum
- occasional linear periosteal new bone: thickened cortex at metaphyseal/ diaphyseal area

g) Chondrocalcinosis
- occurs in triangular cartilage of wrist; knee menisci; symphysis pubis
- seen in about 5% of gout patients

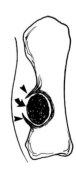

Figure 5.9.

Overhanging margin sign. Reprinted with permission from Yochum TR, Rowe LJ. Essentials of Skeletal Radiology, 2nd ed. Baltimore: Williams & Wilkins, 1996:933.

h) Avascular necrosis (infrequent)
- medullary infarcts, epiphyseal necrosis
- at femoral and humeral heads

i) X-ray signs of gout in the foot
- this is the most common site
- predilection for first metatarsophalangeal joint
- early signs: metatarsal head erosions (medial and dorsal surfaces)
  1) may also affect fifth MTP joint; first PIP joint, adjacent phalanges
  2) swelling, soft tissue tophi at same sites
- late signs: uniform joint space diminution
  1) prominent *"overhanging margins"* adjacent to periarticular erosions
  2) intraosseous tophi produce lytic *"punched out"* lesions
  3) distinctive lack of osteoporosis (except in acute phase)

j) X-ray signs of gout in the hand and wrist
- asymmetric involvement
- erosions, soft tissue swelling, misalignment
- *spotty carpal sign*: multiple carpal erosions (**DDX:** RA and TB)
- ulnar styloid erosions
- distinctive lack of osteoporosis, lack of ulnar drift

k) X-ray signs of gout in the knee
- erosions at medial and lateral condyles
- *"pseudotumor of gout"*: prepatellar tophi
- **diagnostic hallmark**: soft tissue mass (often with calcification), and erosion at superolateral patella

l) X-ray signs of gout at the elbow
- olecranon and adjacent ulnar erosions with soft tissue swelling in forearm
- tophi in olecranon bursa: *"rising sun sign"* on lateral view

m) X-ray signs of gout at the SI joint
- affected in about 15% of cases
- usually bilateral, asymmetric involvement
- articular erosions with adjacent sclerosis

n) X-ray signs of gout in the spine
- 75% of gout patients have back pain, but x-ray manifestations are rare
- cervical spine most likely to be affected:
  1) odontoid erosions
  2) atlantoaxial instability
  3) endplate erosions
- occasionally: lumbar endplate erosions and facet joint degeneration
- may manifest osteophytes, annular calcifications

- epidural tophi may cause compression myelopathy, paresis (these are more likely in thoracic and lumbar areas)

Y. CALCIUM PYROPHOSPHATE DIHYDRATE CRYSTAL DEPOSITION DISEASE (CPPD)
(synonyms: CPPD Crystal Deposition Disease; CPPD)

1. General Considerations

  a) May have gout-like symptoms

  b) Clinical presentations vary (see Table 5.3)

  c) Onset > 30 years of age; peak incidence at 60 years

  d) Often associated with other diseases: diabetes mellitus, DJD, gout, hyperparathyroidism, hemochromatosis, Wilson's disease, neuroarthropathy, ochronosis hereditary factor in some populations: Czechoslovakian, Chilean, Dutch

  2. Clinical Features

  a) Most commonly: similar to DJD; chronic, progressive joint pain, intermittent swelling, crepitus, reduced range of motion

  b) Chronic course interspersed with acute attacks, especially after periods of immobility

  c) Peripheral joints most often involved: (in descending order of incidence) knees, wrists, hands, ankles, hips, elbows

  d) Wrist involvement often includes carpal tunnel syndrome

  e) Occasional pain, loss of motion in cervical and lumbar spine

TABLE 5.3
Clinical Presentations of CPPD

Designation	Clinical Pattern	Percentage of CPPD
Type A: Pseudogout	acute/subacute, self-limited; affects knee, hip, shoulder, elbow, and forefoot	10–20%
Type B: Pseudorheumatoid	continuous acute attacks over weeks, months; stiffness, fatigue, hypomobility, elevated ESR	2–6%
Type C: Pseudoosteoarthritis	chronic, progressive acute episodes; bilateral symmetric in peripheral joints; knee, elbow contractures	35–60%
Type D: Pseudoosteoarthritis	chronic, progressive, but no acute episodes	10–35%
Type E: Asymptomatic	chondrocalcinosis	10–20%
Type F: Pseudoneuropathy	instability, destructive joint disease, relatively pain-free	up to 2%
Type G: Miscellaneous	variable presentation	up to 2%

f) Pathologic process
- mechanism of deposition unknown
- crystals deposit in cartilage, synovium, tendons, ligaments
    1) in cartilage: both hyaline and fibrocartilage, adjacent to chondrocytes; in intermediate cartilage layers, never on surface
    2) in synovium: CPPD crystals are within phagocytes
    3) most commonly affected tendons: Achilles, triceps, quadriceps, supraspinatus
    4) affects capsular ligaments
- produces acute synovitis
- seems to be influenced by age, genetics, and coexisting disease
- pyrophosphate arthropathy
    1) sequel to cartilage degeneration
    2) structural articular changes resembling DJD or neurotrophic arthropathy
    3) cartilage loss or fibrillation
    4) subchondral trabecular thickening
    5) geodes (subchondral cysts)
    6) intraarticular loose bodies
    7) osteophytes
    8) fragmentation, articular cortical collapse

g) Laboratory studies normal, except for pyrophosphate crystals in synovial fluid

☞ **3. Radiologic Features**

a) Major features are calcifications in or around joints; pyrophosphate arthropathy

b) Chondrocalcinosis (cartilage calcification)
- hyaline cartilage: thin, linear either continuous or intermittent calcification parallel to articular cortex; frequently at wrist, knee, elbow, hip, and shoulder
- fibrocartilage: thick, irregular, shaggy calcifications; frequently at knee menisci, wrist triangular cartilage, symphysis pubis; annulus fibrosus
- tends to coexist with arthropathy, but may be asymptomatic
- see Table 5.4: diseases associated with chondrocalcinosis

c) Other calcifications
- synovial calcifications at joint margins
- joint capsule calcification yields linear bridging across joint space
- ligaments and tendons show thin, linear calcifications extending for considerable distance from joint
- vascular calcifications: two parallel linear calcifications (may occur with diabetes)

- *tumorous CPPD*: massive depositions with calcification, usually with adjacent extrinsic bone erosions near a joint

d) Pyrophosphate arthropathy

- similar to DJD: loss of joint space, subchondral sclerosis, cyst formation, osteophytes, loose bodies, joint deformity

e) **DDX:** DJD

- unusual joint distribution, with no antecedent trauma: e.g., wrist, elbow, glenohumeral joints
- unusual intraarticular sites: selective involvement of radiocarpal, trapezoscaphoid, talocalcaneal, patellofemoral compartments
- prominent subchondral cysts (geodes): intraosseous synovial fluid extrusions
- subchondral bone changes: rapid subchondral fragmentation and collapse, forming loose bodies (similar to neuropathic arthropathy)
- may be no osteophytes, or may be very large osteophytes, regardless of the extent of joint space changes

f) X-ray signs of CPPD at the knee

- most frequent site of clinical and radiologic features
- characteristic hyaline cartilage and meniscus calcifications
    1) chondrocalcinosis on femoral condyles; posterior patellar surface
    2) meniscal chondrocalcinosis: AP view shows triangular calcifications with medially-directed apices, in medial and lateral compartments
- medial femorotibial, patellofemoral, and lateral femorotibial compartments involved (in descending order of incidence)
- sign of CPPD: isolated patellofemoral compartment effects
- subchondral sclerosis, cysts, fragmentation with loose body formation

g) X-ray signs of CPPD in the wrist

- ulnocarpal triangular cartilage calcification
- hyaline calcifications adjacent to any carpals
- synovial and ligamentous calcifications: frequently at scapholunate space
- radiocarpal arthropathy: diminished radioscaphoid space, subchondral sclerosis, cysts, osteophytes
- *"Terry Thomas sign"*: scapholunate disassociation

- "stepladder" radiocarpal alignment: proximal movement of scaphoid, with distal movement of lunate
- **SLAC** deformity: **S**capho**L**unate **A**dvanced **C**ollapse
- severe trapezoscaphoid degeneration
- **DDX:** RA—radioulnar joint remains unaffected in CPPD

h) X-ray signs of CPPD in the spine
- infrequent, nonspecific, usually asymptomatic
- most changes in lumbar spine, some in cervical
- diminished disc height, vacuum phenomena
- body sclerosis, osteophytes, facet arthropathy
- marginal syndesmophytes (annular calcification)
- occasionally, nuclear opacification
- crystal deposition in canal: epidural, may simulate disc herniation
- thickened, bulging ligamentum flavum may calcify
- vertebral displacement, angular deformities, atlantoaxial subluxations

---

TABLE 5.4
Diseases Involving Chondrocalcinosis

Diseases	Processes
"The 3 **C**'s"	**c**artilage degeneration diseases **c**ation diseases **c**rystal deposition diseases
Degenerative joint disease (DJD)	degeneration due to mechanical stress
Neurotrophic joint disease	severe mechanical stress, loss of sensory defenses
Acromegaly	mechanical stress, genetic factors
Hyperparathyroidism	deposition of calcium (Ca^{++})
Hemochromatosis	deposition of iron (Fe^{++})
Wilson's disease	deposition of copper (Cu^{++})
CPPD (with pseudogout, diabetes)	deposition of calcium pyrophosphate dihydrate crystals
Gout	deposition of sodium monourate crystals
Ochronosis	deposition of homogentisic acid crystals
Miscellaneous conditions involving chondrocalcinosis: Paget's disease Systemic lupus erythematosus Osteochondritis dissecans Idiopathic chondrocalcinosis	

      i) X-ray signs of CPPD in hands
- second and third MCP joints most often involved
- diminished joint space, sclerosis, fragmentation of metacarpal head

      j) X-ray signs of CPPD in the shoulder
- glenohumeral degeneration, hyaline chondrocalcinosis
- acromioclavicular fibrocartilage calcification (35% of patients)

      k) X-ray signs of CPPD in the hip
- femoral head and acetabular labrum show hyaline calcifications
- superolateral or entire joint degenerative changes
- may progress to protrusio acetabuli

      l) X-ray signs of CPPD in the foot
- dorsal talonavicular osteophytes, sclerosis, fragmentation

      m) X-ray signs of CPPD at the symphysis pubis
- vertical linear calcification in fibrocartilage of joint
- degenerative changes in marginal cortices

Z. HEMOCHROMATOSIS

1. General Considerations

      a) Metabolic disorder: deposition of iron into all body tissues

      b) Male predilection (20:1)

      c) Primary hemochromatosis: genetic defect of GI absorption

      d) Secondary hemochromatosis: caused by alcoholism (cirrhosis), multiple transfusions, anemia, over-ingestion of iron

2. Clinical Features

      a) **Diagnostic triad:** cirrhosis, diabetes, and bronze colored skin (*"bronze diabetes"*)

      b) Cardiomyopathy is also common

      c) Degenerative arthropathy in second and third MCP joints, knees, hips, shoulders

      d) Pathologic process
- iron deposited in all body tissues
- causes dysfunction in liver, pancreas, skin, heart

3. Radiologic Features

      a) Osteopenia

      b) Chondrocalcinosis

      c) Periarticular calcifications

      d) Uniform diminution of joint space

      e) *"Beak"* or *"hook"* osteophytes, usually at second and third metacarpal heads

f) Subchondral cysts

g) sclerosis

AA. WILSON'S DISEASE
(synonyms: hepatolenticular degeneration)

1. General Considerations

a) Rare autosomal recessive disorder of copper metabolism

b) May manifest between 5 and 50 years of age; usually in adolescence

c) Fatal (usually before age 30) unless continuous treatment is given

 ### 2. Clinical Features

a) Acute hepatitis usually is initial manifestation; progresses to cirrhosis

b) CNS symptoms are almost as frequent as initial presenting symptoms
- tremors, dystonia, dysarthria, dysphagia, drooling, incoordination
- grossly inappropriate behavior
- psychosis

c) Corneal deposits: golden or greenish-golden rings or crescents (Kayser-Fleischer ring)

d) Amenorrhea, repeated miscarriages

e) Hematuria; plus urinary hyperexcretion of amino acids, uric acid, phosphate, calcium, glucose

f) Pathologic process
- Cu^{++} metabolism disturbance
- up to 50 times normal copper concentration in liver
- may diffuse from liver into blood: carried and deposited into other organs
- deposition in brain is strongly symptomatic (see above)

3. Radiologic Features

a) Osteopenia

b) Chondrocalcinosis

c) Cysts, irregular cortices

d) Osteophytes

e) Schmorl's nodes; "squaring" of vertebral bodies

BB. HYDROXYAPATITE DEPOSITION DISEASE (HADD)
(synonyms: calcifying tendinitis, calcifying bursitis, peritendinitis calcarea, periarthritis calcarea, hydroxyapatite rheumatism, hydroxyapatite crystal deposition disease)

 ### 1. General Considerations

a) Radiographic findings correlate poorly with clinical manifestations

        b) Ages 40–70 years

        c) Most commonly, single site involvement; may be multiple

☞   **2. Clinical Features**

        a) Acute tendinitis, bursitis, joint pain

        b) Localized symptoms; no systemic involvement

        c) Most commonly affected: shoulder

        d) Other sites: elbow, wrist, fingers, hip, knee, ankle, foot, cervical and lumbar spine

        e) Pain, tenderness, localized swelling, reduced range of motion

        f) In spine: painful stiff neck, muscle spasm, painful dysphagia, globus hystericus
- short-term: 2–5 days worsening, about 2 weeks to resolution

        g) Pathologic process
- primary etiology unknown
- implicated factors: genetic proclivity, aging, biomechanical stress, trauma, vascular and neurologic factors
- calcium hydroxyapatite crystals deposited within a focal area of degeneration in tissue
- histopathologic effects: necrosis, fibrosis, inflammatory cell infiltrate, granular hydroxyapatite deposits
- in supraspinatus tendon, lesions are in the *"critical zone"*: anatomic portion of the tendon which is poorly vascularized

☞   **3. Radiologic Features**

        a) General features
- tendon calcifications
  1) near insertion
  2) not contiguous with cortical bone
  3) early: wispy, ill-defined
  4) later: homogenous, well-defined calcifications
  5) usually round or oval; but may be linear
  6) size and shape alter over time; lesion may resolve completely
  7) tendons most commonly affected: rotator cuff, hip, upper cervical spine
- bursal calcifications
  1) homogeneously dense, round, or oval
  2) similar to calcified tendon, but located in bursae
  3) most commonly affected bursae:
     - subacromial, subdeltoid, ischial bursae

b) X-ray signs of **HADD** in the shoulder
- General considerations
  1) > 50% of shoulder calcification cases are bilaterally affected, but in unilateral presentations, the right side is more often affected (2:1)
  2) **"SITS"** tendons are most often affected; then both biceps heads and the subacromial and subdeltoid bursae
  3) examination must include both internal and external rotation views
- supraspinatus tendon
  1) most commonly involved tendon
  2) optimum view: external rotation
  3) calcification seen in profile adjacent to (not superimposed) greater tuberosity promontory
  4) internal rotation view projects calcification over humeral head
- infraspinatus tendon
  1) external rotation: calcification overlies middle third of greater tuberosity
  2) internal rotation brings calcification into profile
- teres minor tendon
  1) external rotation: calcification is superimposed over lower aspect of greater tuberosity
  2) internal rotation: calcification projected away from tuberosity
- subscapularis tendon
  1) external rotation projects calcification over humeral head
  2) internal rotation: calcification more medially located, in profile adjacent to inner humeral cortex
- biceps tendons
  1) long head: calcification appears adjacent to superior glenoid fossa rim
  2) short head: lesion appears adjacent to coracoid process
- bursae
  1) subacromial: calcification medial to greater tuberosity, beneath acromial process (homogenous, sharply defined density)
  2) subdeltoid: adjacent to greater tuberosity, laterally placed

c) X-ray signs of HADD in the hip
- gluteus maximus tendon
  1) at insertion into linea aspera
  2) may simulate referred sciatic pain
  3) AP projection: calcification just inferior to intertrochanteric line,

superimposed over lateral femoral shaft

4) frog-leg projection: calcification medial to medial surface of lesser trochanter

5) dense, homogenous opacities; may be multiple

6) cortical margin may be irregular

7) **DDX:** malignant transformation of osteochondroma; calcified lymph node; calcified TB infection; liposarcoma; synovioma; synoviochondrometaplasia; scleroderma

- adjacent to trochanters: piriformis and gluteal insertions, bursae
- AIIS
- acetabular margin
- ischial tuberosity

d) X-ray signs of HADD in tendons of the cervical spine

- longus colli insertions
  1) self-limiting, transient but acutely painful depositions in superolateral insertions
  2) seen on lateral view: amorphous calcifications (up to 2 cm diameter) anterior/inferior to anterior atlas tubercle, in retropharyngeal space
  3) may be in lower cervicals (C2–6)
  4) locally increased retropharyngeal interspace (> 7 mm)
  5) diminished lordosis
- MRI shows edema in superior portions of longus colli in acute stage
- radiographic signs disappear as clinical symptoms resolve

e) X-ray signs of HADD in intervertebral discs

- general features
  1) annular deposition most common: calcification in annular fissures and necrotic fibers
  2) nucleus pulposus may appear as a posterocentral, homogenous, round or oval density (as in normal discogram); calcium is deposited in crevices in the nucleus
  3) vertebral endplate cartilage may calcify: thin linear density parallel to cortical endplate
  4) various etiologies: DJD; sequestered disc prolapse; congenital block vertebrae; idiopathic (different process in childhood and adult cases)
- degenerative disc disease
  1) discal calcifications with: loss of disc height, endplate sclerosis, osteophytes

2) varied appearance of nuclear calcification: round, flattened ovoid, fragmented or linear; most common: fragmented oval contour

3) annular calcification more frequent: anterior disc calcifies, sometimes lateral margins; lower cervicals is most common site

4) called *intercalary bones*: < 2 mm thick, curvilinear, vertically oriented, separate from adjacent vertebral bodies

- sequestered disc prolapse (non-contained disc)

1) any discal extrusion may calcify

2) anterior and lateral prolapses seldom calcify; are asymptomatic

3) posterior prolapses may form loose fragments in spinal canal

4) Schmorl's nodes (intrabody herniations) may calcify

- congenital block vertebrae

1) vestigial nucleus may calcify

2) small, homogenous, rounded opacity

3) occurs at any motion segment that fuses: sacrococcygeal segments; or in Klippel-Feil syndrome; AS; JRA; myositis ossificans progressiva; surgical fusions

- childhood idiopathic IVD calcifications (clinical and radiologic features)

1) male predilection (2:1)

2) onset from 6–12 years of age

3) most common in cervical, then thoracic, and least in lumbar spine

4) usually single, but about 30% have multiple discs involved

5) nucleus pulposus is affected: **not** annulus

6) calcified nucleus may prolapse

7) about 70% have symptomatic pain; about 15% totally asymptomatic

8) about 30% also have fever

9) only 4% have neurologic symptoms

10) mild increase of disc height; moderate flattening of adjacent bodies, which may persist after calcification fragments and dissolves

11) associated neck stiffness (**DDX:** meningitis); local tenderness, scoliosis

12) laboratory findings: elevated ESR, leukocytosis

13) self-limiting within a few weeks, or months

14) sequela: loss of disc height,

osteophytes (premature DJD) at site

- adult idiopathic IVD calcifications
    1) appears degenerative, but without osteophytes, endplate sclerosis or disc height diminution
    2) discal calcification is the only sign; and these are asymptomatic unless herniation is involved
- miscellaneous IVD calcification etiologies
    1) biochemical: gout, pseudogout, hemochromatosis, ochronosis, hyperparathyroidism, hypervitaminosis D
    2) other disorders related to discal calcifications: acromegaly, AS, herpes zoster, poliomyelitis

f) X-ray signs of HADD at the elbow
- commonly at common extensor tendon (lateral epicondyle)
- also at common flexor tendon (medial epicondyle), triceps insertion at olecranon process, olecranon bursa

g) X-ray signs of HADD at the wrist
- at pisiform: flexor carpi ulnaris tendon insertion (most common wrist site)
    1) amorphous, poorly marginated opacity
    2) oblique projection gives optimal view
- next most common: abductor pollicus longus and extensor pollicus brevis tendons at radial styloid
    1) possibly related to *deQuervain's disease* (stenosing tenosynovitis)
    2) skin thickened and displaced, even before calcification is evident
- flexor carpi radialis tendon, adjacent to first metacarpal trapezium joint
- additional wrist sites: common flexor tendons, extensor carpi ulnaris tendon

h) X-ray signs of HADD in the hand
- infrequently involved
- MCP joints: flexor surface of metacarpal head where ligaments or tendons insert

i) X-ray signs of HADD at the knee
- knee is a rare site
- quadriceps tendon at patella
- biceps femoris insertion at head of fibula
- calcifications at medial or lateral epicondyles
- *Pellegrini-Stieda disease*: post-traumatic calcification in medial collateral ligament

j) X-ray signs of HADD in the foot
- flexor hallucis brevis and longus tendons at MTP joint

- peroneal tendons near 5th metatarsal base
- sometimes develop painful calcification at dorsal base of second metatarsal

CC. OCHRONOSIS

1. General Considerations

a) Hereditary metabolic amino acid metabolism disorder

b) Absence of homogentisic acid oxidase
- homogentisic acid is excreted in urine: alkaptonuria
- homogentisic acid is deposited in tissues: ochronosis
- deposition in joints: ochronotic arthropathy

c) Familial incidence is common

d) Male predominance (2:1)

2. Clinical Features

a) Blue/brown pigmentation: skin, sclera, cornea, cartilage of nose and ear

b) Arthritis resembles mild AS: progressive stiffness and pain at spine, hips, knees, and shoulders

c) Onset of arthritic symptoms in 30s

d) May present initially with disc herniation

e) Site incidence
- spine: 95% of cases
- knee: 30% of cases
- shoulder: 20% of cases
- hip: 20% of cases

f) Posture shows increased thoracic kyphosis, decreased lumbar lordosis

g) Pathologic process
- tyrosine and phenylalanine not metabolized, due to lack of homogentisic acid oxidase
- homogentisic acid in urine and sweat turns black when exposed to air or alkali
- discoloration is yellow, blue or black macroscopically, yellow (ochre) microscopically
- makes cartilage brittle, so it cracks, fibrillates, erodes, and calcifies or ossifies
- in spine, this affects the IVD (most at inner annular layers): fissuring and fragmentation; multiple vacuum phenomena form

h) Laboratory findings: urinary homogentisic acid; false positive for urinary glucose

3. Radiologic Features

    a) Spinal changes

- lumbar and thoracic areas most prominently affected
- distinctive disc changes:
    1) loss of disc height
    2) "vacuum" phenomenon
    3) thin, wafer-like calcifications parallel to vertebral endplates (calcification of endplate hyaline cartilage)
    4) usually simultaneous involvement of multiple levels
    5) small osteophytes; low level of marginal bony proliferation
    6) can progress to osseous ankylosis across greatly diminished disc space (**DDX:** AS, where disc height remains normal)
- no syndesmophytes form
- severe facet arthrosis, eventual ankylosis
- loss of lumbar lordosis; increased thoracic kyphosis
- severe osteoporosis
- spinal ligaments may ossify

    b) Peripheral joint changes

- usually at shoulder and knee, simulates DJD:
    1) loss of joint space, sclerosis, cysts, osteophytes, chondrocalcinosis
    2) flattened articular surfaces
- in hip uniform joint space loss with minimal osteophyte formation, like AS

    c) Visceral involvement

- kidney and prostate calculi

DD. TUMORAL CALCINOSIS

1. General Considerations

    a) Etiology unknown

    b) Affects children, adolescents: usually 6–25 years of age

    c) Predilection for black population

    d) Masses show increased uptake on isotopic bone scans

2. Clinical Features

    a) Palpable soft tissue mass near joint

    b) Masses enlarge progressively, may ulcerate through skin

    c) Usually adjacent to shoulder, hip, elbow joints

    d) Treatment: excision; recurrence if excision is incomplete

  e) Pathologic process
- localized extracapsular accumulations of calcium
- multiloculated cysts, filled with viscous, semi-fluid suspension of calcium triphosphate or calcium carbonate salts in albumin
- dense, fibrous cyst walls lined with epithelioid and giant cells

  f) Laboratory tests occasionally show elevated serum phosphate and alkaline phosphatase

3. Radiologic Features

  a) Dense calcified mass near a joint

  b) Early: small, discrete nodules that enlarge, become increasingly dense

  c) May be 1–20 cm in diameter

  d) Well-defined, lobulated margins

  e) Upright films may demonstrate a fluid level

  f) Some extrinsic pressure erosions (more likely at posterior distal humerus)
- otherwise, bone and joint structures are normal

EE. SARCOIDOSIS
(synonym: Boeck's sarcoid)

1. General Considerations

  a) Etiology unknown

  b) Predilection for black and Scandinavian populations

  c) Multiple organ systems affected

  d) MRI shows leptomeningeal and bone lesions, even when plain films are normal

2. Clinical Features

  a) Acute onset
- patients usually young adults: 20–40 years of age
- with erythema nodosum: expect self-limiting course with spontaneous resolution
- erythema nodosum over anterior tibia (good prognostic sign)
- high rate of spontaneous remission; rarely has bone lesions

  b) Insidious onset
- heralds relentless, progressive fibrosis; debilitating, often fatal
- starts with older patient (> 40 years of age)
- bone lesions parallel skin lesions in this form
- about 50% have arthralgia, swelling, deformity: especially in hands and feet
- about 50% have asymptomatic skeletal lesions

c) Chest is often first area to have visible abnormalities: chest films should be done early if sarcoidosis is suspected
- unsuspected, mild disease (fibrosis) may be discovered on routine chest film

d) Face, neck and shoulders may have skin rash: discrete red nodules or purple nodules (*lupus pernio*)

e) Effects in the eye: iritis, uveitis, iridocyclitis

f) Systemic effects: fever, persistent coughing, lymphadenopathy, anorexia, weight loss, hepatosplenomegaly

g) *Lofgren's syndrome*: acute sarcoidosis with high fever, arthralgia, lymphadenopathy, and erythema nodosum

h) Pathologic process
- noncaseating granuloma is the **hallmark lesion**
    1) **DDX:** TB—with sarcoidosis there is no caseous necrosis or *Mycobacterium*
    2) compact focus of mostly epithelioid cells, with lymphocytes, giant cells, plasma cells
- mass within bone causes pressure atrophy of surrounding trabeculae
- non-caseating granulomas appear in various tissues, most commonly lymph nodes, spleen, liver
- non-caseating granulomas resolve to be replaced by fibrous tissue, inhibits organ function

i) Laboratory findings
- anemia, leucopenia, eosinophilia
- reversed albumin-globulin (A:G) ratio
- possibly hypercalcemia
- Kviem test: intradermal injection of sarcoid tissue suspension (positive: formation of superficial granulomas)
- often: elevated angiotensin converting enzyme (ACE) levels

j) Definitive diagnosis is via histologic examination of scalene node or by liver biopsy

3. Radiologic Features

a) Chest
- PA view shows bilateral bronchopulmonary lymph node enlargement
    1) *"potato nodes"*: fusiform opaque mass just lateral to hilum
    2) separated from heart by lucent lung
- right paratracheal lymphadenopathy plus bilateral hilar adenopathy: *"1-2-3 sign"* (*pawn broker's sign*)

- alveolar infiltrates, interstitial nodules, fibrosis: "*honeycomb lung*"

b) Distal extremities
- hand is most common site; especially the middle and distal phalanges
- bilateral, asymmetrical involvement
- intraosseous granulomas, or paraosseous masses causing erosions
- wide range of lesion patterns: most common are diffuse reticular lesions and well-circumscribed lesions
- diffuse reticular pattern
  - a) diffuse intraosseous perivascular granulomas infiltrate Haversian canals, erode adjacent fine trabeculae
  - b) medullary trabeculae appear coarse, prominent, and mildly osteoporotic
  - c) as infiltrates increase, distinct "*lacelike*" trabecular pattern develops with more prominent radiolucencies
- well-circumscribed pattern
  - a) localized lytic lesions, alone or with the diffuse reticular pattern
  - b) round to ovoid lesions; central or eccentric, well marginated
  - c) endosteal scalloping without periosteal response
  - d) rarely progress to crippling, deforming bone destruction
- distal phalanx may be sclerotic or may be resorbed
- joints usually normal, but there may be effusion, loss of joint space, subchondral collapse

c) Other skeletal sites
- rarely affects other sites
- bone
  1) long bones may develop reticular or well-circumscribed lesions without periosteal response
  2) lytic skull lesions do occur, but rarely
- muscles may develop tumorlike masses; must be differentiated from neoplasms
- spinal structures
  1) vertebrae rarely affected
  2) when vertebrae are involved: 75% lumbar, 25% cervical
  3) most commonly at thoracolumbar junction
  4) lytic vertebral body lesions with marginal reactive sclerosis
  5) very rare: diffuse or single blastic lesions (*ivory vertebrae*); **DDX:** blastic metastasis
  6) discs unaffected

FF. PIGMENTED VILLONODULAR SYNOVITIS (PVNS)

1. General Considerations

    a) Inflammation of synovial tissue; can affect any synovium

    b) rare; of unknown etiology

    c) classification controversial: inflammatory arthritis or benign synovial neoplasm?

    d) treatments: excision (but recurrence is common), radiation therapy

2. Clinical Features

    a) Young, middle-aged adults

    b) Slightly more likely to occur in men

    c) Most commonly in lower extremities: preference for knee

    d) Also affects hip, ankle, wrist, hand, foot, and rarely the spine

    e) Lumbar facet effects mimic synovial cyst; may cause radicular pain

    f) Joint swelling, stiffness, locking

    g) **DDX:** meniscal injury in knee (often there is no antecedent trauma)

    h) pathologic process
- undefined pathogenesis
- histologic findings
    1) hyperplastic connective tissue with phagocytic cellular infiltrations
    2) hemosiderin deposits
- gross changes
    1) large, folded red and brown masses
    2) close to cortical bone, these may cause extrinsic pressure erosion, especially in hip, ankle, wrist, and hand (tightly compartmentalized joints)

    i) Definitive laboratory findings: brown or serosanguinous synovial fluid aspirate, histologic evaluation for hemosiderin deposits and phagocytic cellular infiltrates

3. Radiologic Features

    a) Soft tissue signs
- intra-articular effusions
- dense, lobulated masses (arthrography, CT, MR give best evaluation)
- overlying fascial displacement

    b) **DDX:** neurovascular soft tissue malignant tumor
- both show on angiogram with hypervascularity, "puddling," tumor "blush"
- arthrography: intrinsic nodular filling defect of joint cavity
- on CT, PVNS does **not** enhance with contrast (malignant neoplasm does)

- MR shows heterogeneous synovial process with edematous foci
- ultrasound shows soft tissue mass with both solid and cystic areas

c) Bone signs
- loose-packed joints (knee, shoulder) are unlikely to show erosive bone lesions
- *"tight"* joints (hip, ankle, elbow, wrist, hand): extrinsic bone erosions are more common
  1) hip: concentric femoral neck erosions ("apple core deformity")
  2) marginal erosions; smooth, well-defined cortical excavations (appear "bubbly") can affect all intracapsular bone surfaces
- **DDX:** gout, RA

REVIEW—STUDY QUESTIONS

1. What is the pathologic process that results in ochronosis?
2. What are the radiologic features of gout, and where do they usually appear?
3. Give differentiating characteristics (pathologic, clinical, and radiologic) between CPPD and HADD.
4. What are the radiologic features of ochronosis in the spine?
5. Explain the biochemical abnormality the causes gout.
6. Where do skeletal manifestations of sarcoidosis most commonly appear? Describe them.
7. Name and describe two prominent signs of sarcoidosis which may appear on a PA chest film.
8. What is Wilson's disease? What are its radiologic features?
9. Name and define three "cation diseases" that might be associated with chondrocalcinosis.
10. What are the "3 Cs" associated with chondrocalcinosis?
11. What is HADD and what are the most common sites for HADD?
12. What processes are associated with a radiologic finding of calcification of the IVD?
13. What populations are most frequently affected by sarcoidosis?
14. Which joints are more likely to show bony effects of pigmented villonodular synovitis, and why?
15. Name and describe three of the seven clinical presentation patterns of CPPD.
16. What is alkaptonuria, and in what arthritis does it appear?
17. Describe two patterns of bone destruction caused by sarcoidosis.
18. What arthritis involves multiple vacuum phenomena and multiple contiguous disc calcifications?
19. What features distinguish CPPD from DJD?
20. What is the Lesch-Nyhan syndrome?

1. An "Andersson lesion" is:
   a) a pathologic fracture through a long bone.
   b) a pseudoarthrosis caused by a pathologic fracture through a previously ankylosed joint.
   c) an ankylosed spinal motion segment.
   d) a cavitation between the spine and the ossified anterior longitudinal ligament.

2. A striking difference between the pathologic process of rheumatoid arthritis and psoriatic arthritis is that the latter does not involve:
   a) pannus.
   b) periarticular osteoporosis.
   c) narrowing of the joint space.
   d) cortical margin erosions.

3. The onset of systemic lupus erythematosus most frequently occurs in:
   a) males above 50 years of age.
   b) females above 40 years of age.
   c) males between 10 and 40 years of age.
   d) females between 10 and 40 years of age.

4. The Lesch-Nyhan syndrome is a rare hereditary clinical syndrome associated with:
   a) rheumatoid arthritis.
   b) ochronosis.
   c) Wilson's disease.
   d) hyperuricemia.

5. Scleroderma has potentially serious effects on all of the following except:
   a) the heart.
   b) the kidneys.
   c) the lungs.
   d) the gastrointestinal tract.

6. Forestier's disease commonly involves calcification and ossification of:
   a) the posterior longitudinal ligament.
   b) the anterior longitudinal ligament.
   c) the ligamentum flavum.
   d) the nuchal ligament.

7. Sjogren's syndrome, seen with various connective tissue disorders, involves:
   a) excessive tearing and serous mucous production.
   b) vasculitis.
   c) scleromalacia perforans.
   d) generalized drying of mucus membranes.

8. Coxarthrosis is a term used to describe:
   a) advanced degenerative joint disease of the hip.
   b) surgical fixation of the hip.
   c) early degeneration of the acetabular joint.
   d) formation of an auxiliary acetabular joint because of congenital dislocation.

9. In the hands, the x-ray appearance of "dot-dash" cortical interruptions is characteristic of:
   a) gout.
   b) psoriasis.
   c) pseudogout.
   d) rheumatoid arthritis.

10. Synoviochondrometaplasia is:
    a) an inflammatory arthritide.
    b) a degenerative arthritide.
    c) a metabolic arthritide.
    d) a tumor-like or neoplastic lesion.

11. The subjective signs of ankylosing spondylitis are frequently aggravated by:
    a) moderate activity.
    b) a posture of slight spinal flexion.
    c) alcohol consumption.
    d) caffeine consumption.

12. Psoriatic arthropathy most commonly affects joints of the:
    a) hands and feet.
    b) lumbosacral spine.
    c) thoracolumbar spine.
    d) cervicothoracic spine.

13. The arthritis associated with Reiter's syndrome is:
    a) relentlessly progressive.
    b) usually self-limiting, but prone to recurrence and may leave residual joint damage.
    c) limited by steroid treatments, and seldom recurs.
    d) apt to recur, but seldom results in residual joint damage.

14. Most frequently, gout develops in:
    a) postmenopausal women on diuretics.
    b) males between 20 and 40 years of age.
    c) males between 40 and 60 years of age.
    d) men or women older than 60 years of age.

15. CREST syndrome is associated with:
    a) premature closure of the iliac crest physis.
    b) scleroderma.
    c) Raynaud's phenomenon.
    d) Thibierge-Weissenbach syndrome.

16. Diabetes mellitus has a recognized correlation with:
    a) ankylosing spondylitis.
    b) Reiter's syndrome.
    c) osteitis pubis.
    d) DISH.

17. A better prognosis is indicated when rheumatoid arthritis:
    a) is asymmetric and its onset is in later years.
    b) is symmetric in distribution.
    c) is clinically recognized before age 30.
    d) involves subcutaneous nodules.

18. Radiologic indications of sacroiliac degenerative joint disease:

    a) usually include sclerosis of the sacral joint surface.
    b) usually involve changes in the lower two-thirds of the joint.
    c) usually include a vacuum cleft.
    d) usually involve changes in the upper third of the joint.

19. Rheumatoid arthritis in the hands often:

    a) spares the distal interphalangeal joints.
    b) spares the second and third metacarpophalangeal joints.
    c) spares the first ray.
    d) spares the proximal interphalangeal joints.

20. Degenerative arthritides include all of the following except:

    a) erosive osteoarthritis.
    b) diffuse idiopathic skeletal hyperostosis (DISH).
    c) neurotrophic arthropathy.
    d) osteitis condensans ilii.

21. An arthritis showing a clear predilection for the axial skeleton in young males is:

    a) seropositive JRA.
    b) classic systemic Still's disease.
    c) Marie-Strümpell's disease.
    d) pseudogout.

22. In the spine, x-ray findings may be identical in cases of ankylosing spondylitis and:

    a) ochronosis.
    b) rheumatoid arthritis.
    c) neurotrophic arthropathy.
    d) enteropathic arthropathy.

23. Reiter's syndrome has clear associations with:

    a) Crohn's disease.
    b) regional enteritis.
    c) ulcerative colitis.
    d) dysentery caused by *Salmonella.*

24. The term *podagra*, associated with gout, refers to:

    a) the belief that poison fell "drop by drop" into the joint.
    b) the chalky urate deposits in joints.
    c) a predilection for the foot.
    d) hyperuricemia.

25. The diagnosis of idiopathic chondrolysis of the hip should be strongly suspected when there is:

    a) a young woman with prolific osteophytic growth at the acetabular joint.
    b) a patient in the fifth decade with osteoarthritis of the hip.
    c) an asymptomatic young woman with protrusio acetabuli.
    d) a young man with a limp and knee pain.

26. The vacuum cleft indicates degenerative joint disease only when it is seen:

    a) in the hip.
    b) in the shoulder.
    c) in the spine.
    d) in the knee.

27. Rheumatoid arthritis generally spares:

    a) the cervical spine.
    b) the lumbar spine.
    c) the shoulder joints.
    d) the carpal joints.

28. Lower costovertebral or costotransverse involvement in osteoarthritis may result in:

    a) gastrointestinal disease.
    b) Maigne's syndrome, which simulates gastrointestinal disease.
    c) Robert's syndrome, which involves pain referred to the lower lumbar spine.
    d) Robert's syndrome, which simulates gastrointestinal disease.

29. Articular lesions typical of rheumatoid arthritis result in the radiographic appearance called:

    a) "mouse ears" sign.
    b) "overhanging margin" sign.
    c) "gull wing" sign.
    d) "rat bite" erosions.

30. Inflammatory processes may lead to ossification of spinal ligaments, causing the development of:

    a) osteophytes.
    b) spondylophytes.
    c) syndesmophytes.
    d) periostitis.

31. X-ray signs of juvenile rheumatoid arthritis in the hands commonly include:

    a) ballooning of the distal interphalangeal joints.
    b) interphalangeal ankylosis.
    c) arachnodactyly.
    d) multiple altered digit lengths.

32. Enteropathic arthritis in the peripheral skeleton usually does not affect:

    a) the hips.
    b) the elbows.
    c) the knees.
    d) the wrists.

33. Reiter's syndrome has been observed to have:

    a) a 50:1 male predilection.
    b) a 2:1 male predilection.
    c) a 2:1 female predilection.
    d) a 25:1 male predilection.

34. The theory of pathogenesis of hypertrophic osteoarthropathy that is most widely accepted involves:

    a) an increased peripheral blood flow (humoral theory).
    b) a decreased peripheral blood flow (humoral theory).

c) autonomic reflex vasodilation (neurogenic theory).

d) visceral lesion produces a substance that increases peripheral blood flow (endocrine theory).

35. Chondrolysis of the hip is most commonly:

a) idiopathic.

b) secondary to slipped femoral capital epiphysis (SFCE).

c) secondary to septic or rheumatoid arthritis.

d) secondary to immobilization, as with paraplegia.

36. Among the "universal" radiologic signs that characterize degenerative joint disease are:

a) inflammation and periarticular periostitis.

b) symmetry of distribution and uniform loss of joint space.

c) eburnation and geodes.

d) syndesmophytes and subchondral sclerosis.

37. Synoviochondrometaplasia is:

a) a malignant neoplastic process.

b) a metabolic process.

c) an ischemic necrosis.

d) a benign arthropathy.

38. An intercalary bone is:

a) calcification of the anterior annulus.

b) calcification of the nucleus pulposus.

c) calcification of the posterior longitudinal ligament.

d) calcification of the nuchal ligament.

39. The inflammatory spondyloarthropathies:

a) frequently result in atlantoaxial hypomobility.

b) may result in complete dissolution of the odontoid process.

c) may affect the synovium between the anterior tubercle and the posterior odontoid.

d) may result in ossification of the transverse ligament.

40. An enthesis is:

a) an essentially immobile joint.

b) an inflammation of the periosteum.

c) a slightly movable joint.

d) the periarticular site of tendon or ligament insertion into bone.

41. Still's disease is:

a) a variant of ankylosing spondylitis.

b) a seronegative chronic arthritis seen in pediatric patients.

c) a transient, monoarticular arthritis.

d) a metabolic arthritis.

42. Seronegative arthritides include all of the following except:

a) enteropathic arthropathy.

b) neurotrophic arthropathy.

c) Reiter's syndrome.

d) ankylosing spondylitis.

43. Marginal syndesmophytes:

a) are typical of psoriatic arthritis.

b) are thin, vertical ossification of the inner annular fibers.

c) are characteristic of ankylosing spondylitis and of enteropathic arthropathy.

d) are usually unilateral, originating from peripheral body-endplate junctions.

44. Hypertrophic osteoarthropathy (HOA) appears to develop most commonly as a sequel to:

a) renal failure.

b) myocardial infarction.

c) bronchogenic carcinoma.

d) cholecystitis.

45. An arthritide that occurs in consequence of rheumatic fever is:

a) rheumatoid arthritis.

b) Still's disease.

c) Jaccoud's syndrome.

d) Reiter's syndrome.

46. Erosive osteoarthritis may involve:

a) positive rheumatoid factor.

b) positive HLA-B27.

c) periarticular osteoporosis.

d) the base of the thumb.

47. Spinal involvement in neurotrophic arthropathy is most often associated with:

a) spina bifida.

b) leprosy.

c) syphilis.

d) syringomyelia.

48. Among the most common spinal sites for degenerative arthritis are:

a) C1-C2.

b) L1-L3.

c) C7-T1.

d) C5-C7.

49. Rheumatoid arthritis may result in:

a) bony ankylosis of synovial joints.

b) bony ankylosis of fibrocartilaginous joints.

c) "carrot stick" fractures in the lower cervical spine.

d) ossification of the posterior longitudinal ligament.

50. A synarthrosis is:

a) a slightly movable joint.

b) a cartilaginous joint.

c) a freely movable joint.

d) an essentially immobile, fibrous joint.

51. Theories regarding the etiology of osteitis pubis include all of the following except:

a) vascular etiology involving venous stasis, engorgement, and local osteoporosis.

b) microfractures caused by unaccustomed vectors of stress.

c) low-grade infection after childbirth or pelvic surgery.

d) Sudeck's atrophy variant.

52. The "Bywater's-Dixon" syndesmophyte, a variety of non-marginal syndesmophyte, may be described as:
    a) a complete syndesmophyte attached to the mid-body of two contiguous vertebrae.
    b) a teardrop syndesmophyte, contiguous with a mid-vertebral body, and tapering distally.
    c) a bagpipe syndesmophyte, with a bulky base attached to the mid-body of a vertebra.
    d) a floating syndesmophyte bridging the disc space but not ossifying at the vertebral body.

53. A vertebral appearance associated with ankylosing spondylitis is:
    a) sail vertebra.
    b) fish vertebra.
    c) barrel vertebra.
    d) spool-shaped vertebra.

54. The "fat-pad sign" at the elbow is:
    a) specific to occult fracture of the elbow.
    b) a reliable indicator of elbow involvement in osteoarthritis.
    c) present in up to 90% of cases involving rheumatoid arthritis at the elbow.
    d) a late indication of elbow pathology.

55. As rheumatoid arthritis progresses, pannus:
    a) creates extensive periostitis.
    b) is resorbed.
    c) undergoes fibrosis.
    d) undergoes liquefaction.

56. The eponym for neurotrophic arthropathy is:
    a) Charcot's joints.
    b) Newman's joints.
    c) Volkmann's joints.
    d) Lisfranc's joints.

57. Osseous nodules at the proximal interphalangeal joints are:
    a) Heberden's nodes, indicative of osteoarthritis.
    b) Bouchard's nodes, indicative of osteoarthritis.
    c) Haygarth's nodes, indicative of arthritis deformans.
    d) Heberden's nodes, indicative of gout.

58. With systemic lupus erythematosus, osteoporosis is:
    a) first seen in the lumbar spine.
    b) a rare occurrence.
    c) severe, and conducive to pathologic fracture in long bones.
    d) mild, and seldom symptomatic.

59. A young adult male with signs of inflammatory spinal arthritis may be suspected to have:
    a) gout.
    b) rheumatoid arthritis.
    c) ankylosing spondylitis.
    d) synoviochondrometaplasia.

60. Globus hystericus is a symptom that may accompany:
    a) ochronosis.
    b) Wilson's disease.

    c) hydroxyapatite deposition disease in the cervical spine.
    d) bronze diabetes.

61. Conditions similar to osteitis condensans ilii may develop at:
    a) the pubic symphysis and the medial clavicle.
    b) the pubic symphysis and the distal clavicle.
    c) the distal clavicle and the ischial tuberosities.
    d) the pubic symphysis and the ischial tuberosities.

62. In the thoracic and lumbar spine, psoriatic arthritis is likely to manifest with:
    a) fine, marginal syndesmophytes.
    b) coarse, asymmetric nonmarginal syndesmophytes.
    c) coarse, symmetrical marginal syndesmophytes.
    d) coarse, asymmetric osteophytes.

63. In ankylosing spondylitis:
    a) the posterior longitudinal ligament ossifies.
    b) the outer annulus and the tissue beneath the anterior longitudinal ligament ossify.
    c) the outer fibers of the anterior longitudinal ligament ossify.
    d) both the inner and outer fibers of the anterior longitudinal ligament ossify.

64. Otto's pelvis is:
    a) malum coxa senilis.
    b) associated with Paget's disease.
    c) protrusio acetabulae.
    d) ischemic necrosis of the femoral head.

65. Pannus is:
    a) vascular granulation tissue.
    b) an inflammatory exudate.
    c) an erosion of subchondral bone.
    d) inflamed collagen tissue.

66. Ossification of the posterior longitudinal ligament may result in:
    a) demyelination of the posterior and lateral white columns in the spinal cord.
    b) flattening of the anterior margins of the spinal cord.
    c) Erb's palsy.
    d) brachial plexus lesions.

67. Osteoarthritis in the shoulder complex most often involves:
    a) the acromioclavicular joint.
    b) the posterosuperior glenohumeral joint.
    c) the anterosuperior glenohumeral joint.
    d) the sternoclavicular joint.

68. An x-ray sign that is distinctively characteristic of systemic lupus erythematosus is:
    a) subchondral bone cysts.
    b) asymmetric loss of joint space.
    c) reversible, symmetric, bilateral deformities.
    d) fluffy periostitis.

69. The intervertebral disc is considered:
    a) an amphiarthrosis.
    b) a synarthrosis.

c) a diarthrosis.

d) none of the above; it is a unique joint.

70. A male patient with diabetes, cirrhosis of the liver, and a "bronze" color to his skin is likely to have a diagnosis of:

   a) Wilson's disease.
   b) CPPD.
   c) ochronosis.
   d) hemochromatosis.

71. An arthropathy with a 9:1 female predominance and a predilection for multiparous women is:

   a) systemic lupus erythematosus.
   b) erosive osteoarthritis.
   c) scleroderma.
   d) osteitis condensans ilii.

72. Sacroiliac involvement in psoriatic patients:

   a) is rare, occurring in less than 10% of cases.
   b) is most commonly unilateral.
   c) is most commonly bilateral and asymmetric.
   d) is most commonly bilateral and symmetric.

73. Radiographic indications of ankylosing spondylitis involving the sacroiliac joints include all of the following except:

   a) syndesmophytes.
   b) subtle widening of the SI joint space early in the disease.
   c) star sign.
   d) ghost joint.

74. Inflammatory arthritis may be indicated by radiographic evidence of:

   a) posterolateral migration of the femoral head.
   b) medial migration of the femoral head.
   c) axial migration of the femoral head.
   d) anteromedial migration of the femoral head.

75. Rheumatoid arthritis involves the cervical spine in:

   a) less than 10% of the cases.
   b) approximately 50% of the cases.
   c) approximately 80% of the cases.
   d) 100% of the cases.

76. Ossification of the posterior longitudinal ligament has been observed to have a predilection for:

   a) Eskimos.
   b) Native Americans.
   c) African Americans.
   d) Japanese.

77. The "movie sign" is:

   a) radiologic evidence of upper cervical hypermobility in extension.
   b) neurologic evidence of brachial plexus lesions caused by pressure on the medial arm.
   c) laboratory evidence of a clotting disorder.
   d) clinical evidence of osteoarthritis of the knee.

78. Conditions known to be associated with systemic lupus erythematosus include:

   a) Raynaud's phenomenon and alopecia.
   b) reflex sympathetic dystrophy and Raynaud's phenomenon.
   c) renal failure and reflex sympathetic dystrophy.
   d) cholecystitis and renal failure.

79. The "bare area" refers to:

   a) the articulating surfaces of bone, where there is no periosteum.
   b) the intracapsular surfaces of bone, where there is no periosteum.
   c) the intracapsular surface of bone, where there is no hyaline membrane.
   d) the periphery of the articular surface, where there is no articular cartilage.

80. The most common clinical presentation of CPPD involves:

   a) bilateral, symmetric arthritis in peripheral joints, with knee and elbow contractures; seen as a chronic condition with progressively severe acute episodes.
   b) a relatively pain-free instability of peripheral joints.
   c) a chronic, progressively severe peripheral arthritis with no acute episodes.
   d) a self-limiting peripheral arthritis affecting the distal lower extremities.

81. *Calcinosis cutis* is the term for:

   a) subcutaneous calcifications.
   b) sheetlike calcifications that appear along myofascial planes.
   c) punctate calcifications in the myofascial tissue of the hands.
   d) punctate calcifications within the joint capsules of the fingers.

82. Lesions of psoriatic arthritis are known to occur:

   a) in a ray pattern.
   b) most commonly in the metacarpophalangeal joints and wrists.
   c) in a symmetric distribution.
   d) rarely in the interphalangeal joints.

83. Enthesopathy at the insertion sites of annular fibers may result in:

   a) Romanus lesions.
   b) a "shiny corner sign."
   c) the radiographic appearance of "rosary beads."
   d) Andersson lesions.

84. The "summation effect" is caused by:

   a) increasing thoracic kyphosis seen with advanced osteoporosis.
   b) cervical disc diminution, osteolysis, and invagination seen with rheumatoid arthritis.
   c) increasing low back rigidity seen with osteophytes and lumbar disc diminution in DJD.

d) increasing rigidity seen with ankylosing spondylitis as the process progresses.

85. Keratoconjunctivitis sicca is:

a) dry eyes (lacrimal gland atrophy).
b) an allergic inflammation of the sclera.
c) a chronic, low-grade infection of the eyes.
d) idiopathic, excessive production of tears and serous mucus.

86. "Carrot stick" fractures caused by AS, which may cause serious neurologic complications, are most common at:

a) C5-C7.
b) T4-T6.
c) T10-L2.
d) L4-S1.

87. Chondromalacia patellae is most common:

a) in adolescents.
b) in osteoporotic females.
c) in geriatric patients.
d) in marathon runners or broad jumpers.

88. All of the following statements about systemic lupus erythematosus are true except:

a) it apparently involves significant immunologic abnormalities.
b) it shows a clear female predilection.
c) almost all SLE patients exhibit the classic pattern of malar erythema.
d) it frequently involves the urinary, cardiopulmonary, nervous, and musculoskeletal systems, and the integument.

89. Synovial joints include:

a) a fibrous capsule, synovium, and hyaline cartilage.
b) fibrocartilaginous tissue with some hyaline cartilage.
c) synovium and fibrocartilage.
d) synovium and fibrocartilage with some hyaline cartilage.

90. Common factors that exacerbate gouty arthritis include:

a) green, leafy vegetables and yogurt.
b) milk and citrus fruits.
c) aspirin and diuretics.
d) apples, oranges, and bananas.

91. Vitiligo, telangiectasia, and *mauskopff* are all features associated with:

a) scleroderma.
b) systemic lupus erythematosus.
c) Still's disease.
d) hemochromatosis.

92. An important clinical consideration associated with psoriatic arthritis patients is:

a) severe early osteoporosis.
b) high likelihood of Otto's pelvis.

c) likelihood of cauda equina syndrome.
d) likelihood of atlantoaxial instability.

93. In a patient with ankylosing spondylitis, posterior vertebral body scalloping may indicate:

a) malignant degeneration.
b) concurrent Hodgkin's disease.
c) early posterior longitudinal ligament involvement.
d) dural ectasia with arachnoid diverticula.

94. The "Terry Thomas sign" is radiologic evidence of:

a) midcarpal ankylosis.
b) lunate luxation.
c) multiple carpal erosions.
d) scapholunate separation.

95. Felty's syndrome is defined as rheumatoid arthritis with:

a) Raynaud's syndrome.
b) leukopenia and splenomegaly.
c) cardiac lesions.
d) CNS lesions.

96. Diffuse idiopathic skeletal hyperostosis shows a clear predilection for:

a) males over 40 years of age.
b) adolescent males.
c) adolescent females.
d) middle-aged females.

97. Osteoarthritis at the knee most often affects:

a) the patellofemoral joint.
b) the medial femorotibial joint.
c) the proximal tibiofibular joint.
d) the lateral femorotibial joint.

98. The most common radiographic sign of Reiter's syndrome in the knee is:

a) the development of a fabella.
b) the development of Pelligrini-Stieda calcification.
c) swelling caused by intraarticular effusion.
d) periostitis at the proximal tibial metaphysis.

99. Poorly defined erosions of bone and osteopenic subarticular bone are characteristic of x-ray findings in:

a) metabolic arthritides.
b) crystalline arthritides.
c) inflammatory arthritides.
d) degenerative arthritides.

100. Waldenstrom's sign is:

a) femoral head anterosuperior migration, with decreased superior and medial joint space.
b) femoral head posterosuperior migration, with decreased superior and medial joint space.
c) femoral head anterosuperior migration, with decreased superior and increased medial joint space.
d) femoral head posterosuperior migration, with decreased superior and medial joint space.

PRACTICE TEST CHAPTER 5—ANSWER KEY

1.	b	11.	c	21.	c	31.	b	41.	b	51.	b	61.	a	71.	d	81.	a	91.	a
2.	b	12.	a	22.	d	32.	a	42.	b	52.	d	62.	b	72.	c	82.	a	92.	d
3.	d	13.	b	23.	d	33.	a	43.	c	53.	c	63.	b	73.	a	83.	a	93.	d
4.	d	14.	c	24.	c	34.	c	44.	c	54.	c	64.	c	74.	c	84.	b	94.	d
5.	b	15.	b	25.	c	35.	b	45.	c	55.	c	65.	a	75.	c	85.	a	95.	b
6.	b	16.	d	26.	c	36.	c	46.	d	56.	a	66.	a	76.	d	86.	a	96.	a
7.	d	17.	a	27.	b	37.	d	47.	c	57.	b	67.	a	77.	d	87.	a	97.	b
8.	a	18.	b	28.	d	38.	a	48.	d	58.	c	68.	c	78.	a	88.	c	98.	c
9.	d	19.	a	29.	d	39.	b	49.	a	59.	c	69.	a	79.	d	89.	a	99.	c
10.	b	20.	d	30.	c	40.	d	50.	d	60.	c	70.	d	80.	a	90.	c	100.	c

Chapter 6

NEOPLASMS
Tumors and Tumorlike Processes:
Benign, Malignant, Quasi-Malignant
Processes

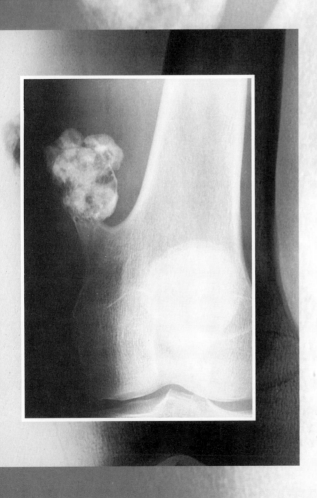

A.   PRIMARY BENIGN BONE TUMORS

1.   Solitary Osteochondroma

a)   General considerations

- nature of the lesion
    1) exostosis from cortical surface
    2) usually with hyaline-lined cartilage cap

- definitions
    1) single lesion is a solitary osteochondroma
    2) multiple osteochondromas: 2 or 3 bones involved, no familial history
    3) hereditary multiple exostosis (HME): familial history, lesions throughout skeleton
- unknown etiology
    1) possibly displaced cartilage from physis leads to solitary lesions
    2) HME may be caused by congenital dysplasia: tumor-like growths at metaphyses

- incidence
    1) most common benign skeletal tumor
    2) 50% of all benign bone neoplasms
    3) 75% discovered before age 20; often incidental discovery of "silent" lesion
    4) 2:1 male predominance
- location
    1) long tubular bones most commonly affected
        - femur: 34%
        - humerus: 18%
        - tibia: 15%
    2) any bone pre-formed in cartilage can host an osteochondroma
        - pelvis: 8%
        - scapula: 5%
        - ribs: 3%
    3) rarely in spine: near secondary ossification centers (neural arch)

b)   Clinical presentation

- lesion itself is "silent" (asymptomatic)
- patient notices a hard, painless mass near a joint (*"lumpy joints"*)
- "stalk" of osteochondroma may fracture: severe pain, swelling
- symptoms of space-occupying lesion:
    1) impingement on adjacent nerves or blood vessels
    2) neurologic symptoms if spinal osteochondroma encroaches upon the foramen
    3) joint abnormalities if

osteochondroma interferes with normal range of motion

4) osteochondroma from distal posterior femur may cause a traumatic rupture, perforating the popliteal artery

5) obstructive uropathy caused by very large pelvic osteochondroma

c) **Pathologic features**

- most commonly, exostoses arise from metaphyseal area of long bones
    1) sessile form: flat, broad stalk; plateau-like
        - seen in proximal humerus and scapula
    2) pedunculated form: elongated stalk, continuous with host bone
        - by far the more common type
        - capped with hyaline cartilage, often has lobulated contour
        - most common at knee, hip, ankle
- size varies: can be 10 cm
- histology
    1) foci of actively proliferating cartilage cells
    2) normally, ceases growth after physis closes
- may undergo malignant degeneration
    1) only about 1% of solitary osteochondromas
    2) as much as 20% of those in HME
    3) convert to chondrosarcoma usually; some to osteosarcoma or fibrosarcoma
- osteochondroma may develop after radiation therapy
- most appear after childhood irradiation for Wilm's tumor or neuroblastoma
- treatment
    1) symptomatic lesions require surgical excision
    2) incomplete excision leads to recurrence; periosteal surface must be excised
- *subungual exostosis*: arises from distal terminal toe phalanx, usually great toe
    1) fibrocartilaginous cap (instead of hyaline cartilage)
    2) may be painful; surgical removal required
    3) female predominance (2:1)

d) **Radiologic features**

- pedunculated osteochondroma
    1) commonly originate from metaphysis (e.g., distal femur or proximal tibia)
    2) long, slender stalk of bone, continuous with host cortex;

projecting away from the joint (*coat hanger exostosis*)

3) osteocartilaginous domed cap, irregular contour, spotty calcification

4) en face: dense ring of cortex around base, superimposed upon cartilage cap

- sessile osteochondroma

    1) very broad-based, creates a long, asymmetrical widening of bone

    2) usually in metaphyseal/diaphyseal region (e.g., proximal humerus, scapula, proximal femur)

- cauliflower osteochondroma

    1) very large, lobulated cartilage cap

    2) flocculent areas of calcification throughout lesion

    3) when in vertebral neural arch: create *cauliflower spine* appearance

    4) common sites: pelvis (near ASIS, ischiopubic synchondrosis), ribs

- Trevor's disease: epiphyseal growth like an osteochondroma (is **not** an osteochondroma), osteochondroma **does not occur** at epiphysis

e) Differential considerations

- malignant degeneration of osteochondroma

    1) pain

    2) rapid growth

    3) MRI shows thickened cartilage; breached perichondrium

- chondrosarcoma

    1) cartilage thickness: 3 cm or greater (osteochondroma has thin peripheral cartilage: as little as 1 mm)

    2) break in cortex

    3) growing soft tissue mass

- parosteal sarcoma

    1) *"cleavage plane"* between normal bone and neoplasm

    2) osteochondroma's cortex and spongiosa are continuous with host bone

2. Hereditary Multiple Exostosis (HME) (synonyms: multiple osteochondromatosis, external chondromatosis, diaphyseal aclasis)

a) General considerations

- nature of lesions

    1) metaphyseal overgrowth with multiple osteochondromas

    2) average of 10 lesions: may be a few, or hundreds

- etiology: hereditary

- incidence
    1) no gender preference, but less severe in females
    2) usually discovered in first decade of life
- location of lesions
    1) metaphyseal area of distal femur, proximal and distal tibia, proximal humerus, distal radius
    2) hands involved in advanced cases
    3) elbow region spared
    4) bilateral, symmetrical distribution

b) **Clinical presentation**
- familial history of HME
- lesions often asymptomatic: painless, lumpy joints
- *bayonet hand* deformity: shortened ulna, outward bowed radius, with subluxation of the radioulnar joint (30% of patients)
- malignant degeneration or fracture cause acute pain, swelling
- surgical excision for malignant degeneration, or cosmetic reasons

c) **Pathologic features**
- metaphyseal overgrowth—see solitary osteochondroma above

d) **Radiologic features**
- multiple small osteochondromas may appear in hands (late in process)
- sessile osteochondromas common at proximal humerus, pelvis, spine
- may be pressure erosions of adjacent bone
    1) common sites: distal tibia or fibula
    2) gives scalloped margin of outer cortex
- cauliflower-like lesions in pelvis
- costochondral junctions may have multiple lesions
- lesions on neural arch of vertebrae
    1) can create neurological symptoms
    2) can cause cord compression

e) **Differential considerations**
- malignant degeneration
    1) pain at site of an osteochondroma
    2) renewed growth of an osteochondroma
- chondrosarcoma: may be radiographically identical to large, cauliflower lesion (osteochondroma)

3. **Hemangioma**

a) **General considerations**
- nature of lesion
    1) primary, benign neoplasm
    2) made up of capillaries; or cavernous or venous blood vessels

☞

- incidence
    1) most common **benign bone** tumor of the spine
    2) about 1% of all primary bone tumors
    3) usually found in adults > 40 years of age
    4) slightly higher incidence in females
- location
    1) most are in spine or skull (75%)
    2) spine
        - usually thoracolumbar area
        - most in vertebral body
        - 10–15% of spinal hemangiomas extend to the neural arch
    3) skull: usually in frontal bone
    4) occasionally found in cervical spine, long tubular bones, mandible, maxilla, patella, metacarpals, soft tissues
- treatment
    1) symptomatic lesions excised
    2) inoperable spinal lesions irradiated

b) Clinical presentation
- usually clinically silent
- may present with pain, local muscle spasm
- neurologic compromise
    1) hypesthesia or hyperesthesia
    2) radiculitis or local pain (caused by spinal stenosis)
- cord compression caused by
    1) hypertrophy and ballooning of vertebral body
    2) extension of hemangioma into epidural space
    3) vertebral compression fracture (very rare)
    4) hemorrhage
- large cord in midthoracic region predisposes to compression there
- long bone lesions: rare, but may present with dull, vague pain
- hemangioma in maxilla or mandible may cause hemorrhage with dental work (extractions, root canal), potentially fatal

c) Pathologic features
- capillary hemangioma
    1) fine capillary loops
    2) spread outward like a sunburst
    3) found in flat bones, metaphyses of long bones
- cavernous hemangioma (more common)
    1) large, thin-walled vessels and sinuses
    2) single-layer of epithelial cells as lining

        3) surrounded by resorbed bony trabeculae

        4) found in vertebrae and skull

- occasionally, reactive new bone may form with either type

d) Radiologic features

- in spine
  1) usually solitary; may be two or three lesions
  2) coarse vertical striations in vertebral body: *corduroy cloth* or *striated vertebra* appearance
  3) slight, overall loss of density
  4) rarely, vertebral body may be expanded
  5) vertebral endplates unaffected
  6) occasionally, paravertebral mass (usually on left) caused by extension of lesion, or compression fracture
- in skull
  1) round or oval lucency (en face) 1–7 cm diameter
  2) most commonly in frontal bone
  3) often has fine, dense spiculae radiating from center: *sunburst* or *spoked wheel* appearance
  4) lesion extends outward, beyond normal bone contour; inner table preserved; outer table eroded or erased
- in other bones
  1) expansile, lytic, fine, lacy network
  2) honeycombing lesion
  3) may also have sunray appearance
- in soft tissues
  1) usually in forearm, lower leg, paravertebral area
  2) spherical calcifications within mass (phleboliths)

e) Differential considerations

- Paget's disease
  1) often expands vertebrae
  2) thickened cortical endplates (*picture frame appearance*)
- osteoporosis
  1) *pseudohemangiomatous appearance*
  2) multiple vertebrae affected (hemangioma is usually solitary on plain films)

4. Osteoma

    a) General considerations

- asymptomatic, benign tumor of membranous bone
- incidence
  1) apparently rare: about 1% of otolaryngology patients

2)   discovered in adults

3)   female predominance (3:1)

- location
  1)   usually in frontal or ethmoid sinuses
  2)   outer or inner skull tables
- treatment: symptomatic osteoma may require excision

b)   Clinical presentation

- clinically silent
- may interfere with sinus drainage, causing chronic sinusitis
- can create retro-orbital pressure, headaches, mucoceles, and (rarely) brain abscess
- giant osteomas can fill sinus cavity
  1)   ocular disturbances
  2)   exophthalmos
  3)   headaches
  4)   recurrent sinusitis
- mandibular osteoma
  1)   mechanical and cosmetic jaw problems
  2)   rarely: pressure on carotid sinus and internal carotid artery may cause bizarre vision and balance effects

- *Gardner's syndrome*
  1)   triad of abnormal growths: (in 45% of cases)
     - multiple osteomas
     - colonic polyps
     - soft tissue fibromas
  2)   autosomal dominant transmission
  3)   these osteomas are distinctive:
     - protuberant, oval, dense masses attached to cortices
     - multiple lesions, attached to various bones
     - sometimes lobulated
  4)   sites of lesions
     - frontal bone, mandible (near mandibular angle)
     - maxilla, sphenoid, ethmoid, zygoma
     - may be in small tubular bones of hands, feet
  5)   bone lesions may be absent
  6)   when present, osteomas precede polyps and fibromas
  7)   polyps should be considered premalignant
     - colons of family members should be examined, too
     - prophylactic bowel resection is treatment of choice

c) **Pathologic features**
- trabecular (spongy) osteoma: originates in cancellous bone
- ivory (compact) osteoma: originates in cortical bone

d) **Radiologic features**
- round or oval, well-circumscribed, very radiopaque
- usually < 2 cm diameter
- giant osteoma
    1) may enlarge to expand sinus walls
    2) may develop off outer skull table
- osteoma associated with Gardner's syndrome
    1) protuberant, dense, oval lesions
    2) attached to cortices
    3) sometimes lobulated
    4) in skull, hands, feet

5. **Bone Island**
   (synonym: enostoma)

a) **General considerations**
- nature of lesions: solitary, discrete sclerotic area
- sites
    1) ilium, ischium, sacrum, proximal femur
    2) less often: humerus, vertebra, talus, scaphoid, ribs
- only site where they do not occur: skull
- etiology unknown

b) **Clinical presentation**
- usually an incidental finding; asymptomatic lesion
- most common in adults, but also found in children
- size
    1) usually unchanging over years
    2) about 30% show active growth
    3) may even decrease in size

c) **Pathologic features**
- focus of compact lamellar bone within normal spongiosa
- metabolic activity continues within lesion

d) **Radiologic features**
- intramedullary lesions
    1) align with long axis of trabeculae
    2) do not protrude from cortical surface of host bone
- round, ovoid, or oblong radiopaque lesions
    1) sharply demarcated margins
    2) may have a *brush border* (radiating spicules that mingle with trabeculae of the surrounding spongiosa)

- skeletal sites
  1) majority of small lesions are in femoral neck, intertrochanteric space of proximal femur
  2) occur in epiphysis or metaphysis; **not** in diaphysis
  3) rare in spine: may be found in lumbar vertebral body or, (even less often) neural arch
  4) larger ("giant") bone islands may occur in pelvis (> 1 cm)
- bone scan
  1) usually does not "light up"
  2) when bone island is growing (metabolically active), it may show slightly increased uptake
  3) rarely, during period of rapid growth, bone island may appear "hot" on bone scan

e) Differential considerations

- osteoblastic metastasis
  1) well-defined, less dense than a bone island
  2) usually polyostotic
  3) no "brush border"
- osteoid osteoma
  1) usually painful
  2) has central nidus within sclerotic area
- osteoma
  1) protrudes from bone surface
  2) mostly in skull, neck area; rare site for bone island
- actively growing bone island
  1) slow rate of growth over years
  2) lack of pain at site
  3) in some cases, biopsy may be required for definitive diagnosis

6. Osteoid Osteoma

a) General considerations

- nature of lesion
  1) painful neoplasm
  2) soft, nodular center; surrounded by reactive sclerosis
- etiology unknown
- incidence
  1) about 11% of benign bone tumors
  2) young people, usually 10–25 years of age or younger
  3) male predilection (2:1)
- location
  1) 50% are in femur or tibia
  2) predilection for femoral neck, trochanters

3) about 10% in spine; usually in neural arch (sclerotic pedicle)
4) can occur in almost any bone: usually cortical, but may be intramedullary or even subperiosteal

- treatment
    1) wide en bloc excision
    2) nidus must be completely removed to avoid recurrence
    3) reactive sclerosis need not be totally removed
    4) entire lesion may regress spontaneously over many years
    5) vertebral body lesions treated by irradiation

b) Clinical presentation

- classic: pain worse at night, relieved by aspirin (65% of cases)
- increasingly severe, deep, aching pain of insidious onset
- vasomotor disturbances: sweating, heat in affected area
- pain may be referred to nearby joint (30% of cases)
- local swelling, point tenderness
- if joint area is involved: painful limp, limited motion, stiffness, weakness, muscle atrophy
- scoliosis, or torticollis
- lumbar or proximal femur lesion may simulate disc lesions

c) Pathologic features

- gross lesion
    1) nidus is a soft, reddish brown, vascularized tumor
    2) usually < 1 cm diameter
    3) surrounded by broad zone of reactive sclerosis
    4) thickened cortex
    5) solid periosteal response
    6) mature nidus may develop a fleck: center *"target calcification"*
- histologically
    1) nidus shows small, spherical nodules of highly vascularized fibrous connective tissue
    2) contains benign giant cells in interlacing network of osteoid trabeculae
    3) trabeculae are thin and variably mineralized

d) Radiologic features

- cortically located lesions
    1) lucent nidus surrounded by reactive sclerosis

2) may have central fleck of calcification in nidus
3) lesion will show earlier on tomogram or bone scan

- intramedullary lesions
  1) when intracapsular, much less sclerosis surrounds them
  2) lucent nidus may be only visible abnormality
- spinal lesions
  1) neural arch is usually the location: most often the lamina
  2) 60% are in lumbar spine
  3) initial lucent nidus may require bone scan and tomogram for detection
  4) mature, sclerotic lesion may present as sclerotic *"ivory pedicle"* or *"ivory lamina"*
  5) apt to cause painful scoliosis, with lesion on concave side
  6) vertebral body lesion may produce ivory vertebra or focal sclerosis near endplate
- bone scan may show *double density sign*: focal area of intense uptake within regional area of increased uptake

e) Differential considerations

- Brodie's abscess
  1) also has pain, **worse at night, relieved by aspirin**
  2) lucent nidus larger than osteoid osteoma's: > 1 cm
  3) sclerotic rim is thicker and more irregular
  4) angiographic study is key: osteoid osteoma shows a *"vascular blush"* not present in Brodie's abscess
- stress fracture
  1) sequential studies reveal callus of healing fracture
  2) tomography clarifies nature of lesion
- sclerotic or ivory pedicle: differentiate from stress reaction to unilateral spondylolysis, congenital contralateral pedicle agenesis, osteoblastoma, or osteoblastic metastatic carcinoma
- pain pattern may simulate disc lesion: tests for sciatica will be negative

7. Osteoblastoma

a) General considerations

- benign osteoblastic neoplasm
  1) usually a solitary lesion
  2) rarely, multicentric
- incidence: rare, about 1% of all primary bone tumors
  1) usually children and young adults (70%)
  2) male predilection (2:1)

- location
    1) most frequently in the spine
        - neural arch most often
        - prime targets: spinous process, transverse process, lamina
    2) vertebral body rarely primary site, but may host extension from neural arch
    3) thoracolumbar is most commonly affected spinal area
    4) cervical spine
        - more likely at C4-C6
        - rarely in the atlas
    5) long bones (30% of cases)
        - lower extremities most often
        - metaphyseal and diaphyseal lesions
        - small bones of hands and feet may host lesions
        - dorsal talus preferential site
    6) other skeletal locations: skull, maxilla, mandible, ribs
- treatment
    1) surgical curettage or simple excision
    2) recurrence rate is low (around 5%)
    3) inoperable spinal lesion may be irradiated

b) Clinical presentation
- moderately severe pain, lasting up to 2 years
- not particularly worse at night, and not relieved by aspirin
- in extremities
    1) local pain and tenderness
    2) gradually enlarging palpable mass
- thoracolumbar lesions
    1) painful scoliosis (>50% of cases)
    2) local muscle spasm, rigidity
- with spinal stenosis
    1) referred pain, paresthesias, weakness
    2) may even progress to paraplegia
- cervical spine lesions
    1) dull, aching pain
    2) slight to moderate cervical tenderness (lasts for months)
    3) fewer neurologic sequelae
        - most cervical lesions are in the spinous process
        - spinal canal is widest in cervical area

c) Pathologic features
- gross lesion
    1) violet red, hemorrhagic, gritty, friable mass
    2) nidus (as compared with that of

osteoid osteoma) is larger (2–10 cm), softer

- histologic lesion
    1) may be nearly identical to osteoid osteoma
    2) prominent, plump osteoblasts around woven bone and highly vascular tissue
    3) orderly pattern of osteoid trabeculae, broader and longer than those in osteoid osteoma
    4) usually: thick trabeculae of osteoid and woven bone with irregular, serrated borders

d) Radiologic features
- appearance in spine
    1) expansile lesion
    2) clearly defined, eggshell-thin cortical rim
        - most are lucent; some may be mottled or opaque; usually 4–6 cm diameter, but may be larger
- appearance in extremities
    1) lytic, expansile lesion in metaphysis or diaphysis
    2) very thin cortex, with lucent nidus (> 2 cm)
    3) most occur around the knee and hip

e) Differential considerations
- osteoid osteoma
    1) clinically
        - pain less severe and not worse at night
        - not particularly relieved by aspirin
    2) radiologically
        - very thin cortex, no halo of sclerosis
- malignant osteosarcoma: no unequivocal cellular anaplasia
- aneurysmal bone cyst (especially in spinous process): ABC is more expansile, with soap bubble appearance

REVIEW—STUDY QUESTIONS

1. What is the most common benign bone tumor of the spine?
2. How can the clinician differentiate between osteoid osteoma and osteoblastoma?
3. What is the most common benign skeletal tumor?
4. What is a brush border, and with what lesions is it identified?
5. Where are osteomas most commonly found?

6. Define and describe HME.
7. Name three entities that are considerations in the differential diagnosis of a benign bone island.
8. Describe the characteristics that enable the clinician to differentiate those three entities from a bone island.
9. Where are osteomas most frequently encountered?
10. Of the seven lesions discussed so far, which have female predilections and which have male predilections?
11. Which are more likely to be found in adults than in children and youth?
12. Why will a bone island sometimes show as "hot" on a bone scan?
13. Describe the radiologic appearance of an osteoid osteoma.
14. Which of the above seven entities occur fairly commonly?
15. Bone islands can occur almost anywhere. Where are they **not** found?

8. **Solitary Enchondroma**
    (synonym: central chondroma)

    a) **General considerations**
        - nature of lesion
            1) tumor arises in islands of cartilage in metaphysis
            2) can occur in any bone preformed in cartilage
            3) proximal lesions are more prone to malignant degeneration
        - incidence
            1) most common benign bone tumor of the hand
            2) 10% of all benign bone tumors
            3) ages 10–30, no gender preference
        - location
            1) 50% in small tubular bones of hand
                - phalanges: 40% (usually proximal end)
                - metacarpals: 10% (usually distal end)
            2) in decreasing order of incidence
                - proximal phalanges, distal metacarpals, middle phalanges, distal phalanges
            3) thumb usually spared
            4) preference for ulnar side of hand
            5) other sites: feet, femur, humerus, ribs, patella
            6) second most common patellar neoplasm
            7) rare in pelvis and sternum, but high potential for malignancy
        - treatment: curettage, then cryosurgery and bone chip packing

b) Clinical presentation
- lesions in hands or feet
  1) painless swelling or lump
  2) pathologic fracture
     - localized pain and swelling
     - usually with trivial trauma
- lesions in long bones
  1) tend to be more symptomatic
  2) active growth with malignant degeneration may cause sudden onset of pain

c) Pathologic features
- cartilaginous lesion: residual cartilage islands left in metaphysis as physis grows away
- small masses or nodules of hyaline cartilage, separated by a scant fibrous stroma
- stroma may be highly vascularized
- about 50% have calcific foci

d) Radiologic features
- expansile geographic lucency with well-defined margins
- intact cortex; may be thinned by endosteal scalloping and expansion
- usually centrally located in metaphysis; occasionally eccentric (creates a large mass)
- defect may be purely lucent; may contain stippled or punctate calcifications (50% of cases)
- *calcifying enchondroma*: enchondroma with heavy calcification
  1) rings, or broken rings
  2) small, rounded calcifications within a lucent matrix

e) Differential considerations
- malignant degeneration of enchondroma
  1) unrelenting pain in previously silent lesion
  2) cortical disruption
  3) focal malignant periosteal reaction
  4) poorly defined zone of transition
  5) large soft tissue mass
- purely lucent lesion, consider: fibrous dysplasia, simple bone cyst, chondroblastoma, giant cell tumor, osteoblastoma
- epidermoid inclusion cyst (a lesion of distal phalanx): will have history of trauma and lack calcification in lesion
- glomus tumor
  1) painful distal phalanx lesion
  2) abnormal dilatation of blood vessels
  3) lucent defect causing pressure erosion of cortical bone

- medullary bone infarct
    1) resembles calcifying enchondroma
    2) infarct calcifications are streaky, rough, with serpiginous borders
    3) infarct may have fibro-osseous margin
        - on one side of lesion, this can form a straight line
    4) infarct does not expand bone

9. **Multiple Enchondromatosis**
   (synonym: Ollier's disease; enchondromatosis)
   a) **General considerations**
      - nature of lesion
          1) cartilage dysplasia of bone
          2) inborn anomaly of enchondral bone formation
          3) unossified cartilage remnants left in diaphyses and metaphyses
      - incidence: most commonly found in patients from 10 to 30
      - location
          1) small bones of hands and feet are most common sites
          2) femur and tibia frequently involved
          3) iliac crest is most common flat bone site
          4) usually bilateral; may be unilateral
          5) centrally situated in bone, but can be eccentric
      - treatment
          1) only deforming or symptomatic lesions require treatment
          2) curettage or en bloc excision

   b) **Clinical presentation**
      - usually painless: pain with pathologic fracture or superimposed trauma
      - very large lesions may cause deformity, loss of limb function

      - *"Maffucci's syndrome"* (very rare)
          1) bone enchondromatosis with soft tissue cavernous hemangiomas
          2) soft tissue masses, with phleboliths (visible on plain film)
          3) malignant transformation of these enchondromas occurs in as many as 25% of cases

   c) **Pathologic features**
      - lesions similar to solitary enchondromas
      - cartilage dysplasia of bone, inborn anomaly of enchondral bone formation
      - malignant degeneration: estimates of incidence vary widely (10–50%)

   d) **Radiologic features**
      - round or oval lucencies
      - symmetrically expand bone

- occasionally eccentric, causing asymmetrical enlargement
- commonly with central matrix calcification
- streak-like or vertical lucencies project toward diaphysis
- multiple lesions: unilateral or bilateral
    1) hands, feet
    2) long tubular bones
    3) iliac crest

    e)   Differential considerations
- malignant degeneration
    1) pain at previously silent lesion site
    2) destruction of cortex
    3) enlarging soft tissue mass

10.   Periosteal Chondroma
(synonym: juxtacortical chondroma)

    a)   General considerations
- benign, slow-growing, cartilaginous tumor
- up to 4 cm diameter
- incidence
    1) rare
    2) no gender predilection
    3) target population: young adults
- location
    1) metaphyseal lesion, within and beneath periosteum of tubular bone
    2) usually in small bones of hands and feet, humerus
    3) occasionally in femur, tibia, radius, ulna, fibula
- treatment: en bloc excision

    b)   Clinical presentation
- painless mass, often with palpable bony lump
- some have long-standing mild pain

    c)   Pathologic features
- cartilaginous matrix, especially in smaller lesions
- lamellar bone between tumor and medullary cavity

    d)   Radiologic features
- classic triad
    1) cortical scalloping
    2) overhanging bony edges
    3) calcified, cartilaginous matrix
- scalloped, saucerized outer cortex
- well-defined inner margin
- both superior and inferior edges may be overhanging
- about one-third of patients have distinct soft tissue mass
- periosteal bone
    1) may extend as a ledge or buttress

from adjacent cortex around part of chondroma

   2)   usually at proximal end

- dense lamellar bone: forms rind separating tumor from medullary cavity (cleavage plane)

      e) Differential considerations

- fibrous cortical defect
- periosteal desmoid
- periosteal chondrosarcoma
- aneurysmal bone cyst

11. Chondroblastoma (synonym: Codman's tumor)

    a) General considerations

- nature of lesion
  1) benign cartilaginous tumor
  2) average 3–6 cm in diameter
  3) may possibly undergo malignant degeneration: this is still unresolved
- incidence
  1) rare: < 1% of all primary bone tumors
  2) majority of patients 10–25 years of age
  3) male predilection (2:1)
- location
  1) epiphyseal region of long tubular bone (before closure)
  2) rarely extend into metaphysis
  3) 90% in medullary cavity; 10% in cortex
  4) metaphyseal/epiphyseal lesions usually eccentric
  5) most common bones: proximal femur (especially trochanters), distal femur, proximal tibia, proximal humerus (especially tuberosities), tarsals, innominates (with marked predilection for triradiate cartilage)
  6) rare sites include skull, mandibular condyle, mastoid, manubrium, finger, rib, patella
  7) most common patellar neoplasm is chondroblastoma
- treatment
  1) curettage with bone chip packing
  2) with expendable bones the treatment of choice may be resection (recurrence 20% or more)

    b) Clinical presentation

- mild, dull pain; often referred to adjacent joint
- possible local swelling and tenderness
- over long term: weakness, muscle atrophy

c) **Pathologic features**
  - uniform, small polyhedral cells with sharp cytoplasmic margins
  - may have multinucleated giant cells (secondary to hemorrhage and necrosis)
  - calcified chondroid material which stains positively with alcian blue; gives a *chicken wire* appearance

 d) **Radiologic features**
  - medullary oval or round lytic lesion in epiphysis (or into metaphysis)
  - sharp zone of transition, with slight marginal rim of sclerosis
  - geographic, lucent lesion
  - usually eccentric, but may be centrally placed
  - matrix calcifications in 50% of cases
    1) punctate or stippled interior
    2) fluffy *cotton wool* appearance
  - apposition of periosteal bone
  - solid periosteal new bone creates metaphyseal buttress
  - older lesions: bone expansion, deformity, peripheral sclerosis, fluffy matrix calcifications
  - pathologic fracture is rare

 e) **Differential considerations**
  - Brodie's abscess: periosteal response is adjacent to lesion, not in nearby metaphysis
  - eosinophilic granuloma
    1) rarely epiphyseal
    2) rarely eccentric
  - ischemic necrosis
    1) step-off defects
    2) early crescent sign
  - giant cell tumor: develops later, after closure of epiphysis

12. **Chondromyxoid Fibroma**

  a) **General considerations**
    - benign tumor of chondroid, fibrous, and myxoid tissues
    - classified as being of cartilage origin
    - incidence
      1) rare: < 1% of all bone tumors
      2) 10–30 years of age
      3) no gender predilection
    - location
      1) 50% occur at the knee: usually proximal tibia
      2) other common sites: femur, humerus, fibula, ribs, ilium, hands, feet
      3) metaphyseal locale in tubular bones, but occasionally may extend into epiphysis or occur in diaphysis

- treatment
    1) excision or curettage
    2) about 10% recurrence rate
        - more likely in patients < 15 years old
        - more likely in tumors with more myxoid material and large, atypical nuclei
    3) recurrences treated by recurettage with cauterization or cryosurgery

b) Clinical presentation
- insidious onset, slowly increasing local pain
- occasional swelling
- may be asymptomatic
- pathologic fracture is rare

c) Pathologic features
- histologic lesion
    1) fibrous tissue
    2) chondroid ground substance
    3) giant cells (sometimes in great numbers)
- chondroid, myxoid, and fibrous patterns vary widely
- minimal pleomorphism

d) Radiologic features
- lucent oval or round geographic lesion; long axis parallel to the bone in long bones
- eccentric, usually metaphyseal location; great majority are in proximal third of the tibia
- scalloped, sclerotic margin; thinner sclerosis on cortical side, thicker on medullary side
- endosteal pressure erosion (scalloped margin)
- frequently trabeculated (chambered, soap-bubbled); incomplete, pseudotrabeculations
- calcification within lesions too small to be seen radiographically

13. Fibrous Xanthoma of Bone

a) Classification: nomenclature and synonyms
- *Non-ossifying fibroma* (*NOF*): known as nonosteogenic fibroma, metaphyseal fibrous defect, solitary xanthoma, xanthogranuloma of bone, fibrous medullary defect
- *Fibrous cortical defect* (*FCD*): known as subperiosteal cortical defect, Caffey's defect
- likely that these are the same lesion at different stages of development

☞ **13. A. Nonossifying fibroma (NOF)**

    a) General considerations
- may not be a neoplasm; may simply be faulty ossification
- incidence
    1) 8–20 year olds
    2) asymptomatic, so true incidence unknown
    3) male predilection (2:1)
- location
    1) diametaphyseal; rarely epiphyseal; may be carried by growth into diaphysis
    2) eccentric
    3) lower extremity: most often the distal tibia; also proximal tibia, distal femur, fibula, proximal humerus
    4) rarely: ribs, ilium
- treatment
    1) spontaneous regression with no treatment is the norm
        - 2–5 years: defect fills with solid bone; dense, sclerotic
        - 4–5 years: loses density, blends with surrounding bone
    2) very large, symptomatic lesions
        - curettage or en block excision
    3) pathologic fracture at lesion site
        - cast, immobilize
        - fracture usually heals with lesion still present
        - if lesion enlarges: surgical intervention indicated
    4) no malignant degeneration

    b) Clinical presentation
- usually silent
- large lesion may cause pain
- lesion may weaken bone, lead to pathologic fracture

    c) Pathologic features
- whorled bundle of spindle-shaped, stromal connective tissue
- varying amounts of intercellular, collagenous material
- foam cells often present: contain lipid and giant cells

    d) Radiologic features
- solitary, ovoid lucent lesion; 2–7 cm in diameter
- eccentric
- thin; often expands cortex
- scalloped margins
- often multilocular, bubbly appearance
- dense, sclerotic medullary border, but thin cortical margin

- may fill entire width of long bone (e.g., in fibula)
- no periosteal response (except with pathologic fracture)

 13. B. Fibrous Cortical Defects (FCD) (Caffey's Defect)

a) General considerations

- may be a non-ossifying fibroma, early identification
- incidence
    1) higher incidence in males (2:1)
    2) commonly discovered in 4- to 8-year-old children
    3) may occur in around 40% of normal, healthy children
- lesion lasts longer in males (4 years, as compared with 2 years in females)
- lower extremity lesions most common
    1) posteromedial distal femur is preferred site
    2) other sites: tibia, fibula, proximal femur, proximal humerus, ribs, ilium
- seldom require treatment; spontaneous regression in 2–5 years is the norm

b) Clinical presentation

- asymptomatic
- usually discovered when x-ray is done for unrelated reasons

c) Pathologic features

- possibly non-neoplastic
- faulty ossification
- theories of origin
    1) fibrous cell rests
    2) defect from adjacent periosteum
    3) may be caused by avulsion fracture at a muscle attachment

d) Radiologic features

- geographic, lytic lesion
- eccentric placement in metaphysis
- usually round or ovoid, extending parallel to long axis of bone
- small lesion, purely lytic; larger lesions may be soap-bubbly
- sclerotic rim, sharp zone of transition
- often multiple lesions

 14. Simple Bone Cyst (SBC)
(synonyms: unicameral bone cyst (UBC), solitary bone cyst, juvenile bone cyst)

a) General considerations

- nature of lesion
    1) not a neoplasm
    2) fluid-filled cyst lined with fibrous tissue
    3) lesion adjacent to growth plate is *"active"*: has growth potential

    4) cysts displaced from growth plate are "*latent*" (may be misnamed, because they can still grow)
- at first thought to be single-chambered, but may be multilocular
- incidence
  1) > 3% of biopsied primary bone tumors
  2) 80% of patients are 3–14 years old
  3) male predilection (2:1)
- location
  1) 50% of lesions are in proximal humerus
  2) 25% are in proximal femur
  3) after growth plate closure, 52% are in pelvis and calcaneus
  4) occasional lesions in ribs, fibula, tibia, sacrum, clavicle, small bones of hand
  5) metaphyseal lesions, adjacent to epiphyseal cartilage plate
  6) central lesions, with long axis parallel to long axis of long bone
- treatment
  1) curettage with cauterization and bone chip packing
  2) high rate of recurrence (30 to 40%)
  3) steroid injection appears to reduce recurrence significantly

b) Clinical presentation
- asymptomatic until there is pathologic fracture
- about two thirds of these are fractured at some time

c) Pathologic features
- fluid-filled cavity in metaphysis
- lined by fibrous connective tissue with mesothelial surface
- reactive bone growth reinforces cavity margin
- may have several small spaces at periphery of large central cyst
  1) embedded in adjacent connective tissue
  2) also lined with single-layered, flattened mesothelium
  3) act as source of recurrent cysts if not completely excised
- lining undergoes metaplasia, becomes an osseous, cementum substance
  1) suggests fibrous dysplasia
  2) may contain myxoid tissue, giant cells, cholesterol clefts
  3) has potential for malignant degeneration
- fluid in cyst: clear, straw yellow, or sanguinous, may contain clots

☞

    d) **Radiologic features**
- lucent geographic lesion
- broad at metaphyseal end, narrowing at diaphyseal end
- longer than wide: truncated cone appearance
- may contain thin septa
  1) bubbly, loculated appearance
  2) pseudo-loculation: septa are incomplete
- endosteal scalloping
- expansile; but expansion does not extend beyond epiphyseal diameter
- **no** cortical disruption, soft tissue mass, nor periosteal response
- matrix calcification is unusual
- *"fallen fragment sign"*: seen with about *10%* of pathologic fractures
  1) small, detached fragment floats in lytic defect
  2) changes orientation with patient's change of position
- *"hinged fragment sign"*
  1) fragment remains attached
  2) may be mobile (swings into cavity)
- calcaneus: characteristic SBC appearance
  1) geographic, completely lytic lesion at base of calcaneal neck
  2) located inferior to the anterior part of posterior facet
  3) straight, vertical anterior margin
  4) curvilinear posterior border
  5) usually lateral to midline (axial projection)

    e) **Differential considerations**
- in calcaneus
  1) chondroblastoma and giant cell tumor: tend to be central lesions as seen in axial projections
  2) vascular nutrient foramen: triangular lucency with superiorly oriented apex

☞ **15.** **Aneurysmal Bone Cyst (ABC)**

    a) **General considerations**
- nature of lesion
  1) non-neoplastic, solitary bone lesion
  2) blood-filled, cystic cavity
  3) named for its roentgen appearance
- etiology is unknown, but:
  1) pressure on osseous structures causes erosion, cyst formation
  2) "secondary" ABC: cyst occurs along with giant cell tumor, osteosarcoma, SBC, NOF, fibrous dysplasia (may display some characteristics of those lesions)

- incidence
  1) about 1% of biopsied primary bone tumors
  2) female predilection (3:2)
  3) 75% of cases found in patients 5 to 20 years old
- location
  1) 80% in long tubular bones and spine
  2) most often found in femur and tibia
  3) most common spinal sites
     - thoracic and lumbar spine
     - usually in neural arch: spinous process, transverse process, lamina, pedicle
     - vertebral body lesions usually associated with neural arch lesions
  4) long bone lesions usually eccentric, metaphyseal (some diaphyseal)
  5) other sites: flat bones, short tubular bones, fibula, patella, calvarium (usually the occiput), and ribs
     - in short tubular bones: central diaphyseal lesions
     - most common benign bone tumor of clavicle
- treatment
  1) curettage with bone chip replacement
  2) almost 50% recurrence rate
  3) rate of recurrence reduced with irradiation
  4) inoperable spinal lesions irradiated

b) Clinical presentation
- often: antecedent trauma
- acute onset of pain at site of lesion
- severity of pain increases rapidly
- frequently subject to pathologic fracture
- neurologic deficits or paraplegia (with spinal ABC)

c) Pathologic features
- cystic, blood-filled cavity
- cut surface: spongelike appearance; non-elastic tissue
- proliferation of marrow's vascular component
  1) anastomosing fibrous-walled channels or lacunae
  2) endothelial cell lining (may be incomplete)
- walls contain RBCs, hemosiderin granules, foreign-body giant cells, reactive bone spicules

d) Radiologic features
- expanding, rapidly-growing, lytic lesion: may reach 8–10 cm in diameter

- very thin sub-periosteal shell; paper thin or *"eggshell"* rim
- long bones
    1) eccentric, usually metaphyseal lesions
    2) creates a saccular protrusion, resulting in a cortical bulge
        - *blown-out appearance*
        - *finger-in-the-balloon sign*
    3) multiple fine internal septae; most appear purely lytic, but soap-bubble appearance does occur
    4) periosteal new bone at margins of lesion give *buttressing* effect
    5) after growth plate closure: lesion extends into epiphyseal end of bone; rarely crosses open growth plate
    6) CT or MR demonstrate **fluid/fluid** levels within lesion; show septated chambers
- spinal lesions
    1) grossly expansile lytic lesion without septae (*inflated spine* appearance)
    2) most commonly in thoracic and lumbar areas
    3) usually neural arch: spinous process, transverse process, lamina, pedicle

e) Differential considerations
- SBC: **no** buttressing (common to ABC)
- osteoblastoma in spine: usually less expansile (biopsy may be required for differentiation)

16. Intraosseous Lipoma

a) General considerations
- incidence
    1) rarest primary benign bone tumor
    2) wide age range (5–70 years) with peak in 40s
    3) no gender predilection
- location
    1) long bone metaphyses
    2) tibia and fibula most often
    3) other sites: calcaneus, rarely in spine
- treatment
    1) curettage and bone packing for symptomatic lesions
    2) asymptomatic lesions best left alone

b) Clinical presentation
- usually asymptomatic
- occasionally painful

c) Pathologic features
- well-demarcated lesion, 2–13 cm diameter
- grossly: bright yellow
- filled with fatty tissue, identical to soft tissue lipoma

d) **Radiologic features**
- lytic lesion; elongated, ovoid, lobulated, with wedge-shaped diaphyseal end
- well-defined, often sclerotic border with narrow zone of transition
- usually metaphyseal
- expands by eroding inner margin of cortex
- "*target sequestrum*" or "*doughnut-shaped sequestrum*"
    1) central necrosis; central, round density
    2) occasionally, this target calcific nidus is absent
- characteristic calcaneal lesion
    1) trapezoidal
    2) broad base, narrow, truncated superior surface
- CT or MRI can identify lesion contents as fatty tissue

e) **Differential considerations**
- cartilage tumors: central calcification appears as rings or broken rings
- infarcts: calcification is peripheral rather than central
- SBC: CT or MRI identifies density of fatty tissue in lipoma

REVIEW—STUDY QUESTIONS

1. What is the apparent relationship between an NOF and an FCD?
2. What is the least common primary benign tumor of bone?
3. What entities must be considered in the differential diagnosis of an ABC, and how can they be differentiated?
4. What is a *fallen fragment sign*, and when is it found?
5. How is this related to a *hinged fragment sign*?
6. What is Ollier's disease?
7. What are the common synonyms for an SBC?
8. What is Codman's tumor?
9. What is the most common benign bone tumor of the hand?
10. Which of the above benign neoplasms are subject to malignant degeneration, and under what conditions is this most prone to occur?
11. Of the last ten neoplasms we have reviewed, which show a marked male predilection? Female?
12. Contrast the radiologic appearance of an ABC and an SBC.
13. A *chicken wire* appearance is a common finding in the histologic examination of what benign neoplasm?
14. What "classical triad" helps to identify the radiologic appearance of a juxtacortical chondroma?
15. What is Caffey's defect?

B. PRIMARY QUASIMALIGNANT BONE TUMOR

    1. Giant Cell Tumor
           (synonym: osteoclastoma, old term should be discarded)

   a) **General considerations**
   - nature of lesion
     1) neoplasm formed from connective tissue in marrow
     2) highly vascular
     3) about 20% of them are malignant
   - incidence
     1) 5–8% of primary malignant bone tumors; 15% of primary benign bone tumors
     2) benign giant cell tumors show female predilection: 3:2
     3) malignant giant cell tumors have male predilection: 3:1
     4) almost always found in ages 20 to 40 years; form after closure of the physis
   - location
     1) most frequently: distal femur, proximal tibia, distal radius, proximal humerus
     2) sacrum, calcaneus, innominate, carpal bones, patella
     3) giant cell tumor at distal radius: invariably malignant (99%)
     4) most common benign tumor of the sacrum
     5) very rare in spine above sacrum: may be in lumbar or cervical spine
     6) third most common patellar neoplasm (almost always benign at this site)
        - patellar malignancies are usually metastatic
        - other patellar neoplasms (usually benign cartilaginous tumors), e.g., chondroblastoma (most common patellar neoplasm) or enchondroma (second most common patellar neoplasm)
     7) very rarely multifocal giant cell tumors occur: **rule out** multiple brown tumors (hyperparathyroidism)
     8) subarticular lesion
        - begins near or within ossified epiphyseal line
        - extends to joint surface and into the metaphysis
   - treatment
     1) curettage combined with liquid nitrogen freezing, bone packing, or grafting
     2) up to 50% recurrence: adjacent structures slowly invaded, tumor

extends beyond inner ridge of trabeculae

3) complete resection sometimes required, especially around the knee

4) inoperable spinal lesions irradiated

5) benign lesion: excellent prognosis

6) malignant lesion: < 10% 5-year survival rate

b) Clinical presentation

• localized swelling and tenderness

• intermittent, aching pain

• restricted motion of adjacent joint

• may remain asymptomatic even if tumor is very large

c) Pathologic features

• plump, ovoid, or spindle-shaped stromal cells among multinucleated giant cells

• benign lesions have preponderance of giant cells

• malignant lesions have few giant cells

• appositional bone growth: produces peripheral reactive trabeculae

• regularity or anaplasia of spindle cells determines clinical behavior of tumor

d) Radiologic features

• metaphyseal, eccentric lesion in long bones

• subarticular lesion in adults (even in flat bones)

• sharply circumscribed, lytic (60%), or soap-bubble (40%) lesion

• thin, expanded cortex

• wide zone of transition at endosteal margins

• lesion may fill bone shaft, especially in thin bones (ulna and fibula)

• sometimes delicate periosteal reaction

• vertebral lesion: expansion, lytic destruction of vertebral body or neural arch

• aggressive malignant tumor: lucent lesion, disrupted cortex, soft tissue mass

e) Differential considerations

• most critical differentiation (between benign and malignant): requires clinical, radiologic, histologic correlation

• osteoblastoma

• aneurysmal bone cyst

C. PRIMARY MALIGNANT BONE TUMORS

 1. Multiple Myeloma
(synonym: Kahler's disease)

a) General considerations

• nature of lesion

1) malignant proliferation of plasma cells infiltrating bone marrow

2) etiology unknown

- incidence
    1) most common primary malignant bone tumor (27% of all biopsied bone tumors)
    2) 75% of cases, patients 50–70 years old
    3) male predilection (2:1)
- location
    1) most common site: lower thoracic and lumbar spine
    2) any red-marrow-filled bone is vulnerable
        - flat bones: pelvis, skull, ribs, clavicle, scapula
        - long tubular bone diaphyses: femur, humerus
        - rarely found distal to knee or elbow (about 10% of cases)
- treatment
    1) poor prognosis: most die within 3 years
    2) palliative treatment: radiotherapy and chemotherapy
    3) management of hypercalcemia, hypercalciuria, hyperuricemia

b) Clinical presentation
- bone pain, intermittent at first but becoming continuous
- pain worse during the day, aggravated by exercise and weight-bearing
- pathologic fracture indicated by rapid onset of severe pain after mild trauma or slight strain (20% of patients suffer pathologic fracture late in the disease)
- weight loss, cachexia, anemia, unexplained osteoporosis
- impaired immune system: increased susceptibility to respiratory infection and other bacterial infections
- quartet of abnormalities commonly seen with multiple myeloma
    1) anemia: proliferation of plasma cells replaces or alters hematopoietic tissues
    2) deossification of bones containing red marrow
    3) abnormal serum proteins and urinary proteins
    4) renal disease
- death caused by pneumonia and respiratory failure most common; kidney failure next

c) Pathologic features
- multiple permeative lesions
- gelatinous, red, soft masses of neoplastic plasma cells (plasmacytoma)

- nuclei of cells: round to oval (classed as a *"round cell disorder"*)
  1) other round cell disorders: Ewing's sarcoma; non-Hodgkin's lymphoma of bone (reticulum cell sarcoma)
- around lesions, osteoclastic activity is increased
- sequelae: bone destruction, pathologic fractures, hypercalcemia
- kidney involvement: tubular damage leading to kidney failure
- amyloidosis: targets kidneys, heart, GI tract, liver, spleen, and sometimes the skeleton
- amyloid arthropathy
  1) severe morning fatigue, stiffness, weight loss, symmetrical joint involvement
  2) *pad sign* of secondary amyloid arthropathy: mass of amyloid around joint
  3) skeletal amyloid masses may calcify
- plasmacytomas in extramedullary sites
  1) usually in the nasopharynx
  2) sometimes occur in the nasal cavity, oral cavity, tonsils, sinuses, or larynx locally invasive tumors; erode adjacent bone

d) Laboratory findings
- blood cytology
  1) normochromic, normocytic anemia
  2) thrombocytopenia
  3) rouleaux formation
  4) elevated ESR
- serum analysis
  1) > 30% of cases show hypercalcemia
  2) serum phosphorus usually normal unless there is kidney disease
  3) hyperglobulinemia
     - reversed A/G ratio
     - plasma proteins elevated in > 50% of myeloma patients
- urinalysis
  1) *Bence Jones protein*
     - first coagulates, then dissolves at temperatures > 60° C
     - > 40% of myeloma patients have Bence Jones proteinuria
  2) hyperuricemia (uric acid in the blood) in about 60% of cases
  3) marrow biopsy
     - columns of plasma cells of varying maturity
     - > 10% plasma cells in marrow is diagnostic for myeloma

e) Radiologic features
- radionuclide bone scan
    1) scan is usually *"cold"* because osteoclastic activity predominates at the lesions
    2) scan is *"hot"* focally at the site of pathologic fracture
- plain film
    1) osteoporosis becomes apparent as disease progresses; especially in spine
        - diffuse loss of density
        - thinning of cortical margins
        - lower thoracic and lumbar regions most severely affected
        - vertebral body may appear to have same density as disc
        - pathologic vertebral collapse is inevitable, single or multiple
            a. vertebra plana
            b. *"wrinkled vertebra"* of myeloma
    2) sharply circumscribed osteolytic defects (*radiologic hallmark of multiple myeloma*)
        - *"punched-out lesions"*: multiple, round, purely lytic
        - most common in skull, pelvis, long bones, clavicles, ribs
        - in long bones, diaphysis is commonly involved
        - humerus and femur most common sites
        - widespread lesions in skull may be called *"raindrop"* skull
        - size of lesions tend to be fairly uniform: round or oval
        - no reactive sclerosis
        - medullary destruction abuts endosteal surface of the cortex
    3) osteoblastic lesions
        - rarely see sclerotic lesions with multiple myeloma
        - $< 3\%$ of cases
        - can occur in ribs, sternum, ilium, and occasionally in vertebrae, skull and long bones
        - very rarely: a solitary "ivory vertebra"
- MRI and CT
    1) both can image soft tissue components
    2) both clearly define marrow lesions

f) Differential considerations
- reversal of A/G ratio: occurs with sarcoidosis, chronic nephritis, chronic cirrhosis, lymphogranuloma venereum

- Bence Jones proteoses: occurs with lymphoma, polycythemia vara, and sometimes in metastatic disease
- hyperuricemia seen also with leukemia and gout
- punched-out lesions in calvarium: DDX metastasis
- sclerotic lesions: DDX metastasis, mastocytosis, lymphoma, myelosclerosis
- diagnostic criteria for multiple myeloma
    1) bone marrow biopsy shows at least 10% abnormal, atypical, or immature plasma cells, plus one of the following
        - serum M-protein spike
        - urine M-protein spike
        - Bence Jones proteinuria
        - characteristic osteolytic bone lesions
        - generalized osteoporosis (with 30% myeloma cells in marrow)
        - biopsy-proven plasmacytoma

2. **Solitary Plasmacytoma**

   a) **General considerations**
   - nature of lesion
       1) localized plasma cell proliferation
       2) about 70% eventually develop diffuse multiple myeloma
   - incidence
       1) wide age range, about half below and half above 50 years
       2) much less common than multiple myeloma
   - location: mandible, ilium, vertebrae, ribs, proximal femur, scapula
   - treatment
       1) local irradiation
       2) surgical excision

   b) **Clinical presentation**
   - patient initially reports localized pain
   - pathologic fracture is common

   c) **Pathologic features and laboratory findings**
   - plasma cells undergo malignant proliferation at a single site
   - laboratory findings: normal, or may show abnormal serum electrophoresis
   - see laboratory findings: multiple myeloma (above)

    d) **Radiologic features**
   - lucent, geographic lesion
   - may be highly expansile
   - soap-bubble internal architecture

   e) **Differential considerations**
   - pseudotumor of hemophilia

- hydatid disease of bone
- fibrous dysplasia
- giant cell tumor
- brown tumor caused by hyperparathyroidism
- blow-out metastasis (renal or thyroid origin)

☞ **3. Central Osteosarcoma**

   a) General considerations
   - nature of lesion
     1) one of the osteogenic sarcomas
        - central osteosarcoma
        - multicentric osteosarcoma
        - parosteal osteosarcoma (juxtacortical osteosarcoma)
        - secondary osteosarcoma
        - extraosseous osteosarcoma
     2) primary malignant bone tumor
     3) in bone affected by Paget's disease, also in apparently normal bone
     4) hematogenous metastasis to the lung (common)
        - *"cannonball metastases"*
        - may lead to hypertrophic osteoarthropathy
        - commonly causes spontaneous pneumothorax
     5) may also metastasize to bone (*"skip lesions"*) and to kidneys
   - incidence
     1) second most common primary malignant bone tumor
     2) 20% of all primary malignant bone tumors are osteosarcoma
     3) 75% of patients are 10–25 years old
     4) male predilection (2:1)
     5) apparently affects people who are taller than average for their age
   - location
     1) long bones in the extremities
     2) distal femur most often affected
     3) proximal tibia and fibula and proximal humerus common sites
     4) 58% of osteosarcoma: around the knee
     5) 75%: in the metaphysis, abutting the physis
     6) occasionally: diaphyseal or epiphyseal lesions
     7) some in: calvarium, sacrum, pelvis, mandible, maxilla, scapula, clavicle, ribs, hand, calcaneus, spine (usually thoracic and lumbar areas)
     8) in spine: vertebral body is target site

- treatment
    1) amputation: treatment of choice before metastasis
    2) irradiation for local containment and pain control
    3) lung resection when there is metastasis
    4) prognosis has been poor: about 20% 5-year survival rate
    5) adding intensive chemotherapy: recently shows 80% 5-year survival rate
    6) sclerotic lesions: progress more slowly, less aggressive

b) Clinical presentation
- usual presentation: painful swelling at site of lesion
- may be antecedent trauma, but its relationship to lesion is questionable
- "*traumatic determinism*": lesion revealed by, rather than caused by, trauma
- initially insidious, transitory; pain becomes severe and persistent
- may restrict joint movement
- may cause limp if lesion is in lower extremity
- occasionally presents with deep venous thrombosis ("*tumor thrombus*": external compression by the tumor)

c) Pathologic features
- gross and microscopic findings depend on degree of ossification
    1) less ossified
        - firm, but not hard to the touch
        - sarcomatous connective tissue stroma
        - yellowish dots and streaks (islands of new bone)
    2) more ossified
        - hard, densely compact mass
- tumor obviously penetrates cortex, extends into soft tissues
- periosteum elevated by tumor
- histologic appearance
    1) spindle-shaped stromal cells
    2) spheroid cells with multiple hyperchromic nuclei: highly anaplastic lesion
    3) collagenous intercellular material enmeshed with sarcomatous stromal cells
    4) normal trabeculae resorbed and destroyed

d) Laboratory findings
- elevated alkaline phosphatase

- highest elevation occurs with sclerotic, densely ossified tumor

   e) Radiologic features
- focal metaphyseal lesion
- three basic lesion appearances
  1) sclerotic lesion (about 50%)
     - dense ivory lesion filling medullary space
     - may have roughened, lobulated margin (*"cumulus cloud appearance"*)
  2) lytic lesion (about 25%)
  3) mixed pattern (about 25%)
     - mottled, permeative lesion
     - poor zone of transition
- cortical disruption is common
- highly irregular periosteal new bone formation: involves extracortical, dense, soft tissue mass with transverse spicules or radiating striations (*"sunburst, sunray"*)
- may show *"Codman's reactive triangle"*
  1) elevation of periosteum by tumor at margins of the lesion, adjacent to cortical breach
  2) can also be seen with benign lesions, e.g., traumatic periostitis, osteomyelitis, eosinophilic granuloma, thyroid acropachy)
- large soft tissue mass: common finding; often has ossification within the mass
- lesion may create bone expansion
- pathologic fracture occurs
- CT and MRI best delineate marrow infiltration, soft tissue mass, and response to therapy

4. Multicentric Osteosarcoma
(synonyms: sclerosing osteogenic sarcomatosis, childhood multifocal osteosarcoma, osteosarcomatosis)

   a) General considerations
- nature of lesions
  1) multiple lesions develop simultaneously
  2) unknown whether these are metastases or simultaneous independent lesions
  3) early pulmonary metastases
  4) rapidly fatal
- incidence
  1) rare; only around 20 known cases
  2) usually between 5 and 10 years old
- location
  1) metaphyses of long tubular bones, rarely involve the epiphysis
  2) spine, pelvis, sternum, skull, and ribs involved
  3) often bilateral and symmetrical

b) Clinical presentation
- child, usually in first decade
- pain begins as an ache
- pain becomes severe and multifocal

c) Pathologic features and laboratory findings
- heavily ossified lesions
- elevated alkaline phosphatase enzyme

d) Radiologic features
- spine: ivory vertebra; or irregular, nodular, opaque mass in vertebral body
- round or large oval sclerotic lesions in metaphyses, eventually fill the medullary canal
- bilaterally symmetric opacities

e) Differential considerations
- bone islands: similar early in disease process; lesions rapidly expand to fill medullary canal
- heavy-metal (lead) poisoning: transverse, band-like opacities
- diaphyseal sclerosis (Engelmann's disease)
- melorheostosis (flowing hyperostosis)
- osteopetrosis (Albers-Schönberg's disease)
- osteopoikilosis (multiple metaphyseal lesions)

5. Parosteal Osteosarcoma (synonyms: juxtacortical osteosarcoma, surface osteosarcoma)

a) General considerations
- nature of lesion
  1) slow-growing tumor
  2) heavily calcified connective stroma
  3) juxtacortical tumor within the periosteum
- incidence
  1) uncommon (about 1% of all primary malignant bone tumors)
  2) most frequently found in patients 30–50 years old
- location
  1) majority on posterior, distal femoral metaphysis (50%)
  2) 25% on proximal tibia or humerus
  3) other sites: ulna, radius, clavicle, metacarpals, phalanges, mandible
- treatment
  1) less aggressive lesions: en bloc resection (< 50% recurrence)
  2) highly aggressive lesions: amputation
  3) survival rate after excision: as high as 70%

b) Clinical presentation
- swelling or mass formation
- dull, aching pain

- occasionally: impaired joint function
- insidious onset: symptoms up to 1 year before detection

c) **Pathologic features**
- lobulated, sessile mass with broad-based attachment to underlying bone
- bony, hard mass
- periosteal fibrous tissue separates tumor from cortex
- some involve the medullary canal, giving a negative prognosis
- average 10 cm in diameter; range from 3 to 25 cm

d) **Radiologic features**
- opaque, homogenous juxtacortical mass
- classically: on popliteal surface of distal femur
- cleavage plane
    1) 1–3 mm wide
    2) separates most of mass from cortex
    3) stops at stalk of tumor
- lobulated peripheral margin
- no periosteal new bone formation

e) **Differential considerations**
- post-traumatic myositis ossificans
    1) usually completely separated from the bone: no connecting stalk
    2) sarcoma: uniformly dense central portions, less dense periphery
    3) myositis: less dense central portion, halo/rim of dense cortical bone
    4) over time: myositis diminishes, sarcoma grows

6. **Secondary Osteosarcoma**

a) **General considerations**
- nature of lesion
    1) malignant degeneration of a benign disorder
    2) may develop from
        - Paget's disease (0.9–2% of cases)
        - polyostotic fibrous dysplasia (0.5%)
        - hereditary multiple exostosis (osteochondromas) (20%)
        - enchondromatosis (Ollier's disease) (up to 50%)
    3) may develop subsequent to ionizing radiation
- incidence
    1) target population varies with pre-existing conditions
    2) post-radiation sarcoma: latent period 5–40 years, average around 15 years
    3) clinical presentation, pathologic features: same as primary sarcoma

b) **Radiologic features**
- permeative, moth-eaten bone destruction
- periosteal reaction as with primary sarcoma
- soft tissue mass

7. **Extraosseous Osteosarcoma**

    a) **General considerations**
- typical sarcoma, but originating in soft tissue rather than bone
- commonly metastasizes to lung
- incidence: usually 30–50 years old
- location
  1) soft tissue of thigh is most common
  2) also in pleura, heart valves, cranial dura, retroperitoneum, buttock, axilla, breast, renal capsule

    b) **Pathologic features**
- histologically identical to osseous osteosarcoma

    c) **Radiologic features**
- nonspecific general appearance
- very large soft tissue mass
- often relatively distant from bone
- may have calcification within the mass

8. **Chondrosarcoma**

    a) **General considerations**
- nature of lesion
  1) chondrogenic, malignant tumor
  2) may be primary or secondary (degeneration of osteochondroma or enchondroma)
  3) may be central (medullary or intraosseous), peripheral, or extraosseous
- incidence
  1) third most common primary malignant bone tumor (10% of all primary malignant bone tumors)
  2) central type is most common (5 times more frequent than peripheral)
  3) extraosseous is rare
  4) usual age range: 40–60 years
  5) male predilection (2:1)

TERMINOLOGY FOR INTRASPINAL TUMOR LOCATIONS

Term	Tissue of Origin
intramedullary	inherent to spinal cord substance
intradural extramedullary	leptomeninges, spinal nerve roots
extradural	vertebral bodies, epidural tissues

- location
  1) may be central or peripheral in bone; may be extraosseous
  2) most commonly in pelvis and proximal femur (50%)
  3) other sites: ribs, proximal humerus, scapula, distal femur, proximal tibia, scapula, craniofacial bones, sternum, hand, foot, spine
  4) in any bone preformed in cartilage
  5) very rare in the hand, but most common primary malignant **bone** tumor of the hand (only 4% of hand malignancies are chondrosarcoma)
     - usually in metacarpals or phalanges
     - rare in carpals
  6) most common primary malignant bone tumor of sternum and of scapula
  7) spinal chondrosarcoma
     - rare in the spine
     - no spinal area especially predilected
     - extramedullary defect and compression fracture may result, with consequent neurologic deficit
- treatment
  1) tumor spreads slowly, by direct extension
  2) treatment of choice: local excision, segmented resection, or amputation
     - lesion farthest from trunk most amenable to excision (rather than amputation)
     - nearer trunk: radical removal indicated
     - recurrence incurable
  3) with early, complete removal: 90% 5-year survival rate
  4) metastasis does occur, usually via venous channels
     - parenchymal metastases most common; usually pulmonary
     - rarely metastasizes to skeleton or regional lymph nodes

b) **Clinical presentation**
- pain, swelling (individually or combined)
- pain may be a late symptom
- only one-third of rib chondrosarcomas initially painful
- peripheral chondrosarcoma especially asymptomatic: swelling only, or very minor pain
- growing tumor: impingement upon adjacent structures may cause symptoms

- spontaneous pathologic fracture
- malignant degeneration of a previously benign enchondroma: persistent, unrelenting pain
- highly aggressive lesion occurs
  1) rapid expansion
  2) early, severe pain
  3) cortical destruction
  4) rapidly growing soft tissue mass

c) Pathologic features

- calcium-laden cartilaginous tissue, gritty to the touch
- faceted gray-white or bluish lobules
- histologic sections show plump, cartilaginous cells; multiple nuclei of various sizes
- significantly hyperchromic
- may have some mitotic figures
- more myxoid tissue and less calcification: higher grade malignancies
- greater calcification density: may indicate lower degree of malignancy
- secondary chondrosarcoma:
  1) usually peripheral
  2) seeded from osteochondroma's osteocartilaginous cap
- secondary chondrosarcoma from malignant degeneration of
  1) enchondromatosis (Ollier's disease): the most common cause of secondary chondrosarcoma (up to 50% of patients experience malignant degeneration)
  2) HME (multiple osteochondromas 20%)
  3) solitary osteochondroma: only 1% suffer malignant degeneration
  4) Paget's disease (0.9–2%)
  5) fibrous dysplasia (0.5%)
  6) irradiation
- generally, proximal lesions more at risk of degeneration than distal lesions

d) Radiologic features

- large, lucent, round, or oval lesion
- poorly defined margins
- expansile
- in long bones: usually in metaphysis or diaphysis (epiphyseal lesions rare)
- endosteal scalloping
- as tumor grows: fusiform expansion of shaft; cortical thickening
- advanced stage: extensive cortical erosion
- proximal femur or humerus: may host purely lytic epiphyseal lesions

- matrix appearance
    1) bubbly, with circular lucencies of uncalcified cartilage
    2) mottled, permeating destructive pattern
    3) about one-third of lesions purely lytic
    4) two-thirds have scattered calcifications (popcorn, cotton wool, stippled, rings and broken rings)
- periosteal response
    1) occasionally: laminated or spiculated appearance of new bone formation
    2) peripheral chondrosarcoma: usually spiculated periosteal response, or Codman's reactive triangle
- soft tissue mass
    1) scattered amorphous calcifications
    2) may be initial radiologic sign (with juxtacortical or extraosseous tumor)

☞ 9. **Ewing's Sarcoma**

    a) **General considerations**
- nature of lesion
    1) primitive primary malignant bone tumor
    2) *round-cell tumor* (as are myeloma and the reticulum cell sarcoma also known as non-Hodgkin's lymphoma)
    3) may originate from marrow stem cell (derived from the primary reticulum)
    4) aggressively malignant
    5) frequently see early metastasis to bone (often spine) and lungs
- incidence
    1) fourth most common primary malignant bone tumor (7% of all primary malignant bone tumors)
    2) 50% of patients < 20 years old; peak age 15
    3) rare if < 5 years of age or > 30
    4) younger patients: usually peripheral lesions
    5) > 20 years old: axial lesions more likely
    6) male predilection (2:1)
    7) less frequent in black population
- location
    1) usually in long, tubular bones and in flat bones
    2) order of incidence: femur, tibia, fibula, humerus
    3) classically in diaphysis; may be metaphyseal or metadiaphyseal
    4) incidence order in flat bones: ilium, ischium, pubis, ribs, scapula
    5) rarely in spine: most in sacrum or lumbar segments

      6) isolated cases in feet and mandible

      7) location within bone: medullary

- treatment
  1) irradiation in conjunction with chemotherapy
  2) amputation, with lesion near knee
  3) 5-year survival rate has been 5%; recently improving (one study: up to 35% 5-year survival)

b) Clinical presentation

- pain and swelling at site of lesion
- initially dull pain, becoming severe and persistent
- slight to moderate fever (may simulate infection)
- localized heat, dilated vessels, tenderness

c) Pathologic features and laboratory findings

- soft, friable, hemorrhagic medullary lesion
- often has cystic necrotic areas
- penetrates cortex to produce extraosseous mass
- sheets of small round or oval cells with prominent, uniformly sized nuclei
- abundant mitotic figures; no tumor giant cells, no pleomorphism
- glycogen granules demonstrated with staining
- anemia, leukocytosis, elevated ESR

d) Radiologic features

- diaphyseal, permeative lesion with wide transition zone
- up to 50%: delicate, laminated, *"onion skin"* periosteal response
- possible periosteal response: spiculated *"sunray pattern,"* fairly short spicules: *"groomed whiskers"* or *"trimmed whiskers"* effect (thinner, more hair-like than in osteosarcoma)
- early characteristic sign: cortical saucerization (in only about 7% of cases)
- sometimes: scalloping of outer cortical margin (if tumor grows through haversian system and presents subperiosteally)
- usually shows mixed lytic and sclerotic pattern; rarely purely lytic
- flat bones: diffuse sclerosis in about one-third of cases
- pathologic fracture relatively infrequent (about 5% of cases)

e) Differential considerations

- biopsy specimen may be impossible to differentiate from
  1) non-Hodgkin's lymphoma
  2) neuroblastoma
  3) leukemia
  4) eosinophilic granuloma

- glycogen granules stain
    1) present in Ewing's sarcoma
    2) absent in non-Hodgkin's lymphoma
- clinically: mimics infection

10.   Fibrosarcoma

    a)   General considerations

- nature of lesion
    1) varying amounts of collagen but no tumor bone, osteoid, or cartilage
    2) medullary (central) or periosteal fibrosarcoma
    3) medullary fibrosarcomas usually arise de novo
    4) fibrosarcoma: may arise from degeneration of preexisting benign lesion
        - fibrous dysplasia
        - Paget's disease
        - chronic osteomyelitis
        - bone infarct
        - post-radiation
    5) infarct: degenerates into malignant fibrous histiocytoma of bone
    6) metastasizes (late) to lung, liver, lymphatic system
    7) metastatic lesions form same type of tumor
- incidence
    1) commonly in adults 30 to 50 years old
    2) wide possible age range: reported from age 4 to age 83
    3) no gender predilection
    4) relatively rare: 2% of primary malignant bone tumors
- location
    1) most commonly: lower extremity long bones in younger patients
    2) in older patients, most commonly flat bones: usually ilium
    3) 50% at the knee: femur, tibia
    4) femur, tibia, and humerus together: ⅔ of fibrosarcomas
    5) classic locations: femoral condyles, humeral epicondyles
    6) frequent sites: innominate, skull, facial bones
    7) rare sites: ribs, clavicles, scapulae, spine, small tubular bones
    8) twice as many medullary lesions as periosteal lesions
    9) usually metaphyseal; eccentric placement
    10) occasionally extends into epiphysis or occurs mid-diaphyseal

- treatment
  1) amputation (usually involves joint disarticulation)
  2) with medullary lesions: 5-year survival rate around 27%
  3) with periosteal lesions: 5-year survival up to 58%

b) Clinical presentation
- local pain and swelling
- pain may be referred to a joint
- pathologic fracture: initial presentation in one-third of cases

c) Pathologic features
- grossly: fibrous, fleshy, firm, gray-white mass
- grow huge
- hemorrhagic, necrotic central areas
- cellular patterns widely variable
  1) less malignant specimens: spindle-shaped fibroblasts interlaced with collagen bundles
  2) more malignant types: irregularity and anaplasia of fibroblasts; multiple nuclei and hyperchromic cells
- tumors contain hemorrhage, necrosis, sometimes secondary calcification
- bony sequestration sometimes encountered (the only primary malignant bone tumor with sequestration as a common feature)

☞ **d) Radiologic features**
- expanding, eccentric, medullary lesion
- highly destructive: cortical thinning, endosteal erosion
- often > 5 cm in diameter when discovered
- lytic lesions: lucent with no matrix calcification
- mixed lesions: permeative destructive pattern, poorly defined, fuzzy margins
- periosteal reaction rare
- huge soft tissue mass common

☞ **e) Differential considerations**
- *Lichtenstein's rule of thumb:* "If a lesion suggests a primary malignant bone tumor but not any one in particular, then think of fibrosarcoma as a possibility, especially if the lesion is in the femur or tibia of an adult."

11. Chordoma

a) General considerations
- nature of lesion
  1) primary malignant bone tumor from vestiges of the notochord persisting in nucleus pulposus; or from

aberrant notochordal cell rests in vertebral bodies

2) seldom metastasizes: direct extension into surrounding soft tissue

- incidence
  1) uncommon: approximately 1% of all primary malignant bone tumors
  2) all ages: most commonly between 40 and 70
  3) male predilection (2:1)

- location
  1) 85% at the ends of axial skeleton: sacrococcygeal or spheno-occipital
  2) about 50% sacrococcygeal
  3) about 35% spheno-occipital (in clivus of Blumenbach)
  4) remainder in vertebrae; most commonly C2 body
  5) usually in vertebral body; rarely intradural

- treatment
  1) sacrococcygeal lesions: surgical resection
  2) intracranial and vertebral lesions irradiated
  3) poor prognosis, low survival rates

b) Clinical presentation
- sacrococcygeal chordoma
  1) expanding mass; insidious onset of perineal pain, numbness
  2) pressure on intestinal tract: constipation, rarely rectal bleeding
  3) pressure on urinary tract: frequency, urgency, hesitancy; eventually incontinence
  4) sciatic motor and sensory signs from lesions infiltrating emerging sacral, pudendal or coccygeal nerves
  5) presacral mass palpable with rectal examination: firm, extrarectal, fixed to sacrum
- spheno-occipital chordoma
  1) headache: most consistent symptom (> 80% of cases)
  2) ocular disturbances: blurred vision, diplopia
  3) hemiparesis (when cerebrum is involved)
  4) ataxia (when cerebellum is involved)
  5) cerebellar pontine angle involvement: possible deafness, dizziness, tinnitus
  6) downward-growing chordoma: nasal discharge, local pain, nasal obstruction (breathing difficulties)

- vertebral chordoma
    1) extrinsic pressure on nerve roots, cord, or extravertebral structures
    2) anterior extension from cervical lesion: dysphagia, breathing difficulties, palpable mass
    3) sensory alterations: numbness followed by pain, usually in arm or leg
    4) motor weakness: not unusual
    5) paraplegia or quadriplegia: very late development

c) Pathologic features

- soft, gray-toned, semitransparent mass
- direct extension, crossing discs into contiguous vertebral bodies
- forms lobulated, well-encapsulated mass in adjacent soft tissues
- discolored by hemorrhage
- small, round, compact cells
- wide range of cytoplasmic vacuolation (from very little to grossly distended, *"physaliphorous,"* vacuolated cells)
- more mature tumors: significant amounts of intercellular mucin
- contain cartilage and ossified cartilage

d) Radiologic features

- sacrococcygeal chordoma
    1) optimal plain film projections
        - AP with 30° cephalad tube angulation
        - lateral (helpful in detecting anterior soft tissue mass)
    2) CT: more sensitive in detecting these irregular, lytic lesions
        - plain film: about 80% of lesions
        - CT: about 90% of lesions
    3) lesions: central or eccentric
    4) oval or circular lesions, with scalloped margins
    5) cortical expansion; AP widening of the sacrum
    6) matrix of tumor
        - incomplete septa, calcifications
        - about 50%: amorphous calcification, visible on plain film
        - CT demonstrates calcification: about 85% of cases
        - soft tissue mass shown in 78% of plain films; 93% of CT studies
- spheno-occipital chordoma
    1) favored sites
        - midline area of clivus of Blumenbach
        - adjacent to sella turcica

2) appearance
- extensive destruction of bone
- large soft tissue mass with flocculent calcification
- appearance varies widely, may simulate more common tumors

- vertebral chordoma
  1) sites
     - vertebral body: common site
     - C2 body: most frequently involved
     - any vertebra can host lesion
  2) appearance
     - radiopaque vertebral body (ivory vertebra)
     - lytic lesions: loss of bone density
     - partial or complete pathologic fracture
     - associated large soft tissue mass
     - extension across joint space, with IVD destruction
  3) **N.B. chordoma: only primary malignant bone tumor that crosses joint space**

e) **Differential considerations**
- sacral lesions
  1) considerations
     - osteolytic metastatic carcinoma
     - chondrosarcoma
     - giant cell tumor
     - aneurysmal bone cyst
     - plasmacytoma
  2) helpful features
     - differentiation from chondrosarcoma may require biopsy
     - others seldom have a soft tissue mass associated with bone destruction
- spheno-occipital lesions
  1) mimic other, more common tumors (meningioma with secondary reactive changes)
  2) radiologic differentiation may not be possible
- vertebral lesions
  1) considerations
     - multiple myeloma
     - metastatic disease
     - infection
  2) helpful features
     - IVD destruction and adjacent vertebral involvement: most likely chordoma (providing infection has been ruled out)

12. **Non-Hodgkin's Lymphoma of Bone (Reticulum Cell Sarcoma)**
    (synonyms: reticulosarcoma, lymphosarcoma, round cell sarcoma)

    a) **General considerations**
- nature of lesion
  1) extranodal lymphoma
  2) initially: localized, solitary bone lesion
- incidence
  1) rare (3–4% of primary malignant bone tumors)
  2) only about 30% of malignant lymphomas involve skeletal system
  3) majority of patients 20–50 years of age
  4) historically, 2:1 male predilection
- location
  1) about 40% of tumors: around the knee
  2) most commonly affected bones: femur, tibia, humerus
  3) other sites: pelvis, ribs, scapulae, vertebrae
  4) usually diaphyseal or metadiaphyseal lesions
- treatment
  1) irradiation with adjuvant chemotherapy
  2) 5-year survival rate 48%; 10-year survival rate 33%

    b) **Clinical presentation**
- intermittent, dull, aching, localized pain
- not relieved by rest
- possibly: palpable mass or soft tissue swelling
- general apparent well-being of patient, despite significant lesion size

    c) **Pathologic features**
- firm, often friable, white or gray-white tumor
- frequently contains hemorrhage and necrosis
- round cells (fairly large ovoid or spherical nucleus, often with nucleoli)
- sparse cytoplasm, commonly with mitotic figures
- varying amounts of intercellular stroma
- staining: may demonstrate delicate strands of reticulum around the tumor cells
- histologic differentiation among various lymphomas very difficult

    d) **Radiologic features**
- permeative, lytic lesion in medullary bone (early in process)

- later: patchy cortical destruction (diaphyseal lesions show cortical disruption later than metaphyseal lesions)
- minimal periosteal response: occasionally laminated new bone formation
- soft tissue mass (later in process)
- pathologic fracture common: more than with any other primary malignant bone tumor
- occasionally the lesion is sclerotic
- vertebral collapse occurs with spinal involvement

e) Differential considerations

- lytic lesions
    1) Ewing's sarcoma
        - has prominent periosteal reaction
        - tends to occur in much younger population
- sclerotic lesions: mimic osteoblastic metastasis
- vertebral collapse
    1) metastasis
    2) solitary plasmacytoma

13. Hodgkin's Lymphoma of Bone

a) General considerations

- nature of lesion
    1) primary bone lesion (rarely)
    2) more commonly: secondary to systemic Hodgkin's lymphoma
    3) primary lesions commonly in chest, liver, spleen, or lymph nodes
    4) bone lesions are lytic, sclerotic, or mixed
- incidence
    1) slightly more frequent in males (1.4:1)
    2) peak incidence in two age ranges
        - 15–34
        - > 60
    3) approximately 10–20% of Hodgkin's lymphoma cases show skeletal lesions
- location
    1) skeletal lesions primarily in vertebral body
    2) thoracolumbar region most commonly affected
    3) other sites: ilium, scapula, sternum, ribs, femur
    4) medullary lesions
    5) polyostotic lesions in two-thirds of patients
- treatment
    1) if discovered early enough: irradiation with chemotherapy
    2) 5-year survival rate close to 80%

b) Clinical presentation
- pain, brought on or intensified by alcohol consumption
- lytic lesions are most symptomatic
- neurologic signs and symptoms, often caused by vertebral collapse and cord compression

☞ **c) Pathologic features**
- tumors contain "*Reed-Sternberg cells*": large, multinucleated reticulum cells
- ratio of these cells to normal lymphocytes varies
    1) lymphocytes predominate, with few Reed-Sternberg cells
    2) moderate number of Reed-Sternberg cells with a mixed infiltrate
    3) similar to "2," but contains dense, fibrous tissue
    4) few lymphocytes, numerous Reed-Sternberg cells, extensive fibrosis

☞ **d) Radiologic features**
- 75% of bone lesions lytic, 15% sclerotic, 10% mixed
- mixed lytic/sclerotic lesions: tendency for periosteal response
- anterior or lateral vertebral body scalloping
- sclerotic lesion: may create ivory vertebra
- tubular bone lesions usually lytic
    1) medullary and cortical destruction
    2) exuberant periosteal response possible with cortical destruction

☞ **e) Differential considerations**
- differentiate between Hodgkin's ivory vertebra and
    1) Paget's disease (tends to expand the vertebra)
    2) blastic metastasis (usually in patients > 60 years old)
- vertebral body scalloping: helps rule these out (present with Hodgkin's)

14. Synovial Sarcoma (synonym: synovioma)

a) General considerations
- nature of lesion
    1) mesenchymal sarcoma mimicking synovial tissue
    2) invariably a solitary lesion
    3) only primary malignant tumor in direct anatomic relationship with joint surface, bursae, tendon sheaths
- incidence
    1) relatively rare
    2) usually in patients 30–50 years old
    3) no gender predilection
- location
    1) most often lower limbs

2) occurs at joints: knee, hip, ankle most commonly
3) also at wrist, elbow, feet
4) rarely midshaft in long bone, caused by dissection of synovium down tendon sheaths

- treatment
    1) surgical excision followed by irradiation
    2) 5-year survival rate:
        - lower extremity lesions: 43%
        - upper extremity lesions: 31%

b) Clinical presentation

- pain and soft tissue mass at tumor site
- may simulate monoarticular arthritis

c) Pathologic features

- nodular soft tissue mass
- often contains calcifications, which may be visible on x-ray
- histology mimics normal synovial tissue

d) Radiologic features

- nodular soft tissue mass near joint
- average size: 7 cm in diameter
- about one-third of cases: tumor shows fine, granular specks of calcification
- 10%: cortical bone erosion from extrinsic pressure
- with true bone invasion:
    1) ragged, ill-defined margins with wide zone of transition
    2) no surrounding sclerotic rim
- MRI: inhomogeneous, septated mass with infiltrative margins

15. Adamantinoma
(synonyms: malignant angioblastoma, dermal inclusion tumor, ameloblastoma, primary epidermoid carcinoma of bone, carcinoma sarcomatodes)

a) General considerations

- nature of lesion
    1) unknown pathogenesis: may be of epithelial or mesodermal origin
    2) theory: from displaced embryonic epithelium of dental enamel germ cells (epithelial cell rests)
- incidence
    1) very rare (about 150 reported cases)
    2) patients 10–30 years of age
- location
    1) almost all cases in tibia (14 in other locations)
    2) other sites: jaw, ulna, humerus, femur, fibula; very rarely in spine
    3) 75% of lesions mid-diaphyseal
- treatment
    1) amputation: treatment of choice
    2) high rate of recurrence with excision

          b) **Clinical presentation**
- pain with swelling around lesion
- no systemic signs

☞   **c)** **Radiologic features**
- may be cortical or medullary
  1) cortical lesions
     - lytic, bone blister appearance
     - sawtooth cortical lesion with ragged margins
     - multichambered, bubbly lesion
  2) medullary lesions
     - large, circumscribed lucent area
     - lesion filled with mottled density
     - sometimes reticulated, honeycombed appearance
- long-standing tumor
  1) significant cortical thinning
  2) spool-shaped, "eggshell" cortical bulges
- expanding tissue disrupts cortex, forms soft tissue mass
- minimal periosteal response, may be laminated

☞   **d)** **Differential considerations**
- fibrous dysplasia
  1) adamantinoma: younger cohort
  2) adamantinoma: periosteal response
  3) adamantinoma: appearance of moth-eaten destruction in tumor matrix
  4) adamantinoma lacks bowing of bone
  5) adamantinoma lacks ground glass appearance

REVIEW—STUDY QUESTIONS

1. Name the three skeletal sites where chondrosarcoma is the most common malignant bone tumor.
2. In what skeletal sites does chondrosarcoma most frequently occur?
3. What is traumatic determinism?
4. Name the four most common primary malignant bone tumors, in descending order of incidence.
5. Describe the radiographic appearance of Ewing's sarcoma.
6. Give the usual age ranges for the four most common primary malignant bone tumors.
7. What bone pathologies may present as an "ivory vertebra," and how may their appearances differ?
8. What tissues or structures are affected by extradural, intradural extramedullary, and intramedullary spinal tumors?
9. With which primary malignant bone tumor does the complication of pathologic fracture most commonly occur?
10. What are five laboratory findings that may be indicative of multiple myeloma?

D. METASTATIC BONE TUMORS

1. General Considerations

    a) Nature of lesions

- majority from extraskeletal lesions; mostly epithelial
- common primary sites: breast, lung, prostate, kidney, thyroid, bowel
- occasionally primary bone sarcoma will metastasize: e.g., Ewing's tumor
- tumors that **do not metastasize to bone**: CNS tumors, basal cell carcinoma of the skin
- marrow-rich bones generally predisposed to metastatic seeding
- metastatic spread distal to the knee or elbow rare
- metastatic spread of any tumor indicates poor prognosis

    b) Incidence

- metastases: the most common malignant skeletal tumors (about 70% of all malignant bone tumors)
- autopsy findings: 20–35% of all primary visceral malignancies metastasize to bone
- 80% of metastases to bone: from breast, prostate, lung and kidney
- females: 70% of bone metastatic lesions from primary breast tumors, the rest from thyroid, kidney and uterus
- males: 60% of bone metastatic lesions from prostate, the rest from lung (25%) and other organs
- patients > 40 years old
- Hodgkin's lymphoma: most common source of metastases in patients 20–35
- common causes in patients 10–20 years old: Ewing's sarcoma and osteosarcoma
- children < 5: most commonly from neuroblastoma

    c) Location

- 40% of all bony metastases: spine
  1) most commonly thoracic and lumbar, less often cervicals; very rarely atlas
  2) vertebral bodies and pedicles specifically targeted
  3) usually polyostotic: solitary lesions less common; difficult to diagnose
- 28% of bony metastases: ribs and sternum
  1) ribs 4 times more commonly involved than sternum
  2) sternal body usually involved, rather than manubrium
  3) multiple ribs often involved
- 12% of bony metastases involve pelvis and sacrum

1) seeded from viscera via Batson's venous plexus
2) thyroid or renal tumors: primary sources for "blow-out lesions" in bony pelvis

- 10% of metastatic lesions to bone involve calvarium
    1) thyroid, breast contribute lytic lesions to calvarium
    2) prostate metastases cause blastic lesions in calvarium
- remaining 10% in long tubular bones of extremities
    1) proximal femur
    2) proximal humerus
    3) scapula and clavicle may also develop metastatic lesions
- rarely: acral metastasis
    1) more likely in foot
    2) occasionally in hand (usually from the lung)

d) Treatment
- metastasis carries poor prognosis
- systemic therapy: generally chemotherapy
- increased sclerosis may be hopeful sign; increased lucency indicates progression of disease
- complications: pathologic fractures, extradural cord compression

 2. Clinical Presentation

a) Systemic signs: recent, unexplained weight loss; cachexia

b) Late in disease: anemia, fever

c) Skeletal pain (initially intermittent) of insidious onset, often worse at night

d) Pathologic fracture

3. Pathologic Features

a) Pathologic process
- tumor cells or fragments liberated from primary neoplasm
- pathway of dissemination available (pathway of metastasis)
    1) direct extension
        - most common with tumors of peritoneal cavity; e.g., uterine tumor extending into ilium
        - mechanical spread by instruments or gloves during surgery
        - rarely: seeded "downstream" from primary lesion in intestines or urinary tract
    2) lymphatic dissemination
        - rarely carry tumor emboli to bone
        - no lymphatic channels in bone marrow

      3) hematogenous dissemination
- most common route for skeletal metastases
- veins vulnerable to tumor penetration (arteries are not)
- lungs, liver, axial skeleton commonly seeded via veins
- prostate carcinoma seeds to pelvis, lumbar spine
  - a. Batson's venous plexus provides route
  - b. intra-abdominal or intrathoracic pressure variations facilitate reflux blood flow toward paravertebral plexus
- requires suitable site for growth of metastatic emboli

☞ **b)** Lesion behavior
- lytic destruction
  1) pressure from proliferating neoplasm on trabeculae and cortices
  2) trabeculae may be resorbed
  3) osteoclasts usually not involved in this process
  4) most metastatic lesions begin in medullary cavity
  5) lytic lesions rarely begin in cortex
  6) cortical lytic lesions usually originate in lung, breast, or kidney
- blastic metastases
  1) increased density caused by deposition of nonneoplastic new bone
  2) osteoid tissue's reactive response to the tumor
  3) represents a futile attempt at bone repair

☞ **4. Laboratory Findings**
- **a)** Elevated ESR
- **b)** Occasionally, elevation of serum calcium (with diffuse lytic lesions)
- **c)** Elevated alkaline phosphatase with blastic metastasis
- **d)** Elevated acid phosphatase, and prostate specific antigen (PSA) with prostatic carcinoma (when spread to skeleton)

☞ **5. Radiologic Features**
- **a)** Imaging modalities
  - nuclear bone scans
    1) detect alterations in metabolic activity of bone
    2) image changes with as little as 3–5% bone destruction

3) agent of choice: technetium-99m methylene diphosphonate (99mTc-MDP); low radiation dose, convenient half-life monoenergetic photon (140 keV)

4) osteoblastic activity (reaction to bone destruction) renders a *"hot spot"* on the scan

5) nonspecific: reflects increased metabolic activity of any etiology

6) lesions with little or no bone reaction (e.g., myeloma) not found with nuclear scanning

- computed tomography (CT)
  1) more sensitive than plain film studies
  2) excellent evaluation of cortical involvement
  3) good detection of soft tissue mass
  4) especially useful for localizing biopsy sites
- magnetic resonance imaging (MRI)
  1) superior definition of both osseous and soft tissue lesions
  2) short tau inversion recovery (STIR) images: optimal for subtle tissue abnormalities
- plain film radiography
  1) basic skeletal survey for suspected metastasis
     a. lateral skull projection
     b. AP and lateral spine (cervical, thoracic, lumbosacral)
     c. AP view of the pelvis
     d. AP view of the ribs
     e. PA view of the chest
  2) 30–50% loss of bone density occurs before lesion is visible on plain film

b) Radiologic signs of metastatic lesions
- alterations of bone density
  1) osteolytic (75% of metastatic lesions)
     a. moth-eaten or permeative pattern of bone destruction
     b. most commonly seen with metastases from lung or breast
  2) osteoblastic (15% of metastatic lesions)
     a. usually lesions from prostate, breast, cecum, bronchi
     b. diffuse, scattered pattern
  3) mixed lesions (10% of metastatic lesions)
     a. combination of lytic destruction and blastic proliferation
     b. most commonly from breast, sometimes from lung

Calcifying Metastases

"BOTTOM"

Breast

Osteosarcoma

Testicular

Thyroid

Ovary

Mucinous adenocarcinoma of the GI tract

- changes in architecture
- only about 10% of metastases solitary
  1) some carcinoma of thyroid, kidney, lung
  2) *"blow-out metastatic lesions"*: bubbly, highly expansile, large lesion **DDX:** solitary plasmacytoma; giant cell tumor
- general differences between primary and secondary tumor appearance
  1) periosteal response: more likely with primary tumors
  2) soft tissue mass: more likely with primary tumors
  3) lesions 10 cm long (and more): usually primary; metastatic lesions more commonly 2–4 cm long
  4) few metastases expand bone (blow-out metastases do); primary tumors often do
  5) primary tumors more often solitary; metastatic tumors usually multiple
  6) no generalizations are definitive: always exceptions

c) Metastatic spinal lesions
- 40% of all metastatic bone tumors: in spine; especially thoracic and lumbar areas
- vertebral body lytic destruction
  1) focal osteoporosis, or comparative lucency of one vertebral body
  2) pathologic fracture: both anterior and posterior body height diminished; vertebra plana
  3) wedge-shaped vertebra
  4) destruction of endplate integrity without disc height reduction
     a. angular endplate deformity
     b. malignant Schmorl's node (with or without significant trauma)
     c. disc rarely invaded by tumor
- vertebral body blastic process
  1) diffuse or localized sclerotic lesion
  2) *"ivory vertebra"*: single vertebral body with homogenous, diffuse increased opacity
- pedicle
  1) most commonly involved neural arch structure
  2) *"one-eyed pedicle sign"* or *"winking owl sign"*: loss of cortical margin of one pedicle; usually in lower thoracic or lumbar spine
  3) best seen on AP projection
  4) most commonly at single level; may be multiple

       5) occasionally occurs bilaterally:
           "blind vertebra"

d) Metastatic lesions in the pelvis
- about 12% of skeletal metastases: to pelvis
- frequent site of renal or thyroid *"blow-out lesions"*
- CT especially useful in detecting pelvic lesions

e) Metastasis to the skull
- calvarium: about 10% of all metastatic bone lesions
- > 90% are lytic, mostly from thyroid or breast
- < 10% are blastic, mostly from prostate and gastrointestinal tract (carcinoid tumors)
- multiple, well-defined holes without sclerotic rims
- usually lesions of varying sizes; present simultaneously

f) Metastasis to ribs and sternum
- about 28% of metastases: to ribs and sternum
- four times as many to ribs as to sternum
- both lytic and blastic lesions
- pathologic rib fracture common
- permeative lesions
- *"extrapleural sign"*: most commonly caused by metastasis to ribs
- **rarely** encounter blow-out lesions here

g) Metastatic lesions in extremities
- proximal femur and humerus most commonly affected extremity sites
- pathologic fracture may occur
- suspect metastasis with non-traumatic avulsion of lesser trochanter
- lung, breast or kidney tumors: may metastasize to feet or hands
  - a. hands: predilection for the distal phalanx
  - b. bronchogenic carcinoma: tends to metastasize to hands (distal phalanx)
  - c. extensive osteolysis of distal phalanx; soft tissue mass
  - d. articular space spared
- acral metastasis: rare, perhaps caused by lack of suitable seeding sites, lower temperatures, sparse red marrow in bones

h) Periosteal responses with metastatic lesions
- with most metastases: no periosteal response
- in adults, lesions from prostate, lung, and breast: some have periosteal response
  - a. about 5% of pelvic metastases from the prostate:

spiculated periosteal
response along inner pelvic
rim, ischial tuberosity,
proximal femoral shaft
- b. reaction to tumor: periosteal
response on side of involved
bone opposite tumor site
- in children, periosteal response with
metastases from neuroblastoma
- spiculation in cranial vault: with
metastatic neuroblastoma

6. **Differential considerations**

a) Osteolytic metastasis differentiated from
- neurofibromatosis
- enchondromatosis
- polyostotic fibrous dysplasia
- brown tumors of hyperparathyroidism
- gout
- osteomyelitis of tubercular or fungal
origin
- Histiocytosis "X"
- Gorham's angiomatosis ("vanishing bone
disease")

b) Osteoblastic metastasis differentiated from
- melorheostosis
- osteopoikilosis
- osteopathia striata
- osteopetrosis
- Paget's disease
- sarcoidosis
- tuberous sclerosis
- sclerotic secondary hyperparathyroidism
- chronic osteomyelitis
- sickle cell anemia
- mastocytosis
- fluorosis

c) Blow-out metastases may resemble giant cell
tumor, or solitary plasmacytoma

d) In spine:
- infection disrupts endplate integrity;
usually involves loss of disc height
- missing pedicle may be agenesis; usually
involves reactive sclerosis, enlargement of
contralateral pedicle
- ivory vertebra may be
1) Paget's disease: tends to enlarge or
"*balloon*" vertebra
2) Hodgkin's lymphoma: may cause
anterior or lateral scalloping (*gouge
defect*) of the vertebral body; usually
seen in younger patients

e) In skull:
- myeloma: most common differential
consideration
- punched-out lesions of myeloma: usually
uniform size; metastases usually of
varying size

E. NEUROBLASTOMA
(synonym: sympathicoblastoma)

1. **General Considerations**
    a) Nature of lesion
       - early-metastasizing abdominal neoplasm
       - metastases may present as plaques on the brain surface
       - commonly metastasizes to bone

    b) Incidence
       - < age 5 years old; 80% in children < 36 months of age

       - second most common childhood abdominal neoplasm (after Wilm's tumor)
       - familial incidence observed

    c) Location
       - primary tumors
          1) adrenal gland (75%)
          2) posterior mediastinum (20%)
          3) paravertebral sympathetic ganglionic chain (5%)
          4) very rarely a primary CNS tumor
       - metastases
          1) > 50% involve skeletal metastases: commonly to spine, pelvis, ends of long bones (spares epiphyses), and skull

    d) Treatment
       - excision of localized primary lesions
       - irradiation with chemotherapy
       - occasionally lesion undergoes spontaneous regression, with hemorrhage and necrosis

2. **Clinical Presentation**
    a) Child with a palpable abdominal mass
    b) With skeletal lesions: bone pain
    c) Pallor or petechiae when marrow is involved

3. **Pathologic Process and Laboratory Findings**
    a) Functional tissue, producing elevated levels of serum or urinary catecholamines
    b) 24-hour urine collections: elevated vanillylmandelic acid (VMA) and homovanillic acid (> 90% of cases)
    c) anemia, thrombocytopenia, leukopenia (when marrow is affected)

4. **Radiologic Features**
    a) Multiple, diffuse, fairly symmetric lesions
    b) Vertebral collapse
    c) Widened paravertebral stripe
    d) Widened skull sutures (caused by plaques deposited on brain surface)
    e) Soft tissue mass and sunburst spiculation of skull tables (**pathognomonic**)

F. TUMORLIKE PROCESSES

 1. **Paget's Disease**
(synonym: osteitis deformans)

a) **General considerations**
- nature of lesion
  1) unknown etiology
     - not generalized to all bone: endocrine or metabolic hypotheses are less likely
     - viral etiology: most current theory
     - environmental factor may be indicated (demographic distribution)
  2) increased number and activity of osteoclasts
  3) osteolysis followed by extensive attempts at repair
  4) bone softening, expansion, deformation
- etiologic theories
  1) inflammatory
  2) endocrine
  3) autoimmune
  4) inborn error of connective tissue metabolism
  5) vascular
  6) metabolic
  7) neoplastic
  8) chronic infection with measleslike *"slow virus"*
- incidence
  1) geographic variations in incidence
     - most prevalent in United Kingdom, Australia, New Zealand
     - least prevalent in Asia, Africa, Scandinavia
     - no difference in prevalence in black and white populations in United States
     - more prevalent in northern than in southern United States
  2) patients usually > 55 years old; rarely < 40
  3) male predilection (2:1)
- location
  1) most commonly polyostotic
  2) diminishing order of frequency: pelvis and sacrum; femur, skull, tibia, vertebrae, clavicle, humerus, ribs
  3) fibula least often involved
  4) occasionally any other bone affected, including sesamoids
  5) in feet, most commonly calcaneus and talus

6) lower extremity involved twice as often as upper

7) right side of skeleton involved more frequently than left

8) preferred spinal sites: third and fourth lumbars, lower thoracics, atlas and axis

9) tubular bones: invariably involves subarticular bone end, extending into mid-diaphysis

- treatment
    1) salmon and human calcitonin to inhibit bone resorption
        - inhibits osteoclastic bone resorption
        - decreases osteoclast activity and numbers
        - pain relief usually within 2–8 weeks
        - usually give 3-month trial
    2) supportive braces to prevent deformity of weight-bearing bones

b) Clinical presentation

- about 90% of cases asymptomatic, especially early in disease; often for many years
- dull pain: most common presenting symptom
    1) low intensity
    2) boring pain
    3) present day and night
    4) not aggravated by exertion
- up to 5° C difference between affected and unaffected sides of the body
- bone expansion: increasing hat size or shoe size
- bone deformities
    1) bowing of weight-bearing bones
    2) femoral neck deformities: "*coxa vara, shepherd's crook*" deformity
    3) tibial bowing: anterior bowed "*saber shin*" deformity; lateral bowed "*genu varum*" or "bowleg" deformity
    4) craniofacial deformities: basilar invagination, "*leontiasis ossea*" (increased frontal and parietal bossing create "*lionlike facies*")
- neurologic abnormalities
    1) palsies involving third, sixth, and seventh cranial nerves
    2) nerve deafness with severe auditory canal stenosis
    3) osseous-induced basilar artery syndrome: headaches, giddiness, vertigo, spinal cord ischemia
- pathologic fracture (most common complication of Paget's disease)

    1) transversely oriented called "*bananalike*" fractures

    2) most frequently in proximal one-third of femur (femoral neck or subtrochanteric)

    3) most occur in sclerotic or mixed (biphasic) phase of disease, not in lytic (destructive) phase

    4) other fracture sites: lumbar vertebrae, tibia commonly affected

- pseudofractures (synonyms: "*Looser's lines, increment fractures, Milkman's syndrome, umbau zonen*")

    1) demineralization and replacement with fibrous tissue in localized areas of bone

    2) may predispose to complete transverse (bananalike) fractures

    3) may remain totally asymptomatic

    4) most commonly at femoral neck and subtrochanteric region, in the scapula, pubic and ischial rami, proximal ulna, proximal tibia

- spinal stenosis

    1) caused by pressure of expanding bone, or pathologic vertebral fracture

    2) most common in upper thoracic spine (area of largest cord, smallest canal)

    3) known to occur in lumbar spine (cauda equina syndrome) and at the axis

    4) signs: weakness of legs, urinary incontinence, sensory disturbance

- anemia, caused by fibrous tissue replacing bone marrow (less common complication)
- acetabular degenerative joint disease

    1) called Paget's coxopathy

    2) secondary to accelerated enchondral ossification, replacement of cartilage by pagetic bone

    3) concentric or symmetric joint narrowing (acetabulum and femur equally affected)

    4) protrusio acetabuli

    5) cartilage necrosis over diseased bone

    6) accelerated subchondral ossification caused by increased underlying bone vascularity

- knee joint degeneration
- spinal intersegmental ankylosis: intradiscal invasion and fusion
- ureteric colic: increased hypercalcemia and hypercalciuria cause urinary calculus formation
- high-output cardiac failure

    1) pagetic bone: 20 times the vascularity of normal bone

2) congestive heart failure (if at least one-third of the skeleton is involved)

3) hyperdynamic circulation rare with less skeletal involvement

c) Malignant degeneration of pagetic bone

- incidence of degeneration
    1) overall, 0.9% to 20% of cases
    2) < 2% of cases with minimal, asymptomatic Paget's disease
    3) up to 20% of cases with advanced, polyostotic, symptomatic disease
    4) rarely occurs < age 40 years; more common in ages 57–66
    5) 2:1 male predilection
- indications of degeneration
    1) severe localized pain, perhaps creating local disability
    2) occasionally, a pulsatile mass
    3) spontaneous pathologic fracture
- site distribution of degeneration
    1) relatively high incidence in humerus
    2) relatively low incidence in vertebrae
    3) femur most commonly involved
    4) in decreasing frequency: humerus, ilia, skull, tibia
    5) malignant degeneration of pagetic bone unusual in: calcaneus, talus, rib, fibula, ulna, and radius; very rare in spine
    6) most commonly affects diaphyseal medullary canal
- histologic findings of degeneration
    1) osteosarcoma: most common tumor type
    2) fibrosarcoma: second most common
    3) less commonly: chondrosarcoma, malignant fibrous histiocytoma, reticulosarcoma
    4) giant cell tumor: a complication (benign or malignant)
    5) metastatic disease very seldom complicates Paget's disease
- radiologic findings of degeneration
    1) 50%: focal lytic subcortical destruction
    2) oval lucent area stands out against background of pagetic bone
    3) 25%: sclerotic lesions
    4) 25%: mixed
    5) frequently: pathologic fracture
    6) usually **no** periosteal response
    7) soft tissue mass common in advanced cases
    8) *"cannonball metastasis"* to lung: frequent consequence

- prognosis
    1) grave: about 8% 5-year survival rate
    2) excision, irradiation, and chemotherapy all employed

d) Pathologic features
- pagetic lesions: significant vascularity and fibrosis
- *four-stage process*
    1) **Stage one:** osteolytic, destructive, or monophasic stage
        - osteoclastic overactivity
        - gross loss of bone density
        - normal bone replaced by fibrous tissue and osteoid
        - hemorrhage and necrosis
    2) **Stage two:** combined, mixed, or biphasic stage
        - simultaneous destruction and reparative efforts
        - cortical thickening, accentuated trabecular patterns, bone expansion
        - "cheap" fibrous bone replaces that destroyed by osteoclasts
    3) **Stage three:** sclerotic or ivory stage
        - uniform thickening of trabeculae
        - possibly bone expansion
        - most commonly in vertebrae or ilia
    4) **Stage four:** malignant degeneration
- second stage: significant cortical accretion, growing into spongiosa until there is no demarcation between cortex and spongiosa
- hypervascularity includes multiple, microscopic arteriovenous malformations

e) Laboratory findings
- elevated serum alkaline phosphatase
- increased urinary hydroxyproline
- serum calcium usually **normal**

f) Radiologic findings
- bone scan: to locate additional sites, if a pagetic lesion is found on x-ray
- general features: depend on stage of disease
    1) bone density changes
    2) coarsened trabeculae
    3) cortical thickening
    4) bone expansion
    5) pseudofractures
    6) bowing deformities
    7) pathologic fracture
- subarticular distribution of lesions
- most often, calvarium, innominates, long bones are affected

- early in process: sharply defined lytic area with narrow zone of transition
- aggressive lesions may cause periosteal reaction
- radiologic signs at specific skeletal sites
  1) skull
     - early: spherical geographic lytic lesions
     - usually starts in frontal, occipital areas
     - inner table spared; outer table destroyed from within
     - destruction crosses sutures
     - *"osteoporosis circumscripta"*: sharply defined lytic area with narrow zone of transition
     - in stage two: sclerosis of inner table begins
     - irregular patches of thickened diploë (seen as opacities): *"cottonwool appearance"*
     - fuzzy, poorly defined margins
  2) spine
     - single or multiple lumbar vertebrae most commonly involved
     - usually seen in second stage (mixed or biphasic stage)
     - enlarged vertebral body
     - thickened cortex: appears squared-off; *"picture frame vertebra"*
     - accentuated trabeculae, especially vertical
     - monostotic form: *"ivory vertebra,"* often with straightened or bulged anterior margin caused by bone expansion and cortical thickening
     - lytic phase: pathologic collapse of vertebra, often involving posterior elements as well as vertebral bodies
  3) pelvis
     - lytic lesions in ilia: usually spherical
     - most commonly, combined stage seen here
     - unilateral or bilateral, and may involve sacrum
     - pubic and ischial cortical thickening and expansion
     - patchy sclerosis, intermittent lucencies, accentuated trabeculae
     - cortical margin thickened along pelvic rim with Kohler's teardrop obliterated (*"rim sign or brim sign"*)

- protrusio acetabuli caused by weakened bone
- commonly: monostotic involvement of the sacrum

    4) long tubular bones

- femur most commonly involved
  - a. usually found in second stage
  - b. subarticular lesion, may extend into diaphysis
  - c. expanded cortices, coarse trabeculae (especially vertical)
  - d. eventual obliteration of marrow cavity subtrochanteric pseudofractures (usually on lateral or convex cortical surface): form bilaterally symmetric lucent bands
  - e. varus deformity of hip ("*shepherd's crook deformity*")
- tibia: second most common site of lytic Paget's disease
  - a. subarticular, elongated lucent defect
  - b. sharp-bordered "V"; "*flame-shaped*" or "*blade of grass*" appearance
  - c. anterior bowing of tibia ("*saber shin deformity*")
  - d. avulsion fracture of tibial tuberosity (rare)

g) Differential considerations

- osteolytic/osteoblastic metastatic carcinoma
  1) appearance very similar to second or third stage Paget's disease
  2) similar age predilections
  3) thickened cortex: common in Paget's disease, not in metastasis
  4) cortical disruption: common in metastasis, not in Paget's disease
  5) significant bone expansion: common in Paget's disease, not in metastasis
  6) long bone subarticular location of lesion: peculiar to Paget's disease
- hemangioma of bone
  1) vertically striated vertebral body, similar to second stage Paget's disease
  2) endplate cortical thickening: common with Paget's disease, not with hemangioma
  3) "squaring" or bulging of vertebral body: common with Paget's disease, only occasionally with hemangioma

- fibrous dysplasia
    1) often features pseudofractures, as does Paget's disease
    2) subarticular long bone lesions: common to Paget's disease, not to fibrous dysplasia
- ivory vertebra: several possible etiologies, most commonly
    1) osteoblastic metastasis: usually does not alter vertebral body contours
    2) Hodgkin's lymphoma: frequently anterior or lateral vertebral body scalloping
    3) Paget's disease: frequently "*squares*" or bulges vertebral body margins
- pseudofractures: in several bone pathologies, including
    1) osteomalacia
    2) florid rickets
    3) fibrous dysplasia
    4) hyperphosphatasia

2. **Fibrous Dysplasia**

    a) **General considerations**
    - etiology unknown
    - nature of lesion

    1) three basic forms of fibrous dysplasia
        - monostotic
        - polyostotic
        - polyostotic with associated endocrine abnormalities
    2) benign condition
    3) slowly progressive disorder of fibro-osseous tissue
    4) locally circumscribed lesions
    5) along with Paget's disease: it is a "*great imitator*" of many bone pathologies
    6) monostotic form
        - does **not transform** to polyostotic form
        - less likely to result in pathologic fracture
        - infrequently disfiguring
    7) polyostotic form
        - tends to affect entire limbs
        - causes severe deformity
        - frequently leads to pathologic fracture, often recurrently
    8) endocrine effects (McCune-Albright syndrome)
        - usually unilateral bone involvement
        - skin pigmentation (café au lait spots)
        - precocious sexual development
            a. onset of female menarche by age 5 or 6
            b. only occasionally affects males

- cherubism: fibrous dysplasia of the jaws
    1) autosomal dominant inheritance
    2) familial
    3) recognized at about 18–24 months of age
    4) spontaneous regression during puberty
- fibrous dysplasia incidence
    1) monostotic
        - most common: about 70% of fibrous dysplasia cases
        - manifests in early teens
        - no gender predilection
    2) polyostotic
        - about 27% of fibrous dysplasia cases
        - manifests around age 11
        - no gender predilection
    3) polyostotic with endocrine disturbances
        - McCune-Albright syndrome
        - about 3% of fibrous dysplasia cases
        - distinct female predilection
        - usually manifests in first 5–6 years of life
- location
    1) monostotic fibrous dysplasia
        - 75% of lesions: rib, proximal femur, tibia, or skull
        - less frequently: pelvis, humerus, maxilla (involved twice as often as mandible), mandible (only 10% of monostotic cases usually involves cranial-facial bones)
        - usually diametaphyseal medullary location
        - rarely affects cortex
        - usually in anterior, proximal tibia
        - most common benign rib lesion
        - rare in clavicle, scapula, tarsals, carpals, other long bones, spine
    2) polyostotic fibrous dysplasia
        - usually in femur, skull, tibia, humerus, ribs, fibula, radius, ulna
        - extends into shoulder and pelvic girdle, vertebrae
        - tends to involve entire limbs (monomelic distribution)
        - infrequent in spine: vertebral bodies (multiple) usually involved
        - usually involve cranial-facial bones
        - asymmetric cranial distribution
        - monomelic (single limb) or bilateral distribution occurs
    3) *"café au lait"* spots: neck, chest, back, shoulder and pelvic girdle

b) **Clinical presentation**
- often totally asymptomatic
- lesions in proximal femur: intermittent pain, limp
- pathologic fracture: persistent pain
- polyostotic lesions: deformities, such as
    1) bowing of bones
    2) leg length discrepancy: coxa vara, bowed femur ("*shepherd's crook*" deformity)
- cranial-facial asymmetric enlargement, deformity
- unilateral cranial hyperostosis: "*leontiasis ossea*" (leonine appearance)
- thoracic localized bony prominence (with rib involvement)
- ethmoid or sphenoid involvement: obstructed nasal cavity
- "*café au lait*" spots of varying sizes
    1) dark brown to yellowish pigmentation
    2) on side of skeletal involvement
    3) usually distributed around midline: lower lumbar area, buttocks, back of neck, shoulders, chest, oral mucosa
    4) "*coast of Maine*" appearance: irregular jagged margins
    5) in all forms; most common in polyostotic with endocrine abnormalities

c) **Pathologic features**
- physiologic absorption of normal bone
- replacement with proliferating isomorphous fibrous tissue
    1) spindle cells make up much of fibrovascular connective tissue matrix
    2) irregular, poorly formed trabeculae with no functional orientation
- hypotheses include
    1) arrest of bone maturation at woven bone stage
    2) disturbed postnatal cancellous bone maintenance
    3) faulty differentiation of bone-forming mesenchyme
- cancellous bone replaced: yellowish-white or gray, resilient tissue containing small cysts filled with amber fluid
- fibrous matrix with poorly ossified bone spicules: elastic, gritty consistency (like sand embedded in putty)
- more bone spicules in skull, maxilla, olecranon: firmer consistency
- older lesions more dense: younger lesions have looser stromal arrangement, less collagen formation

- rarely: malignant degeneration (about 0.5% of cases)
    1) mean age of degeneration: 32 (range 8 to 61)
    2) degeneration slightly more prevalent in males
    3) degeneration more likely in polyostotic than monostotic form
    4) polyostotic: proximal femoral lesions most commonly affected
    5) monostotic: cranial-facial lesions most prone to degeneration
    6) degeneration: fibrosarcoma or osteosarcoma
    7) clinically: pain, swelling, radiographic changes typical of malignancy

☞ **d) Laboratory findings**
- serum alkaline phosphatase: sometimes elevated slightly
- serum calcium and phosphorus: normal
- café au lait spots: melanocytes or Malpighian cells (keratinocytes) **do not** have giant pigment granules

☞ **e) Radiologic features**
- skeletal lesions absent at birth; visible in early childhood; progressive throughout life
- bone scans not helpful: may be "*cold*," "*warm*," or "*hot*" at lesion sites
- monostotic form
    1) most commonly in proximal femur or in a rib
    2) long bone lesions: diametaphyseal (not subarticular) medullary defects
    3) radiolucent lesions, often loculated or trabeculated
    4) "*ground glass*" or smoky opacities within lucent lesion; "*wipe out*" of trabecular patterns
    5) well-demarcated; with thick, sclerotic border (rind of sclerosis)
    6) medullary canal widened; endosteum thinned and scalloped
    7) expansion of bone in fusiform or spherical enlargement
    8) cortex may be markedly thinned, but intact
    9) bone deformity, occasionally with pathologic fracture
    10) no periosteal response (except with fracture or degeneration)
- polyostotic form
    1) bowing of weightbearing bones
    2) "*shepherd's crook deformity*" of the femoral neck

- coxa vara, with femoral angle near 90°
- bowed proximal femur

3) widened medullary canal; may involve entire diaphysis of long bone

4) thinned, scalloped endosteum

5) *"ground glass appearance"* of lesions (rather than lucency of monostotic form)

6) loculated lesion, with incomplete septa or ridges

7) pseudofractures or *"increment fractures"*: infractions at regular intervals along length of bone

8) usually pelvis, lower extremity, upper extremity, ribs, skull involved

9) tends toward unilateral distribution, or asymmetrically bilateral (one side more extensively affected)

10) unilateral pelvic involvement: ipsilateral proximal femur invariably affected

11) rib involvement
   - unilateral or bilateral, often asymmetric
   - *"long lesion"* (> 4 cm)
   - gross expansion and loculation of bone
   - *"extrapleural sign"*
   - subject to spontaneous fracture
   - fibrous dysplasia: most common cause of benign long lesion in ribs

12) pseudoarthrosis may occur in lower extremity

13) skull involvement
   - loculated, expansile, lytic lesions: most often in vertex
   - skull base lesions often sclerotic
   - calvarium broadened, with coexistent sclerotic and lucent lesions
   - thinned external table
   - maxilla and mandible often involved

14) spinal involvement
   - infrequent site; usually in vertebral body, but may affect arch
   - most often in lumbar spine: vertebral collapse
   - vertebral lesions homogeneously lucent
   - disc space may or may not be diminished

 f) Differential considerations
   - Paget's disease
     1) Paget's long bone lesions

subarticular: fibrous dysplasia metadiaphyseal
  2) also features pseudofractures (as do osteomalacia and rickets)
  3) both entities may feature mixed sclerotic/lytic lesions
  4) Paget's thickens cortices: fibrous dysplasia thins them
- neurofibromatosis
  1) pseudoarthrosis in both: especially in the tibia
  2) both feature café au lait spots on skin
     - neurofibromatosis spots usually lighter
     - fibrous dysplasia spots irregularly marginated ("*coast of Maine*")
     - neurofibromatosis spots smoothly marginated ("*coast of California*")
     - histologic exam: giant pigment granules in Malpighian cells or melanocytes in neurofibromatosis; **absent** in fibrous dysplasia
- osteitis fibrosa cystica
- multiple brown tumors of hyperparathyroidism

3. **Neurofibromatosis (NF)**

   a) **General considerations**
      - nature of lesions
        1) autosomal dominant transmission of inherited disorder
        2) two clinical forms delineated
           - neurofibromatosis 1 (von Recklinghausen's)
             a. café au lait spots
             b. neurofibromas
             c. bone changes
           - neurofibromatosis 2: acoustic nerve tumors
        3) lesions of neurofibromatosis 1
           - neuroectodermal and mesodermal dysplasia
           - "*café au lait spots*": pigmented cutaneous lesions
           - "*fibroma molluscum*": soft, elevated cutaneous tumors
           - axial and appendicular skeletal alterations
        4) peripheral nerves usually affected, may involve central nervous system (mental retardation)
      - incidence
        1) familial history of neurofibromatosis in about 60% of cases
        2) 1 in 3,000 births

3) no gender, demographic, or racial predilection
- location of lesions
    1) café au lait spots on back, chest, abdomen
    2) fibroma molluscum nodules anywhere and everywhere on body
    3) neurofibromas on optic nerve, spinal nerves, any peripheral nerves
    4) characteristic deformations in spine, skull, ribs, and long bones

b) Clinical presentation
- *"café au lait"* spots
    1) cutaneous macules: chestnut or yellowish
    2) **second most common** skin manifestation of NF
    3) smoothly marginated (*"coast of California"* appearance)
    4) seen in about 50% of NF patients
    5) diagnosis requires at least six spots > 1.5 cm in diameter (1 or 2 present in about 15% of normal population)
    6) age-related: size, number, pigmentation may increase up to third decade
    7) occasionally fade with age
- fibroma molluscum
    1) multiple, asymptomatic cutaneous nodules
    2) pedunculated, nipplelike, or sessile soft skin tabs
    3) from tiny to > 5 cm in diameter
    4) **most common** skin manifestation of NF, and best diagnostic cutaneous feature
- elephantiasis neuromatosa
    1) diffuse plexiform neurofibromas
    2) large soft tissue masses, create skin folds
    3) may cause massive skin, soft tissue, and bony enlargement (focal giantism)
- symptoms vary depending on site of abnormalities
    1) among effects of skull lesions
        - optic nerve neurofibroma: blurred vision, scotoma, transient blindness
        - posterior superior orbital wall lesion: pulsating exophthalmos, blepharoptosis, dislocation of the eyeball
        - facial asymmetry
    2) among effects of spinal lesions
        - localized pain
        - motor symptoms, up to and including paraplegia

- kyphoscoliosis frequently occurs; may be severe: sometimes asymptomatic; may induce cord compression and paraplegia
- atlantoaxial subluxation (rarely) caused by ligament laxity suboccipital headache, upper extremity motor weakness
- renal artery stenosis may lead to renal hypertension
- adrenal pheochromocytoma often associated with neurofibromatosis (also may cause hypertension)
- malignant degeneration to neurofibrosarcoma: pain and progressive enlargement

c) Pathologic features
- neurofibroma: gray or grayish brown, firm, rubbery mass
- appears exactly like schwannoma (neurinoma) or neuroma
- histologic composition: interlacing strands of elongated foam cells and pigment in a palisading pattern
- about 5% undergo malignant degeneration: more likely with repeated biopsies

d) Radiologic features

- skeletal lesions in about 50% of neurofibromatosis patients
- spinal lesions
  1) scoliosis
     - most common skeletal feature
     - short segment (5–7 vertebrae involved)
     - most commonly kyphoscoliosis: lower thoracic spine
     - acutely angular
     - may lead to paraplegia
  2) cervical kyphosis
     - acutely angular reversal of cervical lordosis
     - usually accompanied by posterior vertebral body scalloping
  3) vertebral body scalloping
     - may be posterocentral or eccentric, unilateral scalloping
     - posterocentral: secondary to dural ectasia; usually multiple levels
     - eccentric unilateral scalloping: usually caused by dumbbell neurofibroma from spinal nerve root; protruding through IVF
       a. usually at a single level
       b. involve cervical or thoracolumbar areas most often

        c.   enlarge IVF due to erosion of posterior body and pedicle

4) paraspinal mass visible on AP thoracic or PA chest projections: intrathoracic meningocele or large dumbbell neurofibroma

- intrathoracic meningocele
  - a. protrusion of dura and arachnoid through thoracic IVF and posterior ribs into extrapleural thoracic cavity
  - b. in about 66% of cases
  - c. from 1 to 6 cm in diameter
  - d. usually asymptomatic posterior mediastinal mass
  - e. usually right lateral
  - f. myelography: fill with contrast material (neurofibroma does not fill)
  - g. may also enlarge IVF: erodes posterior body, pedicle, posterior ribs
- dumbbell neurofibroma
  - a. plain film: may be indistinguishable from meningocele
  - b. myelography: will not fill with contrast (solid tumor)

- skull lesions
  1) orbital defects
     - "*bare orbit*": agenesis or hypoplasia of posterior orbital wall, sphenoid, and orbital plate of frontal bone
       - a. fairly common in neurofibromatosis
       - b. allows direct contact of temporal lobe and meninges with orbital soft tissues; creating pulsating exophthalmos
       - c. most commonly unilateral
     - optic nerve neurofibroma
       - a. enlarges optic foramen
       - b. may require CT for adequate visualization
  2) lambdoidal defect ("*asterion defect*")
     - lucent defect adjacent to lambdoidal suture, posterior to parietal-mastoid and occipital-mastoid sutures
     - usually on left side
     - hypoplastic or agenetic area (not neurofibroma erosion)
     - up to 10 cm in diameter
     - may be associated with hypoplastic ipsilateral mastoid process

3) macrocranium (and macroencephaly)
- frequent finding with neurofibromatosis
- often missed
- prominent in Treves' "elephant man" case

- rib lesions
  1) *"twisted ribbon appearance"*: ribs thin, irregular, scalloped, attenuated
  2) intercostal neurofibromas erode inferior rib surface
  3) sometimes mesodermal dysplasia or hypoplasia
- tubular bone lesions
  1) pseudoarthrosis: pathologic fracture with lack of normal healing
     - tibia most commonly affected
     - usually lower two-thirds of tibia
  2) also deossification and bowing of weight-bearing bones
  3) small tubular extremity bones: twisting (similar to ribs)
  4) multiple non-ossifying fibromas (NOF)
     - multiple cystic, central, or intramedullary lesions
     - usually in metaphysis of long tubular bones of lower extremities
     - infrequent finding
     - usually multiple, bilateral; much larger than typical NOF
  5) focal giantism
     - single bone or entire extremity
     - normal bone shape
     - associated soft tissues proportionately enlarged
     - pathogenesis: chronic hyperemia caused by hemangiomas and lymphangiomatous lesions
- extraskeletal lesions
  1) soft tissue masses (neurofibromas) in various sites
     - intracranial lesions
     - intramural gastrointestinal lesions
     - in lung, mediastinum, kidney, adrenal gland

e) Differential considerations
- with benign polyostotic tumorlike lesions, consider seven bone disorders: (**"TRY" 7**)
  1) Paget's disease
  2) fibrous dysplasia
  3) Histiocytosis "X"
  4) neurofibromatosis
  5) hereditary multiple exostoses (HME)

6) Ollier's disease (multiple enchondromatosis)
7) multiple brown tumors of hyperparathyroidism

- fibrous dysplasia
    1) café au lait spots
        - in fibrous dysplasia: spots are darker, larger, have irregular margins ("*coast of Maine*" appearance)
        - in neurofibromatosis: spots lighter, smaller, have smooth margins ("*coast of California*" appearance)
        - café au lait spots: also seen with tuberous sclerosis
        - 15% of normal population: one or two café au lait spots
    2) may also feature pseudoarthrosis
- rib erosions: may be caused by aortic coarctation or other conditions
- pulsating exophthalmos: may indicate intraorbital aneurysm, vascular anomalies
- vertebral body scalloping: simulates spinal tuberculosis; lymphoma
    1) with infection: diminished disc space
    2) neurofibromatosis: normal disc space
    3) Hodgkin's lymphoma scallops anterior and lateral vertebral bodies
    4) neurofibromatosis scallops posterior body margins

REVIEW—STUDY QUESTIONS

1. What is the clinical picture indicative of metastatic disease?
2. What are the radiologic signs of spinal metastasis?
3. What are the three most commonly encountered causes of an ivory vertebra, and how do we differentiate among them?
4. What is the most common abdominal neoplasm in children? What is the second most common?
5. Name at least five entities that must be considered in differential diagnosis of lytic bone lesions?
6. What are the differentiating features between the café au lait spots of neurofibromatosis and those of fibrous dysplasia?
7. What is a rim sign? A picture frame vertebra? A shepherd's crook deformity? Osteoporosis circumscripta? Increment fractures?
8. What bone disease is most likely to involve subarticular lesions in patients of advanced age?
9. Describe cherubism and explain its etiology and prognosis.
10. List seven entities ("TRY" 7) that must be considered in differential diagnosis of benign polyostotic tumorlike lesions.

1. A periosteal reaction of "trimmed whiskers"—very thin, fairly short spicules of reactive new bone—is most typical of:

   a) parosteal sarcoma.
   b) central osteosarcoma.
   c) Ewing's sarcoma.
   d) chondrosarcoma.

2. In male patients, the primary source of skeletal metastasis is a primary tumor in the:

   a) colon.
   b) kidney.
   c) lung.
   d) prostate.

3. The pathognomonic lesion seen in the metastasis of neuroblastoma to the skull is:

   a) widening of the skull sutures.
   b) multiple, diffuse, symmetric lucencies.
   c) a soft tissue mass with sunburst spiculation of the skull tables.
   d) scalloped geographic lesions in the calvarium.

4. In both the cervical and thoracolumbar spine, neurofibromas may cause:

   a) posterocentral vertebral scalloping.
   b) enlargement of the IVF caused by erosion of the pedicle and posterior body.
   c) multiple level eccentric bilateral scalloping.
   d) single level eccentric bilateral scalloping.

5. Paget's disease may be radiographically distinguished from fibrous dysplasia because Paget's will commonly have:

   a) a hazy, "ground glass" appearance.
   b) pseudofractures.
   c) bowing deformities in the long tubular bones.
   d) subarticular long bone lesions.

6. The typical radiologic appearance of a periosteal chondroma includes a classic triad of:

   a) endosteal scalloping, eccentric expansion of the bone, and a calcified, cartilaginous matrix.
   b) cortical scalloping, overhanging bony edges, and a calcified, cartilaginous matrix.
   c) a distinct soft tissue mass, cortical scalloping, and a calcified, cartilaginous matrix.
   d) eccentric bone expansion, a distinct soft tissue mass, and a calcified, cartilaginous matrix.

7. Clinically, aneurysmal bone cysts:

   a) are usually silent, and are incidental findings on x-rays taken for other reasons.
   b) are discovered only when there is pathologic fracture.
   c) are characterized by acute onset of local pain, which rapidly increases in severity.
   d) are rarely subject to pathologic fracture.

8. The triad of abnormal growths seen in almost half of the cases of Gardner's syndrome consists of:

   a) café au lait spots, soft tissue fibromas, and multiple osteomas.
   b) café au lait spots, colonic polyps, and multiple osteomas.
   c) soft tissue fibromas, multiple osteomas, and colonic polyps.
   d) colonic polyps, soft tissue fibromas, and café au lait spots.

9. Osteosarcoma shows a clear predilection for:

   a) females of childbearing age.
   b) males > 50 years of age.
   c) females < 25 years of age.
   d) males < 25 years of age.

10. A "coat hanger exostosis," projecting away from a joint, describes:

    a) a sessile osteochondroma.
    b) a pedunculated osteochondroma.
    c) Trevor's disease.
    d) a large traction spur.

11. The fourth most common primary malignant bone tumor, Ewing's sarcoma, constitutes approximately:

    a) 20% of all biopsied primary malignant bone tumors.
    b) 15% of all biopsied primary malignant bone tumors.
    c) 11% of all biopsied primary malignant bone tumors.
    d) 7% of all biopsied primary malignant bone tumors.

12. The most common malignant skeletal tumor is:

    a) osteosarcoma.
    b) metastasis.
    c) multiple myeloma.
    d) chondrosarcoma.

13. Neuroblastoma is:

    a) the second most common childhood abdominal neoplasm.
    b) the most common abdominal neoplasm in children < 5 years of age.
    c) an abdominal neoplasm commonly seen in multiparous females.
    d) the second most common abdominal neoplasm in geriatric patients.

14. The most common clinical feature of spinal involvement in neurofibromatosis is:

    a) a "short segment" kyphoscoliosis in the lower thoracic spine.
    b) a long "C curve" thoracolumbar scoliosis.
    c) an acute reversal of the cervical lordosis.
    d) an acute reversal of the lumbar lordosis.

15. The characteristic subarticular lucency in a tubular bone that is characteristic of Paget's disease is:

    a) a punched-out lesion.
    b) a "blade of grass" defect.
    c) a shepherd's crook defect.
    d) a saber shin defect.

16. A purely lucent bone lesion in the hand causes the physician to consider all of the following except:

    a) osteoma.
    b) simple bone cyst.
    c) solitary enchondroma.
    d) osteoblastoma.

17. Aneurysmal bone cyst is:

    a) a non-neoplastic lesion.
    b) a cartilaginous neoplasm.
    c) a collagenous neoplasm.
    d) a fibrous neoplasm.

18. Sinusitis, exophthalmos, headaches, visual disturbances, and balance problems are possible signs of:

    a) hemangioma.
    b) aneurysmal bone cyst.
    c) osteoid osteoma.
    d) osteoma.

19. The second most common primary malignant bone tumor is:

    a) Ewing's sarcoma.
    b) plasmacytoma.
    c) chondrosarcoma.
    d) osteosarcoma.

20. A subungual exostosis is:

    a) a lesion in the great toe, seen with tophaceous gout.
    b) a type of osteochondroma at the distal end of the terminal phalanx of a toe.
    c) a thickening of the tissue beneath the nail of the great toe, seen with psoriatic arthritis.
    d) a nodule beneath the nail of the great toe, seen with rheumatoid arthritis.

21. Non-Hodgkin's lymphoma, myeloma, and Ewing's sarcoma are all:

    a) primary malignancies affecting adolescent patients.
    b) round-cell tumors.
    c) osteosarcomas.
    d) possible products of degeneration of Paget's disease.

22. A painful, lytic, expansile lesion in the mandible, with periosteal new bone response, is most likely to be:

    a) fibrous dysplasia.
    b) giant cell tumor.
    c) aneurysmal bone cyst.
    d) adamantinoma.

23. In differentiating multiple myeloma from lytic metastasis to the skull, a helpful feature is:

    a) multiple myeloma lesions tend to become confluent, geographic lesions.
    b) multiple myeloma lesions tend to be of varied sizes.
    c) lytic metastatic lesions tend to be of varied sizes, and multiple myeloma lesions more uniform.
    d) lytic metastatic lesions are more apt to be round, and multiple myeloma lesions more ovoid.

24. Optic nerve neurofibroma may result in:

    a) irreversible blindness.
    b) scotoma and transient blindness.
    c) pulsating exophthalmos.
    d) dislocation of the eyeball.

25. During the lytic phase of Paget's disease, spinal x-rays may show:

    a) squared-off, picture frame vertebrae.
    b) enlarged ivory vertebrae.
    c) vertebra plana.
    d) rugger jersey vertebrae.

26. Solitary enchondroma:

    a) is equally likely to be either lucent or to have stippled or punctate calcifications.
    b) may occasionally contain a fleck of calcification, but us usually purely lucent.
    c) is usually filled with flocculent calcification.
    d) is densely sclerotic.

27. The "fallen fragment" or "hinged fragment" signs are characteristic of the radiographic appearance of:

    a) pathologic fracture of hemangioma in a lumbar vertebra.
    b) a "carrot stick" fracture.
    c) pathologic fracture with fibrous dysplasia.
    d) pathologic fracture of a simple bone cyst (SBC).

28. Osteoma shows a predilection for:

    a) geriatric males.
    b) pediatric males.
    c) pediatric females.
    d) adult females.

29. The radiologic appearance of a solitary plasmacytoma is most often:

    a) a vertebra plana or "silver dollar vertebra."
    b) an ovoid, sclerotic medullary lesion with a lucent nidus.
    c) an expansile, lucent geographic lesion with soap-bubble internal architecture.
    d) a lucent geographic lesion with punctate calcifications.

30. Osteochondromas are most commonly found in:

    a) the mandible and the sacrum.
    b) the spine.

c) the long tubular bones.

d) the small tubular bones of the hands and feet.

31. The most common primary malignant bone tumor of the hand is:

a) central osteosarcoma.

b) parosteal sarcoma.

c) fibrosarcoma.

d) chondrosarcoma.

32. The only primary malignant tumor in direct anatomic relationship with a joint surface is:

a) a malignant giant cell tumor.

b) a synovioma.

c) a chordoma.

d) plasmacytoma.

33. The list of differential diagnoses for osteoblastic metastasis should include all of the following except:

a) fibrous dysplasia.

b) Paget's disease.

c) brown tumors of hyperparathyroidism.

d) chronic osteomyelitis.

34. Diagnosis of neurofibromatosis requires at least six café au lait spots because:

a) fibrous dysplasia also presents with café au lait spots.

b) at least 15% of the normal population have one or two café au lait spots.

c) at least 25% of the normal population have three or four café au lait spots.

d) patients with fibrous dysplasia may have three to five café au lait spots.

35. Both "osteoporosis circumscripta" and "cottonwool appearance" describe the radiographic appearance of the skull in cases of:

a) lytic metastatic disease.

b) fibrous dysplasia.

c) multiple myeloma.

d) Paget's disease.

36. The most common benign bone tumor of the hand is:

a) a bone island.

b) an osteochondroma.

c) a solitary enchondroma.

d) fibrous dysplasia.

37. The incidence of pathologic fracture with a simple bone cyst is:

a) less than 10%.

b) almost 33%.

c) over 65%.

d) over 90%.

38. Hemangioma in the skull:

a) erodes the outer table, extending outward beyond normal bone contour.

b) preserves the outer table, but erases the inner table of the skull.

c) erodes both inner and outer skull tables, with dense radiating spiculae.

d) expands the outer table, projecting beyond the normal skull contour.

39. "Raindrop skull" describes:

a) occasional lytic lesions of varying size in the skull, with clear sclerotic margins.

b) the signs of hyperparathyroidism in the skull.

c) early lytic metastatic disease in the skull, with geographic lucencies and small lytic lesions.

d) widespread, uniformly sized oval lucencies with no reactive sclerosis, typical of multiple myeloma in the skull.

40. The most common benign bone neoplasm is:

a) hemangioma.

b) nonossifying fibroma

c) osteochondroma.

d) fibrous cortical defect.

41. Intramedullary tumors are those which occur:

a) in the epidural tissues.

b) in the leptomeninges.

c) in spinal nerve roots.

d) within the substance of the spinal cord.

42. "Reed-Sternberg cells" are found in histologic examination of:

a) Non-Hodgkin's lymphoma of bone.

b) plasmacytoma.

c) Hodgkin's lymphoma of bone.

d) adamantinoma.

43. Tumors that occasionally metastasize to the distal extremities are usually from:

a) the gastrointestinal tract.

b) the lungs, breast, or kidneys.

c) skin lesions (such as melanoma).

d) the prostate, uterus, or ovaries.

44. The clinical form of neurofibromatosis known as von Recklinghausen's is apt to include:

a) acoustic nerve tumors.

b) large, "Coast of Maine" café au lait spots.

c) small, "Coast of Maine" café au lait spots and bone changes.

d) small, "Coast of California" café au lait spots and bone changes.

45. In addition to bowing deformities and bone density changes, radiologic signs of Paget's disease include all of the following except:

a) pseudofractures.

b) cortical thickening.

c) bone expansion.

d) thinning of stress-bearing trabeculae.

46. The histologic appearance of an osteoid osteoma may be nearly identical to:

a) an osteosarcoma.

b) an osteoma.

c) an osteoblastoma.

d) an osteochondroma.

47. Treatment for a simple bone cyst (SBC) is usually:

    a) wide en bloc excision.
    b) curettage with irradiation.
    c) curettage with cauterization and bone chip packing.
    d) not necessary, since they are self-limiting and resolve in 2–5 years.

48. The radiologic appearance of hemangioma in the spine is most typically:

    a) a sandwich vertebra.
    b) a corduroy cloth, or striated vertebra.
    c) a rugger-jersey vertebra.
    d) a picture frame vertebra.

49. Extramedullary plasmacytomas, often seen in patients with multiple myeloma, are locally invasive tumors that erode adjacent bone, and most often occur in:

    a) the chest wall.
    b) the retroperitoneum.
    c) the pelvic basin.
    d) the nasopharynx.

50. An exostosis with a hyaline-lined cartilage cap, projecting from a cortical surface is:

    a) a traction osteophyte.
    b) an osteochondroma.
    c) an osteoblastoma.
    d) a chondroblastoma.

51. The café au lait spots of fibrous dysplasia:

    a) are large, with smooth margins.
    b) are small, and have smooth margins.
    c) are large, with jagged, irregular margins.
    d) are small, lightly pigmented, and have jagged, irregular margins.

52. The "blind vertebra" is an x-ray sign representing:

    a) a horizontally "split" vertebra, as in a seat belt (Chance) fracture.
    b) unilateral lytic destruction of the cortical margin of a pedicle.
    c) bilateral loss of the cortical margins of the pedicles.
    d) congenital agenesis of a pedicle.

53. Hodgkin's lymphoma is most often seen in:

    a) two age groups: 15–34, and over 60.
    b) children under 15.
    c) children between 5 and 10.
    d) adults between 35 and 60.

54. Chondrosarcoma represents:

    a) 27% of all primary malignant bone tumors.
    b) 20% of all primary malignant bone tumors.
    c) 10% of all primary malignant bone tumors.
    d) 7% of all primary malignant bone tumors.

55. Multiple myeloma may be detected by:

    a) a "hot" bone scan at the lesion sites.
    b) serum hypocalcemia.
    c) Bence Jones proteinuria.
    d) increased serum phosphorus.

56. The relationship between an FCD and an NOF is:

    a) the fibrous cortical defect probably represents early identification of a non-ossifying fibroma.
    b) the non-ossifying fibroma probably represents early identification of a fibrous cortical defect.
    c) the fibrous cortical defect may resolve, but is likely to predispose the bone to formation of a non-ossifying fibroma.
    d) the non-ossifying fibroma may predispose the bone to formation of a fibrous cortical defect.

57. A benign osteoblastic neoplasm that is seen more often in the spine than in the appendicular skeleton is:

    a) an osteoid osteoma.
    b) an osteoma.
    c) a bone island.
    d) an osteoblastoma.

58. Commonly seen radiologic signs of malignant degeneration in pagetic bone include all of the following except:

    a) cannonball metastasis to the lung.
    b) onion-skin or laminated periosteal response.
    c) oval lucent lesions seen against a background of pagetic bone.
    d) pathologic fracture.

59. Although hemangioma is a benign lesion, it may cause symptoms due to:

    a) periostitis.
    b) bone expansion.
    c) cord compression.
    d) basilar invagination.

60. Approximately half the patients with neurofibromatosis develop osseous lesions, most commonly in the:

    a) skull or facial bones.
    b) spine.
    c) chest wall.
    d) pelvis.

61. The smoky opacity of polyostotic fibrous dysplasia lesions:

    a) is set off from normal bone by a thick rind of sclerosis.
    b) is set apart from normal bone by an egg-shell margin.
    c) blends imperceptibly into normal bone.
    d) is set off from normal bone by a hazy, sclerotic zone of transition.

62. Metastatic tumors are more likely than primary tumors to have:

    a) periosteal response.
    b) soft tissue mass.

c)   polyostotic expression.
d)   expansile lesions.

63.   Reticulum cell sarcoma is also known as:

a)   Hodgkin's disease.
b)   Non-Hodgkin's lymphoma.
c)   Ewing's sarcoma.
d)   synovial sarcoma.

64.   Parosteal sarcoma:

a)   is a highly aggressive lesion of the spine.
b)   is one of the few primary malignancies with a strong predilection for the hands.
c)   is a rapidly fatal sarcoma, occurring primarily in pediatric patients.
d)   is usually a slow-growing malignancy, found in middle-aged adults.

65.   The 5-year survival rate for patients with a malignant giant cell tumor is:

a)   > 80%.
b)   > 50%.
c)   >20%.
d)   < 10%.

66.   Non-ossifying fibroma and fibrous cortical defect are both:

a)   caused by cartilaginous remnants in the metaphysis after the physis closes.
b)   examples of cartilaginous tumors.
c)   examples of fibrous xanthoma of bone.
d)   benign tumors with a high likelihood of malignant degeneration.

67.   On plain film, the osteoid osteoma is seen as:

a)   a sclerotic nidus within a less dense area of reactive sclerosis.
b)   an area of reactive sclerosis containing a lucent nidus.
c)   a uniformly dense, sclerotic lesion with an ill-defined border.
d)   a lucent lesion with a small central calcific fleck and an "eggshell" rim.

68.   Cardiac failure is a possible complication of Paget's disease because:

a)   increased serum calcium results in calcification of the coronary arteries.
b)   pagetic bone has 20 times the normal vascularity and causes high-output cardiac failure.
c)   increasing size of the sternum may cause cardiac tamponade.
d)   anemia because of loss of bone marrow weakens the heart.

69.   In the spine, the most common benign bone tumor is:

a)   osteochondroma.
b)   aneurysmal bone cyst.
c)   hemangioma.
d)   osteoid osteoma.

70.   Skull lesions commonly occurring with neurofibromatosis include all the following **except:**

a)   bare orbit with pulsating exophthalmos.
b)   growing fracture, as sutural margins are eroded.
c)   asterion defect adjacent to the lambdoidal suture.
d)   macroencephaly (macrocranium).

71.   The most common benign rib lesion is:

a)   monostotic fibrous dysplasia.
b)   bone island.
c)   solitary enchondroma.
d)   chondroblastoma.

72.   A serious limitation of plain film radiography, when ruling out skeletal metastasis, is that:

a)   it cannot detect bone density loss < 60–65%.
b)   it cannot detect bone density loss < 55–60%.
c)   it cannot detect bone density loss < 50–55%.
d)   it cannot detect bone density loss < 30–50%.

73.   A lesion that is known to cross discs and spread into contiguous vertebral bodies is:

a)   osteosarcoma.
b)   chordoma.
c)   Ewing's sarcoma.
d)   adamantinoma.

74.   The "cumulus cloud appearance" on x-ray describes

a)   the mottled, permeative lesion with a poor zone of transition, seen in about 25% of central osteosarcoma.
b)   the dense, ivory lesion with rough, lobulated margin seen in about 50% of central osteosarcoma.
c)   the fluffy periostitis caused by early cortical disruption by an aggressive malignancy.
d)   the lobulated soft tissue mass that forms around a chondrosarcoma.

75.   Giant cell tumors in the spine:

a)   are generally in the neural arch of thoracic vertebra.
b)   are rare, but most commonly occur in the thoracic vertebral bodies.
c)   are rare, but most often occur in lumbar or cervical vertebrae.
d)   are commonly seen in the thoracolumbar vertebrae.

76.   Chondromyxoid fibromas appear on plain film as:

a)   opaque, oval, eccentric lesions creating endosteal scalloping.
b)   lucent, eccentric, sometimes "soap-bubbled" oval lesions, with scalloped, sclerotic margins.
c)   lucent, eccentric oval lesions, with fluffy or punctate calcifications and hazy margins.
d)   lucent, eccentric expansile lesions, with thin, egg-shell margins.

77. After excision of an osteoid osteoma, the lesion may recur unless:

    a) the entire nidus has been removed.
    b) the entire area of reactive sclerosis has been removed.
    c) the site is irradiated after excision.
    d) the excision is performed when the lesion is metabolically inactive.

78. Osseous-induced basilar artery syndrome, with vertigo, headaches, and spinal cord ischemia, may be symptomatic of:

    a) multiple myeloma.
    b) osteomalacia.
    c) idiopathic osteoporosis.
    d) Paget's disease.

79. Hereditary multiple exostosis may result in a "bayonet hand" deformity, in which:

    a) the ulna is shortened and bows outward.
    b) the ulna is shortened and the radius bows outward.
    c) the radius is shortened and the ulna bows outward.
    d) the radius is shortened and bows outward.

80. Benign polyostotic tumorlike lesions suggest consideration of seven bone disorders ("TRY" 7), including all of the following except:

    a) fibrous dysplasia.
    b) neurofibromatosis.
    c) fibrous xanthoma.
    d) Ollier's disease.

81. Cherubism is fibrous dysplasia of the jaws that:

    a) regresses spontaneously during puberty.
    b) accompanies severe mental retardation.
    c) includes endocrine abnormalities that significantly shorten the life span.
    d) becomes apparent during puberty

82. With most metastatic bone disease, nuclear bone scan will show "hot spots" where there is:

    a) a minimum of 30% bone destruction.
    b) as little as 3–5% bone destruction.
    c) a minimum of 15% bone destruction.
    d) as little as 1% bone destruction.

83. Chordoma is a primary malignant bone tumor that is usually spread by:

    a) hematogenous routes.
    b) lymphogenous routes.
    c) direct extension.
    d) mechanical spread by instruments or gloves during surgical procedures.

84. Tumor thrombus is:

    a) external compression by a tumor, causing deep venous thrombosis.
    b) hematogenous spread of primary tumor fragments.
    c) pressure on the spinal cord, caused by an expanding lesion.
    d) stroke-like symptoms caused by tumor emboli.

85. Giant cell tumors are:

    a) neoplasms formed from connective tissue in the bone marrow.
    b) non-neoplastic cysts in the epiphysis.
    c) neoplasms formed in the epiphysis, before closure of the physis.
    d) malignant tumors of the epiphysis of pediatric patients.

86. Buttressing by periosteal new bone is a feature common to:

    a) periosteal chondroma and aneurysmal bone cyst.
    b) osteoblastoma and osteochondroma.
    c) osteochondroma and solitary enchondroma.
    d) chondroblastoma and osteochondroma.

87. Osteoid osteoma can be differentiated from a bone island because the former:

    a) protrudes from the bone surface and is found mostly in the skull.
    b) is usually polyostotic and is usually painful.
    c) has a central nidus within a sclerotic area and is usually painful.
    d) is usually lucent, and is often found in the skull.

88. Osteitis deformans may be a painless condition, but may be discovered because of:

    a) associated respiratory symptoms.
    b) associated renal symptoms.
    c) increasing hat or shoe size.
    d) increasingly rigid back with loss of lordotic lumbar curve.

89. Trevor's disease strongly resembles an osteochondroma, except that:

    a) it has no cartilage cap.
    b) it occurs at the epiphysis.
    c) it points toward the joint.
    d) it has no pedunculated stalk.

90. The thin, irregular, scalloped and attenuated ribs seen in neurofibromatosis are described as having:

    a) a paddle rib appearance.
    b) bifurcated appearance.
    c) indurated appearance.
    d) twisted ribbon appearance.

91. The monostotic form of fibrous dysplasia:

    a) does not transform to the polyostotic form.
    b) occasionally progresses to the polyostotic form.
    c) frequently progresses to the polyostotic form.
    d) invariably, relentlessly progresses to the polyostotic form.

92. "Blow-out lesions" in the bony pelvis are likely to represent skeletal metastases from:

    a) the prostate.
    b) the thyroid or kidneys.
    c) the lungs.
    d) the breast.

93. In patients over 60, fibrosarcoma is most frequently found:

    a) in the ilium.
    b) in the spine.
    c) in the facial bones.
    d) in the femur.

94. The treatment of choice for primary central osteosarcoma (before metastasis) is:

    a) irradiation.
    b) chemotherapy.
    c) wide en bloc excision followed by irradiation.
    d) amputation.

95. Aneurysmal bone cysts in long bones:

    a) may extend into subarticular bone after closure of the physis.
    b) typically extend across the open growth plate into the epiphysis.
    c) are typically central lesions, symmetrically expanding the metaphysis until the cortex ruptures.
    d) are typically eccentric, thinning and expanding the cortex, and creating an "onion skin" periosteal response.

96. Chondroblastoma is most often located:

    a) in the medullary cavity of the epiphyseal region of a long tubular bone.
    b) in the medullary cavity of the metaphysis of a long tubular bone.
    c) in the cortex of the metaphysis of a long tubular bone.
    d) in the cortex of the epiphyseal region (before closure) of a long tubular bone.

97. Bone islands do not occur:

    a) in pediatric patients.
    b) in the ribs.
    c) distal to the knees or elbows.
    d) in the skull.

98. Paget's disease is a polyostotic disorder that affects any bone, but is least often found in:

    a) the atlas and axis.
    b) the fibula.
    c) the clavicle.
    d) the carpus.

99. Osteochondroma in a long bone occurs at the:

    a) epiphysis.
    b) physis.
    c) metaphysis.
    d) diaphysis.

100. Osteomas originate in:

    a) cortical bone.
    b) cancellous bone.
    c) both cortical and cancellous bone.
    d) periosteum.

PRACTICE TEST CHAPTER 6—ANSWER KEY

1.	c	11.	d	21.	b	31.	d	41.	d	51.	c	61.	a	71.	a	81.	a	91.	a
2.	d	12.	b	22.	d	32.	b	42.	c	52.	c	62.	c	72.	d	82.	b	92.	b
3.	c	13.	a	23.	c	33.	c	43.	b	53.	a	63.	b	73.	b	83.	c	93.	a
4.	b	14.	a	24.	b	34.	b	44.	d	54.	c	64.	d	74.	b	84.	a	94.	d
5.	d	15.	b	25.	c	35.	d	45.	d	55.	c	65.	d	75.	c	85.	a	95.	a
6.	b	16.	a	26.	a	36.	c	46.	c	56.	a	66.	c	76.	b	86.	a	96.	a
7.	c	17.	a	27.	d	37.	c	47.	c	57.	d	67.	b	77.	a	87.	c	97.	d
8.	c	18.	d	28.	d	38.	a	48.	b	58.	b	68.	b	78.	d	88.	c	98.	b
9.	d	19.	d	29.	c	39.	d	49.	d	59.	c	69.	c	79.	b	89.	b	99.	c
10.	b	20.	b	30.	c	40.	c	50.	b	60.	b	70.	b	80.	c	90.	d	100.	c

Chapter 7

INFECTIONS
HEMATOLOGIC OR VASCULAR
CONDITIONS

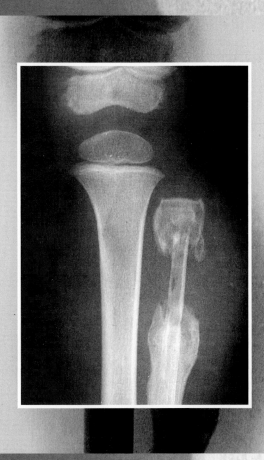

A. INFECTIONS IN BONE

1. Suppurative Osteomyelitis

a) General considerations

- nature of lesions
    1) skeletal sepsis
    2) 90% *Staphylococcus aureus*
    3) weakened bone: predisposed to pathologic fracture
    4) infection extended into joint: septic arthritis
    5) pyemic abscess or focal cellulitis: distant sites seeded through hematogenous spread
    6) *Brodie's abscess*
        - local, aborted form of suppurative osteomyelitis
        - mimics osteoid osteoma: localized limb pain, worse at night, dramatically relieved by aspirin
        - history of recent infection or surgery (often dental)
        - most common in male children
        - usually in metaphyses of tubular bones; occasionally in diaphyses of tubular bones or in flat bones
        - sites in decreasing order of incidence: distal tibia, proximal tibia, distal femur, proximal or distal fibula, distal radius
        - abscess walled off by inflammatory granulation tissue within bone cavity; sclerosis of adjacent spongiosa
        - cavity filled with necrotic debris, purulent or mucoid fluid; may be sterile or contain infectious agent (usually *Staphylococcus aureus*)
        - treated by surgical decompression and curettage
    7) *Garré's sclerosing osteomyelitis*
        - chronic, low-grade, diffuse, nonpurulent osteomyelitis
        - pathogens absent when cultured
        - usually in long tubular bones
        - exuberant fusiform thickening of bone; usually cortical lesions with significant reactive new bone formation
        - no bone destruction, no sequestrum
        - moderate nocturnal pain
    8) chronic osteomyelitis
        - unresolved infection
        - most commonly in tibia, but can occur in any bone
        - sclerosis, cortical thickening, laminated or solid periosteal new

bone, areas of destruction and dense sequestra
- affects long portion of bone; into diaphysis

- incidence
  1) incidence greatly reduced by antibiotics
  2) most patients 2–12 years old; male predilection (3:1)
  3) suppurative spondylitis mostly in patients 40–60 years old; male predilection
  4) immunosuppressed patients more vulnerable to *Hemophilus influenzae, Diplococcus pneumoniae, Mycobacteria, Pseudomonas,* fungal infection, gram-negative organisms
  5) immunosuppressed patients: newborns, alcoholics, AIDS patients, drug abusers, those on corticosteroid therapy
- etiology: four major routes of invasion
  1) hematogenous spread of infection (most common route)
  2) contiguous spread from sinuses, cutaneous or dental primary sites
  3) direct implantation via puncture wounds, penetrating injuries (common in feet), or open fractures; IV drug use (*mainliners' syndrome: Pseudomonas*)
  4) postoperative infection from contaminated surgical sites
- location
  1) extremities: usually metaphyseal; may disseminate to epiphysis or diaphysis; medullary lesions, which may erode cortex
  2) most common in large tubular bones: femur most often affected, then tibia, humerus, radius, and (rarely) clavicle
  3) soft tissues often involved before osseous lesions appear
  4) spine: initial site in children, disc; in adults, anterior vertebral endplate
  5) 2–4% involve the spine; lumbar most often, then thoracic; cervical least often
  6) with *"mainliners' syndrome"*— predilection for axial skeleton's "**S**" joints: **s**pine (often cervical), **s**acroiliac, **s**ymphysis pubis, **s**ternoclavicular joints
- treatment
  1) antibiotic therapy: prevents necrosis, if diagnosed early enough
  2) with significant bone destruction:

surgical drainage and debridement
of sequestered fragments

☞
b) Clinical presentation
- presentation varies significantly with age
of patients
  1) infants and young patients
     - acute process
     - fever, chills, local pain and
swelling
     - often significant loss of limb
function
  2) adult patients
     - process more chronic and
insidious
     - fever, malaise, edema, local
erythema and pain
     - in about 50%: history of previous
infection in skin, respiratory tract,
genito-urinary tract or other
organ system
- spinal infections
  1) history of furunculosis, urinary or
upper respiratory tract infection
  2) recent surgery or instrumentation
(catheterization, cystoscopy)
  3) local tenderness, decreased range of
motion
  4) fever (rare)
- patients with "mainliners' syndrome"
  1) intravenous drug users
  2) diabetics
  3) steroid immunosuppressed patients
  4) hemodialysis patients
  5) culture *Pseudomonas*; sometimes
Aerobacter or *Klebsiella*

☞
c) Pathologic features and laboratory findings
- bone vulnerable to hematogenous spread
of osteomyelitis (Fig. 7.1)
  1) infant bone: first year, vessels
penetrate physis, permit
hematogenous seeding of infectious
agent into epiphysis and joint
  2) physis (growth plate): effective
barrier against hematogenous spread
after first year

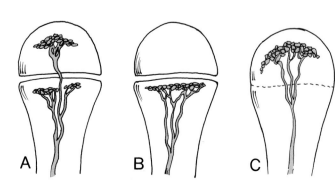

Figure 7.1.

*Blood supply to epiphysis in infant (**A**),
child (**B**), and adult (**C**).*

3) growth plate closure: revascularized subarticular bone again vulnerable to hematogenous seeding
- infectious organism implants in medullary bone
- vascular and cellular reaction: localized suppurative edema
- edema increases intramedullary pressure: capillaries and sinusoids compressed in marrow cavity
- compression: infarction of marrow fat, hematopoietic tissue, and bone
- adjacent to infarction: inflammatory exudate, hyperemia, increased osteoclastic activity
- result is focal osteolysis, regional osteoporosis
- inflammation penetrates endosteum, enters Haversian and lacunar systems, reaches subperiosteal space
- exuberant periostitis (especially in infants, who have fewer Sharpey's fibers to anchor periosteum to bone)
- interruption of blood supply to cortex: necrosis
- *sequestrum* formation: dead bone from medullary and cortical infarcts "set apart" from normal bone (osteoclasts remove smaller sequestered fragments, but larger fragments may require surgical removal)
- pus lifts periosteum: pain and new-bone formation
- *involucrum*: periosteal new bone collar formed around infection (walls it off)
- *cloaca*: defect in the involucrum through which inflammatory products drain; most commonly seen in chronic, antibiotic-resistant osteomyelitis
- *empyema necessitatis*: discharge (decompression) of inflammatory products via cloaca
- *Marjolin's ulcer*: development of squamous cell carcinoma within a cloaca
  1) in chronic osteomyelitis, usually after 20–30 years of chronic infection
  2) most common in femur or tibia
- "pin tract" osteomyelitis may entail a *ring sequestrum*
- culture: usually (90% of cases) *Staphylococcus aureus*
- spinal lesions also caused by: gram-positive *Streptococcus*, Pneumococcus; gram-negative *Escherichia coli*, *Pseudomonas*, *Salmonella*, *Klebsiella*, *Corynebacterium*
- various varieties of *Brucella* (brucellosis): infect spine and sacroiliac joints
- elevated white cell count, Schilling shift to the left, elevated ESR and CRP

- spinal infection: white cell count may be normal; minimally elevated

d) Radiologic features
- radiographic latent period (no signs visible on plain film)
    1) extremity infections: about 10 days
    2) spinal infections: as much as 3 weeks
    3) nuclear bone scan: positive within a few hours of symptoms
- soft tissue radiologic signs
    1) earliest visible signs; within three days of infection
    2) deep soft tissue swelling (around metaphysis in infants and children)
    3) elevation of adjacent fat pad or fat stripe
    4) obliteration of myofascial margins
    5) harder to detect in adults, until swelling creates soft tissue mass
- bone destruction in extremities
    1) *moth-eaten* or *permeative* patterns of bone destruction
    2) first usually focal metaphyseal lesion; disseminates to epiphysis or diaphysis
    3) during first year of life, or after physis closure: may penetrate to subarticular bone; invade joint
    4) over time: osteopenic, moth-eaten lesion with sclerotic rim and sclerotic sequestrum
    5) cortical disruption
- periosteal response
    1) laminated (*lamellar*) pattern of periosteal new bone formation: common in infants and children
    2) Codman's triangle (occasionally)
    3) new bone production: may create large *involucrum* (less dense than *sequestrum*); eventually remodeled and resorbed
- spinal lesions
    1) children and adolescents
        - still have vascular channels to the disc
        - disc infection causes visible signs
            a. disc narrowing
            b. paraspinal edema (abscess formation)
            c. endplate destruction
            d. patchy lytic destruction throughout vertebral body
    2) adult patients
        - vascular channels into vertebral endplate, but disc is avascular
        - infection usually in anterior subchondral endplate

- localized area of lucency and irregularity just beneath endplate
- vertebral destruction progresses, collapse ensues
- paravertebral swelling: widened retropharyngeal, retrotracheal space; displaced paraspinal lines; lumbar paravertebral or psoas abscess
- MR detects epidural abscess
- infection involves disc secondarily
- late in process: possible osseous ankylosis

- *Brucella* spondylitis (various presentations on plain film)
  1) diminished disc height; destruction of vertebral endplate
  2) anterior discovertebral erosions (like Schmorl's nodes) with normal disc
  3) "*ivory vertebra*," peripheral *vacuum phenomenon*, anterior osteophytes
  4) most common in lower lumbar spine
- sacroiliac involvement (common with brucellosis infection)
  1) loss of articular cortex
  2) subchondral erosions
  3) reactive sclerosis

    e) Differential considerations
- periosteal response: may simulate primary malignant neoplasm; traumatic periostitis
- sacroiliac lesions: simulate inflammatory sacroiliitis (e.g., Reiter's syndrome, psoriatic arthritis)

2. Childhood Inflammatory Discitis (synonyms: nonspecific spondylitis, discitis, spondyloarthritis, childhood intervertebral disc infection)

    a) General considerations
- nature of lesion
  1) entity distinct from vertebral osteomyelitis
  2) infectious etiology assumed; organisms may not be isolated
  3) often follows upper respiratory infection, subsequent head or neck infections
  4) traumatic fragmentation of cartilaginous endplate: possible contributing factor
- incidence
  1) ages 1–16 years
  2) male predilection
- location
  1) 75% in lumbar spine
  2) may be thoracic; rarely cervical
- treatment: antibiotic therapy

b) Clinical presentation
- low-grade fever, anorexia, malaise, irritability
- little child may refuse to walk, stand, or sit
- older child complains of back and hip pain

c) Pathologic features and laboratory findings
- hematogenous spread to disc from previous infection site
- infection destroys disc; fragments and destroys adjacent endplate
- elevated ESR; normal leukocyte count
- possible *Staphylococcus aureus* culture

d) Radiologic features
- latent period: 3–4 weeks after symptom onset
- bone scan: most sensitive modality early in process
- first radiologic sign: disc space narrowing
- subchondral endplate fragmentation and destruction
- reactive subchondral endplate sclerosis
- posterior elements spared
- occasional mild spinal flexion deformity
- rarely results in ankylosis

☞ **3. Septic Arthritis**

a) General considerations
- nature of lesion
  1) usually bloodborne pathogens from distant infection; direct implantation
  2) secondary septic arthritis: complicates joint replacement surgery
  3) *Tom Smith's arthritis*
     - septic arthritis in bones in which the metaphysis is enclosed within the adjacent joint capsule
     - predisposed to rapid development of septic arthritis: ruptures metaphyseal cortex, entering joint; spreading via synovial fluid to epiphyseal or subarticular bone
     - affects proximal and distal femur, distal tibia, proximal and distal humerus (hip, knee, ankle, shoulder and elbow)
- incidence
  1) any age patient, but most common < 30 years
  2) no gender predilection
  3) factors influencing incidence and site
     - age of patient
     - specific pathogen involved
     - host resistance

- location
    1) most frequently affected joints: knee and hip
    2) less often: shoulder, hand, foot, ankle
    3) treatment: antibiotic therapy, preferably very early in the process

b) Clinical presentation
- severe, localized articular pain and capsular edema
- restricted range of motion
- erythema, acute fever, sometimes with chills
- altered gait (when weight-bearing joint is infected)

c) Pathologic features
- infectious organisms in vasculature of synovial membrane
- infected synovial membrane contaminates synovial fluid
- purulent exudate distends capsule: increased pressure leads to chondrocyte necrosis
- disintegration of acute inflammatory cells and cartilage cells: releases proteolytic enzymes, destroying articular surface
- if process continues: possible dislocation (especially common in newborn hip; occurs in adult hips too)
- use of affected joint: total loss of articular space
- subchondral bone penetrated, articular cortex destroyed
- possible bony or fibrous ankylosis
- intraarticular or juxtaarticular gas
    1) forms if infectious agent causes gas production
    2) e.g., *Escherichia coli* or *Clostridium perfringens*

d) Laboratory findings
- elevated ESR
- leukocytosis with shift to the left
- positive blood or joint fluid cultures to identify infectious agent
    1) *Staphylococcus aureus*: most common agent
    2) *Hemophilus*
    3) alpha and beta hemolytic Streptococci
    4) Gonococcus
    5) *Escherichia coli*
    6) *Salmonella*
    7) Pneumococcus
    8) *Brucella*
    9) *Serratia*
    10) *Nocardia*

11) *Clostridium perfringens*
12) mycobacterial or fungal pathogens

e) Radiologic features
- earliest diagnosis: nuclear bone scan (1 to 2 days after symptoms appear)
- soft tissue signs on plain film
    1) capsular distension, displacing juxtaarticular fat
        - in hip: displaced fat folds for obturator internus, psoas major, and gluteus medius
        - *Waldenstrom's sign*
            - joint effusion (from any cause) increases distance between the lateral margin of Kohler's teardrop and the medial margin of the femoral head
            - measurement should be close to equal on left and right, with < 2 mm difference between them
    2) rapid loss of joint space (totally obliterated within a few weeks) due to cartilage destruction
- bone alterations on plain film
    1) loss of *subarticular white line*:
        - earliest skeletal sign
        - loss of normal subchondral cortical bone
    2) metaphyseal medullary moth-eaten destruction (progressing to complete resorption of articulating ends of bones)
    3) laminated extracapsular periosteal response (with cortical disruption)
    4) possible bony or fibrous ankylosis
    5) after resolution of infection: articular surface remodeled but deformed: articular spacing not restored

REVIEW—STUDY QUESTIONS

1. What is the most common causative agent of suppurative osteomyelitis?
2. What are the presenting symptoms and radiologic features of childhood inflammatory discitis?
3. In suppurative osteomyelitis, subarticular involvement depends on the age of the patient. Explain why.
4. What is "Tom Smith's arthritis?"
5. What diagnostic modality provides the earliest detection of septic arthritis?
6. What three factors determine patient and site vulnerability to septic arthritis?

7. What is the earliest radiologic skeletal sign of septic arthritis?

8. Describe the clinical presentation of Brodie's abscess. What entity does this mimic?

9. What is "Marjolin's ulcer?"

10. Explain the four major routes of invasion for suppurative osteomyelitis.

☞   **4. Nonsuppurative Osteomyelitis (Tuberculosis) (TB)**

   a)   **General considerations**
      •   nature of lesions
         1)   hematogenous spread into bone from primary respiratory tract infection
         2)   recent resurgence of antibiotic-resistant strains
         3)   respiratory infection primarily due to *Mycobacterium tuberculosis*
         4)   ingested form (*Mycobacterium bovis*) now mostly eradicated in United States
      •   incidence
         1)   leading cause of death in western countries 100 years ago
         2)   almost eradicated during this century, now increasing because of immigration patterns and socioeconomic conditions
         3)   most frequently affects young children (70% are < 5), immunodeficient patients
         4)   spinal tuberculosis: most patients < 30 years old
         5)   tubercular arthritis more likely in middle-aged and elderly
         6)   no gender predilection
      •   location
         1)   infection in spine: tubercular spondylitis (*Pott's disease*): lumbar, thoracic, cervical
         2)   infection in appendicular skeleton (tubercular arthritis): hip, knee, (most often); ankle, shoulder, elbow, pubes, wrist
         3)   *caries sicca* (archaic term, not in current usage)
            •   TB in shoulder joint
            •   destruction of humeral head: multiple large, erosive lesions
            •   small surface contact area for articular cartilage: destruction particularly widespread
         4)   *cystic tuberculosis*
            •   rare form of appendicular TB in diaphyses or metaphyses of long bones, or even in flat bones

- simultaneous appearance of
  multiple, symmetric, well-defined,
  round, or oval lytic lesions
- untreated: becomes aggressive;
  expansile; may generate
  laminated periosteal response
- rarely involves joints

5) *tuberculous dactylitis*
- in small tubular hand and foot
  bones
- most patients < 5 years old
- usually monostotic, with
  consecutive formation of multiple
  lesions
- about 25% have multiple
  simultaneous lesions
- diffuse soft tissue swelling, bone
  expansion with thinned cortex
- described as *spina ventosa*
  (inflated or air-filled thorn)
- very rarely affects joints

6) *Pott's puffy tumor*
- in calvarium
- solitary tubercular focus
- *button sequestrum* with fluctuant
  cold abscess in the scalp

7) tuberculous bursitis (*Weaver's
  bottom*)
- tuberculous infection in
  subgluteal bursae
- synovial membranes of any
  bursae can be infected
- predilection for greater trochanter
  of femur
  a. osseous destruction
  b. with dormancy of infection,
     moderate calcification
     appears around deformed
     trochanter

- treatment
  1) chemotherapy: isoniazid, ethambutol,
     rifampicin
  2) skeletal lesions subject to
     debridement and arthrodesis

b) Clinical presentation
- insidious onset, chronic progression
- spondylitis
  1) insidious onset of back pain,
     decreased range of motion, focal
     tenderness
  2) possible neurologic signs
  3) sudden lower limb paraplegia (*Pott's
     paraplegia*)
  4) advanced disease: pus-draining sinus
     tract
- appendicular
  1) initially mild joint pain, stiffness

2) tenderness, soft tissue swelling, joint effusion, local heat

3) with progression: muscle contractures markedly limit range of motion

4) eventual muscle atrophy, deformity

5) often limp (hip and knee are most common sites)

c) Pathologic features

- *Pott's disease* (*tubercular spondylitis*)

  1) thoracolumbar area most often affected (usually L1)

  2) believed to be disseminated via Batson's venous plexus

  3) implant in anterior subchondral vertebral endplate

  4) caseous necrosis (visible on film in 2–5 months)

  5) weakened endplate: spread of infection to disc

  6) collapsed vertebra: infection transferred to disc by direct extension (in herniated material)

  7) rarely extends into posterior arch (about 2% of cases)

  8) disc height diminishes

  9) paravertebral abscess formation

     - cervical spine: retropharyngeal or retrotracheal abscess

     - thoracic spine: large, bilateral, anterolateral abscesses

     - lumbar spine: psoas abscess—slow-growing, necrotizing abscess (unilateral or bilateral)

     - *empyema necessitatis*

       a. draining sinus from abscess

       b. may surface paraspinally, in inguinal area, or near lesser trochanter (near psoas insertion)

     - abscess: collection of caseous necrotic debris

     - if uncontaminated: may calcify in dense, *snowflake pattern*

  10) subligamentous dissection

      - rare: massive, extensive paraspinal abscess, with little osseous disease

      - between vertebral body and anterior longitudinal ligament

      - disc space initially spared, infection spreads to contiguous segments

      - anterior vertebral body sustains *gouge defects* (shallow cortical erosions)

- eventual disc narrowing, vertebral collapse
- *Pott's paraplegia* (rare)
  1) collapse of multiple vertebrae
  2) infectious disc deterioration
  3) granulation tissue along with osseous debris (sequestra): protrude into spinal canal
  4) mass pressure: paraplegia
  5) neural arch involvement: dura invested with granulation tissue and/ or pressure from liquid abscesses, causing mechanical compression
- tubercular arthritis
  1) usually monoarticular
  2) organism lodged in synovium or in metaphyseal medullary bone
  3) usually start in metaphysis, secondary spread to joint
  4) significant joint effusion early in process
  5) thickened synovium; granulation tissue formed over articular cartilage
  6) cartilage destroyed, cortical bone eroded
  7) initial cortical erosions: in "bare area," similar to process in RA
  8) both joint surfaces eroded: sequestra form (*kissing sequestrum*)
  9) hypervascular inflammation: hyperemic osteoporosis

d) Laboratory findings
- joint aspirates, tissue exudates, or tissue specimens cultured
- *Mycobacterium tuberculosis*: most often identified agent

e) Radiologic features
- tubercular spondylitis
  1) 21-day latent period before plain film can detect bone lesions
  2) earliest sign: lytic destruction in anterior corner of endplate; some loss of disc space
  3) AP projection: can show abscess formation
     - thoracic sites: dense paraspinal mass overlying lucent lung
     - thoracolumbar sites: soft tissue swelling into psoas shadow, often around a focus of vertebral destruction; opaque mass often pear-shaped, frequently calcified
  4) vertebral collapse and loss of disc space
  5) *gibbus deformity*: acutely angulated flexion deformity, usually thoracic

6) *long vertebra*: young patients with open growth plates
   - long-standing gibbus deformity
   - vertical elongation of subadjacent vertebral body (reaction to chronic infection)
   - occurs without infection in quadriplegic patients—known there as a *tall vertebra*

- tubercular arthritis
  1) early signs: joint widening (secondary to joint effusion) and soft tissue swelling
  2) subchondral cortical destruction
  3) moth-eaten bone destruction, often on both sides of joint
  4) juxtaarticular osteoporosis (caused by hyperemia and disuse atrophy)
  5) later, joint space narrowing as cartilage and bone destruction progresses
  6) "*Phemister's triad*"
     - slowly progressive joint space narrowing
     - juxtaarticular osteoporosis
     - peripheral erosive defects of articular cortex (bare areas show erosion similar to RA)
  7) solid or laminated periostitis (rare)
  8) end stage: fibrous ankylosis
  9) "*megacondyle*": focal overgrowth of medial epiphysis at knee caused by hyperemia (more consistently seen with JRA or hemophilia)

- sacroiliac tuberculosis
  1) usually unilateral
  2) "pseudowidening" of sacroiliac joint
  3) early lytic lesions
  4) eventual ankylosis

f) Differential considerations
- pyogenic spondylitis
  1) rapid onset of acute pain
  2) swift progression
  3) frequently with sequestrum, sinus formation, periosteal response
  4) rarely features abscess or sinus formation
  5) causes moderate osteoporosis
  6) bony ankylosis if not treated
- gouge defects in anterior vertebral bodies
  1) suggest aneurysm
  2) simulate lymph node erosion (metastasis, lymphoma, myeloma)
- peripheral erosions in appendicular articulations: simulate rheumatoid arthritis

- megacondyle: seen with Still's disease, hemophilia
- unilateral sacroiliac lesions: psoriatic arthropathy, Reiter's syndrome, or rheumatoid arthritis

☞ **5. HIV (Human Immunodeficiency Virus) Infection**

a) General considerations
- nature of disease entity
  1) deficiency of T lymphocytes (especially T helper cells)
  2) may progress to acquired immune deficiency syndrome (AIDS)
  3) reduces resistance to protozoan infections, fungal infections, bacterial infections, viral infections, helminthic infections, cancer
- incidence
  1) population at risk
     - those with multiple sexual partners
     - intravenous drug users
     - blood transfusion recipients
     - those who come into contact with body fluids
- nature of lesions
  1) with advanced disease, lesions common to various entities appear:
     - infections
     - lymphoma
     - anemia
     - Kaposi sarcoma
     - polymyositis
     - arthritis
  2) soft tissue lesions more common than skeletal lesions characteristic of their specific disorder, such as:
     - osteomyelitis
     - tuberculosis involving peripheral joints
     - lymphoma (non-Hodgkin's particularly prevalent with AIDS)
     - anemia
     - Kaposi sarcoma
     - erosive arthropathy (with exacerbated Reiter's syndrome or psoriatic arthropathy)
- treatment
  1) treatment for HIV/AIDS itself, experimental
  2) other treatment depends on infection or disease entity

6. Syphilitic Osteomyelitis
(synonyms: syphilis, lues)

a) General characteristics
- nature of lesions

1) angiitis (or endarteritis) of vasa vasorum (small arterioles)
2) skeletal syphilis: congenital or acquired
3) neurotrophic arthropathy: common sequela caused by traumatic joint degeneration (not syphilitic invasion of the joint)

- incidence
  1) recent resurgence in the United States
  2) congenital syphilis transmitted via placenta, from mother to child
     - usually in fifth or sixth month of gestation
     - untreated: 25% die in utero, 25–30% die shortly after birth
     - infection usually persists into second year of life
  3) acquired syphilis: sexually transmitted disease (STD)
- location of lesions
  1) congenital syphilis: metaphyses of upper and lower extremity long bones, sometimes the teeth
  2) acquired syphilis: skeletal lesions in skull, tibiae, and clavicles, occasionally other sites (< 10% of patients develop skeletal lesions)
- treatment
  1) penicillin therapy
  2) primary and secondary syphilis: counseling; to avoid sexual contact, minimize disease spread

b) Clinical presentation
- congenital syphilis
  1) 40% of surviving infants develop late symptomatic syphilis
  2) in older children: bilateral, painless joint swellings
     - *Clutton's joints*: sometimes are warm and painful
     - *Hutchinson's teeth*: peg-shaped, hypoplastic, and notched
- acquired syphilis
  1) presentations vary; disease relatively rare, may be missed
  2) primary lesion: "*chancre*"—painless genital ulcer
  3) secondary lesions include
     - cutaneous rash
     - enlarged lymph nodes
     - uveitis
     - periostitis and joint pain
     - glomerulonephritis, liver and spleen involvement
     - malaise, headache, anorexia,

nausea, aching bones, fatigability, fever, anemia, jaundice, neck stiffness
- acute syphilitic meningitis may develop
- *condyloma lata*: infectious papules at mucocutaneous junctions
- *alopecia areata*: patchy hair loss

4) latent syphilis
- during first 2 years after infection: recurring infectious mucocutaneous papules
- later latent period completely asymptomatic, often permanently

5) tertiary syphilis
- stage when skeletal involvement occurs
- "*benign tertiary syphilis*": characteristic lesion is a *gumma*—chronic granulomatous reaction leading to necrosis and fibrosis
- bone involvement: deep, boring pain; worse at night
- palpable or visible swelling or lump at superficial bone sites
- *cardiovascular syphilis*: dilated aneurysm of the ascending aorta, narrowed coronary ostia, or aortic valve insufficiency
- *meningovascular neurosyphilis*: headaches, dizziness, poor concentration, lassitude, insomnia, neck stiffness, blurred vision, mental confusion, epileptic seizures, papilledema, aphasia, hemiplegia or monoplegia; cranial nerve palsies, "*Argyll Robertson pupil*"
- *parenchymatous neurosyphilis*: gradual behavior changes, convulsions, aphasia, transient hemiparesis; irritability, loss of concentration, loss of memory, defective judgment, headaches, insomnia, lethargy, emotional instability, asthenia, depression, delusions of grandeur; tremors of mouth, tongue, hands, body; dysarthria; brisk DTRs; *tabes dorsalis* gives pain, ataxia, sensory changes and loss of DTRs

c) **Pathologic features**
- *Treponema pallidum* spirochete disseminated via lymph and blood systems, lodged in smaller vessels: *endarteritis obliterans*
- metaphysitis: spirochetes beneath fetal growth plates

1) granulation tissue replaces vessels beneath cartilage
2) bone formation in zone of primary ossification prevented

- gummatous ulcerations and necrosis in cutaneous, subcutaneous tissue
- granulation tissue infiltrates bone, periosteum
- periosteal response: thickens cortices, alters bone contours

☞   **d) Laboratory findings**
- VDRL: venereal disease research laboratory serologic test (screening)
- RPR: rapid plasma reagin serologic test
- FTA-ABS: fluorescent treponemal antibody absorption test (specific)
- CSF: cerebral spinal fluid examined to exclude neurosyphilis
- secretions may be examined under darkfield microscope
- *Treponema pallidum* may be cultured or diagnosed on a "Pap smear"

☞   **e) Radiologic findings**
- congenital syphilis
  1) metaphysitis (Phase 1)
     - broad, horizontal, lucent metaphyseal bands
     - *"saw-toothed appearance"*: metaphyseal fragmentation, infractions
     - changes at growth plate junction, usually bilateral and symmetrical
     - may cause epiphyseal separation; do not affect epiphysis itself
     - *"Wimberger's sign"*: symmetrical erosive defects in medial surfaces of proximal tibiae
     - knees, shoulders, wrists most commonly affected
  2) periostitis (Phase 2)
     - solid or laminated reaction
     - diffuse, symmetrical response on nearly all major long bones
  3) osteitis (Phase 3)
     - granulation tissue from metaphysis to diaphysis
     - reactive sclerosis around lytic lesions, with long bone periostitis
     - periostitis with cortical overgrowth: undulating, dense cortex
     - *"saber shin"*: frequently bilateral, anterior bowing of tibiae
     - lytic defects (*gummata*) scattered throughout the bone
- acquired syphilis
  1) most common sign: proliferative

periostitis—diffuse thickening of cortices (both inner and outer cortices)

2) usually solid or laminated periostitis; sometimes "*lacelike*" aggressive periostitis

3) "*saber shin*" (in syphilis): thickened cortex, not true bowing—medullary cavity still vertical, not bowed

4) cortical or medullary lytic "*gummata*" with sclerotic margins

5) skull: usually outer table of frontal bone destroyed by lytic *gummata*

f) Differential considerations

- syphilis: one of the "*great imitators*" of disease

- syphilitic skin rashes simulate a variety of skin conditions: marked and symmetric on flexor and volar surfaces—especially palms and soles

- metaphysitis of congenital syphilis simulates leukemia, metastatic lesions of neuroblastoma, or scurvy

7. Mycotic Osteomyelitis

a) General considerations

- nature of lesions

    1) fungal skeletal infections usually secondary to primary respiratory system infection, or soft tissue focal infection

    3) bone affected by *Coccidioides, Actinomyces israelii* or *Actinomyces bovis* (actually bacteria, not fungi), *Monosporium apiospermum, Monosporium mycetoma, Nocardia madurae, Nocardia brasiliensis, Candida, Aspergillus, Histoplasma, Cryptococcus torula, Blastomyces, Sporothrix, Phycomyces mucor, Phycomyces rhizopus*

    4) *Coccidioides immitis* infections secondary to respiratory infection

    5) bacteria *Actinomyces*: considered and treated as fungi; present in mouth, nose, and bowel of normal individuals

        - cervicofacial infections (most common)

        - pulmonary infections (about 15% of cases)

        - rare abdominal infections (ileocecal area)

    6) "*Madura foot*" caused by soil fungi, chronic granulomatous fungal disease

- incidence

    1) coccidioidomycosis: endemic in southwest United States (San

Joaquin Valley of southern California, southern Arizona, New Mexico)

   2) actinomycosis: high incidence of face and neck infections

   3) maduromycosis: worldwide, most common skeletal fungal infection
- most common in tropics
- usually in men aged 21–40 years
- highest incidence in India
- in United States, agent is *Monosporium apiospermum*
- elsewhere, agents are *Nocardia madurae* and *Nocardia brasiliensis*

- location of skeletal lesions
   1) coccidioidomycosis
- about 20% of cases involve bone
- most common sites: spine, pelvis, ribs, long bones (any bone may be infected)
- bony prominences predilected: tibial tubercle, malleoli, medial clavicle, trochanters, acromion, patella, calcaneus, olecranon
- multiple vertebral bodies, pedicles, laminae and adjacent ribs

   2) actinomycosis
- most commonly in mandible (often at angle of mandible)
- also attacks spine, ribs, pelvis
- thoracic and lumbar spine
- multiple vertebrae: vertebral bodies, neural arch and contiguous ribs

   3) maduromycosis
- tarsometatarsal region most commonly infected
- advanced cases spread to infect all bones of foot
- hand, wrist, arm or leg bones rarely involved

- treatment: pharmaceuticals, excision, or amputation

b) Clinical presentation

- coccidioidomycosis
   1) first stage of disease—respiratory infection: asymptomatic, mild, or acute bronchitis with pleural effusion; or pneumonia
   2) fever, cough, chest pain, chills, sputum production, sore throat, hemoptysis
   3) after dissemination, may mimic tuberculosis: infections in liver, spleen, lymph nodes, skin, kidneys, bone, and meninges

4) *"desert rheumatism"*: conjunctivitis, arthritis, erythema nodosum

5) most often, indolent respiratory infection, low grade, self-limiting

6) aggressive dissemination may be fatal

- actinomycosis
  1) most commonly: recent oral surgery, tooth extraction or socket infection
  2) long-standing soft tissue infection may precede extension into bone
- maduromycosis
  1) bone involvement usually after long-standing soft tissue swelling
  2) visible tumefaction and draining sinuses

c) Pathologic features and laboratory findings
- coccidioidomycosis
  1) fungus spores in dust inhaled
  2) inflammatory consolidation in terminal bronchioles (primary phase)
  3) dissemination phase (secondary phase) follows bronchial ulceration
  4) aspiration of infected exudate from bronchioles; or vascular spread of pathogens
- actinomycosis
  1) resident pathogens (bacteria) in devitalized tissue, or carried into deep tissues via surgical or other penetrating wound
  2) associated factor: poor oral hygiene
  3) direct extension from adjacent soft tissue into bone (e.g., retroperitoneal or mediastinal lymph nodes)
  4) rarely, hematogenous spread
- maduromycosis
  1) direct contact with infested soil
  2) suppurative tissue reaction with microscopic granulomas
- laboratory findings include the identification of causative organisms

d) Radiologic features

- coccidioidomycosis
  1) early: well-defined lytic lesions; laminated periosteal response
  2) later: cortical disruption, sclerosis around lytic lesions
  3) abscess, with draining sinus
  4) rarely joint involvement, but may simulate TB in joints
  5) spinal involvement
     - paraspinal mass (abscess)— often psoas; may calcify
     - lucent lesions: vertebral bodies, neural arch structures, ribs

- disc spaces relatively spared
- multiple vertebrae, but vertebral collapse rare

- actinomycosis
  1) most common: mandibular destruction, often at angle of jaw
  2) lytic lesion, little or no reactive periosteal new bone
  3) spinal involvement: multiple vertebra
     - lytic lesions, occasional sclerosis
     - discs are spared
     - bodies, arches, adjacent ribs involved
     - ribs, vertebral bodies may thicken with periosteal new bone
     - sawtooth outline of vertebral bodies
- maduromycosis
  1) early: poorly defined lytic lesions
  2) later: widespread lytic destruction without clearly-defined margins
  3) bizarre filiform or undulating deformity of bones
  4) fistulae common, but no periosteal new bone formation, and rarely sequestrum
  5) possibly: diffuse intraarticular osseous ankylosis

e) **Differential considerations**
- tuberculous osteomyelitis
  1) psoas abscess of coccidioidomycosis: indistinguishable from that of TB
  2) actinomycosis: small paravertebral abscess, but not calcified
  3) TB: vertebral collapse, loss of disc space; not often present with mycotic osteomyelitis
- neurotrophic arthropathy: destroys tarsal bones, but produces prominent sclerosis (not seen with *Madura foot*)

REVIEW—STUDY QUESTIONS

1. What is the pathogen that causes syphilis, and what is its primary effect in the vascular system?
2. Describe coccidioidomycosis: its pathogen, method of dissemination, effects on the body, and possible prognoses.
3. What is Phemister's triad, and with what disease entity is it associated?
4. What is Pott's' puffy tumor? With what disease entity is it associated?
5. What are the most common locations of paraspinal abscesses? With what disease entities are they associated? Which are most likely to contain calcifications?

6. Describe the radiologic findings of the three phases of congenital syphilis.

7. What is the primary damage done with HIV infection?

8. Describe cystic tuberculosis.

9. Which of the disease entities considered as a mycotic osteomyelitis is really bacterial?

10. Compare and contrast the radiologic features of sacroiliac involvement in suppurative osteomyelitis, tubercular osteomyelitis, ankylosing spondylitis, and Reiter's syndrome.

11. Describe the clinical and radiologic presentation of Madura foot.

12. What are VDRL and FTA-ABS, and with what disease are they associated?

13. What is the most common source of actinomycosis, and where do its infectious lesions most often appear?

14. What are three possible causes of gouge defects in vertebral bodies?

15. What are Clutton's joints?

B. HEMATOLOGIC AND VASCULAR DISORDERS

 1. Sickle Cell Anemia

a) General considerations

- radiologically visible skeletal changes only with severe, chronic anemias
- nature of condition: congenital, hereditary hemolytic anemia
- incidence
    1) almost exclusive to black population and some Mediterranean peoples
    2) homozygous genotype: in up to 3% of black population
    3) sickle cell trait (asymptomatic) in 7–9% of black Americans
- location of lesions
    1) femoral or humeral heads
    2) multiple vertebral bodies
    3) small tubular bones of hands and feet, skull
    4) distal femur and humerus, proximal tibia
    5) diaphyseal destruction in femur, tibia, fibula humerus, radius, ulna
- treatment
    1) prevention and treatment of infections with appropriate antibiotics
    2) hydroxyurea therapy to reduce incidence of pain crisis, increasing hemoglobin content

b) Clinical presentation
- only homozygous individuals symptomatic
- after about 6 months of age, patient develops pallor, weakness
- episodic crises of abdominal pain, jaundice, acute bone pain, dactylitis
- *"hand-foot syndrome"*: bilateral, symmetric, painful swellings of hands and feet (predisposed to sickle-induced infarctions, or to *Salmonella* osteomyelitis)
- hips and shoulders painful—avascular necrosis of humeral or femoral heads (hip prostheses employed, but about 50% fail)
- splenomegaly, later becoming infarcted and filled with fibrosis; may atrophy, leading to autosplenectomy
- cardiomegaly and heart failure
- gallstones caused by hyperbilirubinemia
- painful mesenteric vascular thromboses: *"sickle-cell crisis"*
- renal failure
- homozygous patients rarely live > 30 years

c) Pathologic features and laboratory findings
- erythrocyte sickling caused by abnormal hemoglobin (HbS)
- with local hypoxia, erythrocytes elongate, curve
- increased fragility of red blood cells, increased blood viscosity, increased stasis of flow
- lowered pH
- effort to maintain viable red cell level results in splenomegaly, marrow hyperplasia
- hyperplastic marrow: local ischemia, necrosis
- decrease in trabeculae, thinning of cortices, bone infarcts, growth deformities
- spinal effects: nutrient artery to central endplate obstructed; central endplate growth inhibited, displaces inward
- laboratory tests show normocytic RBCs but in low numbers, and with reduced Hb, elevated serum bilirubin, leukocytosis; "sickle-shaped" erythrocytes

d) Radiologic features
- small tubular bones of hands and feet
    1) earliest radiologic sign of infarction: soft tissue swelling
    2) about 2 weeks later: diaphyseal linear periostitis
    3) rarefaction of involved bone (simulates osteomyelitis)
    4) loss of diaphyseal constriction in medullary cavity

- skull
  1) effects visible only above internal occipital protuberance (marrow-rich area)
  2) widened diploic space
  3) granular texture or (when disease is severe) *"hair-on-end"* trabecular pattern
- long bones
  1) marrow hyperplasia: generalized osteopenia; sparse, coarsened trabeculae; large vascular channels; widened medullary cavity; cortical thinning
  2) chronic endosteal appositional new bone formation: generalized sclerotic pattern of entire skeleton in adult patient
  3) infarction
     - serpiginous medullary infarcts
     - femoral and humeral heads: epiphyseal infarcts
     - femoral head infarcts
       a. 8–20% of cases, often bilaterally
       b. *"crescent sign"*: subchondral fracture of weight-bearing surface of femoral head
       c. *"step defect"*: sharp depression in articular surface
       d. flattened or irregular weight-bearing surface
       e. *"bite sign"*: curvilinear band in superior femoral head
     - bone growth alterations may follow infarcts
       a. cupped metaphyses
       b. shortened bone
       c. tibio-talar slant deformity (when lateral distal tibial epiphysis is affected)
     - protrusio acetabuli (female predilection)
  4) MR: modality of choice for visualizing infarcted areas
  5) late in process, CT will show *"asterisk sign"*: loss of normal starlike pattern of femoral head trabeculae
  6) osteomyelitis
     - *Salmonella* osteomyelitis
       a. frequent complication
       b. 100 times more frequent in sickle-cell patients than in normal population
       c. possible route of entry: via enteric infarcts

- unique presentation: bilateral, symmetric, diaphyseal distribution
- moth-eaten destruction
- periosteal response: solid or laminated
- may occasionally involve spine

7) other overall changes (often widespread, symmetric) in long bones include
- coarsened trabeculae
- patchy medullary sclerosis
- cortical splitting "*bone within a bone appearance*"

- spinal effects
  1) prominent osteoporosis, with accentuation of vertical trabeculae
  2) thinned and prominent cortices
  3) endplate deformities
     - several contiguous vertebrae with identical central depressions in upper and lower endplates "*fish vertebra*" (Fig. 7.2)
     - usually in thoracic or lumbar vertebrae; usually teen-aged patient
  4) vertebral body collapse because of massive infarction, episodic ischemic crises
     - may regain normal vertebral body height
     - visible residual increase in density only remaining sign
  5) midbody anterior vascular notch enlarged
     - seen in children, most notably in thoracolumbar vertebrae

Figure 7.2.

Sickle cell anemia: spinal changes. **A**. Normal circulatory dynamics in a developing vertebral body. **B**. Following thrombosis of the central nutrient vessels, central growth is inhibited, producing the characteristic "H" vertebra. **C**. Initially, the depression is smooth, concave, and shallow. **D**. Later, the configuration becomes more characteristic (arrows).

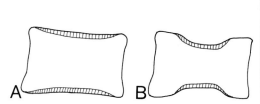

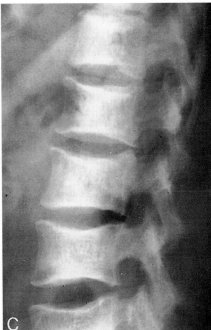

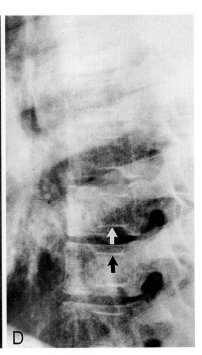

- caused by compensatory marrow hyperplasia
  6) complicating *Salmonella* spondylitis
     - diminished disc height
     - contiguous endplate and vertebral body destruction
     - soft tissue mass (paraspinal abscess)
- mediastinum
  1) intrathoracic extramedullary hematopoiesis (infrequent)
     - lobulated or rounded soft tissue densities
     - in posterior mediastinum at middle and lower thoracic levels
- abdomen
  1) splenic calcifications (30% of homozygous sickle cell patients)
  2) usually punctate, some with diffuse or curvilinear calcifications

e) Differential considerations
- epiphyseal infarcts: identical to idiopathic or posttraumatic ischemic necrosis
- juvenile or adolescent diffuse spinal osteoporosis seen with steroid therapy, also with Cushing's syndrome
- "*fish vertebrae*" with thalassemia and with Gaucher's disease
- intrathoracic extramedullary hematopoiesis much more frequent with thalassemia

2. Thalassemia
(synonyms: Cooley's anemia, Mediterranean anemia)

a) General considerations
- nature of condition
  1) hereditary disorder of hemoglobin synthesis
  2) variable degrees of anemia: most severe is thalassemia major
  3) three general groups: thalassemia major, minor, and intermedia
- incidence
  1) usually in Mediterranean peoples: Greeks, Italians, Turks, Syrians
  2) also in people from India, Philippines, Thailand, and in Native Americans and African Americans
- skeletal sites
  1) involves entire skeleton in infants and children
  2) long bones, skull, spine, ribs, small tubular bones of hands and feet
  3) organs affected: heart, liver, abdominal lymph nodes
- treatment
  1) repeated blood transfusions
  2) consequent hemochromatosis, cardiac failure in teens or twenties at best

b) Clinical presentation
- pallor, lethargy
- retarded growth
- hepatosplenomegaly
- facial features: mongoloid or with maxillary overgrowth "*rodent facies*"
- inhibited sexual development

c) Pathologic features
- thalassemia major: homozygous genotype
- thalassemia minor: heterozygous
- imbalanced globin chain production: ineffective hematopoiesis, hemolysis, anemia
- hypertrophic, hyperactive marrow tissue
- maturation of skeleton: osseous effects of peripheral skeleton **regress** (fatty marrow replaces red marrow); skull, pelvic, spinal lesions progress
- hepatosplenomegaly, posterior mediastinal paraspinal hemopoietic masses (all caused by extramedullary hematopoiesis)
- mediastinal masses: herniation of expanding bone marrow through thinned trabeculae of posterior ribs
- epidural extramedullary hematopoietic masses: cord compression

d) Laboratory findings
- hypochromic, microcytic anemia
- reticulocytosis
- nucleated red blood cells
- target cells
- elevated serum bilirubin

e) Radiologic features
- marrow hyperplasia
  1) osteoporosis with "*honeycomb*" coarse trabecular patterns
  2) enlarged vascular channels
  3) generalized cortical thinning
  4) widened medullary cavity, expanded bone caliber
- growth disturbances
  1) "*Erlenmeyer flask deformity*": diametaphyseal undertubulation because of lack of remodeling within long bones
  2) shortening deformities (especially distal femur, proximal humerus) due to premature fusion of part of the growth plate
  3) growth arrest lines: opaque, transverse bands across metaphyses
- skull changes (above internal occipital protuberance only)
  1) frontal bones earliest and most severely affected
  2) granular osteoporosis
  3) widened diploë

      4) *"hair-on-end"* radiating new-bone spicules
      5) loss of definition of outer table
      6) circumscribed lytic lesions in calvarium (up to 5 cm in diameter)
      7) prominent, enlarged vascular impressions of middle meningeal arteries

- facial bones
  1) frontal, maxillary, sphenoid, and mastoid air cells are not pneumatized
  2) lateral displacement of orbits
  3) *"rodent facies"*: upper incisors displaced forward
- vertebral bodies and neural arches
  1) osteopenia with thinned cortices and coarsened vertical trabecular patterns
  2) slight, generalized endplate concavity
  3) anterior body vascular notch enlargement
  4) growth arrest lines
  5) odontoid hypertrophy
  6) hypotrophic ring apophyses
- changes in sacrum and pelvis
  1) osteopenia
  2) generally thinned cortices
  3) accentuated, coarsened vertical trabecular patterns
- avascular necrosis of femoral heads
- chondrocalcinosis
- hemochromatosis
- fractures
- arthropathy
- soft tissue manifestations
  1) opaque hemosiderin-laden paraspinal lymph nodes
  2) hepatosplenomegaly
  3) cardiomegaly
  4) extramedullary hematopoiesis: posterior mediastinal, bilateral, paraspinal, opaque, lobulated soft tissue masses

  f) Differential considerations
- sickle cell anemia
  1) organized medullary infarcts, rarely seen in thalassemia
  2) vertebral endplates: *"fish vertebrae,"* not found in thalassemia

3. Hemophilia

  a) General considerations
- nature of condition
  1) deficiency of specific clotting factors: blood coagulation disorders
  2) most common varieties
     - hemophilia A—classic hemophilia: lacking factor VIII

- hemophilia B—Christmas disease: lacking factor IX

  3) sex linked, recessive, inherited diseases (carried by females, manifested in males)

- location of lesions

  1) arthropathy most commonly at knee, ankle, elbow

  2) pseudotumors most often affect femur and pelvis

- treatment

  1) prevention of bleeding

     - avoid aspirin (use acetaminophen for analgesia)
     - regular prophylactic dental care to avoid need of dental surgery
     - avoid intramuscular injections: drugs given orally or intravenously
     - vaccination against hepatitis B
     - elevate factor VIII levels in hemophilia A patients before surgeries

  2) replacement therapy

b)   Clinical presentation

- varies with severity of condition
- some almost clinically silent
- some bleed spontaneously, or with very minor injury
- acute and chronic hemarthroses: joint pain, gait changes
- predisposition to joint infection

c)   Pathologic features

- lack of clotting factors: severe, uncontrolled hemorrhage
- repeated hemarthroses: synovial proliferation (pannus) and synovial hemosiderin deposition
- articular adhesions
- progressive fibrosis of subsynovium, capsule, periarticular tissues
- articular cartilage resists degradation, eventually degenerates
- subarticular bone: osteoporotic, develops cysts and epiphyseal overgrowth
- intraosseous or subperiosteal hemorrhage: local resorption, expansion of bone
- reactive periosteal new bone formation

d)   Laboratory findings

- PTT: partial thromboplastin time prolonged
- PT (prothrombin time) and bleeding time: typically normal
- assays of factors VIII and IX: show type and severity of hemophilia

☞

e) Radiologic features

- ischemic necrosis of femoral head (rare)
- bilateral but asymmetric findings of hemophilic arthropathy
- knee (most common site)
    1) femorotibial and patellofemoral joints
    2) joint space maintained until late stages of disease
    3) femoral condyles grossly enlarged, osteoporotic, with irregular and flattened weight-bearing surfaces "*megacondyle*"
    4) widened intercondylar notch due to repeated hemorrhage at cruciate ligament attachments
    5) flattened, usually irregular tibial plateau
    6) tibial and fibular epiphyses enlarged, osteoporotic, with thin cortices and accentuated vertical trabeculae
    8) patella's inferior pole sharply attenuated and squared (due to repeated hemarthrosis inhibiting secondary growth center)
- ankle arthropathy (frequently seen)
    1) fused subtalar joint
    2) "*tibiotalar slant deformity*": premature fusion of medial tibial epiphysis
    3) ischemic necrosis of talus (rare)
- elbow involvement
    1) prominent enlargement of radial head
    2) AP projection displays widened radial and ulnar notches
- dense soft tissue swelling
    1) hemarthrosis
    2) overlying fascial planes, skin lines displaced
    3) MRI: synovial hypertrophy, inflammation, fluid accumulation, articular cartilage destruction
- osteoporosis (especially epiphyseal, caused by hyperemia)
- subchondral cysts: local hemorrhage or escaped synovial fluid
- poorly defined articular cortex
- destructive, expansile, geographic bone lesions: "*pseudotumors*"   "soap bubbly"
    1) intraosseous hemorrhage
    2) rare, but most often involve femur, pelvis, tibia, hand bones
    3) may occur in soft tissues (cystic lesions)
    4) monitored via ultrasound for progression or resolution

- epiphyseal abnormalities
    1) epiphyseal cartilage hyperemia: accelerated epiphyseal growth, maturation
    2) ballooned, enlarged epiphyses
- joint disorganization
    1) complete loss of joint space
    2) significant articular fragmentation
    3) sclerosis
    4) osteophytes
    5) bony misalignment
- pathologic fracture (often spontaneous)
- intramuscular ectopic ossification: most often pelvic gluteal or hamstring tendons
- chondrocalcinosis (possible finding)
- spine: commonly, osteoporosis with no other distinctive findings

f) Differential considerations
- juvenile rheumatoid arthritis (JRA)
    1) ballooned epiphyses (*megacondyle*)
    2) attenuated, squared inferior pole of the patella
- neurotrophic arthropathy: joint disorganization similar to long-standing hemophilic arthropathy

4. Leukemia

a) General considerations
- nature of condition
    1) malignant bone marrow and blood disease
    2) proliferation of white blood cells
    3) varieties of disease with differing clinical and histological pictures
    4) childhood leukemia: acute, rapid onset; usually lymphocytic
    5) adult leukemia: acute or chronic; insidious onset, lengthy course; usually myeloid or lymphocytic
    6) three major histologic varieties: myeloid, lymphocytic, monocytic
- incidence
    1) childhood leukemia, acute lymphocytic leukemia peaks between age 2 and 5 years
    2) most common malignant disease of childhood
    3) acute myeloid leukemia: no age predilection
    4) chronic myelocytic leukemia most frequent in young adults, peaks in 40s
    5) chronic lymphocytic leukemia: usually in middle aged and elderly
- location of skeletal lesions
    1) long bones: bilateral, symmetric involvement of proximal and distal

femur, proximal tibia, proximal
humerus, distal radius

   2) lumbar spine

   3) pelvis

- treatment
  1) complex combinations of drugs
  2) transfusions
  3) marrow transplants

b) Clinical presentation

- childhood acute lymphocytic leukemia
  1) generalized joint pain
  2) weakness and lethargy, pallor and general malaise
  3) lymphadenopathy, splenomegaly
- adult chronic lymphatic leukemia
  1) generalized weakness, fatigue
  2) weight loss
  3) splenomegaly
  4) lymphadenopathy
  5) anemia
- adult chronic myelocytic leukemia
  1) insidious onset: fatigue, weakness
  2) anorexia, weight loss
  3) fever, night sweats
  4) sense of abdominal fullness
  5) advanced stages: pallor, bleeding, marked lymphadenopathy, splenomegaly

c) Pathologic features

- leukemic cells accumulate in bone marrow
- leukemic cells replace normal hematopoietic cells
- blood-borne leukemic cells spread to liver, spleen, lymph nodes, CNS, kidneys, gonads
- lymphocytic form: begins in lymph nodes, spreads to other lymphoid tissues
- myelocytic type: excessive granulocyte production in bone marrow, spleen, and liver
- myelofibrosis in 40% of myelocytic patients
- subperiosteal extension of leukemic cells via Haversian canals (periosteal response)

d) Laboratory findings

- white cell count
  1) acute: may be high, normal, or low
  2) chronic: almost always high
- differential white cell count
  1) acute: high lymphoblasts or myeloblasts
  2) chronic: entire myeloid series, or small lymphocytes

- anemia
  1) acute: severe in > 90% of cases
  2) chronic: mild or absent
- platelets
  1) acute: frequently low platelet count
  2) chronic: may be high (in myelocytic type) or low in some cases

e) Radiologic features
- childhood leukemia:
  1) 50–70% show osseous changes
  2) generalized osteoporosis: decreased density, widened medullary space, thinned cortices
  3) radiolucent submetaphyseal bands
     - beneath and parallel to opaque zone of provisional calcification
     - most prominent at distal femur, proximal tibia, proximal humerus, distal radius
     - bilateral symmetric distribution
  4) lytic lesions
     - early in disease: small, individual, well-defined medullary lesions
     - eventually coalesce to give moth-eaten, mottled density
     - late in disease: become sclerotic
     - endosteal lysis or cortical destruction
  5) periosteal single-layer or multilayered laminated new bone; rarely spiculated
  6) occasionally: sutural diastasis, articular hemorrhage
  7) spinal effects
     - osteoporosis
     - radiolucent sub-endplate bands
     - compression fractures
- adult leukemia
  1) less than 20% show osseous changes
  2) diffuse osteoporosis
  3) radiolucent submetaphyseal bands
  4) lytic lesions: both medullary and cortical
  5) periosteal response

f) Differential considerations
- adult generalized osteoporosis: in multiple myeloma (predominantly in the same age group as patients with chronic lymphocytic leukemia)
- lucent submetaphyseal bands
  1) neuroblastoma
  2) scurvy
  3) syphilis
  4) severe systemic diseases

5. Myelofibrosis

   a) General considerations
- nature of condition
    1) idiopathic disease
    2) complication to chronic myelogenous leukemia or polycythemia vera
    3) usually chronic; occasionally acute or malignant (rapidly fatal)
    4) replacement of normal marrow with fibrosis
- incidence
    1) peak incidence between 50–70 years
    2) no gender predilection
- skeletal sites
    1) bones rich in marrow
    2) liver and spleen
- treatment
    1) no treatment for condition itself
    2) management of complications
        - transfusion or androgens for severe anemia
        - splenectomy
        - chemotherapy and radiation therapy

   b) Clinical presentation
- asymptomatic in early stages
- malaise, weight loss
- fatigue, pallor
- generalized bone pain
- gouty symptoms
- about 50% have hepatomegaly
- splenomegaly is characteristic

   c) Pathologic features
- anemia, leukemic blood changes
- progressive fibrosis of bone marrow
- abnormal myeloid stem cell proliferates
- myelofibrosis: possibly reactive to this, rather than a primary process

   d) Laboratory findings
- normocytic, normochromic anemia
- immature red and white blood cells
- advanced cases
    1) red blood cells misshapen: tear-shaped
    2) thrombocytopenia
- iliac crest biopsy: fibrosis (seldom shown by sternal puncture)

   e) Radiologic features
- osteoporosis initially
- later replaced by diffuse sclerosis
    1) mottled bones early in process
    2) become homogeneously dense

3) complete lack of definition between medullary cavity and cortex
- long bone periostitis
- endosteal thickening
- osteolytic, moth-eaten lesions
- massive splenomegaly
- possible posterior mediastinal extramedullary hematopoiesis (paraspinal masses)

    f) Differential considerations
- osteopetrosis
- blastic metastasis
- Paget's disease
- fluorosis

REVIEW—STUDY QUESTIONS

1. What are the three classifications of leukemia by cell type?
2. What type of leukemia most commonly affects children?
3. What are the radiologic signs of leukemia in children, and why do they appear?
4. Where are the radiologic signs of sickle cell anemia found, and why do they appear?
5. What is Cooley's anemia, and what population groups does it most commonly affect?
6. Where and what are the lesions associated with myeloproliferative diseases?
7. What is the etiology of hemophilia?
8. Tear-shaped red blood cells might suggest the presence of what disease entity?
9. What hematologic disease is characterized by pseudotumors of the bone, and what causes this phenomenon?
10. What populations are most at risk for sickle cell anemia?

6. Arteriosclerosis

    a) General considerations
- nature of condition
  1) *"hardening of the arteries"* (includes three specific entities)
     - *atherosclerosis*: fibrofatty plaque (atheroma) deposited in intimal and subintimal layers of large arteries
     - *Monckeberg's medial sclerosis*: calcification within the muscle wall (media) of medium and small arteries
     - *arteriolosclerosis*: hyaline deposition or hyperplasia of arteriolar wall; luminal narrowing

    2) atherosclerosis and arteriolosclerosis: thickening and reduced elasticity of arterial walls

    3) Monckeberg's medial sclerosis: does not narrow lumina; clinically insignificant

- incidence
  1) atherosclerosis: most common human degenerative disease
  2) especially prevalent after 50 years of age
  3) Monckeberg's medial sclerosis: rare before 50 years of age
  4) arteriolosclerosis: elderly and diabetic patients
- anatomic sites
  1) atherosclerosis: most common in aorta, iliac, subclavian, carotid, coronary, and femoral arteries
  2) Monckeberg's medial sclerosis: most common in femoral, tibial, radial, ulnar, and genital arteries
- treatment
  1) dietary changes
  2) drug therapy (vasodilators)
  3) surgery: thromboendarterectomy, percutaneous transluminal angioplasty, or resection with graft replacement

b) Clinical presentation
- depends on site of occlusion
  1) carotid artery occlusion: visual disturbances
  2) vertebrobasilar occlusion: balance problems
  3) coronary artery occlusion: angina pain or myocardial infarction
- *Monckeberg's medial sclerosis*: asymptomatic; often accompanies diabetes
- arteriolosclerosis: also common with diabetes, peripheral neuropathy, infections, ischemia

c) Pathologic features and laboratory findings
- arteriosclerosis
  1) atheromata accumulate: obstruction, ulceration, thrombus, or aneurysm
  2) fatty streak deposited first, evolves into fibrous plaque
  3) arteriosclerotic calcification (after several years)
- arteriolosclerosis
  1) media hypertrophies
  2) subintimal fibrosis with hyaline degeneration
- laboratory findings
  1) chronic hyperlipidemia, hypercholesterolemia (especially

with the LDL fraction high, HDL
fraction comparatively low)

d) Radiologic features

- arteriosclerosis

    1) unless calcified, atheromata not
    demonstrated on plain film

    2) degree of calcification: not correlated
    with extent of luminal narrowing

    3) calcification rare before age 40;
    increases with advancing age;
    appears correlated with hypertension

    4) angiography: accurately assesses
    presence and extent of occlusion

- calcified atheromata

    1) on plain film: thin, discontinuous,
    linear opacity

    2) two opposing opacified walls:
    "*railroad track appearance*"

    3) visualized end-on, calcified vessel
    walls: circular, ringlike density

- aortic calcification

    1) AP projections

        - abdominal aorta: left of midline,
        superimposed over vertebral
        bodies

        - transverse aortic arch: "*thumbnail
        sign*"—complete or incomplete
        ring of calcification

    2) lateral projections

        - 0–5 mm anterior to anterior
        vertebral body margins

        - > 5 mm anterior to body margin,
        suspect retroaortic pathology
        (e.g., lymphoma, lymph node
        metastasis)

        - normal transverse dimension of
        aorta: not > 3.8 cm

        - earliest plaque: anterior to L3
        and L4

- iliac artery calcification

    1) second most common abdominal
    vessel calcification

    2) frontal projection: linear
    calcification, oriented inferolaterally
    to cross the pelvic inlet near the
    sacroiliac joint

    3) calcified branches of internal iliac
    artery: within pelvic inlet

    4) lateral projection: circular, ringlike
    calcification at bifurcation of iliac
    arteries anterior to L5 body

- femoral artery calcification

    1) may be visible on frontal projection

    2) superimposed over femoral head,
    close to lesser trochanter

- splenic artery calcification
  1) third most often calcified abdominal vessel
  2) frequently tortuous
  3) frontal projection: parallel, curvilinear arcs in upper left quadrant outside splenic silhouette
- carotid artery calcification
  1) frontal projection: calcification at carotid bifurcation
  2) complete or incomplete ring of irregular calcification beneath mandible, lateral to spine
- Monckeberg's medial sclerosis
  1) virtually diagnostic *"coiled"* appearance: circular, ringlike densities along length of vessel
  2) most frequent sites: femoral, tibial, radial, ulnar, and genital arteries
- arteriolosclerosis: no lesions detectable on plain film

7. **Aneurysms**

    a) **General considerations**
    - nature of condition
      1) congenital (rare) or acquired
      2) localized abnormal dilation of any vessel
      3) congenital aneurysm: deficiency in vessel's muscle wall
      4) most common congenital aneurysm: *"berry aneurysm"* in the circle of Willis at base of brain
      5) acquired secondary to various causes (see etiology, below)
    - classifications (by location, etiology, gross appearance)
      1) most common locations
         - aorta
         - iliac arteries
         - splenic artery
         - renal arteries
         - vertebral arteries
         - popliteal arteries (most common peripheral aneurysm)
      2) less common locations
         - cerebral arteries
         - hepatic artery
         - subclavian arteries
         - cardiac aneurysms (usually in left ventricle)
      3) most common etiologies
         - atherosclerosis
         - infection (*"mycotic aneurysm"*)
         - poststenotic dilatation
         - syphilis
         - arteritis

4) less common causes
- cystic medial necrosis with diseases such as Marfan's syndrome
- lead poisoning
- radiation
- diabetes, gout, homocystinuria
- tuberculosis

5) gross morphology
- berry aneurysm
  a. small, spherical dilations, usually < 1.5 cm in diameter
  b. most often at brain base
- saccular aneurysm
  a. spherical lesions > 5 cm in diameter
- fusiform aneurysm
  a. spindle-shaped, sometimes eccentric
- dissecting aneurysm
  a. double lumen vessel (*double barrel*)
  b. may be without dilatation of the vessel
  c. blood diverted into muscle wall for some distance, then returned to lumen
- pseudoaneurysm (traumatic aneurysm)
  a. focal dilatation with no disruption of the adventitia
  b. caused by traumatic injury to the media (muscle layer)

- incidence
  1) most common: abdominal aortic aneurysm (AAA)
     - male predilection (5:1)
  2) second most common: iliac artery aneurysm
     - male predilection (4:1)
     - peak at age 70
  3) third most common: splenic artery aneurysm
     - < age 50, 3:1 female predilection
     - increasing age equalizes gender incidence
     - associations with
       a. multiparous women
       b. cirrhotic patients with portal hypertension
       c. pancreatitis patients
       d. trauma patients

- location of lesion
  1) aortic aneurysm
     - aortic arch predilected site (atherosclerosis, syphilis, trauma)

- traumatic torsion of arch: especially at ligamentum arteriosum attachment
- ascending (proximal) aorta predilected to syphilitic aneurysm (obliterative arteritis of the vasa vasorum)
- descending aorta rarely affected; occasional local dilatation due to atherosclerosis
- abdominal aorta
  a. most common site
  b. usually below renal arteries
  c. usually caused by atherosclerosis
  d. usually fusiform dilatation
  e. prone to rupture through left posterolateral wall

2) iliac artery aneurysm
- second most common aneurysm site
- 75% are extensions of abdominal aortic aneurysm (AAA)
- 90% in common iliac; 10% in internal iliac; < 1 % involve external iliac

3) splenic artery aneurysm
- third most common aneurysm site
- usually solitary, saccular lesions at splenic hilum
- usually about 2–2.5 cm in diameter

4) renal artery aneurysm
- rare site
- usually near renal hilus
- usually 1–3 cm in diameter

5) vertebral artery aneurysm
- rare site
- most often C1-C2 region

6) hepatic artery aneurysm: rare, usually extrahepatic

7) intrinsic heart artery aneurysm
- rare site
- may complicate myocardial infarction
- usually in infarcted area
- most common at left cardiac border

8) popliteal artery aneurysm
- most common peripheral aneurysm (about 70% of peripheral aneurysms)
- male predilection (30:1)
- about 60% bilateral
- about 50% coexist with aortoiliac or femoral artery aneurysms

- diagnostic imaging
  1) plain film
     - aneurysms visible only with sufficient calcification
     - frequently an incidental finding on films taken for other purposes
  2) ultrasound
     - **modality of choice** for evaluating, monitoring progression, confirming diagnosis
     - obesity or excessive bowel gas hamper diagnosis
     - cannot verify suprarenal extension
  3) CT
     - technique of choice for post-surgical evaluations
     - detects extent of aneurysm, degree of thrombosis, site of rupture, distribution and amount of leakage, presence of perianeurysmal fibrosis, ureteral involvement and relationship to renal arteries
  4) MRI
     - eliminates need for angiography
     - allows accurate measurement
     - isolates flow abnormalities
     - identifies clot
     - accurate assessment of visceral branch involvement
     - can fulfill any function that CT provides in this context
  5) angiography
     - often alters surgical approach
     - clarifies arterial anomalies (especially renal arteries)
     - displays suprarenal extension
     - clearly depicts condition of iliac arteries, femoral arteries, mesenteric arteries
     - excellent imaging of aortic complications (occlusion, inferior vena cava lesions)
     - permits identification of horseshoe kidney
- treatment
  1) aortic lesions > 5 cm diameter: usually elective surgery
  2) aortic lesions < 5 cm: monitored with ultrasound 2 or 3 times a year; if enlarging, they go to surgery (resection and graft)
  3) relative risks
     - elective surgery: 5% operative mortality
     - emergency surgery: 80% mortality

b) **Clinical presentation**

☞
- abdominal aortic aneurysm (AAA)
    1) abdominal or low back pain
    2) pulsating pain, worse when supine
    3) palpable pulsations; auscultated bruits
    4) lower limb ischemia
    5) paralysis caused by cord ischemia
    6) bloody diarrhea from ischemic bowel

☞
- coexisting conditions (especially with AAA)
    1) obstructed bowel
    2) obstructed inferior vena cava
    3) obstructed ureters
- additional risk factors
    1) familial incidence
    2) smoking
    3) alcoholism
- dissecting aneurysm
    1) sharp, tearing pain
    2) may be referred to interscapular region
- asymptomatic aneurysms
    1) incidental finding on films taken for other reasons
    2) found by palpation
    3) discovered only when they burst (sudden death)
- leakage
    1) increasing abdominal and back pain
    2) eventual hypovolemic shock
- popliteal artery aneurysm
    1) frequently entails thrombosis
    2) leg ischemia, risk of limb loss

c) **Pathologic features**
- atherosclerosis:
    1) atheromata (subintimal fatty depositions) create fibrosis and calcification
    2) compress the media, causing necrosis and weakened muscle
    3) compress vasa vasorum, leading to medial ischemic necrosis
    4) continuous high pulsatile pressure thins the weakened vessel wall
- infection ("*mycotic aneurysm*")
    1) subacute bacterial endocarditis, intravenous drug use, seeding from local infection
    2) commonly caused by staphylococci and salmonella
    3) often affects abdominal aorta: lobulated, saccular aneurysms (rarely calcify)

- poststenotic dilatation
    1) obstruction causes turbulent flow
    2) distal to obstruction: localized vessel enlargement
- syphilis
    1) ascending aorta predilected to spirochete infiltration
    2) saccular syphilitic aneurysms erode adjacent bone (anterior vertebral body erosions)
    3) far less common since development of antibiotics
- arteritis
    1) inflammation of blood vessels: medial necrosis
    2) idiopathic, or caused by systemic inflammatory conditions: polyarteritis nodosa, rheumatoid arthritis, ankylosing spondylitis, systemic lupus erythematosus
    3) anterior vertebral body erosions due to adherence of inflamed artery to spine

d) Laboratory findings
- with inflammatory conditions: elevated erythrocyte sedimentation rate (ESR)
- renal involvement: raised creatinine level
- leaking aneurysm: anemia; often slight leukocytosis

e) Radiologic features

- aortic aneurysms
    1) most are between renal artery and iliac bifurcation (spinal levels L2 to L4)
    2) frontal projection
        - usually left margin seen to the left of spine
        - soft tissue density (if uncalcified, may not be visible on plain film)
        - thin, curvilinear calcific rim (55–85% have detectable calcification)
        - aortic arch aneurysm enlarges aortic silhouette superiorly and laterally
            a. may displace trachea and esophagus
            b. may have peripheral calcification
        - ascending aortic aneurysm displaces aortic shadow to right and superiorly; thin, curvilinear calcification often at peripheral rim
    3) lateral projection
        - calcified plaque may indicate aneurysm

- posterior extension of aneurysm may overlie the spine
- measure distance between calcified anterior and posterior margins: > 3.8 cm indicates aneurysm
- occasionally: smooth, concave anterior vertebral body erosions
    a. *"Oppenheimer erosions"*
    b. seen especially with inflammatory or syphilitic aneurysms
- optimal view for aneurysm in descending aorta (rare): shows localized dilatation

- iliac artery aneurysms
    1) frontal projection: fusiform shape, overlies sacroiliac joint
    2) lateral projection: large, circular ring of calcification anterior to L5
    3) large saccular aneurysm may simulate pelvic mass
- splenic artery aneurysm
    1) circular, ringlike calcification in left upper quadrant, anterior to spine
    2) usually single, occasionally multiple aneurysms
- renal artery aneurysm
    1) circular, incomplete, ringlike calcification
    2) frontal projection: adjacent to L2-L3
    3) lateral projection: overlies the spine
- vertebral artery aneurysm
    1) extrinsic erosive defect adjacent to C2 pedicle and transverse foramen
    2) mid-cervical spine: tortuosity may cause enlarged intervertebral foramen
- hepatic artery aneurysm: circular extrahepatic opacity in right upper quadrant
- cardiac aneurysm in infarcted area of heart
    1) localized bulge at left cardiac border
    2) may have peripheral rim of calcification
- popliteal artery aneurysm
    1) average popliteal artery aneurysm size: 4 cm
    2) arterial diameter > 7 mm: aneurysm

8. **Phleboliths**

   a) **General considerations**
   - nature of condition
       1) concretions of thrombi attached to venous walls
       2) apparently due to upright posture, not seen in quadrupeds

        3) no recognized factors for predisposition
- incidence
  1) no gender predilection
  2) pelvic phlebolith in at least one third of population by age 40
- anatomic sites
  1) usually within pelvic basin, near superior pubic rami, below ischial spine
  2) frequently within perivesical and perirectal venous plexus
  3) in males: in scrotal veins and dorsal vein of the penis
  4) in females: in veins of the broad ligament

b) Clinical presentation
- completely asymptomatic
- incidental finding on plain films

c) Pathologic features
- thickly packed layers of platelets trapped in network of red blood cells and fibrin
- calcification: predominantly calcium carbonate
- possibly caused by abrupt, intermittent intra-abdominal pressure variations affecting poorly supported, valveless pelvic veins

d) Radiologic features
- dense, round or oval, well-marginated opacity
- often with central lucency
- vary in number from 1 to > 20
- may appear in chains along upper margin of superior pubic ramus
- rarely, chain may overlap sacroiliac joint, ascending parallel to and lateral to spine
- unusual: phleboliths midline in pelvic basin
- phlebolith outside pelvic basin: may indicate soft tissue hemangioma or venous stasis
- apparent change of position of phlebolith: may indicate displacement by prolapse, or by abnormal mass

9. Venous Insufficiency

a) General considerations
- nature of condition
  1) associated with aging and diabetes
  2) predisposing diseases: diabetes mellitus, polyarteritis nodosa, collagen disorders
- incidence
  1) most common between ages 50 and 70

2) incidence increases with advancing age
- anatomic sites
  1) always affects lower extremities
  2) tibia and fibula most obviously affected
  3) femur, metatarsals, phalanges also show effects
  4) diaphyses and metaphyses show periosteal effects

b) **Clinical presentation**
- diminished arterial pulses in lower extremities
- edema
- varicosities
- skin discoloration
- altered temperature
- later in process: ulceration, gangrenous infections

c) **Pathologic features**
- periosteal reaction caused by hypoxia
- sluggish blood flow

d) **Radiologic features**
- most commonly bilateral; in lower legs
- periosteal new bone formed outside cortex
  1) initially as single, thin lamination
  2) later, thickened by subsequent laminations, separation is obliterated
  3) distinctive undulating external contour of laminations
  4) underlying bone unaffected
  5) laminations may obscure the corticomedullary junction
- edematous swelling: increased soft tissue density, obliterated fascial fat planes, displaced skin contours
- skin ulceration: excavation in the skin contour
- calcification
  1) diffuse reticular pattern
  2) phlebolith formation
  3) dense, branching opacity (organized venous thrombosis)
  4) *Monckeberg's arteriosclerosis* in adjacent arteries

REVIEW—STUDY QUESTIONS

1. What are the most common sites of aortic aneurysm, and what are their most common etiologies?
2. What radiologic signs might indicate the presence of aneurysm?
3. What radiologic appearance of phleboliths might be diagnostically significant?

4. What is the characteristic appearance of periosteal reaction caused by venous insufficiency?

5. What arteries are most vulnerable to aneurysm?

6. Name and describe three types of arteriosclerosis.

7. Which of these three types involve radiologic signs visible on plain film?

8. What modalities are optimal for detecting and evaluating aneurysms?

9. What clues help in radiologic differentiation of splenic artery aneurysm from renal artery aneurysm?

10. What is a mycotic aneurysm?

10. **Osteonecrosis**

   a) **General considerations**
   - nature of condition
      1) death of osseous cellular components and marrow
      2) most commonly primary
         - idiopathic or spontaneous
         - usually isolated lesion in femoral capital epiphyses, distal femurs, metatarsal heads, carpal lunate, metadiaphyseal medullary cavities of long bones

      3) epiphyseal ischemic necrosis:
         - self-limiting; eventually heals
         - may be secondary to predisposing factor or condition, including
            a. trauma: fracture, dislocation or subluxation
               - impairs circulation to bone
               - most common in intracapsular epiphyses, e.g., femoral or humeral heads
               - other frequent sites: talus, proximal pole of the scaphoid
            b. alcoholism
               - possible mechanism: fat emboli from fatty liver or increased marrow fat mass
               - usually affects femoral head
            c. corticosteroids
               - clear association between Cushing's disease, corticosteroid therapy, and osteonecrosis
               - mechanism unknown; fat emboli may be implicated
            d. Caisson disease
               - rapid reduction in

environmental pressure
(e.g., deep water diving
releases nitrogen, forms
bubbles in blood vessels)

- epiphyseal and
metaphyseal necrosis: high
fat content in bone
marrow, nitrogen's affinity
for fat
- necrosis often bilateral,
extensive

e. Gaucher's disease

- lipid-laden histiocytes
infringe on marrow
sinusoids
- often bilateral
osteonecrosis, especially
of femoral heads

f. hemoglobinopathy

- sludging, thrombosis,
infarction; usually in
epiphyses and
metadiaphysis of long
bones
- cortical infarctions of
small bones of hands and
feet in infants ("*hand-foot
syndrome*")
- with sickle cell disease,
sickle cell trait, other
hemoglobin structure
disorders

g. collagen diseases

- vasculitis (small vessel
inflammation): vascular
thromboses and tissue
infarction
- rheumatoid arthritis,
systemic lupus
erythematosus, etc.
- corticosteroid therapy
increases the risk

h. radiation

- mechanism unknown:
result is obliterative
endarteritis and cell death
- threshold dose of 3000
rads produces
osteonecrosis
- child's epiphyseal bone
growth affected at 300 to
400 rads

i. pancreatitis

- can produce fatty emboli
- medullary bone infarcts
(rare), also infarction of
peritoneal and mesenteric
fat, brain, kidney

- alcoholism/pancreatitis complications involved

j. gout
- mechanism unknown: may involve increased incidence of diabetes mellitus, hypertension, hyperlipidemia, kidney failure, alcohol intake, and basement membrane thickening in small blood vessel disease
- metaphyseal/diaphyseal medullary infarcts
- epiphyseal center osteonecrosis, often at femoral heads
- about 30% of gout patients show evidence of bone infarction

- incidence: various populations are prey to specific manifestations (see below)
- skeletal sites (most common)
  1) see section "f" for specific epiphyseal necrotic phenomena
  2) predilection for epiphyseal centers
  3) especially femoral head, humeral head, distal femur, metaphyseal and diaphyseal areas of long bones
- treatment varies with location and etiology

b) Clinical presentation
- varies with etiology and location of lesion
- local or referred pain
- antalgia
- reduced, painful range of motion at affected joint
- adjacent muscle atrophy
- metaphyseal or diaphyseal infarcts: asymptomatic, or acutely painful

c) Pathologic process
- subsynovial vessels particularly vulnerable to rupture or compression
- gradual, subtle transition through four phases of disease
  1) **avascular phase**
     - death of osteocytes, marrow cells
     - cessation of epiphyseal growth
     - articular cartilage continues to grow
     - bone not weakened nor deformed
  2) **revascularization phase**
     - new vessels infiltrate necrotic bone
     - new bone deposition around rim of epiphysis at chondro-osseous junction and centrally; ("*creeping*

substitution") new bone deposited
directly onto dead bone

- new bone is "plastic" ("*biological plasticity*"), easily deformed by stresses on the epiphysis: residual deformity
- at this stage, stress fractures can occur beneath cortex
- resorption secondary to phagocytosis, fibrosis, and infiltration by granulation: fragmentation of involved bone

3) **repair and remodeling phase**
- new bone deposition replaces resorbed bone
- still "*plastic*," easily deformed

4) **deformity**
- degree of deformity determined by compressive force on necrotic bone during earlier phases
- the less the deformity, the better the long-term prognosis

- metaphyseal/diaphyseal infarcts: cortical or medullary
  1) cortical infarcts
     - vascular infiltration, with absorption and bone deposition
     - periosteal response: fine lamination of new bone
  2) medullary infarcts
     - most common at diametaphyseal junction
     - central necrotic area within thin, peripheral ischemic zone
     - new vessels and osteoblasts gradually reduce size of necrotic area
     - if healing ceases, peripheral wall becomes fibrous, calcifies and ossifies
     - central necrotic area may also progress to ossification
- rarely, malignant degeneration of infarct to malignant fibrous histiocytoma or fibrosarcoma

   d) Radiologic features
- epiphyseal infarction
  1) collapse of articular cortex
     - at region of maximum mechanical stress
     - local impaction fracture of weakened necrotic bone
     - local loss of normal smooth articular surface: sometimes angular defect in flattened surface, sometimes smooth undulation of the cortical surface

2) fragmentation
- lucent clefts traversing involved bone
- may be numerous enough to appear as though entire epiphysis is gone
- caused by bone resorption and weakening

3) mottled trabecular pattern
- thickened, irregular trabeculae traversing the ischemic bone
- sign of revascularization and repair
- altered orientation, accommodating altered stresses through deformed bone

4) sclerosis
- three patterns occur with revascularization
  a. peripheral cortical margin shows increased density
  b. homogenous, patchy density appears centrally
  c. patches of density may be accentuated by osteoporosis in adjacent metaphysis

5) subchondral cysts
- patchy, well-circumscribed rarefactions
- immediately beneath articular cortex
- in area of most mechanical stress
- most commonly occur in femoral capital epiphysis

6) subchondral fracture
- separates articular cortex from underlying cancellous bone "*rim sign, crescent sign*"
- usually at area of maximum mechanical stress

- metaphyseal/diaphyseal infarction
  1) usually medullary lesions
  2) most frequently in distal femur, proximal tibia, proximal humerus
  3) bone scan visualizes lesion; plain film can't until revascularization phase
  4) MR shows bright area surrounded by serpentine, thin, low signal border
  5) revascularization causes radiographically visible lesion: area of rarefaction
  6) mature infarct shows peripheral rim of calcification
     - lesion longer than it is wide
     - lesion located toward one end of involved bone

- dense, well-demarcated, undulating rim ("*serpiginous configuration*")
- sometimes, internal areas of localized sclerosis
- adjacent cortex is unaffected
- metaphyseal/diaphyseal cortical infarction
    1) most often in small tubular bones of hands and feet
    2) periostitis and localized foci of rarefaction visible within 10 days
    3) cortex appears split longitudinally
    4) later, periostitis thickens, obliterates normal diaphyseal constriction
    5) remodeling restores normal contours

☞ **e) Differential considerations**
- predisposing condition: must be identified and addressed in the treatment protocol
- subchondral cysts: feature of degenerative joint disease

f) Specific entities involving osteonecrosis

I. Spontaneous Osteonecrosis of the Knee (SONK)
- **General considerations**
    1) nature of lesion: ischemic necrosis of unknown etiology
    2) incidence: patients > 60, slight female predominance
    3) skeletal site
        - usually medial femoral condyle; sometimes lateral condyle, occasionally both condyles simultaneously
        - rarely medial tibial condyle
        - rarely superolateral pole of patella or entire patella
    4) treatment is surgical (arthroplasty), often total knee replacement
- **Clinical presentation**
    1) sudden onset of acute pain with no history of trauma
    2) initial plain films usually normal
    3) sharp tenderness over medial femoral condyle
    4) pain increases in severity, becomes chronic and disabling
- **Pathologic features**
    1) focal vascular compromise
    2) necrosis of small condylar fragments
    3) subchondral bone collapse
    4) histiocytic bone resorption
    5) granulomatous tissue
    6) reactive new bone formation
    7) overlying cartilage discoloration, fissuring or total eradication
    8) possibly detached osteochondral fragment
    9) often medial meniscus tears coexist

☞
- **Radiologic features**
    1) bone scan or MRI required for early identification of lesions
    2) plain film findings visible only after weeks or months of symptoms
        - flattened articular surface
        - may show breaks in cortical surface
        - sclerotic foci with surrounding fissures (subchondral fractures) < 1 cm long in subchondral bone (*"crescent sign"*)
        - intraarticular loose osseous fragments, usually with excavated concave defect at site of origin
    3) degenerative changes appear in about one third of cases
        - reduced medial joint space
        - subchondral bone cysts
        - sclerosis
        - osteophytes
    4) meniscal calcifications
    5) varus deformity
    6) extensive necrosis

☞
- **Differential considerations**
    1) steroid therapy
    2) hemoglobinopathies
    3) transplantation

II. **Caisson Disease**
(synonyms: decompression sickness, the chokes, the staggers, the bends; skeletal effects are termed: dysbaric osteonecrosis, pressure-induced osteoarthropathy, barotraumatic osteoarthropathy)
- **General considerations**
    1) nature of lesions
        - accumulation of nitrogen gas bubbles in blood vessels
        - act as emboli; produce infarcts
    2) incidence: patients who have experienced rapid, significant atmospheric pressure changes: e.g., divers surfacing too rapidly; high altitude flyers returning to lower levels
    3) anatomic sites
        - CNS, lungs, muscles, joints, bones
        - especially noted in hips and shoulders, bilaterally
    4) treatment: prevention, and in acute cases, prompt recompression
- **Clinical presentation**
    1) weakness or numbness of extremities
    2) mild paresthesia, severe vertigo
    3) substernal discomfort, coughing on deep inspiration or when smoking

    4) itching, skin rash; rarely: cutaneous edema, mottled skin

    5) exceptional fatigue

    6) abdominal pain in a "girdle" pattern (spinal cord involvement)

    7) late: chronic hip or shoulder pain, leading to disability

- **Pathologic features**
  1) blood-borne nitrogen emboli impair perfusion
  2) fatty tissues (bone marrow, spinal cord, stored fat) absorb up to five times as much nitrogen as other tissue
  3) predisposing factors: obesity, repeated dysbaric episodes, exposure to excessive pressure, extended time under altered pressures
  4) bone changes have extensive latent period: as long as 10 years
  5) nitrogen emboli in bone: in fatty marrow and in metaphyseal/ epiphyseal regions
  6) result in medullary diaphyseal/ metaphyseal infarction; epiphyseal infarctions in femoral and humeral heads

- **Radiologic features**
  1) sites vary: unilateral, bilateral, at any joint or in any marrow-rich bone
  2) plain film scout films should include:
     - both humeri and femora heads and proximal shafts in AP views
     - both knees (including distal two thirds of femur and upper third of tibia) in AP and lateral views
  3) epiphyseal lesions
     - patchy areas of lucency and sclerosis
     - curvilinear subchondral fracture ("*crescent sign*")
     - articular surface collapse
     - secondary degenerative joint disease: osteophytes, reduced joint space
  4) metaphyseal/diaphyseal lesions
     - healed, mature, central medullary infarct
     - elongate lesion, with dense, undulating sclerotic border
     - patchy sclerosis and lucency within lesion

- **Differential considerations**
  1) steroid therapy
  2) hemoglobin disorders
  3) trauma
  4) spontaneous osteonecrosis

III. Radiation-induced Injury to Bone
(synonyms: radiation osteitis, radiation necrosis, osteoradionecrosis)

- **General considerations**
  1) nature of lesions
     - post-radiation atrophy, producing osteoporosis
     - osteitis
     - epiphyseal avascular necrosis
     - arrested bone growth
  2) incidence
     - people who have ingested radioactive substances (usually radium or strontium), e.g., those who painted luminous watch dials
     - people injected with radioactive contrast agents (such as thorium)
     - those with surgical implants of radioactive substances as treatment for local malignancy
     - those treated with radiation therapy, or otherwise exposed to high levels of radiation
  3) location of lesions
     - any bone exposed to radiation affected
     - spine, pelvis, mandible, upper ribs, clavicle, scapula, and proximal humerus: common sites caused by proximity to commonly irradiated malignant lesions
- **Clinical presentation**
  1) signs appear months or years after exposure
  2) pain often caused by complications: epiphyseal avascular necrosis, infection, fracture, malignant degeneration
  3) radiation-induced sarcoma in 1–2% of these patients, most commonly in pelvis and shoulder girdle
- **Pathologic features**
  1) bone and cartilage affected by retarded cellular division, cell death, cellular transformation, and vascular obliteration
  2) inflammation in marrow after irradiation leads to local necrosis
  3) radiosensitive bone cells often die
  4) obliterative endarteritis and periosteal damage
  5) fracture or infection often superimposed
  6) regeneration occurs via *"creeping substitution"* (new bone deposited on trabeculae as dead bone is removed)

7) radiation to growth plate arrests longitudinal growth
   - 300–400 rads, temporary arrest
   - 1800–2600 Gy, permanent arrest
8) irradiated bone shows necrosis, marrow fibrosis, thickened trabeculae
9) adults: bone cell death threshold of 3000 Gy

- **Radiologic features**
  1) 3–12 months latent period before lesions visible on plain film
  2) general features: altered growth patterns, moth-eaten destruction, patchy sclerosis, trabecular thickening, periostitis
  3) less commonly: bone resorption, epiphyseal avascular necrosis, widened sacroiliac joints, soft tissue calcification, neoplasm
  4) earliest sign: osteopenia; then trabecular thickening
  5) lytic lesions, initially small, enlarge gradually
  6) spine
     - immature spine: mild concave scoliosis with vertebral body hypoplasia, lateral wedging
     - endplate irregularity
     - *"bone within a bone"* (rare)
     - patchy lucency and sclerosis of vertebral bodies
     - pathologic fractures
     - intravertebral vacuum cleft sign
  7) pelvis
     - hypoplastic ilium (when immature crest is irradiated)
     - regional moth-eaten destruction with patchy, dense sclerotic foci and trabecular thickening
     - widened sacroiliac joints
     - insufficiency fracture of sacrum
     - protrusio acetabuli
     - calcified soft tissue masses
     - femoral head osteonecrosis
  8) mandible
     - moth-eaten destruction
     - cortical destruction
     - pathologic fracture
     - commonly complicated by infection
     - teeth are removed prior to irradiation
  9) shoulder girdle
     - changes in upper ribs, clavicle, scapula, proximal humerus
     - moth-eaten destruction

- patchy reactive sclerosis
- bone resorption
- painless, slow-healing fractures
- rare: avascular necrosis of humeral head

☞
- **Differential considerations**
  1) Paget's disease
     - radionecrosis: no bone expansion
     - radionecrosis: localized
     - cortical thickness: normal with radionecrosis
     - alkaline phosphatase levels: normal in radionecrosis
  2) osseous metastasis
     - elevated alkaline phosphatase with metastasis
     - low likelihood of involved sites distant to irradiated bone

11. **Epiphyseal Osteonecrosis (synonyms: osteochondritis, osteochondrosis, epiphysitis, aseptic necrosis, avascular necrosis)**
    a) **General considerations**
       - nature of lesions: osteonecrosis—primary or secondary bone death at an epiphysis
       - incidence: varies with specific site and etiology
       - skeletal sites (some of the more common entities)
         1) hip
            - immature femoral head (Legg-Calvé-Perthes disease)
            - weight-bearing surface of medial femoral condyle (spontaneous osteonecrosis of the mature femoral head)
         2) foot: metatarsal head (Freiberg's disease)
         3) wrist: lunate (Kienböck's disease)
    b) Specific entities

☞
    I. **Spontaneous Osteonecrosis of the Mature Femoral Head (synonyms: Chandler's disease, osteochondritis dissecans of the hip, adult avascular necrosis)**
       - **General considerations**
         1) nature of lesion: ischemic necrosis of unknown cause
         2) proposed mechanism: occlusion of lateral circumflex epiphyseal and superior retinacular vessels, which perfuse most of weight-bearing area of femoral head
         3) incidence
            - male predilection (4:1)
            - wide age range: 30–70
         4) skeletal site: 50% are bilateral but asymmetric

5) treatment: replacement prosthesis, or *"core decompression"* early in disease

   - core of bone removed from femoral neck and head
   - reduces intraosseous compression
   - may improve perfusion and promote healing
   - must be done before subchondral fracture occurs

- **Clinical presentation**
  1) buttock, groin, thigh, or knee pain: gradually increasing intensity over years
  2) decreased motion, especially rotation and abduction
  3) eventually, limping gait and muscle atrophy

- **Pathologic features**
  1) notable absence of previous trauma or predisposing conditions
  2) as disease progresses, wedge-shaped necrotic area with centrally directed apex involves the anterosuperior weightbearing area of the femoral head
  3) fovea and inferior femoral head unaffected
  4) area between necrotic bone and sclerotic margin of adjacent normal bone becomes fibrous

- **Radiologic features**
  1) required projections: AP and frog-leg
  2) bone scan and MRI identify lesions earliest
  3) lesions involve anterosuperior femoral head, in wedged or semilunar pattern (*"bite sign or segmental pattern"*)
  4) impaction fracture of necrotic bone with collapse of supported cortex gives early sign: articular cortex collapses in sharp, steplike defect or in mild, concave undulations

     - arclike, curvilinear lucency under the superior weight-bearing surface
     - called *"crescent sign or rim sign"*
     - frog leg projection, or tractioned AP view are optimal

  5) degenerative joint disease ensues: loss of joint space; osteophytes, sclerotic subchondral bone with subchondral cysts
  6) fissures and cysts within necrotic bone

7) articular cortex and attached degenerating articular cartilage: sometimes separated from necrotic segment

- **Differential considerations**
  1) alcoholism
  2) trauma
  3) hemoglobin abnormalities
  4) collagen disease

☞ II. **Legg-Calvé-Perthes Disease**
- **General considerations**
  1) nature of lesions
     - avascular necrosis of femoral capital epiphysis before growth plate closure
     - self-limiting, resolving in 2–8 years
  2) incidence:
     - ages 3–12 years, peak incidence in 5–7 age group
     - male predilection (5:1)
     - few have familial incidence, and condition is rare in blacks
  3) skeletal site: bilateral involvement occurs, but rarely in females
  4) treatment
     - management to minimize deformity (the younger the patient at onset, the better the prognosis; older children tend to suffer more severe deformity)
     - surgical intervention if lateral displacement of femoral head has "uncovered" a large portion of the head
       a. femoral varus derotation osteotomy
       b. iliac osteotomy ("*roof procedure*") to alter acetabular angle
  5) prognostic considerations
     - *Catterall's classification*: predict outcome based on proportion of epiphysis affected
       a. factors indicating poor prognosis
          - extensive epiphyseal involvement
          - lateral displacement of femoral head
          - necrotic fragments beyond lateral metaphyseal margin
          - early closure with horizontal orientation of growth plate

- extensive metaphyseal lucent defect
- elevation of greater trochanter

- **Clinical presentation**
  1) vague groin pain
  2) pain may extend to anteromedial knee
  3) hip abduction and internal rotation produce pain (symptoms may be intermittent)
  4) with time, atrophy of thigh muscles
  5) may have antecedent trauma
  6) Fabere-Patrick test, Trendelenburg test may be positive
  7) adult with history of Legg-Calvé-Perthes disease: evident hip DJD

- **Pathologic features**
  1) primary etiologies vary: evident avascular necrosis
  2) disturbance of venous drainage, intraosseous hypertension
  3) femoral head vasculature particularly vulnerable between ages 4 and 7
     - during most of life, femoral head has three sources of perfusion
       a. epiphyseal vessels: from lateral (mostly) and medial circumflex branches of profunda femoris artery
       b. foveal vessels through ligamentum teres
       c. metaphyseal vessels from bone marrow
     - ages 4–7, epiphyseal vessels provide almost all perfusion
  4) epiphyseal vessels: subsynovial, vulnerable to traumatic insult
  5) disease seems to be initiated with a double infarction within a short time
  6) disease process: (usual osteonecrosis pattern)
     - ischemic death of osteocytes and marrow elements
     - infiltration of new vessels and osteogenic elements (as long as a year after initial infarct)
     - revascularization; absorption and creeping substitution (as long as 4 years)
     - remodeling to residual deformity
  7) articular cartilage unaffected throughout process

- **Radiologic features**
  1) "*hot*" bone scan before lesions are visible on plain film
  2) MRI also facilitates earlier diagnosis

3) soft tissue swelling: convex pericapsular fat lines on lateral femoral neck (compare with contralateral side)

4) increased medial joint cavity width: femur displaced laterally (evaluated by "*Waldenstrom's sign,*" "*teardrop distance*")

5) "smaller" obturator foramen on affected side secondary to antalgic flexion, external rotation and slight abduction (occurs with any painful hip)

6) reduced femoral head size (possibly caused by reduced blood supply)

7) lucent clefts cross epiphysis, indicating fragmentation: usually a curvilinear defect parallel to superior weight-bearing articular surface ("*crescent sign, rim sign*"); frog leg projection may show nitrogen gas in these defects

8) with revascularization: three possible patterns of sclerosis
   - peripherally, cortical sclerosis: "*head-within-a-head appearance*"
   - sequestered areas with patchy, segmented sclerosis
   - homogenous sclerosis of entire epiphysis ("*snowcap appearance*")

9) metaphysis widened and shortened: lateral cortical margin convex

10) cysts with uncalcified growth plate cartilage in lateral or medial femoral neck (late in disease)

11) "*Gage's sign*": lucent defect at lateral epiphysis and adjacent metaphysis early in disease (often indicates poorer prognosis)

12) enlarged greater trochanter: elevates attachments of abductor muscles, reducing their efficacy

13) widened, lucent physis: metaphyseal side appears irregular

14) may see linear lucent submetaphyseal band

15) relatively horizontal orientation of growth plate

16) lateral margin of acetabular roof irregular

17) detached osteochondral fragment (osteochondritis dissecans) with loss of joint space (chondrolysis) requiring early surgery: rare complication occurring only with males

18) various residual deformities include
   - *coxa magnum*: overall femoral head enlargement

- *coxa plana*: flattened femoral head
- *mushroom deformity*: flattened femoral head, transversely enlarged
- *coxa vara*: femoral angle decreased to < 120°; may show *"sagging rope sign"*—curvilinear concave opacity superimposed over the metaphysis
- **Differential considerations**
    - metaphyseal cysts: simulate benign neoplasm
    - adult with deformed femoral head: DDX congenital hip dysplasia
    - congenital dysplasia: no *"sagging rope sign"*
    - congenital hip dysplasia: acetabular dysplasia involved

REVIEW—STUDY QUESTIONS

1. Name and describe the phases characterizing the pathologic and healing process in ischemic necrosis.
2. Correlate the radiographic appearance of the bone with these stages.
3. What is SONK and what population does it usually affect?
4. What treatments are given for spontaneous osteonecrosis in the adult femoral head?
5. Describe the vascular supply that renders the epiphysis vulnerable to ischemic necrosis at the femoral head and at the humeral head.
6. Describe Legg-Calvé-Perthes disease: its clinical, pathologic, and radiologic features.
7. What is Gage's sign, and what is its clinical significance?
8. Where is the "crescent sign" or "rim sign" seen, and what does it indicate?
9. List five conditions that predispose to the development of osteonecrosis.
10. In what age cohort is the femoral head most vulnerable to avascular necrosis and what may predispose it?

III. **Freiberg's Disease (synonyms: osteochondrosis, Kohler's number 2 disease)**
- **General considerations**
    1) nature of lesions: avascular necrosis
    2) skeletal site: metatarsal head— most commonly second metatarsal, occasionally third
    3) incidence: young, adolescents; female predilection (5:1)
    4) treatment
        - management via reduced activity, cast, crutches

- phased return to activity with metatarsal pads, orthoses
- unresponsive cases: surgical excision of metatarsal head

- **Clinical presentation**
  1) usually 13–18 years old, with pain and tenderness over affected joint
  2) pain exacerbated by activity or various footwear
  3) pain, palpable swelling, possibly mild hyperextension of digit
  4) later: crepitus, stiffness, reduced motion, bony enlargement, callus formation

- **Pathologic features**
  1) etiology of avascular necrosis obscure: may involve displacement of physis
  2) may be predisposed by "*Morton's syndrome*": congenitally elongated second metatarsal or shortened first metatarsal
  3) usual osteonecrosis process
  4) weight-bearing on necrotic bone: complications
     - fractures
     - articular cortex deformity
     - intraarticular loose bodies
  5) alterations of joint: thickened capsule, synovitis, cartilage and bone fragments, osteophytes, and fibrocartilage on metatarsal surface
  6) with resolution: degenerative changes and compensatory thickening of adjacent metatarsal cortex

- **Radiologic features**
  1) articular cortical changes: minimal cortical flattening of metatarsal head, progressing to flattened, concave, or undulating surface
  2) density changes: patchy sclerosis during active phase of process; sometimes lucent subchondral fracture parallel to articular surface ("*crescent sign*")
  3) joint space changes: widened joint cavity during active phase; possible loose bodies
  4) thickened metaphysis and diaphysis of involved metatarsal
  5) with healing: metatarsal head and base of opposing phalanx enlarged and bulbous; normal density returns; joint space may narrow with subsequent DJD

☞   **IV. Kienböck's Disease**
       (synonyms: lunate osteochondrosis, lunate
       malacia)
- **General considerations**
    1) nature of lesion: avascular necrosis, idiopathic or related to antecedent trauma or repetitive microtrauma
    2) skeletal location: carpal lunate, occasionally bilateral
    3) incidence: male predilection (9:1); age group 20–40 years
    4) treatment: various surgical interventions, depending upon individual presentations: shorten radius, silastic implant to replace lunate
- **Clinical presentation**
    1) local and radiating wrist pain
    2) swelling
    3) gradually worsening disability
    4) may lead to severe pain, entrapment neuropathy, degenerative arthritis
- **Pathologic features**
    1) possible vascular vulnerability to traumatic insult
    2) negative ulnar variance (short ulna) associated in 75% of cases; may exacerbate vascular vulnerability
    3) process typical of osteonecrosis
- **Radiologic features**
    1) bone scan or MRI: show lesions several months before plain film; MRI shows indications of process
    2) disuse osteoporosis of adjacent bones: accentuates density of normal or sclerotic lunate
    3) cortical changes: articular margin irregular, flattened, or collapsed, especially at radial surface
    4) size changes: small lunate, caused by compression and impaction
    5) density changes: initially, density uniformly increased; later, patchy sclerosis; occasionally linear subchondral fracture in surface adjacent to the radius
    6) after resolution: separation of scaphoid and lunate; secondary DJD of radiocarpal and midcarpal joints

V. Hass's Disease
- **General considerations**
    1) skeletal location: humeral head
    2) nature of lesions: avascular necrosis
       - vascular supply via three major perfusing vessels
           a. arcuate artery (traversing bicipital groove)

      b. branches of posterior circumflex artery

      c. rotator cuff artery (at insertions of rotator cuff insertions)

- supply at muscular insertions disrupted, precipitating necrosis
- predisposing factors: fractures, dislocations, corticosteroid therapy, hemoglobin disorders

- **Radiologic features**
  1) patchy sclerosis and lucency
  2) curvilinear subchondral fracture (*"crescent sign"*)
  3) articular cortical depression

VI. Kohler's Disease

- **General considerations**
  1) skeletal site: tarsal navicular
  2) incidence: predominantly males around 5 years old
  3) nature of lesion: possible ischemic necrosis (vascular deficiency) or may represent a normal growth variation in some cases
  4) resolves with complete reconstitution of navicular to normal appearance

- **Clinical presentation**
  1) local pain, swelling, tenderness, decreased motion
  2) same radiologic picture bilaterally, with asymptomatic lesions

- **Radiologic features**
  1) patchy or homogenous sclerosis of the navicular
  2) collapse and fragmentation
  3) joint spaces preserved
  4) bone scan helps differentiate growth variation from ischemic necrosis

VII. Panner's Disease

- **General considerations**
  1) skeletal site: elbow, in humeral capitellum
  2) incidence: almost exclusively males, 4–10 years old
  3) nature of lesion
     - caused by repetitive trauma
     - associated with pitching or throwing activities

- **Clinical presentation**
  1) local pain, swelling
  2) stiffness, flexion contracture

- **Radiologic features**
  1) sequential sclerosis, fissuring, fragmentation, collapse, and reossification

2) entire epiphysis involved

3) enlarged radial head caused by hyperemia

4) possible premature closure of the physis

5) infrequently, similar lesions in trochlear epiphysis

- **Differential considerations**

    1) osteochondritis dissecans: only a small, local site on the capitellum involved, rather than entire epiphysis

VIII. Preiser's Disease

- **General considerations**

    1) skeletal site: scaphoid

    2) nature of lesion

        - at first believed to be ischemic necrosis not associated with fracture

        - now recognized as caused by ununited fracture of scaphoid

- **Radiologic features**

    1) proximal pole or entire scaphoid necrotic

    2) often, an ununited fracture line

12. Epiphyseal Traumatic Injuries

☞

a) Osgood-Schlatter's disease

- **General considerations**

    1) nature of lesion

        - tendinitis, caused by trauma or repetitive microtrauma

        - may involve partial disruption of patellar ligament attachment

        - self-limiting, but painful and disabling

    2) skeletal location

        - tibial tubercle, at patellar tendon insertion

        - bilateral in up to 50% of cases

    3) incidence

        - adolescents between 11–15 years of age

        - male predilection

    4) treatment: symptom relief via limiting stress to area, brace

- **Clinical presentation**

    1) antecedent history: single violent injury, or activity requiring repetitive knee flexion and extension

    2) local pain, tenderness, soft tissue swelling

    3) pain exacerbated by contracting quadriceps against resistance

    4) recurrent, chronic course, usually resolving with maturation

- **Pathologic features**
  1) inflammation at distal patellar tendon insertion:
     - increased cellularity and vascularity
     - intratendinous fibrocartilage
     - edema of chronic inflammation
  2) cartilage, bone, or both may be displaced
  3) heterotopic new bone: forms in inflamed patellar ligament
- **Radiologic features**
  1) optimal view: lateral
     - done bilaterally for comparison
     - done once with high kVp and once with low kVp on each knee (for optimal assessment of soft tissue as well as osseous elements)
     - about 5° internal rotation of leg to place tuberosity in profile
  2) soft tissue
     - displaced overlying skin contour (swelling of edema)
     - thickened patellar ligament, poorly defined margins
     - infrapatellar fat-pad: blurred margin, increased density; may be obliterated at inferior angle
  3) bone
     - isolated, irregular ossicles toward anterior margin of tuberosity
     - anterior surface irregularities: possible chondro-osseous avulsion
     - after healing: persisting ossicles usually asymptomatic
     - possible complicating factors: genu recurvatum and patella alta
     - some residual osseous deformity to be expected

 b) Scheuermann's disease (synonyms: vertebral epiphysitis, juvenile kyphosis, osteochondrosis juvenilis dorsi)
- **General characteristics**
  1) nature of lesions: currently favored suspected etiology—traumatic growth arrest and Schmorl's nodes (endplate fractures) during adolescent growth period
  2) skeletal site: middle and lower thoracic vertebrae
  3) incidence
     - slight male predominance
     - patients usually 13 to 17 years old
     - increased familial incidence
     - as much as 8% of general population affected

4) treatment
  - reduction of weight-bearing stress by restricting activities while disease is active
  - supportive bracing

- **Clinical presentation**
  1) postural effects
     - increased thoracic kyphosis
     - increased cervical and lumbar lordoses
     - increased anterior pelvic tilt
  2) in some cases: mild scoliosis
  3) protuberant abdomen
  4) mobility in intersegmental extension reduced almost to fixation
  5) tenderness to palpation or percussion on spinous processes
  6) reduced range of motion and reduced strength in trunk extension
  7) asymptomatic, or with pain and fatigue

- **Pathologic features**
  1) mechanism not clear, several suggested
     - secondary ring epiphysis avascular necrosis
     - low-grade infection
     - deformity secondary to disc extrusion
     - hereditary
     - vitamin deficiency or malnutrition
     - endocrine abnormalities
     - muscle imbalance
     - osteoporosis
     - traumatic disc extrusion with growth inhibition (current theory)
  2) discovertebral junction shows histologic abnormalities
     - thinning, foci of degeneration in cartilaginous growth plate
     - subsequent herniation of disc substance into adjacent vertebral body
     - vertical growth potential inhibited
     - growth plate adjacent to herniation displaced anteriorly
     - vertebra sagittally elongated
     - herniated material may separate peripheral ring epiphysis from vertebral body ("*limbus bone*")
  3) no evidence of osteonecrosis
  4) pathologic picture: multiple Schmorl's nodes, anterior vertebral body wedging, irregular endplates,

loss of disc height, thickened, contracted anterior longitudinal ligament

5) occasionally: osseous fusion across intervertebral disc spaces

- **Radiologic features**

1) 5° or more of anterior wedging in at least three contiguous segments: trapezoidal vertebrae due to inhibited anterior development

2) reduced disc height, most severe anteriorly

3) irregular endplates: multiple Schmorl's nodes, usually in anterior two thirds of vertebral body (may resemble infectious process)

4) increased kyphosis, > 40° (most thoracic, some thoracolumbar)

5) possible *"limbus bones"* (also called *"Scheuermann's ossicle"*)

6) possible anterior interbody fusion

7) sagittal elongation of vertebral bodies, with increased anterior concavity

8) mild scoliosis

9) additionally: spondylolysis and degenerative changes
   - disease centered in thoracolumbar spine: early L4 and L5 degenerative changes
   - sometimes termed *"juvenile discogenic disease"*

10) about 25% of cases have persistent venous channels: thin linear lucencies parallel to endplates in center of vertebral bodies

Schmorl's Nodes Seen in
"SHOOT"
Scheuermann's disease
Hyperparathyroidism
Osteoporosis
Osteomalacia
Trauma

c) **Osteochondritis dissecans**
- **General considerations**

1) nature of lesions
   - etiology unknown
   - small, localized necrotic segment of subchondral bone
   - may heal, or may separate and form intraarticular loose body
   - no inflammation: condition more appropriately termed *"osteochondrosis dissecans"*

2) skeletal location
   - most common in knee: lateral aspect of medial condyle
   - occurs at inferior aspect of lateral condyle, medial patellar facet
   - hip: femoral head
   - ankle: lateral and medial aspects of the talus
   - foot: metatarsal head (rare)
   - shoulder: humeral head (rare)

- elbow: capitellum
- wrist: proximal pole of scaphoid (rare)
- temporomandibular joint (rare)
3) incidence
   - usually between ages 11–20 years
   - male predominance
   - at talus, frequent in active individuals between 20–40 years
   - at elbow, capitellar lesions in children who do repetitive, forceful throwing
4) treatment
   - varies with site and symptom severity
   - may require surgical excision of fragment, curettage

- **Clinical presentation**
  1) sometimes entirely asymptomatic
  2) sometimes acute pain
  3) joint effusion
  4) painful joint motion, clicking, locking
  5) tenderness over site of lesion
  6) sometimes familial history (especially: knee lesions in short people)

- **Pathologic features**
  1) mechanical forces involved: shearing, rotatory, or tangential force upon cartilage and subchondral bone
  2) furrow or defect in cartilage (< 2 cm)
  3) lesion may adhere to underlying bone
  4) may have fragmentation of sequestered segment
  5) loose body may be cartilage or osteochondral (cartilage and bone)
  6) overlying cartilage viable, but separated fragment necrotic
  7) site of origin covered with fibrous tissue: surface osseous metaplasia and peripheral deposition
  8) fibrous and fibrocartilaginous tissue between loose body and adjacent bone
  9) resolution: loose body may
     - reattach (if remaining *in situ*)
     - displace and embed in synovium
     - displace and remain free in joint cavity ("*joint mouse*")
     - continue to grow via cartilage growth and calcification
     - be completely resorbed

- **Radiologic features**
  1) fragment *in situ*: opposed and

aligned with small cortical defect marking its site of origin; separated from defect by arclike lucent cleft

2) displaced fragment may be visible, or may resorb; concave defect remains at site of origin

3) sequestered, necrotic fragment: dense, elliptical opacity

4) sclerotic, concave border marks defect at site of origin

5) osteochondritis dissecans at the femoral condyles
   - 30% of cases bilateral
   - 85% affect lateral aspect of medial condyle
   - 15% at weight-bearing surface of lateral condyle
   - required views: AP, tunnel, and lateral projections
   - at site of origin
     a. concave femoral defect < 2 cm
     b. sclerotic margin may be frayed, irregular
     c. later, defect remodels, becomes shallower
   - at zone of interposition between origin and fragment:
     a. lucent arc (with *in situ* fragment, may be very thin)
     b. CT may be required to see very small cleft
     c. can demonstrate attachment, or lack thereof
   - at sequestered fragment
     a. oval opacity
     b. margin smooth, irregular, or even laminated
     c. matrix sclerotic and fragmented, or with normal density and architecture
     d. may be mobile within joint, removed from site of origin
   - secondary degenerative joint disease:
     a. premature onset
     b. high incidence of additional loose bodies
     c. involves all three joint compartments of the knee

6) osteochondritis dissecans at the talus
   - lateral and medial talar dome: most common sites
   - views must include AP, 30° oblique, and lateral projections
   - optimal AP view: foot in plantar flexion

- lesions at medial talar dome
  a. most common talar site; mechanism is inversion, combined with rotation and plantar flexion
  b. posterior lip of tibia separates fragment from medial posterior talar dome
  c. 2–5 mm excavation at medial corner of talar dome
  d. may be no cavity, but 2–5 mm cystic lucency
  e. fragment: small flake, not easily visible
- lesions at lateral talar dome
  a. mechanism: inversion compressing talus against fibula
  b. disruption of lateral collateral ligaments correlates with greater probability of displaced fragment
  c. depression, or cystic lucency (1–2 mm)
  d. wafer thin fragment may not be visible

7) lesions at the hip
   - superior weight-bearing surface of femoral head
   - lucent concave defect visible
   - Legg-Calvé-Perthes disease: may predispose to hip osteochondritis dissecans about 8 years after onset

8) lesions at the patella
   - rare, but most often at medial facet
   - axial (sunrise) and lateral projections optimal
   - lateral view: concave defect adjacent to the convexity of the femoral condyle
   - may involve single or multiple fragments

9) lesions in the foot
   - most often in first or second metatarsal head
   - dorsiplantar view optimal
   - small, cuplike lucent depression, 1–3 mm, at apex of convex articular surface

10) lesions at the shoulder
    - humeral head: small separated subchondral fragment at convex margin, opposed to glenoid cavity
    - may precede complete epiphyseal ischemic necrosis

- after anterior dislocation: small subchondral fragment from impact of humeral head on inferior glenoid rim ("*Hill-Sachs lesion*")
11) lesions at the elbow
    - usually at capitellum
    - cystic lucency on convex surface
    - fragment may displace distal to capitellar defect, become more symptomatic
12) lesions at the wrist
    - proximal pole of scaphoid
    - very rare
13) lesions at the temporomandibular joint
    - also a rarely affected site
    - fragment usually entirely cartilaginous
    - calcified fragment sometimes visible on plain film
    - MRI optimal for definitive diagnosis

- **Differential considerations**
    1) at femoral condyles, normal variations in ossification in patients 4–12 years old: simulate osteochondritis dissecans
    2) epiphyseal growth variants: major differential concern

d) Blount's disease
   - **General considerations**
      1) skeletal site: medial proximal tibial epiphysis
      2) incidence: two age cohorts identified
         - infantile (1–3 years)
            a. 5 times more common than adolescent type
            b. commonly bilateral
         - adolescent (8 to 15 years)
            a. may begin as early as 3 years of age
            b. unilateral presentation
      3) nature of lesion
         - infantile: possibly caused by compression inhibition of growth plate development
         - adolescent most likely secondary to traumatic growth inhibition

☞

   - **Radiologic features**
      1) infantile form
         - medial epiphysis wedge shaped, fragmented, or absent
         - adjacent metaphysis depressed
         - medially-oriented, osteopenic, beaklike metaphyseal protuberance

2) adolescent form
- medial tibial epiphysis wedge shaped
- growth plate locally narrowed
- diaphysis angulated medially

e) Diaz's disease
- **General considerations**
    1) skeletal site: body of talus (beneath tibiotalar articulation)
    2) nature of lesion
        - posttraumatic necrosis, usually 1–3 months after fractures of the talar neck, or dislocations
        - induced by oral corticosteroid therapy
- **Radiologic features**
    1) articular surface collapse
    2) patchy lucency
    3) increased density
    4) secondary avascular necrosis less likely when there is:
        - talar disuse osteoporosis simultaneous with osteoporosis in other bones
        - early formation of a subarticular lucent band ("*Hawkin's sign*")

f) Kummel's disease
- **General considerations**
    1) skeletal site: vertebral body
    2) nature of lesion
        - complete collapse of vertebral body
        - posttraumatic: believed secondary to additional trauma or due to unrecognized fracture
        - other possible causes suggested: nutritional, vascular, or healing abnormalities
- **Radiologic features**
    1) several weeks after trauma: rapid, severe vertebral body compression
    2) usually without intravertebral vacuum cleft sign, which would suggest ischemic necrosis

g) Sinding-Larsen-Johansson disease
- **General considerations**
    1) skeletal site: inferior pole of the patella
    2) incidence: usually in males between 10–14 years old
    3) nature of lesion
        - traction-avulsion of inferior pole developmental nucleus
        - posttraumatic patellar ligament ossification

- may coexist with Osgood-Schlatter's disease
- **Clinical presentation**
  1) pain and tenderness
  2) soft tissue swelling
  3) limping; inability to run
  4) usually resolves within 1 year
- **Radiologic features**
  1) bone fragments adjacent to inferior patellar pole
  2) overlying soft tissue swelling
  3) resolution: fragments remain as free ossicles or are incorporated into patella

13. **Epiphyseal Growth Variants and Miscellaneous Conditions**

   a) **General considerations**
   - nature of lesions: conditions which have been erroneously attributed to ischemic necrosis
   - skeletal sites: almost any epiphysis

   b) Specific entities

   I. **Calvé's Disease**

   a) **General considerations**
   - skeletal site: vertebral body
   - incidence: children
   - nature of lesion
     1) collapsed vertebral body
     2) Calvé believed this was caused by avascular necrosis
     3) lesion proven to be eosinophilic granuloma: term should be eliminated

   b) **Radiologic features**
   - single vertebral body, uniformly compressed, uniform density
   - *"coin-on-end vertebra"*, *"silver dollar vertebra"*, *"wafer thin vertebra"*, *"vertebra plana"*
   - see also Chapter 8 (section B, metabolic disorders; #4, Histiocytosis X; specific entity III) for further discussion of eosinophilic granuloma

   II. **Sever's Disease**

   a) **General considerations**
   - skeletal site: calcaneal apophysis
   - nature of lesion
     1) normal developmental variant
     2) several nuclei of ossification during years between ages 4 and 10
     3) may evidence heel pain
   - still sometimes used: term *Sever's disease* should be eliminated

---

Causes of Vertebra Plana

"FETISH"

Fracture
Eosinophilic granuloma
Tumor (metastatic or myeloma)
Infection
Steroids
Hemangioma

    b) **Radiologic features**
- fragmented, irregular sclerotic calcaneal apophysis
- calcaneal apophysis normally very dense

III. **Van Neck's Disease**

    a) **General considerations**
- skeletal site: ischiopubic synchondrosis
- nature of lesion: normal developmental variant, not osteonecrosis

    b) **Radiologic features**
- irregular adjacent ends of ischium and inferior pubic ramus
- simulates expansile destruction of bone
- usually bilateral and asymmetric

REVIEW—STUDY QUESTIONS

1. What epiphyseal condition may be seen at the knee simultaneously with Osgood-Schlatter's disease?

2. What is the skeletal site of Panner's disease, and who is most likely to get it?

3. Explain what "Calvé's disease" really is, and describe its appearance on plain film.

4. What etiologies have been suggested for Scheuermann's disease, and which is currently most favored?

5. What is "Hawkin's sign", and what is its significance?

6. What is Blount's disease? Is it only found in one joint?

7. Where does "Sever's disease" occur, and why should the name be eliminated?

8. What age cohorts are vulnerable to Blount's disease? How do the manifestations of this condition differ between the two cohorts?

9. In the wrist, where is osteochondritis dissecans most likely to occur?

10. Generally, which gender and age group are most likely to suffer from osteochondritis dissecans?

1. When radiologic findings in a child between 2 and 5 years old include lucent submetaphyseal bands, the differential diagnoses should include (among others):

   a) thalassemia, hemophilia, and lymphocytic leukemia.
   b) leukemia, syphilis, and hemophilia.
   c) hemophilia, neuroblastoma, and leukemia.
   d) lymphocytic leukemia, scurvy, and neuroblastoma.

2. Gout, pancreatitis, hemoglobinopathy, collagen diseases, Caisson disease, Gaucher's disease, alcoholism, trauma, and treatment with corticosteroids or radiation therapy may all predispose a patient to:

   a) hyperparathyroidism.
   b) renal osteodystrophy.
   c) osteonecrosis.
   d) hypophosphatasia.

3. A male patient, aged 7, reports pain in the anteromedial knee and vague groin pain. This is a typical presentation for:

   a) thalassemia.
   b) leukemia.
   c) Osgood-Schlatter's disease.
   d) Legg-Calvé-Perthes disease.

4. Blount's disease is most commonly seen in:

   a) infants, 1–3 years of age.
   b) children, 3–7 years of age.
   c) adolescents, 8–15 years of age.
   d) adolescents and young adults, 15–20 years of age.

5. Scheuermann's disease is believed to affect:

   a) up to 8% of the general population between 13–17 years of age.
   b) up to 25% of the general population < 15 years of age.
   c) up to 5% of the general population < 15 years of age.
   d) up to 3% of the general population between 13–17 years of age.

6. "Megacondyle," seen in tubercular arthritis, is more commonly an x-ray sign of:

   a) suppurative osteomyelitis.
   b) leukemia or sickle cell anemia.
   c) Still's disease, or hemophilia.
   d) thalassemia, or hypervitaminosis A.

7. The most commonly seen radiologic sign of acquired syphilis is:

   a) saber shin appearance due to cortical thickening.
   b) proliferative periostitis (solid or laminated, and sometimes lacelike).
   c) cortical lytic lesions caused by pressure erosion by gummata.
   d) medullary lytic lesions caused by pressure erosion by gummata.

8. Tom Smith's arthritis is:

   a) a variety of spinal osteomyelitis.
   b) septic arthritis in joints in which the metaphysis is within the joint capsule.
   c) a variety of septic arthritis in the spine.
   d) a variety of non-suppurative discitis.

9. The effects of sickle cell anemia in the skull are radiographically demonstrated only:

   a) in the occiput.
   b) in the frontal bone.
   c) below the external occipital protuberance.
   d) above the internal occipital protuberance.

10. A chronic, low-grade, diffuse, nonpurulent osteomyelitis, Garré's sclerosing osteomyelitis is seen on x-ray as:

    a) a lytic destructive lesion, with a sequestrum.
    b) a lytic destructive lesion, with no sequestrum.
    c) cortical disruption with minimal reactive new bone formation.
    d) exuberant cortical fusiform bone thickening, with significant reactive new bone formation.

11. The ballooned epiphyses (megacondyle) and attenuated, squared inferior pole of the patella in a young patient are common characteristics of:

    a) sickle-cell anemia and thalassemia major.
    b) thalassemia major and hemophilia.
    c) juvenile rheumatoid arthritis (JRA) and hemophilia.
    d) childhood leukemia and hemophilia.

12. A "chain" of dense, round or oval, well-marginated opacities on an x-ray, located along the upper margin of the superior pubic ramus, is most likely to be:

    a) undissolved calcium tablets.
    b) phleboliths.
    c) arteriolosclerosis in the internal iliac artery.
    d) a calcified chain of lymph nodes.

13. Bilateral involvement of Legg-Calvé-Perthes disease:

    a) rarely occurs in females.
    b) rarely occurs in males.
    c) does not occur.
    d) occurs in most cases.

14. Osteochondritis dissecans at the talus most commonly involves:

    a) the talar neck.
    b) the talonavicular articulation.
    c) the talocalcaneal articulation.
    d) medial talar dome.

15. Osgood-Schlatter's disease is:

    a) avascular necrosis of the tibial tuberosity.
    b) avulsion fracture of the tibial tuberosity.
    c) mycotic osteomyelitis at the tibial tuberosity.
    d) tendinitis at the tibial insertion of the patellar tendon.

16. Tubercular arthritis causes a constellation of typical radiographic signs known as:

    a) the 1–2-3 sign.
    b) "Phemister's triad."
    c) "TRY-7."
    d) "The Six Ds."

17. Bilateral "saber shin" bowing is a radiologic sign characteristic of:

    a) the metaphysitis phase of congenital syphilis.
    b) Paget's disease.
    c) tubercular osteitis.
    d) the osteitis phase of congenital syphilis.

18. A toddler who has become uncharacteristically irritable, runs a low-grade fever, and refuses to walk, stand, or sit, should be examined to rule out:

    a) Wilm's tumor.
    b) leukemia.
    c) congenital syphilis.
    d) childhood inflammatory discitis.

19. Radiologically, the effects of sickle-cell anemia on the small tubular bones of the hands and the feet may simulate:

    a) osteomyelitis.
    b) hypertrophic arthropathy.
    c) neurotrophic arthropathy.
    d) Tom Smith's arthritis.

20. Skeletally, Brodie's abscess shows a predilection for:

    a) the radius.
    b) the fibula.
    c) the femur.
    d) the tibia.

21. Long-standing hemophilic arthropathy produces effects that simulate:

    a) neurotrophic arthropathy.
    b) rheumatoid arthritis.
    c) psoriatic arthropathy.
    d) septic arthritis.

22. Low back pain that is exacerbated by lying supine may indicate the presence of:

    a) myelofibrosis.
    b) leukemia.
    c) abdominal aortic aneurysm.
    d) metastatic bone disease.

23. The peak incidence of Legg-Calvé-Perthes disease occurs in the age group:

    a) 1–5 years.
    b) 5–7 years.
    c) 12–15 years.
    d) 14–18 years.

24. The radiographic appearance of osteochondritis dissecans may include any of the following features except:

    a) a concave defect in the mother bone, and a thin, arclike lucent cleft between the mother bone and the displaced fragment.
    b) a dense, elliptical opacity, representing a sequestered, necrotic fragment.
    c) a thin, onion-skin periosteal response.
    d) a frayed, irregular, sclerotic, concave border at the site of origin in the mother bone.

25. Panner's disease, occurring almost exclusively in 4- to 10-year-old males, is:

    a) osteonecrosis of the calcaneus, caused by repetitive trauma of running and jumping.
    b) osteonecrosis of the talus, caused by repetitive trauma of running and jumping.
    c) osteonecrosis of the humeral capitellum, caused by repetitive trauma of throwing or pitching.
    d) osteonecrosis of the lateral humeral condyle, caused by repetitive trauma of throwing or pitching.

26. Tubercular arthritis is usually:

    a) polyarticular, with symmetric distribution bilaterally.
    b) polyarticular, with asymmetric bilateral distribution.
    c) pauciarticular, with monomelic distribution.
    d) monoarticular.

27. "Wimberger's sign" is:

    a) an increased distance between the medial margin of the femoral head and the lateral margin of Kohler's teardrop.
    b) symmetrical erosions in the medial surfaces of the proximal tibiae.
    c) broadened, discolored appearance of the epiphyseal line in infants dying from hereditary syphilis.
    d) loss of the knee jerk in tabes dorsalis.

28. Epidural abscess is optimally imaged by:

    a) MRI.
    b) myelography.
    c) scintigraphy.
    d) contrast CT.

29. Typical effects of sickle-cell anemia on vertebral bodies include:

    a) central body bulging ("barrel-shaped vertebra"), "corduroy cloth" vertical striations due to accentuation of vertical trabeculae, and thinning of the cortices.
    b) thinned, prominent cortices, anterior notching of the central vertebral bodies (enlarged anterior vascular notch), and generalized osteopenia.
    c) central endplate depressions (fish vertebra), transient vertebral body collapse, prominent osteoporosis.

d) silver-dollar vertebrae; thickened, sclerotic cortices; vertically striated vertebral bodies.

30. Brodie's abscess shows a predilection for:

    a) adolescent females.
    b) young adult males.
    c) male children.
    d) obese females.

31. The "pseudotumors" of hemophilia are caused by:

    a) intraosseous hemorrhage acting as a space-occupying lesion.
    b) sequestered infectious foci.
    c) engorged and calcified lymph nodes.
    d) paraspinal abscesses.

32. The most common site of aortic aneurysm is:

    a) in the ascending aorta.
    b) below the renal arteries.
    c) in the aortic arch.
    d) between the diaphragm and the renal arteries.

33. Adult avascular necrosis (spontaneous osteonecrosis) at the mature femoral head is probably precipitated by occlusion of:

    a) the profunda femoris artery.
    b) the foveal vessels.
    c) the lateral circumflex vessels from the profunda femoris.
    d) the medial circumflex vessels from the profunda femoris.

34. The loose body typical of osteochondritis dissecans:

    a) must be surgically removed.
    b) may undergo malignant degeneration.
    c) may be completely resorbed, may reattach, or may become a "joint mouse."
    d) continues to grow because it is composed of viable bone.

35. Ischemic necrosis or a normal growth variation may be responsible for alterations at the tarsal navicular, called:

    a) Hass's disease.
    b) Blount's disease.
    c) Kohler's disease.
    d) Kummel's disease.

36. In the earlier stages of Pott's disease, spinal films usually show:

    a) mild to moderate loss of disc space, and endplate disruption.
    b) anterior vertebral body "gouge defects," with little or no disc space loss.
    c) rarefaction of the entire vertebral body, with little or no disc space loss.
    d) superoanterior vertebral body cortical disruption with moderate disc space loss.

37. VDRL is a screening test for:

    a) HIV infection.
    b) previous exposure to tuberculosis.

c) active tuberculosis infection.
d) syphilis.

38. Spinal infection in children or adolescents is most likely to seed first:

    a) in the vertebral endplate.
    b) in subperiosteal bone of the anterosuperior vertebral body.
    c) in the intervertebral disc.
    d) in subarachnoid vascular structures.

39. Sickle cell anemia is:

    a) always symptomatic, but shortens the life-span only in those who are homozygous for the trait.
    b) inevitably a life-shortening condition, although it is markedly more symptomatic in homozygous individuals.
    c) symptomatic only during a "sickle-cell crisis."
    d) asymptomatic, except in homozygous individuals.

40. Brodie's abscess is a localized form of:

    a) suppurative osteomyelitis.
    b) septic arthritis.
    c) nonsuppurative osteomyelitis
    d) mycotic osteomyelitis.

41. Christmas disease is:

    a) a synonym for thalassemia minor.
    b) a synonym for hemophilia B, lack of clotting factor IX.
    c) a synonym for hemophilia A, lack of clotting factor VIII.
    d) a synonym for thalassemia intermedia.

42. The aneurysm that shows a 3:1 predilection for women in patients younger than 50, is the:

    a) aortic arch aneurysm.
    b) renal artery aneurysm.
    c) splenic artery aneurysm.
    d) carotid artery aneurysm.

43. Three to twelve months after radiation therapy, radiation necrosis may be visible on plain film as:

    a) patchy sclerosis, moth-eaten destruction, and periostitis.
    b) lytic medullary lesions with "popcorn calcifications," and thickened, expanded cortices.
    c) lytic cortical lesions, and widened medullary canals with thickened, irregular trabecular patterns.
    d) "licked candy stick" resorption of the articular ends of bones, and calcified articular cartilage.

44. Active individuals between 20 and 40 years of age are most likely to develop osteochondritis dissecans:

    a) at the knee.
    b) at the shoulder.
    c) at the talus.
    d) at the elbow.

45. Kienboch's disease shows a predilection:

    a) for females (5:1) age 12–18 years.
    b) for females (3:1) age 20–40 years.
    c) for males (9:1) age 20–40 years.
    d) for males (2:1) age 15–20 years.

46. A draining sinus from a psoas abscess may surface paraspinally, in an inguinal area, or near the lesser trochanter, and is called:

    a) empyema necessitatis.
    b) Weaver's bottom.
    c) Pott's puffy tumor.
    d) spina ventosa.

47. Endarteritis obliterans is caused by:

    a) *Actinomyces israelii.*
    b) *Treponema pallidum.*
    c) *Aspergillus.*
    d) *Mycobacterium tuberculosis.*

48. Depending on the site of infection, the radiographic latent period for osteomyelitis may be:

    a) up to 6 months.
    b) 10 to 21 days.
    c) up to 7 days.
    d) up to 3 days.

49. Sickle cell anemia almost exclusively affects:

    a) northern European and Scandinavian populations.
    b) Central and South American populations.
    c) Asian and Australasian populations.
    d) Mediterranean and black populations.

50. The most common pathogen (90% of cases) causing suppurative osteomyelitis is:

    a) *Diplococcus pneumoniae.*
    b) *Klebsiella.*
    c) *Streptococcus.*
    d) *Staphylococcus aureus.*

51. The patient population most frequently seen with osteochondritis dissecans at the knee is:

    a) adolescent.
    b) geriatric.
    c) pediatric.
    d) middle-aged.

52. Caisson's disease affects the shoulders and hips bilaterally, appearing on plain film as:

    a) medullary pseudotumors and soft tissue masses.
    b) endosteal scalloping of subarticular cortical bone.
    c) epiphyseal and metaphyseal/diaphyseal infarcts, and secondary degenerative joint disease.
    d) diffuse osteopenia, and softening of bone with bowing of weight-bearing bones.

53. The two most common causes of aneurysm are atherosclerosis and:

    a) infection (mycotic aneurysm).
    b) syphilis.

    c) arteritis.
    d) diabetes.

54. "Rodent facies," with upper incisors displaced forward, is characteristic of:

    a) gargoylism.
    b) fetal alcohol syndrome.
    c) thalassemia.
    d) Hurler's syndrome.

55. Tubercular spondylitis may be differentiated radiographically from mycotic osteomyelitis because:

    a) TB does not exhibit calcification of paravertebral abscesses.
    b) TB often causes vertebral collapse, which is not characteristic of mycotic osteomyelitis.
    c) TB does not affect the intervertebral discs.
    d) TB does not involve prominent sclerosis, which is characteristic of mycotic infections.

56. *Condyloma lata* and *alopecia areata* are secondary clinically evident lesions of:

    a) syphilis.
    b) tuberculosis.
    c) tuberous sclerosis.
    d) systemic lupus erythematosus.

57. Pott's disease is most commonly seen at:

    a) T1 and T2.
    b) T6-T8.
    c) L1.
    d) L4-S1.

58. Freiberg's disease is epiphyseal osteonecrosis at:

    a) the humeral head.
    b) the calcaneus.
    c) the second or third metatarsal head.
    d) the lunate.

59. The involucrum seen in osteomyelitis is:

    a) a collar of new bone walling off an infection.
    b) a defect in the "wall" around the infection, allowing it to drain.
    c) a necrotic bone fragment, isolated from normal bone.
    d) an ulceration into a fibrous "wall" around an infection.

60. Epiphyseal disorders that affect the spine include:

    a) Kummel's disease and Scheuermann's disease.
    b) Diaz's disease and Panner's disease.
    c) Mauclaire's disease and Scheuermann's disease.
    d) Calvé's disease and Mauclaire's disease.

61. Osteochondritis dissecans:

    a) is due to mycotic infection.
    b) is not associated with inflammation.
    c) is an inflammatory arthritide.
    d) is most often caused by *Staphylococcus aureus.*

62. The site most commonly affected by spontaneous osteonecrosis of the knee (SONK) is:
    a) the medial tibial condyle.
    b) the medial femoral condyle
    c) the lateral femoral condyle.
    d) the superolateral pole of the patella.

63. The third most frequently calcified abdominal artery is:
    a) the renal artery.
    b) the splenic artery.
    c) the hepatic artery.
    d) the iliac artery.

64. The long bones of children with thalassemia display:
    a) narrowed, undertubulated metaphyses, shortening, with growth arrest lines.
    b) general osteopenia, narrowed metaphyses with thin cortices, and repeated pathologic fractures.
    c) shortening, with growth arrest lines, and Erlenmeyer flask deformity.
    d) Erlenmeyer flask deformity, and elongation with thinned cortices.

65. The most common site for mycotic osteomyelitis due to Actinomycosis is:
    a) the proximal femur.
    b) L1, caused by hematogenous spread via Batson's plexus.
    c) the ribs and sternum, via lymphogenous spread.
    d) the mandible, at the angle of the jaw.

66. Clutton's joints and Hutchinson's teeth are clinical indications of:
    a) gargoylism.
    b) congenital syphilis.
    c) epiphyseal dysplasia multiplex.
    d) rickets.

67. Pott's puffy tumor appears as:
    a) a "button sequestrum" with a fluctuant cold abscess in the scalp.
    b) a lucent geographic lesion in the calvarium with an "eggshell" rim of sclerosis.
    c) a moth-eaten calvarial lesion with a thick rind of sclerosis.
    d) a cortical lesion in the outer table of the calvarium, with spiculated periosteal response.

68. Freiberg's disease affects adolescents, with a:
    a) 5:1 male predilection.
    b) 2:1 male predilection.
    c) 2:1 female predilection.
    d) 5:1 female predilection.

69. Sequestra are:
    a) collars of new bone walling off an infection.
    b) defects in the "wall" around the infection, allowing it to drain.
    c) necrotic bone fragments isolated from normal bone.
    d) ulcerations into a fibrous "wall" around an infection.

70. A radiologic sign that suggests a favorable prognosis in Diaz's disease is:
    a) Hawkin's sign.
    b) Wimberger's sign.
    c) Klein's sign.
    d) Rim's sign.

71. Scheuermann's ossicle is a synonym for:
    a) an unfused spinous process.
    b) a teardrop fracture.
    c) a limbus bone.
    d) a nuchal bone.

72. Longitudinal splitting of cortical bone is a feature of:
    a) osteochondritis dissecans.
    b) a medullary osteonecrotic infarct.
    c) hypertrophic pulmonary osteoarthropathy.
    d) metaphyseal/diaphyseal cortical infarction.

73. The "thumbnail sign" is a radiographic finding signifying:
    a) chondrocalcinosis at the humeral head, with CPPD.
    b) the cortical rim of an unfused apophysis, usually a spinous process.
    c) a ring of calcification in the transverse aortic arch, with arteriosclerosis.
    d) the small bulge of bone at the site of a torus (incomplete) fracture.

74. "Fish vertebra" are characteristic of:
    a) Cushing's syndrome, sickle-cell anemia, and Gaucher's disease.
    b) Gaucher's disease, Paget's disease, and thalassemia.
    c) thalassemia, sickle-cell anemia, and Gaucher's disease.
    d) congenital syphilis, Gaucher's disease, and Cushing's syndrome.

75. "Desert rheumatism," with symptoms of conjunctivitis, arthritis, erythema nodosum, and respiratory infection, is:
    a) histoplasmosis.
    b) maduromycosis.
    c) actinomycosis.
    d) coccidioidomycosis.

76. The most common skeletal site for acquired syphilitic osteomyelitis is:
    a) the metaphyses of long tubular bones.
    b) the vertebral bodies.
    c) the skull, clavicles, and tibiae.
    d) the pelvic bones.

77. Tuberculous bursitis in subgluteal bursae is called:
    a) Cossack's disease.
    b) Weaver's bottom.

c) spina ventosa.
d) Pott's puffy tumor.

78. In addition to Waldenstrom's sign, radiographic evidence of Legg-Calvé-Perthes disease may include:

a) an abnormal Klein's line.
b) a curvilinear "crescent sign."
c) fraying of the metaphyseal margin.
d) medial and lateral buttressing on the femoral neck.

79. Sub-articular bone is not vulnerable to hematogenous seeding of osteomyelitis:

a) in neonates.
b) in children from about age 1 year until full growth is achieved.
c) in young and middle-aged adults.
d) in the geriatric population.

80. Blount's disease commonly has a radiographic appearance of:

a) a fragmented tibial tuberosity.
b) a fragmented lateral tibial epiphysis.
c) a wedge-shaped medial femoral epiphysis.
d) a wedge-shaped, sometimes fragmented medial tibial epiphysis.

81. Theories for the mechanism causing Scheuermann's disease include all of the following except:

a) avascular necrosis of the secondary ring epiphyses.
b) vitamin or mineral deficiencies.
c) traumatic disc extrusion with growth inhibition.
d) slow-growing, benign lytic neoplasm.

82. In epiphyseal osteonecrosis, a subchondral fracture, seen on plain film as a "rim sign" or "crescent sign":

a) represents the compacted bone of an impaction fracture.
b) represents an avulsion at the site of an enthesis.
c) represents the separation of the articular cortex from underlying cancellous bone.
d) represents the separation of the epiphysis from the physis.

83. The differential considerations, when the radiologic appearance suggests myelofibrosis should include (among others):

a) multiple myeloma, Paget's disease.
b) osteopoikilosis, hemophilia.
c) fluorosis, thalassemia.
d) Paget's disease, blastic metastasis.

84. Patients who have sickle-cell anemia are predisposed to *Salmonella* osteomyelitis with a unique distribution:

a) in the "S" joints of the axial skeleton.
b) in the carpal and tarsal bones, exclusively.
c) in a bilateral, symmetric, diaphyseal pattern.
d) in metaphyses of the small tubular bones of

hands and feet, with symmetric, bilateral distribution.

85. A chronic, granulomatous fungal disease of the foot is:

a) actinomycosis.
b) histoplasmosis.
c) maduromycosis.
d) coccidioidomycosis.

86. A common sequela of syphilitic infection is:

a) fibrous ankylosis.
b) empyema necessitatis.
c) Brodie's abscess.
d) neurotrophic arthropathy.

87. Tubercular infection in the spine (tubercular spondylitis) is called:

a) Tom Smith's arthritis.
b) Clutton's joints.
c) Pott's disease.
d) Maduromycosis.

88. Early identification of Legg-Calvé-Perthes disease is best accomplished via:

a) plain film.
b) ultrasonography.
c) scintigraphy and MRI.
d) CT.

89. The most common route of invasion for osteomyelitis is:

a) instrumentation (contaminated surgical sites).
b) puncture wounds or penetrating injuries (e.g., open fractures).
c) hematogenous spread of infection.
d) contiguous spread of infection (from dental, cutaneous, or sinus infections).

90. The likely etiology of Blount's disease is:

a) ischemic necrosis.
b) normal growth variant.
c) traumatic inhibition of growth plate development.
d) chronic, low-grade infection at the growth plate.

91. Scheuermann's disease is treated with:

a) surgical insertion of Harrington rods.
b) nutritional therapy, stretching, and specific exercises.
c) bracing and restriction of weight-bearing stresses.
d) massage, extension exercises, and light weight lifting.

92. Radiologic manifestations of epiphyseal infarction include all of the following except:

a) solid or laminated periosteal new bone formation.
b) articular cortical collapse in an angular defect or as a smooth undulation.
c) fragmentation of the entire epiphysis.
d) mottled bone caused by patchy sclerosis, thickened trabeculae, and subchondral cysts.

93. A clear association exists between chronic myelogenous leukemia and:

    a) hemophilia.
    b) thalassemia.
    c) myelofibrosis.
    d) systemic lupus erythematosus.

94. X-ray signs in the long tubular bones that suggest a diagnosis of sickle-cell anemia include:

    a) "bone within a bone" appearance, frayed metaphyses, "blade of grass" appearance.
    b) "asterisk sign" in the femoral head, "cupped metaphyses," and "Codman's triangle" of new bone.
    c) tibio-talar slant deformity, frayed metaphyses, and "crescent sign" in the femoral head
    d) "bone within a bone" appearance, "cupped metaphyses," and "asterisk sign" in the femoral head.

95. Metaphysitis is a characteristic of:

    a) tuberculous osteitis, scurvy, leukemia, and sickle cell anemia.
    b) leukemia, sickle cell anemia, metastatic neuroblastoma, and metastatic carcinoma.
    c) leukemia, scurvy, congenital syphilis, and metastatic neuroblastoma.
    d) scurvy, leukemia, sickle cell anemia, and congenital syphilis.

96. Patients with diagnosis of AIDS may have skeletal lesions due to:

    a) osteomyelitis, non-Hodgkin's lymphoma, or anemia (among others).
    b) the effects of the HIV infection itself.

    c) neuropathic arthropathy, if the disease is in late stages.
    d) they do not develop skeletal lesions, but have soft tissue lesions instead.

97. The earliest skeletal radiologic indication of septic arthritis is:

    a) subarticular geodes.
    b) laminated periosteal response, with cortical disruption.
    c) metaphyseal "moth-eaten" medullary lesions.
    d) loss of the subarticular white line (normal subchondral cortical bone).

98. The hip movements which usually exacerbate the pain of Legg-Calvé-Perthes disease are:

    a) hip adduction and external rotation.
    b) hip extension and adduction.
    c) hip abduction and internal rotation.
    d) hip flexion and adduction.

99. Middle-aged male patients who develop suppurative osteomyelitis are most often affected:

    a) in the spine.
    b) in the skull.
    c) in the pelvis.
    d) in the distal extremities, usually the tibia.

100. The joints vulnerable to "Tom Smith's arthritis" are:

    a) the "S" joints of the axial skeleton.
    b) "tightly packed" joints, such as the small joints of hands and feet.
    c) slightly movable joints, such as the symphysis pubis.
    d) the hip, knee, ankle, shoulder and elbow joints.

PRACTICE TEST CHAPTER 7—ANSWER KEY

1. d	11. c	21. a	31. a	41. b	51. a	61. b	71. c	81. d	91. c
2. c	12. b	22. c	32. b	42. c	52. c	62. b	72. d	82. c	92. a
3. d	13. a	23. b	33. c	43. a	53. a	63. b	73. c	83. d	93. c
4. a	14. d	24. c	34. c	44. c	54. c	64. c	74. c	84. c	94. d
5. a	15. d	25. c	35. c	45. c	55. b	65. d	75. d	85. c	95. c
6. c	16. b	26. d	36. b	46. a	56. a	66. b	76. c	86. d	96. a
7. b	17. d	27. b	37. d	47. b	57. c	67. a	77. b	87. c	97. d
8. b	18. d	28. a	38. c	48. b	58. c	68. d	78. b	88. c	98. c
9. d	19. a	29. c	39. d	49. d	59. a	69. c	79. b	89. c	99. a
10. d	20. d	30. c	40. a	50. d	60. a	70. a	80. d	90. c	100. d

Chapter 8

NUTRITIONAL, METABOLIC, AND ENDOCRINE DISORDERS

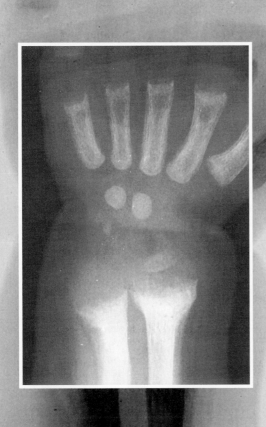

A. NUTRITIONAL DISORDERS

1. **Scurvy (synonyms: hypovitaminosis C, Barlow's disease)**

   a) **General considerations**
   - nature of condition: long-term vitamin C (ascorbic acid) deficiency
   - incidence
     1) infants (usually 8–14 months)
     2) elderly patients with inadequate nutrition
   - skeletal site: epiphyses of long bones
   - vitamin C therapy: reverses almost all findings

   b) **Clinical presentation**
   - infant fed on pasteurized or boiled milk formulas
   - elderly person with compromised diet
   - spontaneous hemorrhage caused by capillary fragility (**hallmark**)
     1) petechiae
     2) bleeding gums
     3) melena, hematuria
   - joint swelling and pain
   - irritability
   - tendency to lie supine and motionless with thighs abducted ("frog-leg" position)
   - bulging at costochondral junctions

   c) **Pathologic features and laboratory findings**
   - intercellular collagen, osteoid and endothelial linings friable
   - vascular fragility
   - inadequate proliferation of cartilage cells
   - inadequate osteoblastic activity
   - laboratory tests may show low serum ascorbic acid levels (< 0.6 mg/100 ml)

   d) **Radiologic features**
   - generalized osteopenia
     1) decreased bone density
     2) loss of trabecular definition
     3) thinned cortices
   - hyperdense metaphyseal zone of calcified cartilage
     1) "*White line of Frankel*"
     2) dense zone of provisional calcification
   - dense peripheral margin of epiphysis, with osteopenic central portion
     1) ring epiphysis
     2) "*Wimberger's sign*"
   - infractions of epiphyseal/metaphyseal junction
     1) cause irregular metaphyseal margins
     2) "*corner sign*," or "*angle sign*"
   - bony protuberances at metaphyseal margins

        1) at right angles to long axis of bone shaft

        2) *"Pelken's spur"*

- lucent band of disordered osteoid directly beneath zone of provisional calcification

        1) *"scorbutic zone"*

        2) *"Trümmerfeld zone"*

- subperiosteal hemorrhages; periosteal new bone forms with healing
- note: radiologic signs evident in infants; not apparent in adult patients
- residual of Frankel's line: growth arrest line visible after healing

2. **Hypervitaminoses**

    a) **General considerations**

- nature of lesions

        1) excessive vitamin A: extensive periosteal new bone formation

        2) excessive vitamin D: ectopic calcifications

- anatomic sites

        1) hypervitaminosis A

          - shafts of long bones, cranial sutures
          - skin and hair
          - liver

        2) hypervitaminosis D

          - blood vessel walls
          - kidneys
          - periarticular tissues

    b) **Clinical presentation**

- hypervitaminosis A

        1) dermatitis, pruritus, jaundiced skin

        2) alopecia

        3) hepatosplenomegaly

- hypervitaminosis D

        - nausea, anorexia
        - polyuria and polydipsia

    c) **Radiologic features**

- hypervitaminosis A

        1) solid, periosteal new bone along the shafts of long bones

        2) diastasis of cranial sutures (especially at the bregma)

- hypervitaminosis D

        1) extensive calcification in blood vessel walls

        2) periarticular calcifications

        3) calcifications in kidneys

3. **Heavy Metal Poisoning**

    a) **General considerations**

- lead, phosphorus, and bismuth: radiographically visible in the body

- lead poisoning: most frequent of these, but still rare
- lead ingested, inhaled, or implanted
- people working with polymerization of polyvinyl chloride (PVC) risk PVC poisoning

b) Clinical presentation
- sudden onset abdominal pain
- encephalopathy, paralysis

c) Radiologic features
- lead, phosphorus and bismuth: similar radiologic changes
- transverse linear sclerosis at metaphyses (*"lead lines"*)
- remodeling abnormalities at sites of metal deposition
- PVC poisoning: acroosteolysis

4. Fluorosis

a) General considerations
- fluorosis: chronic ingestion of fluorine
- used to reduce dental caries: excesses entail negative effects
  1) 1 ppm: reduced incidence of dental caries
  2) > 2 ppm: mottled tooth enamel
  3) 8 ppm: may cause osteosclerosis (10% of individuals)
  4) > 100 ppm: growth disturbances, kidney damage, death
- incidence
  1) endemic fluorosis in India, China, and some other areas because of heavily contaminated drinking water
  2) wine fluorosis, due to habitual intake of fluorine-containing wine
  3) industrial, laboratory exposures
  4) fluorine medications
- skeletal sites
  1) axial skeleton most noticeably
  2) less prominent findings in appendicular skeleton

b) Radiologic features
- initial osteopenia, followed by sclerosis
- growth arrest lines
- exuberant vertebral hyperostosis, spinal exostoses
- sacrotuberous and sacroiliac ligament calcification
- periostitis
- genu valgum

5. Rickets

a) General considerations
- nature of condition
  1) deficiency of vitamin D, calcium, or phosphorus

2) refractory rickets (vitamin D resistant rickets): caused by renal tubular defects; not responsive to supplementary vitamin D

3) renal rickets: with simultaneous hyperparathyroidism secondary to chronic renal disease

4) other causes: dietary deficiencies, inadequate sunlight exposure, intestinal malabsorption, metabolic defects, chronic acidosis, aluminum intoxication, chronic administration of anticonvulsants (Dilantin)

- incidence
   1) infants: 6–12 months of age
   2) rare in western countries
- skeletal sites
   1) growth plates, especially in long bones
   2) costochondral junctions
- treatment: usually administration of deficient nutrients

b) Clinical presentation
- muscle tetany
- irritability
- weakness
- delayed development and small stature
- bone deformities
- soft tissue swellings around growth plates
- costochondral bumps

c) Pathologic features
- rachitic bone has less calcified osteoid, and increased uncalcified osteoid ("*osteoid seams*")
- at physis, normal cartilage cells fail to calcify; degenerate
- physis fills with masses of overgrown cartilage
- metaphyseal osteoid does not mineralize either

d) Laboratory findings
- elevated serum alkaline phosphatase levels
- normal or slightly low serum calcium and phosphorus

e) Radiologic features
- general relative lucency of all bones
- coarsened trabecular patterns
- growth plate abnormalities
   1) "*paintbrush metaphysis*": widened growth plate with irregular, frayed and cupped metaphyseal margins (Fig. 8.1)
   2) absence of zone of provisional calcification
- frayed epiphyseal borders

Paintbrush Metaphysis

"CHARMS"

Congenital infections (syphilis, rubella)

Hypophosphatasia

Achondroplasia

Rickets

Metaphyseal dysostosis

Scurvy

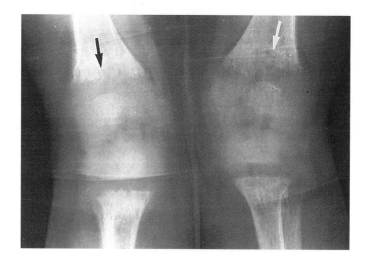

Figure 8.1.
Rickets: growth plate abnormalities in the knee.

- bowing deformities
- fractures and pseudofractures
- decreased length of bones
- scoliosis
- *"rachitic rosary"*: bulbous enlargement of costochondral junctions adjacent to cupped anterior rib ends
- pleural interface or thymic shadow indented by rachitic rosary

B. METABOLIC DISORDERS

1. Osteoporosis

a) General considerations

- nature of condition
  1) reduced **quantity** of normal quality bone
  2) generalized, regional, or localized
     - generalized
       a. majority of skeleton shows decreased bone density
       b. most commonly postmenopausal or senile osteoporosis
     - regional
       a. decreased bone density in one limb, or portion of a limb
       b. most commonly, disuse osteoporosis after injury
       c. Sudeck's atrophy: transient regional osteoporosis
     - localized
       a. focal bone density diminution
       b. with local disease, such as inflammatory arthritis, neoplasm, infection

- incidence
  1) most common metabolic bone disease
  2) generalized osteoporosis usually in elderly population
  3) regional or localized in any age cohort, depending on etiology
☞
- osteoporosis and osteopenia **not** synonymous
  1) *osteopenia*: denotes "poverty of bone," whether reduced **quantity** of bone or reduced **quality**, with normal quantity

X-RAY SIGN

b) Specific conditions

☞
I. **Senile and postmenopausal generalized osteoporosis**
   (synonyms: senile osteoporosis, senescent osteoporosis, old-age osteoporosis)

a) **General considerations**
   - nature of condition
     1) reduced bone quantity throughout much of the skeleton
     2) bone mass decreases after age 35 years
        - earlier and more rapidly in females:
          - 1% per year loss in cortical bone
          - loss of 20–40% by age 65
          - 2% per year loss of trabecular bone
          - with menopause, accelerated loss (to 6% per year in lumbar spine)
   - incidence
     1) 15–20 million Americans
     2) predilection for women (4:1) in patients 40–70 years old
     3) after age 80, ratio equalizes
   - skeletal site (in this case, most common site for fractures)
     1) spinal compression fractures, thoracic and lumbar vertebrae
     2) proximal femur (after age 60, incidence of hip fracture in females doubles every five years)
     3) ribs, humerus, radius
   - generalized osteoporosis is associated with
     1) congenital disorders
        - osteogenesis imperfecta
        - mucopolysaccharidoses
        - hemolytic anemias
        - idiopathic juvenile osteoporosis
     2) vascular disorders
        - sickle cell anemia
        - thalassemia

3) nutritional disorders
- scurvy
- rickets
- hypervitaminosis A
- alcoholism

4) metabolic and endocrine disorders
- hyperparathyroidism
- hyperthyroidism
- diabetes mellitus
- Cushing's disease

5) neoplastic disorders
- multiple myeloma
- metastasis
- leukemia

6) therapies
- long-term steroid therapy
- heparin (> 15,000 units/day)

b) Clinical presentation
- often totally asymptomatic
- pain and disability caused by complications: most commonly, fractures
- shortened stature
- increased thoracic kyphosis
- spinal rigidity

c) Pathologic features
- preferential resorption of trabeculae, sparing the major stress-bearing trabeculae
- thinning of cortices
- associated factors include
  1) hormonal imbalances (often associated with aging)
  2) calcium intake and dietary factors
  3) activity levels
  4) viability of osteoblasts and osteocytes (also related to aging)

d) Laboratory findings
- serum calcium levels vary
  1) senile osteoporosis: normal levels
  2) primary hyperparathyroidism: greatly elevated
  3) some neoplastic conditions: somewhat elevated
- urinary calcium levels normal or somewhat elevated
- urinary hydroxyproline levels elevated

e) Assessment methods
- radiogrammetry measures cortical thickness in peripheral bone
  1) usually uses second metacarpal
  2) compares measurement to accepted standard
  3) does not assess axial skeleton
- single-photon absorptiometry assesses density of bone

> 1) measures transmission count rate
> 2) uses calcaneus, distal radius, or radial shaft
> 3) high rate of false negatives
- dual photon absorptiometry also assesses bone density
  > 1) photons emitted at two different energy levels
  > 2) soft tissue influence eliminated
  > 3) measures density of spine and proximal femur
  > 4) errors caused by osteophytes, sclerosis, facet disease, scoliosis, vascular calcifications
- quantitative computed tomography measures density
  > 1) single or dual photon beam through vertebral body
  > 2) transmission compared with a calibration phantom
  > 3) correlates well with prevalence of vertebral fracture
  > 4) moderately high radiation dose (200–250 mrad)

f) Radiologic features
- increased lucency
  > 1) visible on plain film only after 30–50% reduction of bone mass
  > 2) indicates osteopenia (poverty of bone)
- cortical thinning
  > 1) "*pencil thin*" cortices
  > 2) marrow cavity size correspondingly increased
  > 3) early in process: possible endosteal scalloping
  > 4) altered trabecular patterns
  >   - remaining trabeculae accentuated, especially along stress lines
  >   - eventually, trabecular patterns disappear ("*washed-out*" appearance)
- appearance at specific skeletal sites
  > 1) spine
  >   - altered spinal curves
  >   - a. increased kyphosis caused by anterior wedging of compression fractures, loss of disc height, remodeling of anterior body margins
  >   - b. scoliosis
  >   - c. these increase risk of future fractures
  >   - decreased bone density
  >   - a. internal body density appears similar to density of surrounding soft tissues

      b. radiographic techniques for normal bone yield overexposed film

- altered trabecular patterns
  a. vertical trabeculae accentuated
  b. may simulate hemangioma: (*pseudohemangiomatous appearance of osteoporosis*)
  c. later, no trabeculae visible (*"washed-out appearance"*)
- cortical thinning
  a. bodies and neural arch affected
  b. especially body endplates, pencil thin
- altered vertebral body shape
  a. rarely affect cervical or upper thoracic spine
  b. midthoracic and thoracolumbar spine most often affected
  c. various shape types in same patient
     - *vertebra plana (pancake vertebra, coin on end vertebra, silver dollar vertebra)*
     - wedged vertebra: trapezoidal
     - biconcave vertebra: central depression of both vertebral endplates with normal disc height (*fish vertebra, codfish vertebra, fishmouth vertebra, hourglass vertebra*)
  d. endplate deformities: peripheral or central fractures (most often at L1 and L4) indicated by altered endplate orientation, sharp offset defect, sclerosis adjacent to fracture site
  e. Schmorl's nodes in thoracic and upper lumbar segments, often small and with irregular borders

2) pelvis and proximal femora
   - decreased bone density
     a. most prominent at iliac fossa, pubis, supraacetabular area, femoral neck, greater trochanter
     b. may simulate more aggressive processes
   - trabecular changes
     a. trabeculae in proximal femur: good indicator of degree of osteoporosis

b. normal trabecular patterns in proximal femur:
- principal compressive group: major weight-bearers
  - normally thickest and last to be obliterated
  - accentuated in osteoporosis
  - extend from medial metaphyseal cortex to superior femoral head
- secondary compressive group:
  - usually thin, widely separated
  - originate adjacent to cortex near lesser trochanter, curve laterally upward toward greater trochanter and upper femoral head
- principal tensile group
  - originate from lateral cortex below greater trochanter, arch upward and medially, end in inferior femoral head
- "*Ward's triangle*": lucent triangle formed by confluence of these groups in femoral neck (Fig. 8.2)
  - early in process, more prominent lucency
  - later: opens laterally with regression of principal tensile group
  - may eventually disappear as femur is devoid of visible trabeculae

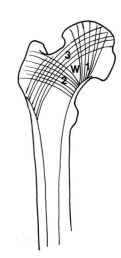

Figure 8.2.
Normal trabecular patterns. #1-principal compressive group. #2-secondary compressive group. #3-principal tensile group. W-Ward's triangle.

- cortical thinning
  a. all cortices in pelvis and femora thinned
  b. most distinctive at iliac crests, pubic rami, ischia, femoral head and neck
  c. distinction between cortex and medullary cavity eventually disappears
- fracture deformities
  a. most frequent at pubic rami and proximal femur
  b. spontaneous or from minor trauma
  c. normal healing time and quality
    - exception: femoral neck fracture

- may precipitate femoral head avascular necrosis
- with concurrent osteoporosis and DJD: pubic rami or medial femoral neck may fracture
- hip DJD (degenerative joint disease)
  a. low incidence with osteoporosis (< 5% of osteoporosis cases have concurrent DJD)
  b. hip DJD correlates with diminished incidence of spinal compression fractures
- insufficiency fractures
  1) axial skeleton: most common in spine, femoral neck, pubic rami
  2) appendicular sites: distal radius (Colles' fracture), humeral neck, ankle malleoli
  3) seen with osteoporosis (any cause), radiation necrosis, osteomalacia, Paget's disease, fibrous dysplasia (any process reducing elastic strength of bone so it cannot withstand normal physiologic stress)
  4) radiologically similar to stress fractures
     - initial films (when pain appears) often negative
     - local solid periosteal response
     - transverse opaque callus zones
     - fracture line rarely visible (usually metaphyseal)
     - often simultaneous at multiple, symmetrical sites
  5) early detection via bone scan
  6) differential diagnosis via CT
  7) sacral insufficiency fractures
     - usually caused by fall to buttocks, patient with senile or postmenopausal osteoporosis
     - often after pelvic irradiation coupled with corticosteroid therapy
     - other precipitating conditions: alcoholism, multiple myeloma, osteomalacia, osteogenesis imperfecta, recent hip replacement
     - incidence
       a. female predilection (5:1)
       b. usually > 65 years old
       c. predisposed by increased pelvic tilt
     - clinical presentation varies: asymptomatic; debilitating pain

over lumbosacral junction, sacrum or buttocks

- 75% have coexisting insufficiency fracture in pelvic ring, usually pubic ramus
- >65% have coexisting extrapelvic insufficiency fractures: e.g. lower ribs, thoracic or lumbar vertebrae, femoral neck
- three patterns of sacral insufficiency fracture (shown on bone scan)
  a. "H" pattern (*butterfly sign* or *Honda sign*): bilateral vertical fractures through sacral ala, connected by transverse fracture through S2, S3, or S4 body
  b. "I" pattern: single vertical fracture through the sacral ala
      - most common sacral insufficiency fracture
      - pattern seen in at least 70% of cases
      - misinterpreted as sacroiliitis due to proximity to SI joint
  c. arc pattern: linear or curvilinear transverse fracture crossing the sacrum horizontally
- barriers to recognition and accurate diagnosis include
  a. low index of clinical suspicion
  b. background osteopenia
  c. absence of displacement
  d. low-grade callus formation
  e. overlying soft tissues obscuring fracture site
  f. inappropriate views
- radiologic indications of sacral insufficiency fracture
  a. lateral view may show offset anterior sacral cortex
  b. axial CT images show displacement of anterior sacral cortex within 1 cm of sacroiliac joint
  c. axial CT will show linear sclerosis or fracture line parallel to sacroiliac joint and lateral to sacral foramina
  d. MRI helps detect fractures through sacral ala
8) pubic insufficiency fractures
- most often through body near symphysis

- may also occur through rami
- often bilateral, frequently concurrent with other pelvic insufficiency fractures, especially through sacral ala
- radiologic appearance simulates destructive neoplasm
    a. patchy sclerosis
    b. irregular lysis
    c. cortical disruption
    d. articular cortex collapse

9) acetabular insufficiency fractures
- hazy, linear band of sclerosis at lateral supraacetabular margin
- may arc parallel to medial acetabular cortex
- may extend to pelvic inlet
- up to 20% bilateral
- often concurrent with other pelvic ring insufficiency fractures

10) femoral neck insufficiency fractures
- indistinct sclerotic streak at medial femoral neck
- vertically oriented, perpendicular to axis of femoral neck
- interrupted trabeculae
- cortical fracture line
- endosteal and extracortical callus
- incomplete fracture line through femoral neck

11) insufficiency fracture of tibia, fibula
- outer margins of distal or proximal tibia and fibula
- distal tibia: sclerotic band parallel with talar dome, about 2 cm above joint line
- proximal insufficiency fractures with significant knee arthritis: exacerbated by varus-valgus deformity

12) insufficiency fracture of posterior calcaneus
- posterior third of calcaneus involved
- commonly seen with diabetes
- hazy, curvilinear sclerotic band, curves obliquely upward and posterior

13) insufficiency fractures of metatarsal necks: usually at junction of head and shaft

14) insufficiency fractures of the sternum
- complaints of pain and swelling over upper sternal body
- usually fractures transversely through upper sternal body
- rarely buckles

- more than two-thirds of patients have spinal compression fractures, increased thoracic kyphosis

g) Differential considerations
- compression fractures (various etiologies)
  1) "*fish vertebrae*" are simulated by nuclear impressions
     - frontal view of notochordal remnants: "*Cupid's bow*"
     - lateral view, notochordal remnants involve posterior two-thirds of endplates
     - CT: parasagittal depressions posterolaterally ("*owl's eyes*")
  2) concave endplates caused by other bone-weakening processes
     - osteomalacia
     - Paget's disease
  3) confused with Schmorls' nodes: these are delineated by cortical bone, are more focal
  4) traumatic fractures
     - usually normal bone density
     - loss of anterior vertebral body height
     - pedicles usually spared, except in severe trauma
  5) pathologic fractures
     - osteopenic, vertebra plana, with pedicle destruction
     - may have intrabody vacuum sign
  6) wedge deformities
     - common developmental deformity at T11, T12, L1
     - anterior Schmorl's nodes precipitate wedging
     - normal physiologic wedging up to 5° per segment
  7) signs of acute or healed fractures
     - trabecular impaction: sclerosis beneath endplate, lasting 8–10 weeks after fracture (callus perpetuates this appearance)
     - "*step sign*": acute angular offset at anterior cortex
     - displaced paraspinal soft tissues may indicate hematoma (with acute fracture)
     - excessive air in small bowel (ileus) may indicate acute fracture, especially in lumbar spine
     - old, healed fractures: no sub-endplate sclerosis, no "*step sign*"
     - healed fracture often accompanied by signs of DJD
       a. osteophytes

    b. vacuum phenomenon
    c. reduced disc height
- hemangioma: simulated by trabecular changes of osteoporosis
  1) osteoporosis: multiple contiguous segments
  2) hemangioma: usually solitary
- vertebra plana: differentiate from far more common causes:
  1) metastatic carcinoma
  2) multiple myeloma
  3) eosinophilic granuloma

REVIEW—STUDY QUESTIONS

1. Name three nutrients which, in excess, result in radiologically visible bone pathology.

2. What causes the disease known as scurvy, and what populations are at risk for scurvy?

3. Name five diseases frequently associated with osteoporosis.

4. What is the difference between osteoporosis and osteopenia?

5. Describe the normal trabecular patterns of the femoral neck.

6. What are the radiologic signs of heavy metal intoxication?

7. Name the three radiologic changes common to osteoporosis of any etiology in most skeletal sites.

8. What is the most common complication of osteoporosis, and where does it most commonly occur?

9. Name at least two causes of each: generalized, regional, and localized osteoporosis.

10. List at least three named radiologic signs associated with scurvy. Three associated with rickets?

II. **Reflex Sympathetic Dystrophy Syndrome (RSDS) (synonyms: Sudeck's atrophy, posttraumatic osteoporosis, acute bone atrophy, causalgia)**

 a) **General considerations**
- nature of condition
  1) a regional osteoporosis
  2) usually follows trivial trauma
- incidence
  1) no gender predilection
  2) most common in patients >50 years old
- skeletal sites: most common in hand and shoulder
- self-limiting, but recovery is slow (many months) and may never be complete
- residual effects: atrophy, contracture, joint stiffness

b) Clinical presentation
- progressive pain
- stiffness
- swelling
- gradually develops atrophy
- symptoms are distal to site of trivial trauma
- condition progresses over 3–6 months

c) Pathologic features
- possibly sympathetic nervous system overactivity in response to trivial mechanical insult
- hyperemia augments osteoclastic resorption of bone

d) Radiologic features
- rapidly appearing, progressing osteoporosis
- bone at first mottled
- may see metaphyseal osteoporosis, tunneled cortices, endosteal resorption
- later, homogenous diminution of density
- normal cortical margins and joint spaces

e) Differential considerations
- osteomyelitis (mottled medullary appearance in early stages)
- rheumatoid arthritis (periarticular osteopenia)

III. Immobilization or Disuse Osteoporosis

a) General characteristics
- nature of condition
  1) a regional osteoporosis
     - most commonly caused by immobilization of traumatic injury, motor paralysis, or inflammation of bones or joints
     - limb amputation or polio: regional osteoporosis due to absence of mechanical stress
  2) resolution: if function is restored, normal appearance may be restored
- pathologic features
  1) immobilized region shows radiographic changes in 7–10 days
  2) changes reach their extreme in 2–3 months

- **radiologic features**
  1) four common patterns of osteoporosis
     - uniform osteoporosis (most common form)
     - spotty osteoporosis
        a. features localized circular lucencies
        b. most prominent at epiphyses
     - bands of osteoporosis: linear

transverse subchondral or metaphyseal lucent bands

- cortical lamination or scalloping: outer and inner cortical margins are no longer clearly defined

2) superior cortex of the acetabulum may appear doubled ("*double cortical line sign*")

IV. Transient Regional Osteoporosis

a) General considerations

- nature of condition
  1) regional osteoporosis which has sudden, idiopathic onset, affects periarticular bone, and is reversible
  2) two specific varieties recognized
     - transient osteoporosis of the hip
     - regional migratory osteoporosis
  3) incidence
     - both entities exhibit male predilection
     - transient osteoporosis of the hip in females: associated with pregnancy
- transient osteoporosis of the hip: most common in patients between 20–40 years old
  4) sites
     - transient osteoporosis of the hip in females: invariably left-sided
     - regional migratory osteoporosis: knee, ankle, foot, and hip

b) Clinical presentation

- sudden onset of pain
- limping and antalgia
- transient osteoporosis of hip: self-limiting course, usually resolved fully in 3–12 months
- regional migratory osteoporosis: signs and symptoms regress over about 9 months; reappear in another joint

c) Radiologic features

- transient osteoporosis of the hip
  1) marked femoral head osteoporosis
  2) less severe osteoporosis of adjacent femoral neck and acetabulum
  3) normal joint space, although MRI may show joint effusion
  4) no bone erosions, cartilage defects, or synovial masses are present
- regional migratory osteoporosis
  1) localized osteoporosis of intraarticular bone
  2) this sign "*migrates*" to another joint, as it resolves in the first

☞   2. **Osteomalacia**
      (synonym: adult rickets)

   a) **General considerations**
      • nature of condition
        1) metabolic disorder, altering the
            quality of bone
        2) osteomalacia is literally translated
            "soft bones"
        3) various causes, mostly due to errors
            in metabolism of calcium,
            phosphorus, or vitamin D, as well as
            the form simply resulting from
            inadequate vitamin D intake
            • deficiency of vitamin D, calcium,
              phosphorus, or dietary chelators
            • inadequate absorption due to
              gastric, biliary, or enteric
              abnormality
            • renal tubular lesions (proximal
              and/or distal)
            • renal osteodystrophy
            • secondary to other diseases or
              conditions
              a. fibrous dysplasia
              b. neurofibromatosis
              c. some neoplastic processes
            • side effect with anticonvulsant
              drugs (Dilantin)
      • incidence
        1) fairly common among Asian
            immigrants to England because of
            traditional diet and lack of exposure
            to sunlight
        2) some conditions are familial because
            of an X-linked metabolic anomaly
      • skeletal sites: affects all bones
      • treatment
        1) dietary supplements of calcium,
            vitamin D, phosphorus
        2) corrective osteotomy for residual
            bone deformities

   b) **Clinical presentation**
      • with abdominal malabsorption conditions
        (e.g., sprue): abdominal pain, bloating,
        diarrhea
      • osteomalacia itself results in
        1) general muscle weakness
        2) bone pain on palpation
        3) deformities in weight-bearing bones
            (spine, pelvis, femur, tibia)

   c) **Pathologic features**
      • relative increase in uncalcified osteoid
        coating trabeculae and the linings of
        Haversian canals (*"osteoid seams"*)
      • net decrease in the quality of the bone
      • bilateral, symmetric apparent fractures at
        right angles to the bone margin: linear

regions of unmineralized osteoid (pseudofractures) which may be caused by insufficiency fracture or by vascular pulsations on softened bone

d) **Laboratory findings** vary with etiology; possible findings include
- increased serum parathormone
- increased serum alkaline phosphatase
- increased serum hydroxyproline
- slight decreases in serum calcium and phosphorous

e) **Radiologic features**
- general decrease in bone density
- coarsened trabecular pattern: spongiosa looks mottled
- loss of cortical definition
    1) thinned cortex
    2) blurred, indistinct endosteal surface
    3) possible intracortical striations
- pseudofractures
    1) bilaterally symmetrical linear lucencies
    2) over time: widen, are bordered by sclerosis
    3) common sites: femoral necks, pubic and ischial rami, ribs, axillary margins of scapulae
    4) called: *"increment fractures," "Looser lines," "Milkman's syndrome," "umbau zonen"*
- deformities in weight-bearing bones
    1) inferior sacral displacement (pelvic canal becomes triradiate)
    2) protrusio acetabulae
    3) bowing of femur and tibia
    4) kyphoscoliosis, increased endplate concavities
    5) "bell-shaped" thoracic cage
    6) platybasia

f) **Differential considerations**
- Paget's disease
- fibrous dysplasia
- hyperphosphatasia

3. Gaucher's Disease

a) **General considerations**
- nature of condition
    1) lipid metabolism abnormality
    2) deficient liposomal enzyme activity (acid beta glycosidase)
- incidence: predominantly affects Ashkenazic Jews
- anatomic sites
    1) liver and spleen
    2) bone marrow

3) femoral and humeral heads
4) hips, knees, spine

b) Clinical presentation
- splenomegaly
- yellowish-brown skin
- scleral pigmentations

c) Pathologic features and laboratory findings
- three presentations
    1) Type 1: chronic adult form: in young adults
    2) Type 2: acute infantile form: manifest in first 3 months of life, fatal within 2 years
    3) Type 3: subacute juvenile form: varied in severity and presentation
- abnormal accumulation of glycosyl ceramide in reticulo-endothelial cells (in bone marrow, spleen, liver)
- Gaucher cell: 20–200 microns; pale pink cytoplasm resembling "crumpled tissue paper," lipid and iron deposits
- Gaucher cells infiltrate and replace normal marrow elements; swell reticulum
- act as a space-occupying lesion; applying pressure on blood vessels, increasing intramedullary pressure
- marrow necrosis and fibrosis; avascular necrosis
- laboratory findings
    1) leukopenia
    2) sometimes: elevated acid phosphatase and alkaline phosphatase

d) Radiologic features
- femur
    1) avascular necrosis of femoral head
    2) *"Erlenmeyer flask deformity"*
    3) osteoporosis
    4) medullary expansion
    5) cortical thinning
    6) periostitis
    7) lytic lucencies
- hips and knees: degenerative joint disease (DJD)
- Gaucher cell deposits: soft tissue masses beyond bone cortex
- occasionally: intraosseous hemorrhagic cyst
- spine
    1) diffuse osteopenia
    2) vertebral body collapse (single or multiple)
    3) kyphosis
    4) endplate *"step defects"* (*"H"-shaped vertebra*)

        5)   biconcave endplates (*"fish vertebra"*)
        6)   intravertebral vacuum cleft sign

  e)   **Differential considerations**
- malignancy (soft tissue masses)
- sickle cell anemia (*"H"-shaped vertebra*)

4. **Histiocytosis X**
    (synonym: Langerhans' cell histiocytosis)

  a)   **General considerations**
- nature of condition
  1) disorder of immune regulation
  2) abnormal proliferation of reticuloendothelial cells
- three entities considered
  1) Letterer-Siwe disease
  2) Hand-Schüller-Christian disease
  3) eosinophilic granuloma
  4) may overlap, or change from one to another

  b)   Specific entities

I.   **Letterer-Siwe disease**

  a)   **General considerations**
- nature of condition: acute, fulminating; fatal without therapy
- incidence: toddlers < 3 years old
- skeletal sites: calvarium, sometimes long bones
- treatment: corticosteroids

  b)   **Clinical presentation**
- high fever
- skin rash
- bleeding gums
- malaise
- lymphadenopathy
- hepatosplenomegaly
- respiratory symptoms

  c)   **Pathologic features and laboratory findings**
- Langerhans' histiocytes proliferate
- infiltration by eosinophilic granulocytes
- skin, lymph nodes, bone, liver, spleen most affected
- commonly complicated by pneumothorax
- laboratory findings: possibly slightly elevated ESR and slight leukocytosis

  d)   **Radiologic features**
- most common finding: calvarial lytic lesions
- rarely: aggressive irregular lysis in long bone diaphyses, with surrounding laminated periosteal new bone

  e)   **Differential considerations**
- long bone lesions simulate Ewing's sarcoma

II. Hand-Schüller-Christian disease

a) General considerations

- nature of condition: chronic, intermittent disease, occasionally fatal
- incidence: manifests any time from early childhood through middle age
- skeletal sites: skull, pelvis and long bones most notably affected
- treatment: corticosteroids; radiation (when there is only a solitary lesion, or very few lesions)

b) Clinical presentation

- pain
- anorexia, weight loss
- malaise
- lymphadenopathy
- hepatosplenomegaly
- respiratory symptoms
- painful soft tissue nodules on the skull
- classic triad, although it occurs rarely:
  - exophthalmos
  - diabetes insipidus caused by a pituitary lesion
  - lytic skull lesions

c) Pathologic features and laboratory findings

- infiltration of affected tissues by granulomatous lesions
- possibly: slightly elevated ESR and mild leukocytosis

d) Radiologic features

- polyostotic destructive foci in immature skeleton (**radiologic hallmark**)
- skull
  1) multiple lytic lesions coalesce: form "*geographic lesions*"
  2) peripheral beveled edge gives "*hole within a hole*" appearance
- long bones
  1) entire bone may have multiple lytic defects (5–10 mm in diameter)
  2) lesions coalesce, create larger defects with endosteal scalloping, beveled cortex ("*hole within a hole*")

III. Eosinophilic granuloma

a) General characteristics

- nature of condition: least severe of the histiocytoses
- incidence
  1) most common histiocytosis (60–80% of all cases)
  2) peak incidence between ages 5 and 10
  3) 75% in patients < 20 years old

- skeletal sites
    1) monostotic involvement three times more common than polyostotic, but about 20% progress to become polyostotic
    2) >50% involve skull
    3) 25%, mandible
    4) 20%, pelvis
    5) 15%, femur
    6) 8%, humerus
    7) 7%, ribs
    8) 6%, spine
    9) hands and feet rarely affected
- treatment: corticosteroid injection, radiotherapy, chemotherapy, or surgery (en-bloc excision or curettage)
- may undergo spontaneous resolution
- heals in 6–24 months

b) **Clinical presentation**
- no systemic effects
- localized pain and swelling
- pathologic fracture may be presenting problem
- spinal lesions may involve pain and/or myelopathy secondary to cord or nerve root compression

c) **Pathologic features**
- proliferation of Langerhans' histiocytes (containing organelles called Birbeck granules) in a granuloma
- inflammatory response dominated by eosinophils
- eosinophilic microabscess: clumped eosinophils within the granuloma

d) **Radiologic features**
- bone scan: check for polyostotic involvement when a lesion has been found
- CT or MRI: help define soft tissue mass (especially in spinal involvement) and periosteal response
- generally: round or oval geographic lytic lesion
- sharply demarcated border and prominent endosteal scalloping
- usually solid or occasionally laminated periosteal response
- skull
    1) round or oval lytic lesion, 1–4 cm in diameter
    2) sharply demarcated
    3) one table more widely lysed than the other: causes "*beveled edge*" lesion with hole in a hole appearance
    4) "*button sequestrum*": isolated central

focus of bone within lesion, may require CT to visualize

   5) lesion can cross suture lines

- mandible
  1) expansile, lytic lesion
  2) teeth displaced, isolated (*"floating teeth sign"*)
  3) teeth themselves unaffected
  4) usually begins near last molar, enlarges forward
  5) inferior mandibular border usually spared

- spine
  1) usually solitary vertebra; occasionally multiple
  2) >50% of spinal lesions thoracic
  3) about 35% lumbar
  4) <15% cervical
  5) neural arch structures usually spared
     - when involved, cortices are spared
     - internal matrix destroyed
     - *"ghostly appearance"* of neural arch
  6) pathologic fracture (most prominent feature)
     - dramatic loss of vertebral height (*"vertebra plana," "silver dollar vertebra," "coin on edge vertebra"*)
       a. as thin as 2 mm (both anterior and posterior surfaces)
       b. > 90% of cases experience 48–95% restoration of body height within 1 year
       c. especially good prognosis for patients < 15 years old at onset
     - before collapse: destruction visible within body centrum
     - short-segment kyphosis
     - may have prominent paravertebral swelling
     - occasionally: *"bone within a bone"* appearance
     - heal with residual sclerosis and trabecular accentuation
     - rarely, after radiotherapy: interbody fusion

- pelvis
  1) usually: supraacetabular lesion in the ilium
  2) relatively large, slightly expansile lesion
  3) usually has sclerotic, beveled edge
  4) may begin with small, moth-eaten/permeative multiple lesions

5) lesions coalesce, forming large, "*geographic defects*"
6) lesions in pubic bone may have laminated periosteal response along the superior pubic ramus
7) ischial lesions also provoke periosteal response

- long bones
  1) usually femur, tibia, or humerus
  2) rarely hands or feet
  3) 60% in the diaphysis
  4) metaphyseal lesions may cross the physis
  5) rarely in the epiphysis
  6) lesions elongate along long axis of the bone
  7) lytic, usually geographic (may be permeative or moth-eaten)
  8) endosteal scalloping, cortical thinning, slightly expansile
  9) "*hole within a hole*" appearance due to beveled edges and undulating margin
  10) solid or laminated periosteal reaction in about 10% of cases
  11) occasionally, pathologic fracture
  12) soft tissue mass (< 10% of cases)

e) Differential considerations
- lytic destruction may simulate aggressive neoplasm, especially in the spine
- epiphyseal lesions mimic chondroblastoma without calcification
- major considerations
  1) osteomyelitis
  2) Ewing's sarcoma
  3) leukemia
  4) lymphoma
  5) fibrous dysplasia

REVIEW—STUDY QUESTIONS

1. *Osteomalacia* and *osteoporosis* both result in *osteopenia*. Define these three underlined terms.

2. What skeletal site is most commonly involved with eosinophilic granuloma?

3. List three specific entities which are manifestations of histiocytosis "X."

4. What is the basic nature of histiocytosis "X," in any of its forms?

5. What is RSDS, and what are some proposed mechanisms to explain its occurrence?

6. What condition is associated with geographic lytic lesions with a "hole in a hole" appearance?

7. What causes the "hole in a hole" appearance of these lesions?

8. What is the classic triad of the Hand-Schüller-Christian disease?

9. What are osteoid seams, and with what condition are they associated?

10. List three synonyms for "pseudofractures." What conditions are associated with them?

C.   ENDOCRINE DISORDERS

1.   Hyperparathyroidism

a)   General considerations

- nature of condition: overactivity of parathyroid gland
- three basic forms of hyperparathyroidism
  1) primary
     - 90% are caused by parathyroid adenoma
     - other causes: carcinoma, hyperplasia, ectopic parathormone-producing tumors
  2) secondary
     - persistent calcium and phosphorous loss
     - caused by chronic renal disease
  3) tertiary
     - parathyroid acting independently of serum calcium levels
     - seen in dialysis patients
- incidence: most common in women (3:1), ages 30–50 years
- anatomic sites
  1) subperiosteal bone, especially at ligament and tendon insertions
  2) tertiary form: lesions at peripheral joints (DRA—dialysis-related arthropathy) and in spine (DRSA—dialysis-related spondyloarthropathy)
  3) subcutaneous, articular, muscular, vascular, and visceral calcifications
  4) predilected sites: hands, skull, spine, pelvis, and shoulder
- treatment: surgery for removal of tumors or ectopic parathyroid tissue

b)   Clinical presentation

- weakness, lethargy
- polydipsia, polyuria
- muscle hypotonia
- renal calculi
- bone tenderness

c)   Pathologic features

- primary

1) increased osteoclastic resorption due to elevated serum parathormone
2) constant release of calcium and phosphorus into bloodstream
3) phosphorus excreted readily, calcium retained
4) imbalance: hypercalcemia and hypophosphatemia

- secondary
  1) calcium loss and abnormal renal vitamin D formation
  2) continuous hypocalcemia
  3) increased parathormone release
  4) bone resorption
- osteoclastic and osteocytic resorption lead to replacement by fibrous tissue ("*osteitis fibrosa cystica*;" "*Recklinghausen's disease of bone*")
- hypodense bone with defective lamellae and defective Haversian systems
- bones are soft, fragile
- "*brown tumors*"
  1) cystlike fibrous accumulations with osteoclastic giant cells
  2) may hemorrhage, undergo liquefactive necrosis, create true cysts
- "*pathologic hallmark*": subperiosteal outer cortical bone resorption at ligament and tendon insertions

d) Laboratory findings
- laboratory findings vary with different forms of hyperparathyroidism:
- primary: intermittent hypercalcemia with hypophosphatemia
- secondary: normal to low serum calcium
- with bone disease, increased alkaline phosphatase
- elevated parathormone

e) Radiologic features
- primary and secondary: cannot be differentiated radiologically
- hyperparathyroidism in general: can be diagnosed radiologically
- secondary form: greater tendency toward osteosclerosis
- "*subperiosteal resorption*" (most definitive radiologic sign)
  1) most common sites
     - radial margins, middle and proximal phalanges of second and third fingers
     - medial metaphyses of humerus and tibia
     - inferior surface of the distal clavicle

2) subligamentous resorption: especially at trochanters, humeral and ischial tuberosities, inferior calcaneal surface

3) appearance
- irregular, frayed, lace-like appearance of external cortex
- apparently widened joint spaces
- osteolysis, especially at acromioclavicular, symphysis pubis, and sacroiliac articulations (wide joint spaces)

- generalized loss of bone density (bone appears granular)
- accentuated trabecular patterns
- endosteal, intracortical and subperiosteal resorption reduce cortical definition
  1) cortical and medullary bone lose clear demarcation
  2) outer surface of cortex blurred, irregular
  3) second metacarpal cortex: subtle longitudinal striations caused by intracortical resorption within Haversian canals
- brown tumors ("*osteoclastoma*")
  1) central, geographic lucencies
  2) slightly expansile
  3) lightly septated
  4) densely sclerotic when healed
  5) most common at mandible, pelvis, ribs, femora
- dialysis-related arthropathy (DRA):
  1) highly destructive, throughout skeleton
  2) caused by amyloid (beta-2 microglobulin) deposits in articular tissue
  3) peripherally
     - chronic, progressive, symmetric polyarthropathy
     - occurs in 40% of dialysis patients
     - periarticular cysts, erosions
     - diminished joint space
     - destruction of articular surface
     - periarticular osteopenia
  4) axially
     - dialysis-related spondyloarthropathy (DRSA)
     - component of DRA found in up to 15% of dialysis patients
     - rarely occurs in absence of peripheral DRA
     - rarely seen before 2 years of dialysis, usually after 3–5 years
     - multiple segments involved, most commonly in cervical spine

- about 30% of DRSA patients asymptomatic
- about 20% with potentially fatal cord compression
- loss of disc height, subchondral cysts, endplate erosions, vertebral collapse with vertebral body erosion, facet erosion with spondylolisthesis (usually at C3 and C4), peridiscal calcification
- soft tissue changes
  1) subcutaneous, articular, muscular, vascular, and visceral calcifications
  2) nephrocalcinosis, renal calculi (in 75% of patients)
  3) chondrocalcinosis within joint cartilages (in 20% of primary hyperparathyroidism patients): usually in knee menisci, triangular wrist cartilage, shoulders, and hips
  4) periarticular calcification in blood vessels, ligaments, tendons, muscles, subcutaneous tissues (especially in secondary hyperparathyroidism)
  5) calcifications in salivary gland, pancreas, lungs, prostate
- hands
  1) **hallmark sign** (*"subperiosteal resorption"*) first shows in the hands
  2) most conspicuous at radial margins of proximal and middle phalanges of second and third fingers
  3) outer cortex frayed and irregular
  4) generalized osteopenia with tapered, and sometimes total tuftal osteolysis
- skull
  1) mottled calvarium (*"salt and pepper skull"* or *"pepper pot skull"*) caused by diffuse granular deossification
  2) definition of inner and outer tables blurred
  3) **lamina dura** resorbed around the tooth socket (characteristic sign)
  4) rare complication: basilar invagination
- spine
  1) vertebral osteopenia, trabecular accentuation
  2) increased endplate concavities; Schmorl's nodes
  3) sub-endplate sclerosis: *"rugger-jersey spine"*
  4) rare presentation: uniform homogenous sclerosis (*"ivory vertebra"*)
  5) DRSA
- pelvis
  1) sacroiliac and pubic articular resorption

2) apparent widening of articulations
- shoulders
    1) bilateral, subchondral, distal clavicle resorption (an early, definitive sign of hyperparathyroidism)
    2) indistinct, frayed articular surface

☞   **f)   Differential considerations**
- brown tumors mimic neoplasm
- DRSA simulates infection, or ankylosing spondylitis (especially SI involvement)
- distal clavicle osteolysis simulates infection or posttraumatic osteolysis, but is **bilateral**

☞   **2.   Acromegaly**

a)   General considerations
- nature of condition
    1) pituitary eosinophilic adenoma
    2) secretes excessive growth hormone
    3) result is excessive **adult** intramembranous bone growth, subcutaneous hypertrophy
    4) excessive growth hormone before skeletal maturity results in gigantism
- incidence: most commonly, onset between ages 20 and 50 years
- skeletal sites
    1) skull and jaw
    2) hands and feet
    3) spine

b)   Clinical presentation
- prominent forehead
- prognathic jaw with dental malocclusion
- broad, large hands with long fingers
- large feet with long toes
- thickened tongue, thickened heel pads
- headache, bitemporal hemianopia (hemianopsia)
- carpal tunnel syndrome (often bilateral)
- scoliosis, degenerative disease of weight-bearing joints
- thickened and darkened skin
- increased perspiration and offensive body odor
- deepened, husky voice
- impotence; menstrual irregularities or amenorrhea

c)   Pathologic features and laboratory findings
- eosinophilic adenoma in anterior pituitary gland: produces excessive growth hormone
- all musculoskeletal tissues affected
- periosteal appositional new bone activated: cortical bone irregularly thickened

Clavicle Resorption
"SHIRT POCKET"
Scleroderma
Hyperparathyroidism
Infection
Rheumatoid arthritis
Trauma
Progeria

- enhanced ectopic bone formation (e.g., bone spurs)
- proliferation of articular cartilage (quickly degenerates)
- hyperplastic subcutaneous tissues, with fatty replacement
- elevated plasma growth hormone (GH) levels

d)   Radiologic findings
- thickened heel pad (>20 mm suggests acromegaly)
- skull
  1) sella turcica enlargement
  2) sinus enlargement (especially huge frontal sinus)
  3) occipital protuberance overgrowth
- jaw
  1) malocclusion
  2) widened mandibular angle
- hand
  1) widened phalangeal and metacarpal shafts
  2) "*spade-like*" ungual tufts
  3) increased width of joint spaces (cartilage overgrowth)
- spine
  1) sagittal and transverse vertebral enlargement (gives appearance of platyspondyla)
  2) premature DJD with exuberant osteophytes
  3) widened disc heights
  4) posterior body scalloping (caused by dural ectasia)
  5) spinous process hyperostosis
  6) thickened laminae and articular processes
  7) thickened, calcified spinal ligaments
  8) cartilage hypertrophy: widened ADI and facet joints

☞   **3.   Cushing's Syndrome**

a)   General considerations
- nature of condition
  1) excessive glucocorticoids released from adrenal cortex
  2) primary Cushing's disease caused by adrenal cortical malfunction
  3) secondary Cushing's disease caused by anterior pituitary neoplasm
  4) iatrogenic Cushing's syndrome caused by administration of corticosteroids ("*steroid-induced osteonecrosis*")
- anatomic sites
  1) face and upper thorax: accumulate fat (redistribution of fat)

Thickened Heel Pad

"MAD COP"

Myxedema
Acromegaly
Dilantin therapy
Callous
Obesity
Peripheral edema

2) bone: general osteopenia

3) femoral heads, humeral heads, femoral condyles, proximal tibiae, talus and spine: subject to steroid-induced osteonecrosis

4) spine and ribs: frequent fracture sites

5) joints: increased vulnerability to arthropathy, septic arthritis, osteomyelitis

6) tendons and subcutaneous tissues: more subject to rupture, atrophy

b) Clinical presentation

- obesity, with *"moon facies"* (round, chubby face)
- *"buffalo hump"*: fatty tissue accumulation over upper thoracic spine
- purple striae on abdomen and in axilla
- accelerated hair growth; sometimes temporal balding
- hypertension
- renal calculi
- osteoporosis
- glucose intolerance
- reduced resistance to infection
- psychiatric disturbances
- relatively painless rib and vertebral fractures

c) Pathologic features

- ACTH possibly elevated: adrenal cortical hyperfunction
- adrenocortical adenoma: produces excess cortisol
- exogenous cortisol: given as therapeutic measure
- fat cell mass increase: fatty emboli from fatty liver may contribute to osteonecrosis
- steroid therapy: decreases fibrous content of tendons, reduces tendon strength, inhibits healing of injury, delays regeneration, promotes fatty degeneration and collagen necrosis

d) Radiologic features

- osteopenia
  1) generalized osteopenia (similar to postmenopausal osteoporosis)
  2) thin cortices
  3) diminished density
  4) bone deformities
  5) biconcave vertebral endplates
  6) multiple vertebrae with hazy endplates due to heavy callus over small, healing endplate fractures
  7) spontaneous fractures: vertebrae, ribs, pubic rami
- osteonecrosis (avascular necrosis):
  1) rare with Cushing's disease (primary

or secondary) but common with long-term corticosteroid therapy (onset after 2–3 years of therapy)

2) most common at
   - femoral and humeral heads
   - femoral condyles
   - proximal tibia
   - talus

3) femoral heads bilaterally affected: 30–50% of cases (not necessarily simultaneously)

4) epiphyses
   - subchondral fractures ("*crescent sign*")
   - weight-bearing surface of femoral head: "*bite sign*"
   - subchondral collapse ("*step sign*")
   - patchy sclerosis

5) metaphyseal/diaphyseal infarctions: rare

6) vertebrae
   - vertebral body collapse, sometimes with "*intravertebral vacuum cleft sign*"
   - about 50% thoracolumbar
   - not known to occur cervically

- fractures
  1) spine
     - "*marginal condensation sign*": hazy band of sclerosis in sub-endplate zones (heavy callus around repeated endplate microfractures)
     - anteriorly wedged compression fractures
     - *vertebra plana*: complete vertebral collapse
     - central fractures (Schmorl's nodes)
     - biconcave endplates ("*fish vertebrae*")
  2) ribs
     - multiple anterior or posterolateral costal fractures
     - hypertrophic callus at site of healing fracture

- corticosteroid arthropathy
  1) linked to long-term corticosteroid therapy
  2) also with NSAIDs such as phenylbutazone and indomethacin
  3) fragmentation and collapse of subchondral bone, sclerosis, loss of joint space
  4) "*bite sign*": gouged-out lesions at articular margins (resemble animal bites)

- osteomyelitis and septic arthritis
    1) long-term corticosteroid: patient more vulnerable to infections
    2) septic arthritis: most common at knee
    3) usually caused by *Staphylococcus aureus*
- altered soft tissue contours
    1) caused by tendon rupture
    2) most often at Achilles tendon or patellar tendon

e) Differential considerations

- "*intravertebral vacuum cleft sign*" also seen in: osteoporosis, multiple myeloma, metastatic carcinoma, alcoholism, Gaucher's disease, Kummel's disease, irradiation therapy
- corticosteroid arthropathy simulates neuropathic joints

4. Thyroid Disorders

a) General considerations

- nature of conditions
    1) hyperthyroidism
    2) hypothyroidism
    3) thyroid acropachy
- incidence
    1) hypothyroidism in a newborn: "*cretinism*"
    2) thyroid acropachy: occasionally in patients successfully treated for a hyperthyroid condition (1% of cases)

b) Clinical manifestations

- hyperthyroid: "*Graves' disease*" (one manifestation), goiter, weight loss, increased appetite, tachycardia, widened pulse pressure, nervousness, increased sweating, palpitations, fatigue, hypersensitivity to heat, insomnia, weakness, frequent bowel movements
- hypothyroid: insidious onset of dull facial expression; hoarse, slow speech; periorbital swelling and puffiness; cold intolerance; drooping eyelids; sparse, coarse, dry hair; coarse, dry, thick, scaly skin; modest weight gain; forgetfulness and personality changes; bradycardia; constipation; paresthesias of hands and feet; brisk contraction and slow relaxation of deep tendon reflexes; anemia, especially with menorrhagia
- thyroid acropachy: painless, progressive digital swelling

c) Radiologic features

- hyperthyroidism: generalized osteopenia
- hypothyroidism
    1) growth inhibition in infants
    2) delayed closure and fragmentation of epiphyses ("*cretinoid epiphyses*")

3) *"wormian bones"* (occasionally)
4) wedging of thoracolumbar vertebra
   (*"sail vertebra"*)

- thyroid acropachy: thick, dense periostitis on radial aspect of the metacarpals and phalanges and the tibial aspect of the metatarsals and phalanges.

REVIEW—STUDY QUESTIONS

1. Describe the clinical and radiologic appearance that may be seen in a patient with acromegaly.

2. What is DRA? What is DRSA? How are they related? What are their radiologic signs?

3. What are the three forms of hyperparathyroidism, and what are their radiologic signs?

4. What are "brown tumors," and with what disease are they associated?

5. What skeletal manifestations may result from inadequate exposure to sunlight?

6. What are the pathologic and radiologic hallmarks of hyperparathyroidism?

7. List three etiologies of excessive corticosteroids in the body.

8. What term is applied to hypothyroidism in a newborn? What are its radiologic signs?

9. What condition is associated with the clinical appearance of *moon facies* and *buffalo hump*?

10. List five conditions which may manifest the intravertebral vacuum cleft sign.

1. With eosinophilic granuloma, a periosteal response:

   a) may be spiculated.
   b) often involves "Codman's triangles."
   c) is usually solid.
   d) is not produced.

2. A destructive, progressive, symmetric polyarthropathy occurs in 40% of patients:

   a) with diabetes.
   b) with psoriasis.
   c) on dialysis.
   d) with syphilis.

3. Patients with Cushing's disease experience a redistribution of body fat, which accumulates:

   a) on the hips and abdomen.
   b) on the hips and chest.
   c) on the face and upper thorax.
   d) on the buttocks and abdomen.

4. Scurvy is manifested in the skeleton by:

   a) reversible signs, such as a metaphyseal, densely calcified, transverse band.
   b) irreversible thickening of the cortices and loss of medullary cavity area.
   c) reversible thickening of the cortices and loss of medullary cavity area.
   d) irreversible osteoporosis, thinning of cortices, and loss of trabeculae.

5. Thyroid acropachy is:

   a) erosion of the distal clavicles.
   b) spade-like ungual tufts.
   c) painless, progressive digital swelling.
   d) subperiosteal erosions in the distal phalanges.

6. For osteoporosis to be detected on plain film, bone loss must reach:

   a) 3 to 5%.
   b) 10 to 30%.
   c) 30 to 50%.
   d) 50 to 65%.

7. Nuclear impressions may be differentiated from the "fish vertebrae" seen with bone-softening conditions by the fact that:

   a) the pathologic concavities occur in both superior and inferior endplates.
   b) the pathologic concavities are smooth, uninterrupted lines.
   c) the pathologic concavities are in the posterior two-thirds of the endplates.
   d) the notochordal remnants involve the posterior two-thirds of the endplates.

8. "Osteoid seams" are a feature of:

   a) hyperparathyroidism.
   b) osteomyelitis.
   c) rickets.
   d) osteoporosis.

9. Osteomalacia does **not** cause:

   a) increased serum alkaline phosphatase.
   b) increased serum calcium and phosphorous.
   c) increased serum hydroxyproline.
   d) increased serum parathormone.

10. Pelken's spurs are:

    a) bony excrescences on the calcaneus caused by stress at the Achilles tendon insertion.
    b) bony protuberances at the metaphyseal margins of the long bones, seen with scurvy.
    c) "chisel fractures" at the epiphyseal/metaphyseal margins of the proximal tibia.
    d) bony "horns" from the posterior surface of the ilium, seen in Fong's disease.

11. Eosinophilic granuloma is most often seen in patients:

    a) with osteomalacia.
    b) over 60 years of age.
    c) under 20 years of age.
    d) 40 to 60 years of age.

12. The pathologic hallmark of hyperparathyroidism is:

    a) a "hole within a hole" appearance caused by a beveled cortical lesion.
    b) subperiosteal outer cortical bone resorption at entheses.
    c) subarticular permeative lesions.
    d) subarticular lucent lesions.

13. Primary Cushing's disease is caused by:

    a) a hypothyroid condition.
    b) an anterior pituitary tumor.
    c) a pancreatic malfunction.
    d) an adrenal cortical malfunction.

14. Heavy metal poisoning may have radiographically visible skeletal effects, if the metal involved is:

    a) lead, copper, or mercury chloride.
    b) iron, lead, or mercury chloride.
    c) lead, phosphorus, or bismuth.
    d) copper, bismuth, or lead.

15. Sensitivity to cold, bradycardia, and deep tendon reflexes that contract briskly but relax slowly are clinical signs that may indicate:

    a) a hypothyroid condition.
    b) heavy metal poisoning.
    c) Letterer-Siwe disease.
    d) Cushing's disease.

16. Conditions that may result in a sharp increase in serum calcium include all of the following except:

    a) hyperparathyroidism.
    b) multiple myeloma.
    c) hyperthyroidism.
    d) postmenopausal osteoporosis.

17. There is a high correlation between insufficiency fractures of the sternum and:

    a) spinal compression fractures with increased thoracic kyphosis.
    b) hip degeneration with a military spine.
    c) hip degeneration with lumbar compression fractures.
    d) spinal compression fractures with thoracic scoliosis.

18. Rickets is:

    a) exclusively a vitamin D deficiency.
    b) a deficiency of calcium, phosphorus, or vitamin D.
    c) a deficiency of vitamin C.
    d) a deficiency of vitamin D, potassium, or calcium.

19. Osteomalacia is a bone-softening condition associated with:

    a) the "leaching" of calcium from the skeleton.
    b) inadequate intake, absorption, or metabolism of vitamin D, calcium, or phosphorus.
    c) malfunction of osteoblasts or osteoclasts.
    d) lack of weight-bearing or tensile stress on bone.

20. The residual density following the healing of the zone of provisional calcification is:

    a) the white line of Frankel.
    b) the scorbutic zone.
    c) the umbau zonen.
    d) the growth arrest line.

21. The most common form of histiocytosis is:

    a) monostotic eosinophilic granuloma.
    b) polyostotic eosinophilic granuloma.
    c) Hand-Schüller-Christian disease.
    d) Letterer-Siwe disease.

22. Lesions particularly characteristic of hyperparathyroidism are:

    a) pseudotumors.
    b) brown tumors.
    c) involucrum.
    d) sequestrum.

23. Corticosteroid therapy may create:

    a) an eosinophilic granuloma.
    b) iatrogenic osteomalacia.
    c) iatrogenic hyperparathyroidism.
    d) iatrogenic Cushing's syndrome.

24. Regional osteoporosis is usually the result of:

    a) disuse after an injury.
    b) infection.
    c) an inflammatory arthritic condition.
    d) hormonal changes of menopause.

25. Grave's disease is a manifestation of:

    a) a hyperthyroid condition.
    b) a cortical adrenal malfunction.
    c) a hypothyroid condition.
    d) an anterior pituitary neoplasm.

26. Serum calcium levels in a patient with senile osteoporosis are usually:

    a) normal.
    b) somewhat elevated.
    c) somewhat depressed.
    d) greatly elevated.

27. The most common sacral insufficiency fracture is:

    a) a single vertical fracture through the sacral ala.
    b) a single transverse fracture through the lower sacral segments.
    c) a bilateral vertical fracture through the sacral ala.
    d) a curvilinear transverse fracture crossing the sacral ala and sacral segments.

28. Fluorosis may result from drinking excessive amounts of:

    a) distilled water.
    b) wine.
    c) cranberry juice.
    d) colas.

29. All of the following are true about transient regional osteoporosis except:

    a) it has a strong male predilection.
    b) in females, it is invariably left-sided, and is associated with pregnancy.
    c) it has two forms: regional migratory form, and a form occurring only in the hip.
    d) it is most common in adolescents.

30. The "white line of Frankel" is a radiographic indication of:

    a) hypervitaminosis A.
    b) rickets.
    c) heavy metal poisoning.
    d) scurvy.

31. The clinical "classic triad," which is *sometimes* seen with Hand-Schüller-Christian disease, consists of:

    a) hepatosplenomegaly, respiratory symptoms, and lytic skull lesions.
    b) exophthalmos, diabetes insipidus, and lytic skull lesions.
    c) diabetes insipidus, hepatosplenomegaly, and painful soft tissue nodules on the skull.
    d) respiratory symptoms, hepatosplenomegaly, and exophthalmos.

32. Primary and secondary hyperparathyroidism create osseous lesions:

    a) in subperiosteal bone, especially at entheses.
    b) in subarticular bone, especially in the peripheral joints.
    c) in the medullary cavities of long bones.
    d) in cancellous bone, especially within the carpus and the small tubular bones of the hands.

33. A diagnosis of acromegaly is suggested by the radiographic finding of:

    a) "floating teeth."
    b) a heel pad > 20 mm thick.
    c) Erlenmeyer flask deformity bilaterally in the long tubular bones.
    d) endosteal cortical thickening, with gradual occlusion of the medullary cavities of long bones.

34. When an osteoporotic patient has greatly elevated serum calcium levels, the differential diagnosis should consider:

    a) senile osteoporosis.
    b) PTH deficiency.
    c) hyperparathyroidism.
    d) hypovitaminosis D.

35. Hypothyroidism in a newborn creates:

    a) osteogenesis imperfecta.
    b) achondroplastic dwarfism.
    c) cretinism.
    d) Morquio's syndrome.

36. All of the following factors associated with senile osteoporosis may be mitigated except:

    a) calcium intake.
    b) viability of osteoblasts and osteocytes.
    c) hormonal balances.
    d) activity level.

37. Patients with pathologic hip fractures:

    a) always have severe, debilitating pain in the affected hip.
    b) always have severe pain in the buttocks.
    c) always have pain referred to the lumbosacral junction.
    d) may be completely asymptomatic.

38. A skeletally visible effect of polyvinylchloride (PVC) poisoning is:

    a) osteonecrosis at the femoral head.
    b) ectopic calcification.
    c) acroosteolysis.
    d) thick, undulating layers of periosteal new bone.

39. The "double cortical line sign" at the superior cortex of the acetabulum is a radiographic indication of:

    a) occult fracture.
    b) early protrusio acetabulae.
    c) early degenerative joint disease.
    d) disuse osteoporosis.

40. Scurvy is caused by long-term deficiency of:

    a) vitamin A.
    b) vitamin E.
    c) ascorbic acid.
    d) calcium.

41. Hand-Schüller-Christian disease is:

    a) an acute, fulminating, often fatal condition.
    b) an acute, benign and self-limiting condition.
    c) a chronic, intermittent disease, which may prove fatal.
    d) a chronic, benign, intermittent condition.

42. Tertiary hyperparathyroidism results in osseous lesions that characteristically appear:

    a) at the iliac margins of the sacroiliac joints.
    b) in the ribs and sternum.
    c) in the skull and shoulder.
    d) in peripheral joints and in the spine.

43. Headaches, dental malocclusion, bitemporal hemianopsia, and bilateral carpal tunnel syndrome might be typical of the clinical presentation of a patient with:

    a) hyperparathyroidism.
    b) gargoylism.
    c) hyperthyroidism.
    d) acromegaly.

44. Trabeculae in the proximal femur develop in characteristic patterns. The major weight-bearers:

    a) extend laterally upward in a curve from the lesser to the greater trochanter.
    b) extend medially upward in an arc from the lateral cortex below the greater trochanter to the inferior part of the femoral head.
    c) extend from the medial metaphyseal cortex to the superior femoral head.
    d) extend from the lateral metaphyseal cortex to the superior femoral head.

45. The intravertebral vacuum cleft is an x-ray sign which is **not** seen in:

    a) Grave's disease.
    b) Kummel's disease.
    c) Cushing's disease.
    d) Gaucher's disease.

46. Generalized osteoporosis is associated with all of the following except:

    a) skeletal trauma.
    b) congenital conditions.
    c) neoplastic diseases.
    d) nutritional or metabolic disorders.

47. Hip fracture in patients with senile osteoporosis has a female predilection of:

    a) 2 : 1.
    b) 3 : 1.
    c) 4 : 1.
    d) 5 : 1.

48. Heavy metal poisoning results in:

    a) transverse linear sclerosis at the metaphyses.
    b) patchy sclerosis in the medullary cavities of long bones.
    c) dense, homogenous sclerosis of medullary bone.
    d) multiple, discrete round or oval concretions throughout all areas of cancellous bone.

49. The most common radiographic appearance of immobilization osteoporosis is:

    a) spotty osteoporosis, with localized circular lucencies at epiphyses.
    b) bands of osteoporosis across the metaphyses of long bones.
    c) uniform, subtle decrease in bone density.
    d) cortical scalloping.

50. Barlow's disease is commonly known as:

    a) osteomalacia.
    b) scurvy.
    c) histiocytosis X.
    d) rickets.

51. The "butterfly sign" ("Honda sign") is a radiographic indication of:

    a) a pathologic fracture of the femoral neck.
    b) bilateral vertical fractures through the sacral ala, with a transverse fracture through a sacral segment.
    c) a vertical fracture through a lumbar vertebra.
    d) a vertical fracture through the center of the sacrum.

52. An early, definitive radiologic sign of hyperparathyroidism is:

    a) apparent widening of the sacroiliac joints.
    b) loss of disc height.
    c) bilateral, subchondral, and distal clavicle resorption.
    d) "rugger jersey" spine.

53. Tertiary hyperparathyroidism is seen in:

    a) patients with parathyroid adenomas.
    b) patients with chronic renal disease.
    c) kidney patients on dialysis.
    d) patients experiencing persistent calcium and phosphorous depletion.

54. Eosinophilic granuloma, Hand-Schüller-Christian disease, and Letterer-Siwe disease are all forms of:

    a) metabolic disorders.
    b) neoplastic disorders.
    c) histiocytosis "X."
    d) endocrine disorders.

55. Immobilization causes local osteoporosis that makes radiographically visible changes in bone within:

    a) 1 week to 10 days.
    b) 2 to 3 weeks.
    c) 1 month to 6 weeks.
    d) 2 to 3 months.

56. Except for femoral neck fractures, pathologic fractures caused by osteoporosis:

    a) heal normally, but require two to three times the normal healing time.
    b) heal in the normal time, but do not follow normal healing patterns.
    c) heal with normal quality and in normal healing time.
    d) require twice the normal healing time, and do not follow normal healing patterns.

57. After age 60, there is a doubling every 5 years in the incidence of:

    a) pathologic lumbar or thoracic vertebral fracture in females.
    b) metastasis to the lumbar spine from primary prostatic cancer in males.
    c) pathologic hip fracture in osteoporotic females.
    d) diagnosed multiple myeloma in patients of both genders.

58. The osseous lesions characteristic of corticosteroid arthropathy are also known to occur with:

    a) some anticonvulsants.
    b) injection of some iodine-based contrast agents.
    c) some NSAIDs (e.g., indomethacin, phenylbutazone).
    d) some antihypertensive medications.

59. A patient who complains of polydipsia, polyuria, and poor appetite, and whose plain films show excessive renal, vascular, and perivascular calcifications may be experiencing the effects of:

    a) hypervitaminosis D.
    b) fluorosis.
    c) hyperparathyroidism.
    d) Cushing's disease.

60. Thyroid acropachy may result after a patient has been successfully treated for:

    a) breast cancer.
    b) bronchogenic carcinoma.
    c) hypothyroidism.
    d) hyperthyroidism.

61. Small bowel ileus may be a radiographic indication of:

    a) spinal degenerative joint disease.
    b) inflammatory arthritis in the lumbar spine.
    c) an occult spinal fracture.
    d) neuropathic arthropathy.

62. Primary or secondary hyperparathyroidism cause vertebrae to have a characteristic radiologic appearance called:

    a) "heaped-up" vertebrae.
    b) "wasp-waist" vertebrae.
    c) "corduroy cloth" vertebrae.
    d) "rugger jersey" vertebrae.

63. Eosinophilic granuloma in a long bone is usually:

    a) in the epiphysis.
    b) in the metaphysis.
    c) in the diaphysis.
    d) in the articular cortex.

64. The effects of Gaucher's disease on vertebral bodies may create the radiographic appearance of:

    a) "heaped-up" vertebra.
    b) "bullet-nosed" vertebra.

c) "barrel-shaped" vertebra.
d) "H"-shaped vertebra.

65. Of the following, the least common cause of vertebra plana is:

a) osteoporosis.
b) multiple myeloma.
c) eosinophilic granuloma.
d) metastatic carcinoma.

66. The most frequent sites of pathologic fracture caused by osteoporosis are at the femoral neck and:

a) the lumbar vertebrae.
b) the thoracic vertebrae.
c) the pubic rami.
d) the ribs.

67. After approximately 35 years of age, females generally lose **trabecular** bone at a rate of:

a) 2% per year.
b) 1.5% per year.
c) 1% per year.
d) 0.5% per year.

68. The "marginal condensation" sign signifies:

a) sclerosis around a healing "umbau zonen" in a patient with osteomalacia.
b) evidence of growth arrest caused by rickets in an infant.
c) periarticular sclerosis in patients with early osteoarthritis.
d) hypertrophic callus over small endplate fractures in patients with Cushing's disease.

69. The radiographic manifestation of skeletal effects of hypervitaminosis A is:

a) "split cortices" of long bones.
b) bulging at the costochondral junctions, similar to the "rachitic rosary."
c) ectopic renal, vascular and perivascular calcifications.
d) prolific solid, periosteal new bone along long bone diaphyses; diastasis at the bregma.

70. Gaucher's disease does **not** create a radiographic appearance of:

a) expansile cortical thickening.
b) Erlenmeyer flask deformity in the femur.
c) medullary expansion in long bones.
d) avascular necrosis of the femoral head.

71. After approximately 35 years of age, females generally lose **cortical** bone at a rate of:

a) 2.5% per year.
b) 2% per year.
c) 1.5% per year.
d) 1% per year.

72. A characteristic radiologic sign of hyperparathyroidism is:

a) "hole-within-a-hole" appearance.
b) "hair-on-end" periosteal reaction.
c) basilar invagination.
d) resorption of lamina dura around tooth sockets.

73. More than 90% of patients who experience eosinophilic granuloma in a vertebral body, causing vertebra plana:

a) require surgical removal of the crushed segment.
b) suffer neurologic deficits.
c) have 48–95% restoration of vertebral body height within a year.
d) require radiation therapy and suffer permanent loss of the affected segment.

74. Gaucher's disease is essentially an abnormality of:

a) calcium deposition.
b) calcium absorption.
c) lipid metabolism.
d) osteoid deposition.

75. Radiographic differentiation between hemangioma and osteoporosis in the vertebrae is aided by the fact that:

a) hemangioma may create a "vertebra plana."
b) hemangioma may create an appearance of vertical striations in the vertebrae.
c) hemangioma usually occurs at multiple spinal sites.
d) hemangioma is usually solitary.

76. The confluence of the major trabecular groups in the femoral neck form a lucent area known as:

a) the iliofemoral triangle.
b) von Weber's triangle.
c) Codman's triangle.
d) Ward's triangle.

77. By age 65, senile osteoporosis entails a bone mass loss of:

a) 30–45% of bone.
b) 20–40% of bone.
c) 10 to 25% of bone.
d) up to 55% of bone.

78. The osteopenia that is a feature of Cushing's disease appears similar to that seen in:

a) rheumatoid arthritis.
b) Sudeck's atrophy.
c) transient regional osteoporosis.
d) postmenopausal osteoporosis.

79. The clinical hallmark of scurvy is:

a) an infant who lies supine and motionless with the thighs flexed and abducted.
b) vascular fragility, evidenced by petechiae, bleeding gums, hematuria, and melena.
c) bulging at the costochondral junctions.
d) an irritable infant with swollen joints.

80. Eosinophilic granuloma is most frequently found in:

a) the spine.
b) the skull.
c) the hands and feet.
d) the mandible.

81. Radiographic evidence of thyroid acropachy is characterized by:

    a) spade-like ungual tufts.
    b) sub-periosteal erosions on the radial sides of the distal and middle phalanges of the second and third digits.
    c) dense periostitis on the radial aspects of the distal and middle phalanges of the second and third digits.
    d) dense periostitis on the radial aspects of the metacarpals, or the tibial aspects of the metacarpals.

82. Skull lesions typical of hyperparathyroidism give an appearance of:

    a) geometric lesions > 5 mm diameter, with beveled edges.
    b) ill-defined lucencies caused by destruction of in inner table and sparing of the outer table.
    c) diffuse granular deossification, creating a "pepper pot skull" appearance.
    d) "hair on end" spicules radiating from expansile lesions of mottled density.

83. Eosinophilic granuloma in the spine most frequently occurs in:

    a) the thoracic vertebrae.
    b) the cervical segments.
    c) the first two sacral segments.
    d) the lumbar vertebrae.

84. A "bell-shaped" thoracic cage may result from:

    a) pectus carinatum.
    b) pectus excavatum.
    c) osteomalacia.
    d) osteoporosis.

85. Traumatic vertebral fractures usually appear on plain film as:

    a) wedge fractures with intact pedicles.
    b) vertebra plana.
    c) crushed vertebra with intrabody vacuum sign.
    d) crush fractures with pedicle destruction.

86. Senile osteoporosis is known to cause all of the following vertebral radiographic appearances except:

    a) barrel-shaped vertebra.
    b) fish vertebra.
    c) wedged vertebra
    d) vertebra plana.

87. The most commonly encountered metabolic bone disease is:

    a) histiocytosis X.
    b) osteomalacia.
    c) osteoporosis.
    d) hyperparathyroidism.

88. The radiologic appearance of vertebrae in a patient with Cushing's disease may feature:

    a) heaped-up vertebrae.
    b) "corduroy cloth" vertebrae.
    c) "fish" vertebrae.
    d) "picture frame" vertebrae.

89. Wimberger's sign is:

    a) a widened "teardrop distance" seen in Legg-Calvé-Perthes disease.
    b) an increased ADI, seen with trisomy 21.
    c) a dense epiphyseal cortical margin with osteopenic central portion, seen with scurvy.
    d) a lucent subcortical band, seen as a sign of good prognosis in the healing of a talar dome fracture.

90. The most common pelvic site of eosinophilic granuloma is:

    a) supraacetabular in the ilium.
    b) at the superolateral iliac crest.
    c) near the anterior inferior iliac spine.
    d) in the ilium, adjacent to the inferior third of the sacroiliac joint.

91. The most notable skeletal effect of a hyperactive thyroid is:

    a) generalized osteopenia.
    b) periarticular osteopenia.
    c) subchondral geodes.
    d) general thickening of cortical margins throughout the skeleton.

92. The radiologic hallmark sign of hyperparathyroidism is:

    a) spondyloarthropathy, with marked loss of disc height.
    b) subperiosteal resorption, which is discernible first in the hands.
    c) nephrocalcinosis.
    d) "salt and pepper" skull lesions.

93. The radiologic appearance of eosinophilic granuloma in long bones or in the skull may be described as:

    a) a round or oval, sharply demarcated geographic lytic lesion with endosteal scalloping.
    b) a poorly demarcated ovoid geographic lesion with a "ground glass" appearance.
    c) an expansile, lucent lesion with "soap bubble" pseudotrabeculations.
    d) a round, sharply demarcated geographic sclerotic lesion, which slowly expands the bone.

94. Osteomalacia does **not** cause:

    a) increased serum alkaline phosphatase.
    b) increased serum calcium and phosphorous.
    c) increased serum hydroxyproline.
    d) increased serum parathormone.

95. The "Cupid's bow" describes the radiographic appearance of:

    a) giant Schmorl's nodes on lateral spinal views.
    b) notochordal remnants on frontal views.
    c) notochordal remnants on lateral views.
    d) significant L5 anterolisthesis on frontal views.

96. In the spine of an elderly patient, a pseudohemangiomatous radiologic appearance is often caused by:

    a) Calvé's disease.
    b) non-Hodgkin's lymphoma.
    c) osteoporosis.
    d) Paget's disease.

97. When there is a reduced quantity of bone, but that bone is of normal quality, the correct term for the condition is:

    a) osteopenia.
    b) osteomalacia.
    c) osteoporosis.
    d) osteochondrosis.

98. The effects of Cushing's disease on bone are most notably:

    a) cortical thickening and gradual expansion of long bones.
    b) osteopenia and pathologic fracture.
    c) subperiosteal resorption and periosteal new bone stimulation.
    d) destruction of marrow as it is replaced by fatty tissue.

99. Scurvy and rickets are best diagnosed radiographically with what views?

    a) shoulder and wrist.
    b) knee and wrist.
    c) knee and hip.
    d) wrist and ankle.

100. The metaphyses of patients with rickets tend to appear:

    a) narrowed, with a compressed and sclerotic growth plate.
    b) expansile (cupped), with a widened and lucent growth plate.
    c) frayed and cupped with a narrowed and irregular growth plate.
    d) cupped, frayed, and irregular, with a widened growth plate.

PRACTICE TEST CHAPTER 8—ANSWER KEY

1.	c	11.	c	21.	a	31.	b	41.	c	51.	b	61.	c	71.	d	81.	d	91.	a
2.	c	12.	b	22.	b	32.	a	42.	d	52.	c	62.	d	72.	d	82.	c	92.	b
3.	c	13.	d	23.	d	33.	b	43.	d	53.	c	63.	c	73.	c	83.	a	93.	a
4.	a	14.	c	24.	a	34.	c	44.	c	54.	c	64.	d	74.	c	84.	c	94.	b
5.	c	15.	a	25.	a	35.	c	45.	a	55.	a	65.	a	75.	d	85.	a	95.	b
6.	c	16.	d	26.	a	36.	b	46.	a	56.	c	66.	c	76.	d	86.	a	96.	c
7.	d	17.	a	27.	a	37.	d	47.	d	57.	c	67.	a	77.	b	87.	c	97.	c
8.	c	18.	b	28.	b	38.	c	48.	a	58.	c	68.	d	78.	d	88.	c	98.	b
9.	b	19.	b	29.	d	39.	d	49.	c	59.	a	69.	d	79.	b	89.	c	99.	b
10.	b	20.	d	30.	d	40.	c	50.	b	60.	d	70.	a	80.	b	90.	a	100.	d

Chapter 9

PLAIN FILM IMAGING OF CHEST AND ABDOMEN
Technical Considerations, Normal Anatomy, Chest Lesions, Abdominal Lesions

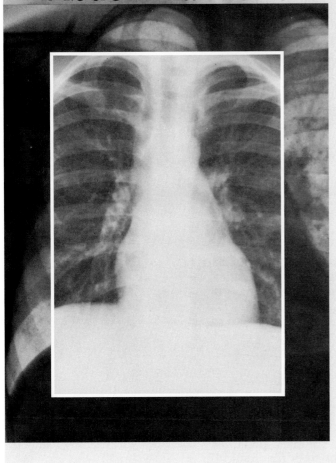

A.   TECHNICAL CONSIDERATIONS (CHEST)

1.   **kVp settings**

   a)   increase kVp over settings for skeletal imaging

   b)   120 kVp or more

   c)   lower mAs settings give better lung detail

2.   **Chest Film Positioning (PA vs. AP; upright vs. supine or lateral recumbent, apical lordotic)**

   a)   Frontal chest film is done PA

   b)   To further evaluate a questionable finding in lung apices, use apical lordotic view (this does not visualize extreme apex, so overpenetrated PA is preferable for this area)

   c)   Lateral (usually left lateral projection)—gives good visualization of posterior lung bases, retrosternal and retrocardiac areas; permits localization of lesions seen on PA projection

   d)   Oblique projections show mediastinal and hilar contours; tracheal bifurcation, etc.
   - RPO and LAO project trachea to right of spine
   - LPO and RAO project trachea to left of spine
   - rotate patient 45° to view heart and great vessels (LAO)
   - rotate patient 30° to view lung fields and hilar structures (RAO or LAO)

   e)   Lateral decubitus: patient side-lying; x-ray beam parallel to floor
   - optimal position (in most instances): abnormal side up
   - view is named by the side the patient lies on: e.g., patient lying on the right side: "*right lateral decubitus*" projection
   - with affected side dependent: shows free pleural effusion, air-fluid levels

   f)   Cross-table lateral: patient supine, x-ray beam parallel to floor
   - can also demonstrate air-fluid levels

3.   **Mobility or Stability of Visualized Masses**

   a)   Respiration may move radiopacities
   - maximum inhalation for chest films (anterior end of right sixth rib should be visible, posterior ends of 10 ribs visible above right hemidiaphragm)
   - on expiration, lungs "*cloud up*" (appear more dense) and heart appears larger ("*pancaked*")
   - expiration view helpful in detecting emphysema (especially unilaterally)

because air is not expelled from affected lung
- pneumothorax appears larger on expiration; small pneumothorax may be visible only on expiration

b) Tension pneumothorax: may shift mass to *opposite side*

c) Gravity may cause shift of unattached masses when patient position is changed

B. ANATOMIC CONSIDERATIONS IN THE THORAX

1. Normal Anatomy and Position of the Heart and Great Vessels

a) Right and left heart borders and ascending aorta are in *anterior* thoracic cavity

b) Most of the right heart border contacts the middle lobe of the right lung
- on lateral view, right ventricle is retrosternal; forms anterosuperior heart border

c) Uppermost right heart border and ascending aorta contact upper lobe of the right lung
- right atrium is posterior to right ventricle but not clearly defined on plain film

d) Majority of left heart border contacts the lingula (analog of middle lobe) of the left lower lung
- left ventricle is posteroinferior on the lateral projection; or lower left on the PA projection

e) Uppermost left heart border contacts upper lobe of the left lung

f) left atrium is *posterior* on the lateral projection

g) aortic knob and descending thoracic aorta: in posterior thoracic cavity

h) the aortic knob contacts the apical posterior upper lobe of left lung

i) left hilum: slightly higher than right hilum

j) "*aortic window*" created by the arch of the aorta

k) Trachea usually slightly to right of middle; bifurcates at the carina (around T4)

2. Normal Anatomy of Lungs: Lobes and Septa

a) Right lung
- three lobes: upper (RUL), middle (RML), lower (RLL)
- two septa (fissures)
  1) major (oblique) fissure separates lower lobe from upper and middle lobes
  2) minor (horizontal) fissure separates upper lobe from middle lobe (runs

from anterior lung to intersect major
fissure posteriorly)

b) Left lung

- two lobes and lingula: upper (LUL),
  lower (LLL), lingula (middle lobe
  homologue)

- LUL and LLL separated by major
  (oblique) fissure, running from approx. T5
  level (posteriorly) to level of anterior
  costophrenic angle (anteriorly)

c) Accessory lobes and septa

- right lung may have azygos lobe (caused
  by anomalous position of azygos vein),
  indicated by azygos fissure in medial right
  upper lung field (in about 0.5% of
  population)

- right lung may have inferior accessory
  fissure: sets apart medial basal segment of
  lower lobe (seen in about 5% of
  population)

- either lung may have superior accessory
  fissure: sets apart superior segment of
  lower lobe (present in about 5% of
  population); indistinguishable on plain
  film from minor (horizontal) fissure of
  right lung

☞ **3. Boyden's Numbering System for Segmental Bronchi
(Supplying Each Lobar Segment)**

a) RUL: three segmental branches of upper
bronchus

- apical RUL bronchus (Boyden #1)
- anterior RUL bronchus (Boyden #2)
- posterior RUL bronchus (Boyden #3)

b) RML: two segmental branches from the
intermediate bronchus

- lateral RML bronchus (Boyden #4)
- medial RML bronchus (Boyden #5)

c) RLL: five segmental branches from lower
bronchus (one superior and four basal)

- superior RLL bronchus (posterior
  superior) (Boyden #6)
- medial basal RLL bronchus (medial and
  anterior) (Boyden #7)
- anterior basal RLL bronchus (anterior
  and lateral) (Boyden #8)
- lateral basal RLL bronchus (lateral and
  posterior) (Boyden #9)
- posterior basal RLL bronchus (posterior
  and medial) (Boyden #10)

d) Lateral and posterior RLL segments are
lowest, anterior and medial are slightly
higher (segments overlap in all projections)

e) To minimize overlap of right lung segments,
use left lateral and left oblique projections

f) LUL bronchus: two main branches, upper

and lower (lingular); upper division supplies two lobar segments

- apical posterior LUL bronchus (Boyden #1 and 3)
- anterior LUL bronchus (analogue of Boyden #2 in left lung)
- superior lingular bronchus (analogue of RML's lateral bronchus) (Boyden #4)
- inferior lingular bronchus (analogue of RML medial bronchus) (Boyden #5)

g) LLL bronchus: five branches, similar to RLL

- superior LLL bronchus (Boyden #6)
- medial basal LLL bronchus (Boyden #7)
- anterior basal LLL bronchus (Boyden #8)
- lateral basal LLL bronchus (Boyden #9)
- posterior basal LLL bronchus (Boyden #10)

☞ **4. Preferential Lesion Sites**

a) Fissure (septum) displacement is reliable sign of lobar collapse; also seen in extensive pneumonias

b) Upper lobe anterior segment shows predilection for lung carcinoma

c) RLL superior segment shows predilection for lung abscess

d) Lung apices: classic site for reinfection TB

e) Lung apices: predilected to silicosis

f) Lower lung fields: site of fibrosis, diaphragmatic plaques common in asbestosis

5. Anatomy of Mediastinum

a) Conventionally divided into anterior, middle and posterior mediastinum, but specific anatomic borders of the divisions not universally defined

- anterior mediastinum
    1) generally includes the area between the anterior border of the trachea and the posterior border of the sternum
    2) some include heart and pericardium
- middle mediastinum: usually includes trachea and esophagus, heart and pericardium
- posterior mediastinum: area posterior to a line constructed superior to inferior, about 1 cm behind the anterior border of the thoracic vertebrae

b) Also divided into superior and inferior portions (as seen on lateral projection)

- superior mediastinum: defined as mediastinal area above a line from the sternomanubrial junction to the fourth thoracic vertebral body or as the mediastinal area above the aortic arch

- inferior mediastinum: from level of sternomanubrial joint down to the diaphragm
- lateral boundaries (seen on PA projection): formed by apparent pleural margins adjacent to mediastinal structures

6. **Anatomy of Right and Left Hemidiaphragms**

   a) Deep sulcus peripherally around dome of each hemidiaphragm: *"costophrenic angle"*
      - posterior angle (sulcus) is deepest, visualized only on lateral view
      - PA projection demonstrates lateral angles

   b) Lateral projection: entire right hemidiaphragm and posterior half of left diaphragm are visible; anterior left hemidiaphragm normally is obliterated by the heart shadow

---

REVIEW—STUDY QUESTIONS

1. How do kVp and mAs settings for chest and abdomen studies differ from those for skeletal exams?
2. Describe the bronchial tree and its pattern of supply to the pulmonary lobes and segments.
3. Describe the divisions of the mediastinum and their contents.
4. What is the costophrenic sulcus? The costophrenic angle?
5. With oblique views, how will you adjust patient positioning to best demonstrate heart, or to see the hilar regions?
6. What is the preferential site for lung carcinoma? For lung abscess?
7. What are two means of obtaining good visualization of the lung apices?
8. How is the lateral decubitus projection labeled (as to which side is named)?
9. Describe the normal anatomic position of the heart borders, including the structures they contact.
10. Compare right and left lung anatomy, using Boyden's numbering system.

C. CHEST LESIONS

1. **General Concepts and Definitions**

   a) **Silhouette sign**
      - loss of normal roentgen silhouette caused by obliteration of visible borders along zone of anatomic contact between a lesion of water density and the diaphragm, aorta, or heart
      - common cause: pneumonic infiltrate adjacent to heart, aorta, or diaphragm
      - water density not in physical contact with

heart; aorta or diaphragm will not obliterate borders; silhouette sign will be absent

☞   **b)   Air bronchogram sign**
- air in bronchi appears as branching black lines (not visible normally)
- caused by air-filled bronchus surrounded by water density
- denotes dense area of infiltrate with air-filled bronchus within it
- most commonly caused by pneumonia; also may indicate pneumonia with pulmonary edema, pulmonary infarcts, or certain chronic lung lesions
- air bronchogram sign indicates lesion in lung, not in mediastinum

☞   **c)   Extrapleural sign**
- lesion with a sharp border convex towards the lung, with distinct tapering margins
- lack of air bronchogram sign indicates a lesion in extrapleural space (rather than in lung parenchyma)
- rib destruction may be present or absent
- most common cause: metastatic lesions in the ribs
- other causes: plasmacytoma of ribs, mediastinal masses, mesothelioma, neurofibroma, pleural or extrapleural hematoma
- should actually be called *"extraparenchymal sign"* since pleural lesions can cause this sign

2.   Interstitial Lung Disease

a)   Interstitium includes walls of: alveoli and their ducts, blood and lymphatic vessels, and bronchi; also interlobular septa and connective tissue accompanying all these structures

b)   *"Miliary nodules"*: small, rounded opacities in the interstitium of the lungs; also called reticulonodular, reticular, network, or fibrotic appearance

☞   **c)**   *"Honeycomb lung"*: diffusely disseminated small air cysts seen with pulmonary emphysema; air-filled sacs 1–10 mm diameter in clusters

☞   **d)**   *"Kerley's lines"* (signs of lymphatic dilation)
- **Kerley's A lines:** thin, nonbranching; several inches long; radiate from bronchi but do not follow bronchi or blood vessels
- **Kerley's B lines:** thin, faint lines 1–3 cm long, 1–2 mm wide; form a horizontal *"stepladder"* pattern, usually in the lateral lung bases, perpendicular to the nearest pleural surface
- **Kerley's C lines:** *"spiderweb"* of fine lines throughout the lungs

☞ **3. Alveolar Infiltrates (Air-space Disease)**

    a) Opacities with fluffy, wispy edges

    b) Lesions often coalesce

    c) Distribution may be segmental or lobar

    d) Bilateral, symmetric infiltrations may be more dense around the hilar regions, fading at the peripheral areas: "*butterfly*" or "*bat-wing*" pattern

    e) often shows an "*air bronchogram sign*"

    f) *Acinus*: a terminal bronchiole and its subdivisions (may fill with exudate)

☞ **4. Solitary Pulmonary Nodule (Coin Lesion)**

    a) Calcified solitary pulmonary nodule is usually benign
- calcified granuloma of resolved tuberculosis
- calcified lesions of resolved infections, e.g., histoplasmosis
- calcified pulmonary hamartoma: uncalcified solitary pulmonary nodule is presumed malignant until proven otherwise

☞ **5. Atelectasis**

    a) General considerations
- nature of condition
    1) loss of pulmonary volume without fluid-filled air spaces; incompletely expanded, shrunken, collapsed, or airless lung
    2) obstruction: most common cause of collapse
- central atelectasis is lobar or segmental collapse and may be caused by
    1) intrinsic lesion: airway plugged by neoplasm (bronchogenic carcinoma), mucous plug (from inflammatory bronchial disease, such as asthma or tuberculosis), foreign body, etc.
    2) extrinsic lesion: airway invaded by adjacent neoplasm or constricted by pressure from a mass adjacent to the airway (e.g., enlarged left atrium, mediastinal masses, enlarged lymph nodes, aneurysm)
    3) constricted airway (e.g., postinflammatory constriction, as in "*middle lobe syndrome*")
- peripheral atelectasis is caused by pressures from the periphery of the parenchyma, such as
    1) compression caused by pneumothorax or pleural effusions
    2) inflammatory exudate (caused by pneumonia)
    3) trauma to the chest wall

    4) emphysema

    5) fibrosis (from granulomatous disease, "*round atelectasis*," peripheral interstitial fibrosis)

    6) mucus plugs (caused by asthma, or infections)

    7) loss of surfactant

    8) frequent post-surgical complication

- "*round atelectasis*": associated with asbestosis; appearance is caused by folded, collapsed lung tissue
- "*plate-like atelectasis*": ("*discoid atelectasis*," "*platter atelectasis*," "*Fleischner lines*") almost always in lung base, 1–3 cm above diaphragm; single or multiple linear densities; unilateral or bilateral; occurs with diseases that reduce diaphragmatic excursion; true etiology and clinical significance unknown
- contraction collapse: with chronic tuberculosis, silicosis, extensive pulmonary fibrosis
- may also be congenital or iatrogenic

b) **Clinical features**

- rapid occlusion and massive collapse: pain on affected side, sudden onset of dyspnea, cyanosis, hypotension, tachycardia, fever, sometimes shock
- in massive collapse: dullness to percussion over affected lung, diminished or absent lung sounds and reduced chest excursion with deep inspiration
- gradually developing atelectasis: usually asymptomatic
- "*middle lobe syndrome*": by definition; chronic right middle lobe collapse caused by granulomatous infection (same mechanism can affect other segments or lobes, and RML collapse can be caused by other mechanisms)
- "*middle lobe syndrome*" may be asymptomatic or may involve a severe nonproductive cough and signs seen in rapid occlusion
- chronic atelectasis usually develops infection, regardless of etiology of collapse
- collapse often occurs during the early stages of lobar pneumonia resolution

c) **Radiologic features**

- three **direct** radiologic signs of lung collapse:

    1) displaced fissures or interlobar septa

- most reliable sign of atelectasis
- greater displacement with more rapid collapse

2) increased opacity of lung
- may be very subtle, undetectable on standard views

3) vascular or bronchial crowding
- crowded bronchial or vascular channels
- vessels in adjacent lobes may curve toward collapsed lobe

☞
- six **indirect** radiologic signs of lung collapse:
   1) hilar displacement
      - upper lobe collapse results in hilar elevation
      - lower lobe collapse usually causes downward displacement
      - middle lobe collapse usually does not displace the hilum
   2) unilateral elevation of a hemidiaphragm (occasionally)
   3) shift of mediastinal structures towards the side of collapse
      - upper lobe collapse may cause tracheal deviation to affected side (unreliable sign)
   4) compensatory emphysema
      - hyperlucency and overdistention of unaffected lung
   5) narrowed rib cage on collapsed side
   6) herniation of lung tissue

☞
- *"silhouette sign"*: in middle lobe syndrome (or any RML collapse) the right cardiac border usually is obliterated

☞
- *"round atelectasis"*: so-called because folded, collapsed tissue gives rounded appearance on film; has *"comet-tail sign"* comma-shaped opacity caused by compressed pulmonary vessels and airways leading from the hilar region

- lower lobe collapse
   1) *"mediastinal wedge"*: opacity on PA projection, as lobe collapses down, back, and medially (with LLL, this may be obscured by cardiac shadow but can be visualized on right oblique view)
   2) LLL collapse: left border of descending aorta, diaphragm, posterior heart are obscured; and upper portion of major septum may displace down and medially
   3) RLL collapse: looks like RML involvement, but without silhouette sign
   4) lateral view shows major septum's posterior displacement and obliteration of part of diaphragmatic shadow

- lingula or middle lobe collapse
    1) "*silhouette sign*"; obliteration of adjacent heart border
    2) RML collapse may involve inferior displacement of minor fissure (lordotic view may be optimal for this)
    3) lateral view shows approximation of major and minor fissures
- upper lobe collapse
    1) RUL collapse
        - minor fissure is elevated (PA view)
        - increased opacity of upper lung area with somewhat triangular outline
        - right hilar elevation and sometimes tracheal shift
        - lateral projection shows superior portion of major septum displaced anteriorly, minor septum elevated
        - part of anterior ascending aorta border obscured
    2) LUL collapse
        - PA view shows increased opacity of medial portion of lung, but with no sharply defined border
        - "*silhouette sign*": adjacent border of aortic knob is obscured by collapsed apicoposterior segment; upper left cardiac border is obscured by collapsed anterior segment
        - lingula collapse often seen with LUL collapse; may be discerned on PA view; may obscure more of left cardiac border
        - tracheal deviation, hilar elevation, vertically oriented vascular markings in LLL
        - lateral projection shows major septum anterior displacement; border of collapse (often including lingula) may extend along sternum to diaphragm
        - may see opaque mediastinal wedge
    3) entire lung collapse (most often left): heart displaced posterior; posterior cardiac border obscured; opposite lung herniated across thorax; sometimes scoliosis develops (convex to affected side)

d) **Differential considerations**
- lobar consolidation: does not displace septa
- encapsulated pleural effusions: thickened pleura, rounded contours, normally

positioned septa, lack of air bronchogram signs

- bronchogenic carcinoma: *reverse "S" curve* seen with carcinoma may also appear in PA view with RUL collapse (also with lymphadenopathy, mediastinal tumor, or lobar collapse caused by bronchial metastasis); (bronchogenic carcinoma may cause atelectasis)
- helpful signs for ruling out bronchogenic carcinoma
  1) *"open bronchus sign"*: indicates peripheral etiology for collapse (bronchus supplying collapsed segment is normal)
  2) *"double lesion sign"*: bronchogenic carcinoma is unlikely to cause certain combinations, such as RUL with RML, LLL with LUL (key is whether a single lesion could simultaneously block airways to the collapsed segments)
- lobar enlargement: septa will bulge outward from the affected lobe

6. **Pleural Lesions**

a) **Free pleural effusion results in two radiographic patterns**
- *"meniscus sign"*: concave upper border (meniscus) appears to extend higher laterally than medially, obliterating the costophrenic angle
  1) more common with larger amounts of fluid
- *"subpulmonary pattern"*: with patient upright, fluid trapped between lung and diaphragm
  1) radiologic appearance resembles elevated hemidiaphragm (diaphragm is in normal position but is obscured by parallel layer of free fluid)
  2) more common with small amounts of fluid
  3) decubitus film helps confirm subpulmonary fluid: fluid gravitates to dependent side of pleural cavity
  4) three radiographic signs of subpulmonary fluid (upright films)
     - high hemidiaphragm
     - shallow costophrenic angles
     - separation of gastric air bubble from diaphragm

b) **Encapsulated (loculated) pleural effusion**
- caused by pleural adhesions
- four radiographic signs of encapsulated fluid
  1) no shift of fluid with positional change (*"lava"* appearance)
  2) absence of *"air bronchogram sign"*

3) pleural thickening elsewhere in same hemithorax
4) "pseudotumor" with convex borders

- "*vanishing tumor*" or "*phantom tumor*": rapid disappearance of "pseudotumor" of encapsulated pleural effusion in patient with congestive heart failure as cardiac compensation is restored

7. **Congenital Anomalies and Variants**

   a) **Aortic anomalies**

   - may be asymptomatic, incidental findings, or may form a vascular ring, with resultant dysphagia or dyspnea
   - aberrant right subclavian artery: from left aortic arch (most common arch anomaly)
   - radiographic signs of aberrant right subclavian artery
     1) PA shows oblique shadow through descending aorta
     2) lateral may show anterior displacement of trachea
     3) posterior right arch may dilate: diverticulum of Kommeral
     4) aneurysm may develop from enlarging diverticulum of Kommeral
   - mirror-image branching
     1) PA shows arch shadow to right of trachea
     2) descending aorta is on right
   - circumflex left ligamentum arteriosum (retroesophageal)
   - circumflex descending aorta: on side opposite aortic arch
     1) retroesophageal segment, often symptomatic
     2) best diagnosed via CT or MRI
   - double aortic arch
     1) common arch anomaly, most frequent symptomatic vascular ring
     2) both arches visible on PA view
     3) lateral view shows anterior compression of trachea
     4) barium swallow shows esophageal indentation
     5) definitive delineation of anomaly via CT or MRI
   - aortic coarctation
     1) narrowing or constriction of the lumen, usually restricting left ventricular outflow
     2) common anomaly, more frequent in males
     3) clinical sign: blood pressure differences between right and left sides
     4) increased incidence of other cardiovascular abnormalities,

especially bicuspid valve abnormalities, tubular hypoplasia of the aortic arch, patent ductus arteriosus, ventricular septal defect, subaortic stenosis, hypoplastic left heart, transposition of great vessels, and berry aneurysms (intracranial)

5) predisposes to aneurysm, dissection, infectious aortitis distal to coarctation

6) plain film
- PA view may show "*3 sign*": focal indentation (stenosis) of lateral border of aorta
- enlarged ascending aorta (prestenotic dilatation)
- dilation of descending aorta distal to coarctation (poststenotic dilatation)
- rib notching (after several years): focal scalloping of inferior rib surface (unilateral or bilateral)
- esophageal indentation clearly shown with barium swallow

7) CT and MRI optimally display anomaly

8) corrected via surgery or balloon angioplasty

9) aberrant innominate artery (retroesophageal)

10) aberrant left subclavian artery
- may occur with "*tetralogy of Fallot*," or other congenital heart conditions
- retroesophageal, and similar to the aberrant right subclavian
- originates from right sided descending aorta
- usually asymptomatic

11) "*situs inversus*": mirror image of normal position
- *situs inversus totalis*: abdominal and thoracic viscera reversed
- *situs solitus*: abdominal viscera normal, thoracic viscera reversed (dextrocardia)

8. **Traumatic Lesions**

a) **Lungs and pleura**
- lung contusion
    1) **General considerations**
        - mechanism is usually blunt trauma, with three mechanical "effects":
            a. inertia of sudden deceleration: mobile tissue is torsioned at interface with stable tissues, resulting in

shearing forces, tears, bleeding

   b. **spallation:** energy shock wave affects liquid-gas interface (e.g., at alveoli)

   c. **implosion:** low-pressure afterwave, expanding gas bubbles on rebound after a high-pressure shock wave

- nature of injury
  - a. parenchyma of lung is bruised
  - b. alveolocapillary membranes rupture, spilling blood and lymph into interstitial and alveolar air spaces usually in lung tissue adjacent to solid structures (ribs, vertebrae) or other organs (heart, liver)
  - c. parenchyma is suffused with blood; may bleed into bronchial tree; pleural space effects may develop over 24 to 72 hours
- incidence
  - a. most common consequence of blunt chest injury
  - b. estimate: occurs in up to 75% of chest trauma patients
  - c. major determinant of morbidity and mortality in chest trauma

2) **Clinical features**
- often asymptomatic in mild cases, or in early stages
- hemoptysis
- bronchorrhea
- tachypnea
- hypoxemia
- decreased cardiac output
- diffuse contusion may cause adult respiratory distress syndrome (ARDS)
- respiratory failure and death

3) **Radiologic features**
- lung opacity (with or without air bronchogram signs)
- diffuse enlargement of a lobe of the lung
- focal bulging of lung border
- consolidation of lung may be focal, multifocal, diffuse

- lung laceration
  - 1) **General considerations**
    - mechanism
      - a. penetration of lung by sharp object (rib fragment, knife)

        b.   inertial shearing stress

- nature of injury
    - a.   slit or tear in lung parenchyma
    - b.   bronchopleural fistulae (frequently)
    - c.   tear may be filled with air ("*pneumatocele*")
    - d.   tear may be filled with blood ("*hematoma*")
    - e.   blood and air in tear form a "*hematopneumatocele*"

2) **Clinical features**
    - respiratory failure
    - sometimes, dark blood in sputum

3) **Radiologic features**
    - not visible initially
    - air-filled space (pneumatocele) may expand rapidly with high-pressure mechanical ventilation treatments
    - tend to form round or ovoid gas pockets (mediastinal gas collections often are more elongated)
    - adjacent to dense parenchymal contusion

- "*hemopneumothorax*" (pneumothorax plus hemothorax)
    1) **General considerations**
        - mechanism
            - a.   any trauma that ruptures lung vessels
            - b.   alveolar compression
            - c.   lung laceration
            - d.   barotrauma
            - e.   lung laceration may cause bronchopleural fistulae, which can result in tension pneumothorax
        - incidence
            - a.   extremely common
            - b.   occurs with a wide variety of injuries
            - c.   about half of hospital patients with chest trauma have hemothorax
            - d.   hemopneumothorax is often bilateral

    2) **Clinical features**
        - small pneumothoraces may collect along medial and inferior ventral chest wall
        - respiratory difficulties (dyspnea)
        - may be associated with pneumomediastinum

☞

    3) **Radiologic features**
- lateral decubitus is optimum view for pneumothorax visualization
- spontaneous pneumothorax indicated by:
  - a. mediastinal displacement
  - b. airlessness (relative increase of opacity) of affected lung
- these signs decrease with lung consolidation, mechanical ventilation

☞

- atelectasis
  1) **General considerations**
     - mechanism
       - a. trauma in unconscious patient may result in aspiration
       - b. attempts at resuscitation may cause aspiration
       - c. bronchial occlusion from any cause may result in atelectasis
       - d. contributing factors: inactivated lung surfactant (neonates), shallow breathing (caused by pain), splinting by intercostal muscles, lung stiffness
     - incidence: frequently seen after blunt chest trauma, infection, or neoplasms
  2) **Clinical features**
     - respiratory difficulty (dyspnea)
     - may have bronchorrhea

☞

  3) **Radiologic features**
     - well demonstrated on lateral decubitus projection (pneumothorax)
     - increased opacification
     - loss of volume
     - air bronchogram signs may be visible on well-penetrated film
     - restored lung capacity after bronchoscopy and chest physiotherapy
     - displaced lung fissures
     - hilar elevation
     - elevated hemidiaphragm

b) Mediastinum
- traumatic rupture of the aorta (TRA)
  1) **General considerations**
     - mechanism
       - a. tearing with rapid deceleration caused by traction at ligamentum arteriosum was once thought to be main mechanism

    b. "osseous pinch" between
       compressed sternum and
       spine is now favored theory
  - incidence
    a. fairly common in motor
       vehicle accident victims
    b. > 85% of these die at scene
       of accident
    c. with prompt diagnosis,
       > 50% of those who reach a
       hospital survive

2) **Clinical features**
   - more than half of victims have no
     clinical manifestations
   - many show no external signs of
     trauma
   - usually signs are identical to any
     thoracic injury signs

3) **Radiologic features** (some of these
   are very specific, but not very
   sensitive, while others are quite
   sensitive but not specific)
   - depressed left mainstem bronchus
     (specific)
   - widened right paraspinal stripe
     (specific)
   - right displacement of superior
     vena cava (specific)
   - right displacement of a
     nasogastric tube (specific)
   - aortic arch distorted or indistinct
     (sensitive)
   - loss of aorticopulmonary window
     (sensitive)
   - tracheal shift to the right
     (sensitive)
   - widened left paraspinal line in the
     absence of fracture (sensitive)
   - prominent left apical cap
     (sensitive)
   - increased mediastinal width
     (sensitive)

4) **Diagnosis**
   - aortogram is required for positive
     identification
   - contrast-enhanced CT used on
     stable patients only; optimal study
     is a spiral/helical CT scan from
     above aortic arch to the carina
   - venous hemorrhage may mimic
     aortic rupture

- cardiac tamponade
  1) **General considerations**
     - mechanism
       a. pneumopericardium
       b. hemopericardium
  2) **Clinical features**
     - low systemic arterial pressure

- tachycardia
- dyspnea, orthopnea
- increased venous pressure
- accentuation of the normal inspiratory drop in systemic systolic blood pressure (*pulsus paradoxus*) to > 10 mm Hg (not specific to tamponade)

☞   3) **Radiologic features**
- small cardiac silhouette surrounded by a lucent border (indicates pneumopericardium)
- hemopericardium or pericardial effusion causes a large, amorphous cardiac silhouette; increasing diffuse cardiomegaly
- in patient with significant amounts of epicardial fat, a lucent fat stripe may be visible within the enlarged cardiac shadow

9. Neoplasms

☞   **a) General concepts**
- characteristic radiologic appearance of hematogenous pulmonary metastasis
  1) rounded nodules
  2) 1–10 cm in diameter
- characteristic radiologic appearance of lymphangitic metastasis: small, well-defined nodules, diffuse throughout both lung fields
- solitary pulmonary nodule with calcification: usually benign (tubercular granulomatous disease)
- cavitation within a parenchymal mass: central necrosis; occurs in metastatic nodules and in squamous cell primary bronchogenic carcinoma
- peripheral margins of parenchymal lung mass may be smooth or jagged; does not indicate benign or malignant nature of lesion
- solitary pulmonary nodule that doubles in size in 280 days or less: almost certainly malignant; should be investigated aggressively

☞   **b) Metastatic carcinoma**
- **General considerations**
  1) nature of lesion
     - two types of metastatic lung tumors
       a. *hematogenous metastasis*
          - usually multiple
          - smooth, rounded nodules scattered throughout both lung fields
          - sizes may be uniform or varied: range from 1–10 cm in diameter in same lung

- solitary lesions usually from kidney, but may arise from any organ
- renal or thyroid tumors may metastasize to lungs as a few large lesions

b. *lymphangitic metastasis*
- areas of small, granular nodules throughout lung fields
- string-like opaque networks from hila into lung parenchyma
- may resemble interstitial sarcoidosis or miliary tuberculosis
- usually spreads to lymph nodes
- primary lesion often is in breast or lung

2) incidence: common
3) primary sources
- adults: tumors in breast, colon, prostate, kidney, thyroid, stomach, cervix, rectum, testes, bone, skin (melanoma)
- children: Wilms' tumor, embryonic tumor, liver, thyroid, Ewing's sarcoma, osteogenic sarcoma

- **Clinical features**
  1) persistent coughing, often nonproductive (caused by bronchial obstruction)
  2) hematogenous spread may cause symptoms to appear first in liver, bone, brain, or adrenal glands before lungs are symptomatic

- **Radiologic features**
  1) *hematogenous spread*
     - "*cannonball metastasis*": round or oval opacities; fairly large, fluffy, ill-defined, unevenly distributed
     - may produce actual bone in the lung parenchyma
     - osteosarcoma is most common primary source
     - sometimes a solitary nodule may become large (usually a metastatic lesion from the kidney)
  2) *lymphogenous spread*
     - multiple scattered small nodules, sharply defined and fairly evenly distributed (metastases from thyroid malignancies usually take this form)
     - hilar node enlargement

- irregular strands of density from hilar region extending into parenchyma
- unilateral or bilateral pleural effusions

c) **Primary malignant tumors**
- bronchogenic carcinoma
  1) **General considerations**
     - nature of lesions
       a. malignant neoplasms in **four** histologic types
          - *squamous cell*: arising in large bronchi; spreads by direct extension and lymph node metastasis; more apt to cavitate
          - *undifferentiated small cell carcinoma* (oat cell cancer): spreads by hematogenous metastases or by lymphatics; usually forms large mass
          - *undifferentiated large cell carcinoma*: also hematogenous or lymphatic spread
          - *adenocarcinoma*: arising peripherally, solitary pulmonary nodule; hematogenous or lymphatic spread; female predilection may obstruct bronchus and look like pneumonia
     - incidence
       a. > 90% of all primary lung tumors
       b. primary cause of cancer **death** in men (35%)
       c. causes 20% of female cancers, and 30% of cancer deaths in women
     - etiology
       a. > 90% of male patients, and about 70% of female patients: primary bronchogenic carcinoma attributed to cigarette smoking
       b. other known etiologies: asbestos, radiation, arsenic, chromates, nickel
     - location
       a. most are endobronchial (central)
       b. apical primary carcinomas: "*Pancoast tumors*" (squamous cell)

      c. oat cell cancer: typically in hilar or mediastinal lymph nodes

2) **Clinical features**
- cough, localized wheezing
- sputum may be bloody
- beware of pneumonia that clears with antibiotic treatment and recurs (obstructive pneumonitis)
- pneumonia may fail to clear with treatment: inflammatory disease in lobe or segment caused by obstruction of bronchus
- atelectasis: mediastinal shift, reduced expansion, localized loss of breath sounds, dullness to percussion
- weight loss and weakness are common, late signs

3) **Radiologic features**
- atelectasis
  - a. probably most common radiologic sign
  - b. may be segmental, lobar, or massive (entire lung)
  - c. opacity of non-aerated lung tissue
  - d. may cause displacement of lung fissures
  - e. may alter size and shape of lobes or segments
  - f. may cause an elevated hemidiaphragm
- mediastinal widening
- altered mediastinal contours (*Reverse "S" sign of Golden*)
- localized emphysema
- tissue consolidation: usually confined to a segment or lobe
- unilateral hilar enlargement and increased hilar density
- large parenchymal mass
  - a. lobulated, generally rounded or oval
  - b. may be peripheral or central
  - c. range from 4 cm to >12 cm diameter
  - d. associated unilateral hilar enlargement and hilar node enlargement
- abscess or cavitation
  - a. usually squamous cell carcinoma
  - b. may cavitate with thick, irregular, nodular wall
- solitary mass or nodule
  - a. almost always without calcifications

        b.   uncalcified nodule > 4 cm diameter should be considered bronchogenic carcinoma until proven otherwise

        c.   often associated with unilateral hilar enlargement

        d.   should always do CT scan of solitary pulmonary nodules to verify presence or absence of calcium

- *Pancoast tumor* (superior pulmonary sulcus tumor)

        a.   best demonstrated by apical lordotic view

        b.   usually squamous cell carcinoma

        c.   Pancoast syndrome has four major features

- apical pulmonary mass
- Horner's syndrome
- pain down the arm
- 50% of these patients have destruction of adjacent ribs or vertebrae

- hypertrophic (pulmonary) osteoarthropathy

        a.   digital clubbing

        b.   sequela: solid periosteal new bone in distal long bones

- plain film usually cannot visualize masses < 5–6 mm in diameter
- optimum evaluation

        a.   initial study: PA and lateral views

        b.   apical lordotic

        c.   oblique films

        d.   CT

        e.   fluoroscopy to identify diaphragm paralysis

        f.   ventilation and perfusion lung scans assess function

        g.   bone scan and liver scan may be advisable if metastasis is suspected

- carcinoid
  1) **General considerations**
     - nature of lesion

        a.   primary or metastatic tumor

        b.   also called "*argentaffinoma*"; gram examination finds yellow tissue

        c.   functioning tissue: produces various amines, polypeptides, or vasoactive substances

    - incidence

        a.   no particular age or gender predilection

        b. fairly common entity
- location
  - a. most commonly in the ileum
  - b. also occur elsewhere in the GI tract, pancreas, gonads, and bronchi

2) **Clinical features**
- features depend upon what substances are being produced by the tumor
- possible symptoms include: uncomfortable cutaneous flushing, abdominal cramps, recurrent diarrhea, wheezing, decreased libido, impotence
- may develop right-sided endocardial fibrosis
- pulmonary stenosis and tricuspid regurgitation

3) **Radiologic features**
- may cause atelectasis: lobar or segmental collapse, displacement of fissures, opacity of non-aerated lung segment
- well-defined mass may be visible on plain film
- malignant masses rarely contain calcifications

- alveolar cell (bronchiolar, bronchoalveolar) carcinoma

  1) **General considerations**
  - consolidates airspaces
  - most commonly multifocal, usually peripheral
  - does not extend beyond lungs
  - less common than carcinoid or bronchogenic carcinoma

  2) **Clinical features**
  - cough that produces nonpurulent sputum
  - most often presents as an asymptomatic mass

  3) **Radiologic features**
  - homogenous, confluent densities with fluffy margins
  - poorly defined peripheral infiltrate or mass
  - may be unilateral or bilateral
  - apt to be found in lung apices

  4) **Differential considerations**
  - lymphoma: most commonly non-Hodgkin lymphoma
  - other causes of alveolar consolidation: metastatic disease, pulmonary edema, hemorrhage, or infection

☞

d) Primary benign neoplasms
- bronchial adenoma
    1) **General considerations**
        - various types: carcinoid, cylindroid, or mucoepidermoid
        - most common benign tumor of the lung
    2) **Clinical features**
        - mean age: 30; 90% of patients < 50 years old
        - may cause bronchial obstruction, atelectasis, obstructive emphysema
        - patient may develop pneumonia, bronchiectasis distal to the tumor
        - occasionally undergoes malignant degeneration
    3) **Radiologic features**
        - rounded tumor mass within a bronchus, usually a large bronchus, near the hilum (80% central); occasionally in lung periphery (20% peripheral)
        - should not calcify
        - occasionally visible on plain film, usually too small; requires CT
- pulmonary hamartoma
    1) **General considerations**
        - remnant of embryonic pulmonary tissue
        - largely composed of cartilage with fibrous connective tissue, epithelial elements
    2) **Clinical features:** usually asymptomatic
    3) **Radiologic features**
        - sharply defined lesion
        - some with "*popcorn-like*" calcification, but often too small to see without CT
        - without calcifications, appearance is identical to granuloma
        - usually peripheral
- bronchogenic cysts
    1) **General considerations**
        - developmental anomaly
        - may become infected
        - contain various secretions
        - may contain air, if communicating with bronchial tree
    2) **Radiologic features**
        - homogenous, sharply defined radiodense rim
        - usually contiguous with mediastinum

- sometimes peripheral
- air-filled cyst may resemble pneumatocele
- sometimes with associated rib or vertebral anomalies: rib fusions, hemivertebrae, block vertebrae
- laryngeal papilloma
  1) **General considerations**
     - originates as juvenile papilloma of the larynx
     - may transfer to lung via aspiration
  2) **Clinical features:** lung lesions may result in cystic bronchiectasis
  3) **Radiologic features:** nodular density in lung

REVIEW—STUDY QUESTIONS

1. Describe the radiologic appearance of pulmonary metastatic carcinoma.
2. Contrast the radiologic appearance of cardiac tamponade caused by pneumopericardium versus hemopericardium.
3. What is the most common anomaly of the aortic arch?
4. List five common primary sources of pulmonary metastatic carcinoma in adults. In children?
5. What are the most common sites for bronchogenic carcinoma, and what is its typical appearance?
6. What is a carcinoid, and what is its typical radiologic appearance in the lungs? Where else is it found?
7. What projection or view best demonstrates atelectasis, and what are the signs of atelectasis?
8. Name four specific radiologic signs, and four sensitive radiologic signs, of traumatic rupture of the aorta.
9. What are the three mechanical effects of blunt trauma that may cause lung contusion?
10. What is the radiologic appearance of alveolar cell carcinoma in the lung?

10. **Infections**
    a) Bacterial infections
       - infectious aortitis (bacterial aortitis)
         1) **General considerations**
            - may be bacterial or mycotic
            - abdominal aorta more often involved, but also affects thoracic aorta (usually ascending arch)
            - incidence: male predilection, usually 50–70 years old
            - with salmonella infection, affected population may be younger

2) etiology
- classical cause was tertiary syphilis
- now more apt to be caused by staph, strep, salmonella, *E. coli*, or pseudomonas

3) imaging
- no definitive plain film findings
- CT and MRI preferred: show air in aortic wall, periaortic thickening, haziness, or nodularity, saccular aneurysm without atherosclerosis, and unexplained change in aortic size

4) treatment
- antibiotic therapy
- surgery: excision, bypass, grafts

 • lobar pneumonia

1) **General considerations**
- infection of alveolar epithelium
- may spread to include entire lobe
- up to 75% of cases caused by *Streptococcus pneumoniae*
- other bacterial agents: *Klebsiella, Legionella pneumophila, Hemophilus influenzae, Mycoplasma pneumoniae* and *Chlamydia pneumoniae*

2) **Clinical features**
- acute onset (a few days to a week)
- cough usually productive; may produce purulent sputum
- hemoptysis common
- pleuritic chest pain, chills, high fever
- often features tachycardia, as high as 120 beats per minute
- commonly accompanied by empyema, bronchopleural fistula (BPF)
- laboratory findings: polymorphonuclear leukocytes, positive sputum or blood cultures
- responds well to antibiotic therapy

3) **Radiologic features**
- confluent airspace opacification
- often see "*air bronchogram sign*" (helps differentiate from tumor)
- focal, spherical consolidation ("*round pneumonia*") is occasional finding, more frequently seen in children
- lobar enlargement (caused by edema) may involve complications, such as pulmonary necrosis, cavitation, gangrene

- fissure bulges away from involved lobe (often seen with *Klebsiella*)
- lobar pneumonia superimposed on emphysema resembles necrotizing pneumonia (numerous small lucencies within consolidated area of lung)

- bronchopneumonia (lobular pneumonia)
  1) **General considerations**
     - epithelial infection of bronchi or bronchioles
     - may begin as acute bronchitis or bronchiolitis
     - soon involve adjacent alveoli; seldom crosses septa
     - usually multifocal
     - most common causative agents: *S. aureus,* Gram-negative bacilli, anaerobic bacteria, *L. pneumophila* (organisms involved in lobar pneumonia may also cause bronchopneumonia)
     - aspiration of fluids is significant etiologic factor (predisposing lung to infection)
  2) **Clinical features**
     - often preceded by an upper respiratory infection
     - sudden onset of shaking chill followed by fever
     - pleuritic pain on affected side with respiration
     - productive cough (blood-streaked or rusty sputum)
     - dyspnea
     - tachycardia
     - may include nausea, vomiting, malaise, myalgia
     - percussion dullness, tactile fremitus, bronchial breath sounds
     - laboratory tests show signs of infection
  3) **Radiologic features**
     - peribronchial thickening and accentuated bronchovascular markings can be seen early in process
     - multiple, poorly defined, patchy nodules ("*acinar nodules*")
     - progressively become confluent, causing multifocal, diffuse airspace opacifications
     - progresses to segmental and lobar opacification, often with cavitating necrosis
     - **DDX:** pulmonary edema, metastatic disease

- interstitial bacterial pneumonia
  1) **General considerations**
     - causative organism is most commonly *M. pneumoniae*
     - may clinically resemble a viral pneumonia
  2) **Clinical features**
     - bronchitis, bronchiolitis
     - headache
     - fever
     - myalgia
     - productive cough
  3) **Radiologic features**
     - miliary, micronodular pattern
     - diffuse, reticulonodular shadows
     - peribronchial thickening, with accented bronchovascular markings
     - progresses toward a bronchopneumonia pattern
- septic bacterial pneumonia
  1) **General considerations**
     - hematogenous spread to the pleura and peripheral parenchyma
     - bacterial emboli lodge in these tissues, producing septic, hemorrhagic edema
     - usual organisms involved are: *S. aureus*, Gram-negative bacilli, anaerobic bacteria, streptococci
  2) **Clinical features**
     - signs typical of pneumonia, but with increased edema
     - pleuritic pain is prominent feature
  3) **Radiologic features**
     - multiple nodules, usually cavitated
     - rarely appear as a diffuse miliary pattern
     - multifocal; most common in lower two-thirds of lungs
- miscellaneous bacterial pulmonary infections
  1) lungs also incur infection with:
     - *Nocardia*, actinomycosis, *Mycobacterium tuberculosis*, *Legionella*, tularemia, Q fever, plague
  2) cause multiple, rounded nodules; sometimes cavitated
- lung abscess
  1) **General considerations**
     - pyogenic abscess caused by liquefaction necrosis
     - causative organisms most often

Staphylococcus, Klebsiella, or
Streptococcus pneumoniae

2) **Radiologic features**
- poorly defined round or oval mass; water density
- may have air-fluid level (if it communicates with the bronchial tree)
- CT shows thickened, irregular wall
- **DDX:** primary or metastatic tumor

- pleurisy
1) **General considerations**
- bacteria or pus may be found in pleural fluid (empyema)
- early in course of infection, pleural effusions are mobile
- later diffuse fibrosis of both visceral and parietal pleura occurs
- adhesions develop, loculating the pleural effusions
- empyema may contain *S. aureus,* anaerobic bacilli, Gram-negative bacilli, and sometimes *S. pneumoniae* or actinomycosis
- with parenchymal necrosis, bronchopleural fistulas (BPF) may develop

2) **Clinical features**
- sudden onset of pleuritic pain
- may be a vague discomfort, or sharp, stabbing pain
- respiration and coughing aggravate the pain
- pain may be referred to the abdomen or to the neck and shoulder
- rapid, shallow breathing
- pleural friction rub: crackles, grating, creaking, or leathery sounds
- pleural effusion reduces the pain of dry friction rub

3) **Radiologic features**
- loculated pleural effusion (late finding)
- BPF must be differentiated from lung abscess
- CT shows smooth wall of empyema and separation of thickened visceral and parietal pleura ("*split-pleura sign of empyema*")
- CT shows diffuse, smoothly thickened parietal pleura, which enhances with IV contrast
- extrapleural fat usually is thickened

REVIEW—STUDY QUESTIONS

1. What is the most common etiology of infectious aortitis?
2. What is "round pneumonia"?
3. List the usual clinical signs and symptoms of pleurisy.
4. What is the "split pleura" sign, and with what condition is it associated?
5. Where is bronchial adenoma usually located, and what is its radiologic appearance?
6. What is PBF, and from what other process must it be differentiated? Describe the differing radiologic signs for these two entities.
7. What are the clinical and radiologic signs of bronchopneumonia?
8. List five common agents of pulmonary infection.
9. Describe the radiologic appearance of pulmonary hamartoma.
10. Contrast the radiologic appearance of pulmonary hamartoma, laryngeal papilloma, and bronchial cysts.

b) Viral infections
- viral pneumonia
  1) **General considerations**
     - about 25% of community-acquired pneumonia is thought to be viral
     - must be a clinical diagnosis; radiologic diagnosis is unreliable
     - viral effects usually confined to airway walls, but may spread to interstitial tissues and lung septa
     - produces alveolar edema, hemorrhage
     - six distinct pathologic patterns produced
       a. acute interstitial pneumonia: edema and mononuclear clear cell infiltrates around bronchi and bronchiolar walls
       b. lobular (or sublobular) inflammation: patchy airspace filling in secondary pulmonary lobules
       c. localized hemorrhagic pulmonary edema: involves a segment or entire lobe; hemorrhagic pulmonary edema, hyaline membrane formation; some polymorphonuclear cell infiltration

      d. generalized hemorrhagic pulmonary edema: polymorphonuclear cell infiltration and hyaline membrane formation is extensive

      e. pleural effusion and exudates: small effusions are common; occasionally shows significant exudation

      f. chronic interstitial fibrosis: diffuse pulmonary fibrosis known to occur (rarely) after viral pneumonia

2) **Clinical features**
- gradual onset with malaise
- often follows upper respiratory infection (URI)
- cough (usually nonproductive)
- low grade fever, no chills
- rarely; pleuritic chest pain
- laboratory findings
  - a. leukopenia
  - b. mild leukocytosis or a normal white cell count
  - c. sputum smear or culture and blood culture non-contributory

3) **Radiologic features** (vary with pathologic patterns)
- thickened end-on bronchial walls
- reticular pattern may radiate from the hila
- diffuse miliary pattern
- patchy airspace filling may result in peribronchiolar or acinar nodular pattern (common with varicella pneumonia)
- confluent opacification of lobe or segment, resembling bacterial lobar pneumonia
- perihilar distribution of acute, disseminated alveolar pattern
- blunting of costophrenic sulci by pleural effusion

- respiratory viruses
  1) influenza A and B viruses
     - **General considerations**
       - a. usually in wintertime epidemics
       - b. at risk: chronic cardiovascular or pulmonary disease patients and elderly patients
     - **Clinical features**
       - a. systemic symptoms: headache, chills and fever, myalgia, malaise

      b.   respiratory symptoms: cough, sore throat

      c.   most serious: primary influenza viral pneumonia; most often seen in patients compromised by mitral stenosis, chronic lung disease, or the stress of pregnancy; often leads to respiratory failure

- **Radiologic features**
  a.   unilateral or bilateral multifocal, patchy infiltrates
  b.   thickened bronchial walls
  c.   diffuse acinar nodular densities, mixed with areas of consolidation
  d.   diffuse alveolar opacification bilaterally
  e.   peribronchial infiltration
  f.   may mimic bacterial pneumonia radiologically

  2) parainfluenza virus

- **General considerations**
  a.   most often seen in children
  b.   usually occurs as a URI
  c.   sometimes progresses to lower respiratory organs in children, although seldom in adults
  d.   some children have superimposed bacterial pneumonia

- **Clinical features**
  a.   coryza and sometimes croupy cough
  b.   sore throat, hoarseness
  c.   wheezing, tachypnea, intercostal retractions

- **Radiologic features**
  a.   diffuse hyperinflation of lungs
  b.   thickened bronchial walls
  c.   peribronchial and interstitial infiltrates, sometimes with patchy alveolar infiltration in two or three lobes
  d.   hilar lymphadenopathy

- nonrespiratory viruses
  1) enteroviruses

  - **General considerations**
    a.   group of viruses including: enterovirus, poliovirus, coxsackievirus, echovirus

  - **Clinical features**
    a.   may result in paralysis, encephalitis or meningitis, specific febrile illness

- **Radiologic features**
  a. when viral pneumonia results, films may show nodular or patchy infiltrates

 2) cytomegalovirus (CMV)
- **General considerations**
  a. newborn infants and immunodeficient patients are at risk
- **Clinical features**
  a. in neonates
    - petechiae
    - jaundice and hepatosplenomegaly
    - microcephaly
    - diarrhea, with pyloric and duodenal ulcerations, necrosis and thickening of muscle wall
  b. with interstitial pneumonia: lymphadenopathy, rash, hepatitis, anemia
    - may see atypical lymphocytosis
  c. in older patients
    - mononucleosis with high fever, chills, fatigue, malaise, myalgia, headache
    - segmental or interstitial pneumonia
    - myocarditis, pleuritis, arthritis, encephalitis
- **Radiologic features**
  a. in neonates
    - diffuse consolidation
    - reticulonodular interstitial infiltrate
  b. in older patients
    - early findings: diffuse miliary pattern or bilateral diffuse reticulonodular interstitial infiltrates
    - later findings: diffuse consolidation, diffuse hemorrhagic pulmonary edema
    - rarely: patchy consolidation with acinar nodules
3) varicella-zoster virus
- **General considerations**
  a. varicella is chickenpox; its reactivation as zoster is shingles
  b. cutaneous chickenpox is sometimes accompanied by pneumonia; most commonly seen in adults

c. particularly at risk: pregnant females, for whom it may be fatal

d. pneumonia resolves as chickenpox resolves

- **Clinical features**
    a. pneumonia develops after 3–5 days of chickenpox

    b. tachypnea, dyspnea, cough, cyanosis, hemoptysis, pleuritic chest pain

- **Radiologic features**
    a. early: thickened bronchial walls, peribronchial infiltrates, diffuse miliary or reticulonodular pattern

    b. later: diffuse, patchy consolidation with acinar nodules

    c. may have pleural effusion

    d. often leaves residual fibrosis, multiple punctate calcifications

    e. **DDX:** "*snowstorm*" calcifications of histoplasmosis (with residual varicella pneumonia there will be no splenic calcification)

 4) Epstein-Barr virus (EBV)

- **General considerations**
    a. infectious mononucleosis

    b. up to 70% of young adults with EBV develop clinical syndrome

    c. ubiquitous virus is most commonly subclinical

- **Clinical features**
    a. fever, sore throat, lymphadenopathy

    b. hepatic tenderness

    c. splenomegaly

    d. up to 5% have pulmonary involvement

- **Radiologic features**
    a. hilar and mediastinal lymphadenopathy

    b. bronchial and/or tracheal deviation or compression

    c. reticulonodular interstitial pulmonary infiltration

    d. pleural effusion

    e. visible splenomegaly

    f. immunocompromised patients may suffer hypertrophic (pulmonary) osteoarthropathy

    g. may have diffuse nodular or reticulonodular infiltrates in lung bases

5) measles virus

- **General considerations**
  - a. most common in infants, non-immunized children
  - b. may occur in older, and immunized, populations
- **Clinical features**
  - a. red, maculopapular rash: moves from forehead, down over face and body, all the way to the feet
  - b. prodrome: malaise, fever, conjunctivitis, photophobia, eyelid edema, irritability, cough, rhinorrhea (up to a week preceding rash)
  - c. respiratory problems: bronchitis, bronchiolitis, croup, or pneumonia (giant cell pneumonia)
  - d. ineffectively immunized individuals are at risk for atypical measles
    - high fever, headache, myalgia, abdominal pain, high fever, extremity edema
    - maculopapular rash, but pattern is different: moves from hands and feet into body and head
    - pneumonia is a more common complication of atypical measles
- **Radiologic features**
  - a. measles giant cell pneumonia
    - reticular pattern throughout lungs
    - thickened bronchial walls, with peribronchial infiltrates
    - diffuse nodular pattern throughout lungs
    - enlarged hilar lymph nodes
  - b. superimposed bacterial pneumonia (more common than giant cell pneumonia with measles)
    - segmental or lobar pneumonia
    - diffuse consolidation
  - c. atypical measles pneumonia
    - dense lobar or segmental consolidation

- hilar and mediastinal lymphadenopathy
- pleural effusion
- pulmonary nodules: sometimes cavitated; may persist as long as 2 years; may calcify

---

REVIEW—STUDY QUESTIONS

1. What type of pneumonia features persistent nodules, sometimes calcified or cavitated?

2. What population is most prone to parainfluenza virus, and what are its clinical and radiologic signs?

3. What are the clinical and radiologic signs of respiratory effects of the measles virus?

4. What are the pulmonary effects of RSV, and what is its radiologic appearance?

5. Describe the six pathologic patterns of viral pneumonia.

6. What is EBV and what are its radiologic features?

7. What is CMV and what two populations are most vulnerable to it?

8. Describe the clinical symptoms of CMV in both these populations, and its radiologic characteristics.

9. What viral infections mimic bacterial pneumonia in radiologic appearance?

10. Why may histoplasmosis resemble varicella virus radiologically, and how are they differentiated?

---

   c) Granulomatous (mycobacterial)

   - tuberculosis (TB)
       1) **General considerations**
          - infectious agent is a mycobacterium, an "*acid-fast bacillus*"
          - specific agents in tuberculosis: *Mycobacterium tuberculosis,* or *Mycobacterium bovis* (the latter rarely seen now)
          - incidence declined until the 1980s; since then has slowly increased
              a. children particularly vulnerable to primary tuberculosis
              b. elderly and immunocompromised populations vulnerable (e.g., patients with AIDS)
              c. reactivation tuberculosis (after initial infection) secondary to immune compromise: malignancy, renal disease, diabetes, alcoholism, aging, or surgery
          - airborne infection

- favored sites for primary tuberculosis
  a. in lungs: lower lobes first, then spread to apices
  b. in skeleton: long bone metaphyses, vertebral bodies
  c. in other organs: kidney cortex, brain cortex

2) **Clinical features**
- often asymptomatic
- general malaise
- night sweats
- cough (usually a minimally productive, early morning cough)
- dyspnea may result from spontaneous pneumothorax or pleural effusion
- hemoptysis: late manifestation

3) **Radiologic features**
- primary TB
  a. parenchymal consolidation (usually in lower lobe)
  b. hilar and mediastinal lymphadenopathy
  c. pleural effusion (in adult patients, but rarely in children)
  d. with healing: consolidation may regress to a clearly-defined nodule, which may be resorbed, or may calcify
  e. *"Ghon tubercle"*: calcified tubercular granuloma in the lung field (*"coin lesion"*)
  f. *"Rhanke complex"*: enlarged hilar lymph node with ipsilateral calcified granuloma (*"Ghon tubercle"*) in the peripheral lung field
- reactivation TB
  a. alveolar consolidation, with or without cavitation
  b. upper lobes (especially apical and posterior segments) and the superior segment of lower lobes usually involved
  c. fibronodular infiltration, often with calcification
  d. miliary pattern (multiple, tiny nodules) which may progress to alveolar consolidation (more common with systemic TB)
  e. less commonly: lymphadenopathy, pleural effusion, pneumothorax, atelectasis
  f. occasionally, a tuberculoma

(smooth, spherical mass that may contain calcification) develops, simulates carcinoma

  g. patients with AIDS commonly present with both lungs involved, and no cavitation

  h. pleural effusions may be loculated with bronchopleural fistula, which are seen as a loculated hydropneumothorax

☞

- sarcoidosis (noncaseating granulomatous disease)

  1) **General considerations**

  - nature of condition

    a. multisystem granulomatous disorder

    b. multiple noncaseating epithelioid granulomas

    c. idiopathic

  - incidence

    a. predilection for American black population (incidence is 17 times higher than in Caucasians) and northern Europeans

    b. most common: 20–40 years of age

    c. slightly more common in females

  - sites

    a. 90% of patients have pulmonary lesions

    b. skeletal: spine, ribs, sternum, hands, and feet

    c. cardiovascular system

    d. CNS

    e. liver, spleen

    f. skin

  2) **Clinical features**

  - may be asymptomatic
  - fever, weight loss, arthralgia
  - peripheral lymphadenopathy
  - cough, dyspnea
  - skin plaques, papules, subcutaneous nodules, erythema nodosum
  - hepatosplenomegaly, and (rarely) jaundice
  - granulomatous uveitis (bilateral), sometimes with secondary glaucoma
  - lacrimal gland involvement
  - angina, conduction abnormalities

- polyarthritis (especially in phalanges)
- cranial nerve palsies
- diabetes insipidus
- hypercalcemia, hypercalciuria; renal calculi, nephrocalcinosis
- leukopenia
- hypergammaglobulinemia (especially in American blacks)

3) **Radiologic features**
- thoracic disease classified by presence of lymph node enlargement, pulmonary lesions, and fibrosis: (typical **Radiologic features**)
  a. Stage 0: plain film appears normal
  b. Stage I: hilar lymphadenopathy bilaterally; lungs appear normal
  c. Stage II: bilateral hilar lymphadenopathy; pulmonary lesions
  d. Stage III: pulmonary lesions without lymphadenopathy
    - Stage IIIA: no pulmonary fibrosis
    - Stage IIIB: pulmonary fibrosis present
- hilar lymph nodes: potato-shaped (*potato nodes*); often separated from cardiac borders (**DDX:** lymphomatous lymphadenopathy: nodes abut cardiac borders; anterior mediastinal node involvement more common with lymphoma)
- pulmonary lesions may be fine or coarse; may be fluffy alveolar confluent opacities with prominent "*air bronchograms*" (caused by confluent interstitial granulomas)
- radiologic pulmonary fibrosis findings range from single linear densities to honeycombed pattern ("*Swiss cheese pattern*") of bullous, fibrocystic disease
- with severe fibrotic lesions, possible: spontaneous pneumothorax, hilar and fissure displacement, mediastinal shift
- 75% of cases show bilateral hilar and paratracheal lymphadenopathy; about 50% include parenchymal involvement
- "*Garland's Triad*": enlargement of hilar, azygos, and right paratracheal lymph nodes

- symmetric bilateral hilar node enlargement is typically seen with right paratracheal node enlargement: "*1-2-3 sign*"; or "*Pawn Broker sign*" (similar to the "3-balls" symbol for pawn shops)
- less common radiologic signs may include
  a. pleural effusions
  b. pleural thickening
  c. apical cyst with fibrotic cap (*Aspergillus* infection)
  d. occasionally, isolated paratracheal, subcarinal, and aorticopulmonary lymphadenopathy are seen (in the absence of hilar involvement)
  e. unilateral hilar lymphadenopathy
  f. calcification of hilar or mediastinal nodes; occasionally with "*eggshell*" peripheral calcification
  g. **DDX:** silicosis (extensive apical lung disease)

- Wegener's granulomatosis
  1) **General considerations**
     - nature of condition
       a. systemic, necrotizing granulomatous process
       b. destructive angiitis
     - sites
       a. lungs and upper respiratory tract
       b. kidneys (necrotizing glomerulonephritis)
       c. heart and pericardium
       d. eyes
       e. destructive lesions in paranasal sinuses
     - incidence
       a. female predilection
       b. all ages are vulnerable
  2) **Clinical features**
     - pulmonary effects may be completely asymptomatic
     - hemoptysis
     - **no** history of asthma or respiratory allergies
  3) **Radiologic features**
     - early: lung bases may show interstitial or reticulonodular infiltrates
     - later: multiple nodular masses of varied sizes, some with cavitation (sharply defined, smooth-walled, and usually in lung bases)

- occasionally: pleural effusions, irregular peripheral infiltration

d) Nongranulomatous (fungal) infections
- actinomycosis
    1) **General considerations**
        - nature of condition
            a. *Actinomyces*: slow-growing, filamentous, Gram-positive bacteria
            b. resemble fungi, with their branching mycelia
            c. *Actinomyces israelii* is most common human pathogen
            d. breach in oral mucosa, human bite, or aspiration from oropharynx: main routs of infection
            e. may be spread from primary dental infection
        - sites
            a. thoracic involvement in only about 15% of cases
            b. face and neck involved in about 55% of cases
            c. pelvic/abdominal infection in about 20% of cases
    2) **Clinical features**
        - cervicofacial form
            a. *"lumpy jaw"*: small, flat, hard swelling
            b. may or may not be painful
            c. may be under oral mucosa, under skin of neck, or a subperiosteal mandibular lesion
        - abdominal form
            a. pain and fever
            b. vomiting, diarrhea, or constipation
            c. abdominal mass, partial intestinal obstruction
        - thoracic form
            a. chest pain, fever, productive cough: late signs
            b. lesions may create sinuses, drain from chest wall

    3) **Radiologic features**
        - alveolar infiltrate may resemble pneumonia
        - cavitated masses
        - pleural effusion
        - rarely, hilar lymphadenopathy
        - extension of mass into chest wall, ribs, vertebral bodies (with bone destruction and reactive periostitis) is possible, but not common

- lesions may invade superior vena cava, esophagus, pericardium, or myocardium

- aspergillosis
    1) **General considerations**
        - three presentations
            a. mycetoma (noninvasive or semiinvasive aspergillosis)
                1) *"fungus ball,"* or ball of matted hyphae
                2) may be mobile within a cavity in the lung parenchyma
            b. invasive aspergillosis
                - causes pulmonary infiltration
                - local infarction of blood vessels leads to dissemination to brain and other organs
                - may cause a fatal fungal pneumonia
            c. allergic bronchopulmonary aspergillosis
                - almost always occurs in asthmatic patients
                - tracheobronchial infestations cause mucoid impaction of the bronchi
                - may lead to atelectasis, cavitation, or obstructive pneumonia
        - nature of condition
            a. most infections caused by *Aspergillus fumigatus*
            b. ubiquitous dimorphic fungus; in soil, water, grain, hay
            c. spores normally present in mouth and airways
            d. become pathogens in immune compromised host
        - incidence
            a. noninvasive or semiinvasive mode is seen in fairly immunocompetent hosts
            b. invasive aspergillosis seen in patients with severely compromised immune systems
            c. allergic bronchopulmonary aspergillosis develops in those with allergies or hypersensitivity
    2) **Clinical features**
        - mycetoma
            a. may be asymptomatic
            b. may lead to massive hemoptysis, requiring

surgical removal of affected
lung
- invasive aspergillosis
    a. patient with acute leukemia,
       granulocytopenia, or AIDS
    b. normal host may also have
       invasive aspergillosis
    c. patient is neutropenic
    d. fever, pulmonary infiltrate
    e. unresponsive to antibiotic
       therapy
- allergic bronchopulmonary
  aspergillosis
    a. asthmatic patient
    b. eosinophilia (>1000/cubic
       millimeter) in blood or
       sputum
    c. skin test positive for
       reactivity to *Aspergillus*
       antigens

3) **Radiologic features**
- mycetoma
    a. cavity (usually apical)
    b. cavity sometimes contains
       mass (fungus ball), a crescent
       of air, or pulmonary infiltrate
    c. extensive pleural thickening
       at lung apex
- invasive aspergillosis
    a. variable appearance
    b. often, bilateral multiple
       nodular infiltrates (40% of
       cases)
    c. may see solitary infiltrates,
       solitary nodules, diffuse
       alveolar infiltrates
    d. often, cavitation with a
       necrotic mass (may simulate
       a mycetoma)
    e. pleural effusion may
       accompany pulmonary
       infiltration
- allergic bronchopulmonary
  aspergillosis
    a. characteristic: *"finger in
       glove"* or *"V"* pattern of
       mucoid impaction with
       bronchial plugging
    b. may see lobar consolidation,
       sometimes with cavitation,
       rarely with fungus ball mass
- blastomycosis
    1) **General considerations**
       - nature of condition
           a. lung is portal of entry, but
              skin infection may ensue
              from dog bite or other
              puncture

- incidence
    a. organism is endemic in southeast, south-central, and Midwestern North America
    b. grows in soil in wooded areas: infection often seen in hunters

2) **Clinical features**
   - acute upper respiratory infection
   - may be self-limiting
   - may progress to chronic, tuberculosis-like pulmonary disease
   - may develop into bilateral pneumonia and adult respiratory distress syndrome
   - often involves skin: chronic skin ulcer
   - may involve bones, prostate, meninges

3) **Radiologic features**
   - acute blastomycosis
       a. segmental or nonsegmental consolidation
       b. pulmonary nodules (solitary or multiple)
       c. pleural thickening, without pleural effusion
       d. may show diffuse nodular or micronodular lesions (poor prognosis)
   - chronic blastomycosis
       a. parenchymal consolidation
       b. lesion may (rarely) invade chest wall
       c. rib lesions with a soft tissue mass
       d. cutaneous fistulas

- coccidioidomycosis ("San Joaquin Valley fever")
    1) **General considerations**
       - nature of condition
           a. *Coccidioides immitis*: dimorphic, soil-dwelling fungus airborne fragments of its hyphae are inhaled by host
       - incidence
           a. endemic to North America's southwestern deserts, Central and South America
           b. human inhabitants and visitors to the Southwest are at risk
    2) **Clinical features**
       - pneumonitis
           a. disease may become reactivated

b. chronic disease presents as fever, weight loss, cough, hemoptysis, chest pain

c. disseminated disease may involve skin lesions, lungs, osteomyelitis

d. disseminated disease may be fatal

3) **Radiologic features**
- alveolar consolidation, usually in lower lobes (may be patchy, segmental, or nonsegmental)
- about 20% of cases show hilar lymphadenopathy
- pleural effusions (usually small and unilateral)
- chronic: single or multiple nodules; or localized alveolar consolidation
  a. may cavitate
  b. may cause pleural effusion
  c. mediastinal adenopathy may be present
  d. 10–15% of cases feature a single, thin-walled cavity
  e. symptomatic cases: may involve alveolar infiltration, or multiple nodules
- disseminated coccidioidomycosis: may have miliary pattern
- can spread to bone and joints

- histoplasmosis
  1) **General considerations**
  - nature of condition
    a. diamorphous fungus of the *Ascomycetes* class
    b. mycelial phase in soil; spores inhaled by host
  - incidence
    a. prevalent in Ohio, Mississippi, and St. Lawrence river valleys
    b. found in soil containing bird or bat feces, so bat caves, chicken houses, etc. may have heavy infestation

  2) **Clinical features**
  - frequently asymptomatic (as high as 95% of cases)
  - primary acute form
    a. fever, cough, malaise
  - progressive disseminated disease
    a. where T-cell immunity is depressed: fever
    b. hepatomegaly (granulomatous lesions, may calcify)
    c. lymphadenopathy
    d. splenomegaly

    e. sometimes, oral or
        gastrointestinal ulcers
    f. can cause Addison's disease
        (hypoadrenal symptoms)
 • chronic cavitary disease
    a. cough
    b. progressive dyspnea
    c. fibrosing mediastinitis may
        develop
3) **Radiologic features**
 • primary acute form
    a. single or multiple focal
        alveolar infiltrations
    b. hilar lymphadenopathy
    c. bilateral multiple nodules
        (discrete, or poorly defined)
        when organism is *H.
        capsulatum*
 • disseminated form
    a. single, sharply marginated
        granuloma (or
        histoplasmoma) sometimes
        with central calcification, up
        to 4 cm in diameter
    b. multiple calcified granulomas
        bilaterally
    c. mediastinal
        lymphadenopathy, with or
        without pulmonary infiltrates
        or nodules
 • chronic cavitary disease
    a. rare manifestation: sclerosing
        mediastinitis (extensive
        fibrosis of the mediastinum)
    b. constricting encapsulation,
        narrowing, obstruction of
        mediastinal structures:
        e.g., superior vena cava,
        esophagus, trachea, right
        mainstem bronchus
    c. gradual, diffuse mediastinal
        widening
    d. *"broncholiths"* (calcified hilar
        lymph nodes)
    e. with *H. capsulatum*, alveolar
        infiltrate, or distinctly-walled
        cavity resembling pulmonary
        tuberculosis or primary
        carcinoma

REVIEW—STUDY QUESTIONS

1. What is Garland's Triad, and with what disease is it
    associated?

2. Describe Wegener's granulomatosis and name its effects
    in the heart, kidneys, and lungs. In what lung areas is it
    most manifest radiographically?

3. What is the Rhanke complex? With what disease is it associated?

4. What areas in the lungs are usually affected by tuberculosis?

5. Describe the radiologic appearance of three presentations of histoplasmosis.

6. Describe the stages of sarcoidosis and the radiologic features of each stage.

7. What is a mycobacterium? What types of lesions do they cause, and what is their radiographic appearance?

8. How do people get actinomycosis? Describe its cervicofacial, thoracic, and abdominal forms. What are the radiologic signs of thoracic actinomycosis?

9. List, compare, and contrast the three presentations of aspergillosis.

10. Fully describe coccidioidomycosis: agent, distribution, route of contamination, effects, and radiologic appearance.

11. Compare and contrast the radiologic appearance of primary and reactivated tuberculosis in the lungs.

12. What is a Ghon tubercle, and with what disease is it associated?

☞ **11. Inhalation Disorders (pneumoconioses)**
   a) Asbestosis
   - **General considerations**
     1) nature of condition
        - pulmonary fibrosis caused by inhalation of asbestos fibers
        - risk is related to cumulative exposure
        - fibers retained in lung parenchyma lead to diffuse alveolar and interstitial fibrosis (fibrous pneumoconiosis)
        - development of malignant mesothelioma (pleural and peritoneal) or bronchogenic carcinoma is related to asbestos exposure combined with smoking
     2) incidence
        - disease develops about 20 years after exposure
        - risk is clearly dose-related
        - cigarette smokers with asbestos exposure (especially > 1 pack a day) are at greatly enhanced risk of lung cancer
   - **Clinical features**
     1) insidious onset exertional dyspnea, dry cough
     2) in heavy smokers: productive cough, wheezing

3) bloody effusion with chest wall pain may indicate malignancy

4) 20–25% of heavily exposed asbestos workers develop bronchogenic carcinoma

5) about 10% of asbestos workers develop mesothelioma

- **Radiologic features**

1) interstitial fibrosis

2) diffuse irregular or linear small opacities, mostly in lower lobes

3) progresses to coarse linear streaks with "*honeycombing*"

4) eventually, heart border may be partially obscured: "*shaggy heart sign*"

5) diffuse or localized pleural thickening
   - uniform, homogeneous density
   - smooth contours
   - often, costophrenic angle is obliterated

6) pleural plaques (smooth plateaus and nodular areas of thickened pleura)
   - in profile: sharply marginated, dense soft-tissue band, up to 10 mm thick, parallel to the lateral thoracic inner wall margin
   - *en face*: poorly-defined, vague, irregular opacity
   - plaques are usually symmetric, bilateral, and more prominent in lower thorax (between sixth and ninth ribs)

7) small pleural effusions

8) small pleural calcifications (along chest wall, diaphragm, cardiac border)
   - *en face*: irregular, unevenly dense (fringed)

9) "*rounded atelectasis*" may develop
   - rounded, sharply marginated mass abutting pleura
   - acute angle between it and pleura indicates intrapulmonary location
   - pleura is most thickened near this mass
   - mass may have curvilinear tail (*comet tail sign*) caused by compressed bronchi and vessels between mass and hilum

10) benign fibrotic masses
    - lentiform or wedge-shaped
    - adjacent pleura is thickened

11) malignant mesothelioma
    - moderate or large pleural effusion with or without a pleural mass

- may appear as diffuse pleural thickening, with or without effusion
- eventually: envelopment of pleura and lung; encasement causes mediastinal shift toward side of disease

b) Coal workers' pneumoconiosis (CWP)
- **General considerations**
  1) nature of condition
     - up to 30% of underground coal miners in the United States affected
     - two forms of the disease
       a. simple CWP affects about 27.4% of miners
       b. complicated form affects about 2.5%
     - simple CWP results from coal dust retention in lungs:
       a. pathologic hallmark is coal macule: dust aggregation around dilated respiratory bronchioles
     - complicated CWP (progressive massive fibrosis: PMF):
       a. inhalation of coal dust along with silica
  2) **Clinical features**
     - simple CWP patients are usually asymptomatic, without significant respiratory impairment
     - PMF presents with respiratory impairment severe enough to cause total disability and, eventually, premature death
  3) **Radiologic features**
     - simple CWP
       a. small, rounded nodules, predominantly in upper lobes
       b. CT shows that early involvement is mainly in right upper lobe, with micronodules that eventually involve all lobes bilaterally
       c. "pseudoplaques" sometimes caused by confluence of subpleural micronodules along visceral pleura and along the fissures
     - complicated CWP (progressive massive fibrosis: PMF)
       a. considered present when any single nodule exceeds 1 cm diameter
       b. lesions concentrate in upper lobes and apical portion of lower lobes

    c. lesions are solid, large opacities, sometimes with cavitation

    d. hilar elevation secondary to scarring

    e. *"angel wing"* pattern of fibrosis

    f. straight stretched lower lobe caused by adjacent fibrosis in lung

    g. CT shows two types of lesions
- irregular borders, with gross parenchymal destruction and typical scar emphysema
- massive fibrosis with regular borders and no scar emphysema

c) Rheumatoid pneumoconiosis (Caplan's disease)

- **General considerations**
  1) nodular pulmonary disease associated with rheumatoid arthritis
  2) serologic evidence of rheumatoid disease may be found even in the absence of arthritis
  3) more common in Europe and Great Britain than in the United States
- **Clinical features**
  1) often asymptomatic, incidental finding on chest film
  2) may occur with or without clinical manifestations of rheumatoid arthritis
  3) dyspnea, productive cough are not distinctive
- **Radiologic features**
  1) may see groups of dense, round nodules
  2) nodules may become confluent
  3) may find mild/moderate interstitial pneumonitis
  4) usually affects upper lungs, apical portions
  5) most often peripheral

d) Silicosis

- **General considerations**
  1) nature of condition
     - fibrotic lung disease caused by inhalation of silicon dioxide dust
     - particles lodge in alveoli, where macrophages try to destroy them, but are destroyed
     - hyalinized collagen is produced
     - four types of silicosis are recognized

a. simple silicosis
b. complicated silicosis
c. acute silicosis
d. Caplan's syndrome (rheumatoid nodules over the silicosis pattern)

2) incidence
- occupations at risk: mining, quarrying, tunneling, sandblasting, foundry work, stone masonry, pottery making
- dose-related: thought to affect about 3% of Americans who have worked at least 20 years in heavy metal mining

- **Clinical features**
  1) simple silicosis usually is asymptomatic; no pulmonary impairment
  2) complicated silicosis involves development of emphysema, often further complicated by superimposed TB
  3) acute silicosis is caused by heavy exposure to high concentrations of respirable silica; rare; requires less than 5 years exposure
     - superimposed mycobacterial infection (25% of cases)
     - rapidly progressing respiratory failure and death
  4) Caplan's syndrome features superimposed large, necrobiotic, rheumatoid nodules (with or without actual rheumatoid arthritis) with simple silicosis

- **Radiologic features**
  1) simple silicosis
     - apical and posterior areas of upper and lower lobes
     - multiple small rounded opacities (1–10 mm in diameter)
     - nodules may calcify
     - hilar and mediastinal nodes may enlarge and develop peripheral calcification ("*eggshell calcification*")
  2) complicated silicosis
     - nodules become confluent (> 1 cm in diameter)
     - progressive, massive fibrosis; usually in periphery or midzone of upper lobes
     - overinflated, emphysematous surrounding lung, especially in the lung bases
     - as fibrosis enlarges, nodularity in the remaining lung diminishes

- masses cavitate, secondary to ischemic necrosis
- staging is done by size of the conglomerate masses:
  A = 1 to 5 cm
  B = > 5 cm but less than one-third of the lung
  C = one-third (or more) of the lung

3) acute silicosis
- ground "*glass appearance*" of diffuse airspace disease
- perihilar distribution
- air bronchogram signs

4) Caplan's syndrome
- nodules (0.5–5.0 cm) that may cavitate and calcify superimposed on background of simple silicosis

12. Mediastinal Diseases and Neoplasms

☞
a) Anterior mediastinum
- sometimes termed "4-Ts" because most lymphomas are T-cell lymphomas
- lymphoma

1) **General considerations**
- most common lesions are caused by Hodgkin lymphoma
- diagnosed by presence, in blood, of Reed-Sternberg cells
- isolated mediastinal involvement occurs with up to 10% of patients with Hodgkin disease
- Lukes and Butler classification system (modified by Rye) has four subtypes:
  a. NS: nodular sclerosis: few Reed-Sternberg cells
  b. MC: mixed cellularity: frequent Reed-Sternberg cells
  c. LP: lymphocyte predominance: few Reed-Sternberg cells
  d. LD: lymphocytic depletion: frequent Reed-Sternberg cells
- non-Hodgkin lymphoma: less likely to involve mediastinal nodes

2) **Clinical features**
- NS
  a. most common (almost 75% of cases)
  b. more advanced involvement than LP subtype
  c. mediastinal involvement is common, with fibrotic response

Most Common Anterior Mediastinal Diseases

3-Ts and an L

Thymoma

Thyroid

Teratoma

Lymphoma

        d. less favorable prognosis than LP, but better than MC or LD
- MC
  - a. second most common subtype
  - b. more advanced involvement than LP or NS
  - c. usually involves older patients
  - d. less favorable prognosis than NS or LP, but better than LD
- LP
  - a. fewer than 5% of cases
  - b. usually involves young patients
  - c. seems to be an early stage of the disease
  - d. most favorable prognosis
  - e. involves both nodular and diffuse forms of involvement
- LD
  - a. fewer than 5% of cases
  - b. usually involves older patients, with systemic symptoms
  - c. disease process is well advanced
  - d. carries the poorest prognosis
- *"Pel-Ebstein fever"* pattern may be seen: a few days of high fever, alternating regularly with a few days or weeks of normal or subnormal temperature
- drinking alcohol may result in immediate pain in diseased areas of the body

3) **Radiologic features**
- bulky mediastinal and hilar lymphadenopathy (mediastinal widening)
- clearly defined, isolated anterior mediastinal masses
- massive disease: mediastinal tumor burden > one-third of the thoracic diameter
- thymic cysts seen in children, or in adult patients after radiation treatment
- thymoma
  1) **General considerations**
     - incidence
       - a. most common adult anterior mediastinal neoplasm
       - b. usually occurs in people > 20 years old
     - nature of lesion

a. usually benign

b. 25–50% may be invasive, but metastasis is rare

- location
  a. usually at level of junction of heart and great vessels
  b. may be midline, visible only on lateral or oblique projection

2) **Clinical features**

- 44–50% of thymomas are in patients with myasthenia gravis; 15% of patients with myasthenia gravis have thymic tumors
- clear associations with red cell aplasia and hypogammaglobulinemia

3) **Radiologic features**

- PA and lateral chest projections used for screening
- lateral film shows small mass, usually at base of heart
- up to 20% may show mottled calcifications
- mass may be oval, round, or lobulated
- sometimes cystic, with peripheral calcium
- mass > 4 cm may alter mediastinal contours on PA film
- adult thymus > 13 mm (with CT imaging) is suspect for either benign hyperplasia or pathology

4) **DDX**

- malignant thymic tumor has identical location and early appearance, but:
  a. is invasive (blurred margins)
  b. grows to reach both sides of midline
  c. may be a carcinoma or a sarcoma
- **DDX:** teratoma, substernal thyroid, lymphoma

- sub-sternal thyroid (intrathoracic goiter)

1) **General considerations**

- location
  a. generally extend from thoracic outlet into mediastinum
  b. usually in superior anterior mediastinum, may extend far downward into inferior posterior mediastinum
  c. most are anterior, but may be retrotracheal (almost always on the right and at the lower tracheal level)

- incidence: female predilection (3:1)

2) **Clinical features**
- history of hyperthyroid
- usually euthyroid when goiter becomes evident
- mass may move with swallowing, or may be fixed

3) **Radiologic features**
- soft tissue mass at thoracic outlet
- usually connected to the thyroid gland by an isthmus of tissue
- trachea deviated, possibly compressed
- may displace both trachea and esophagus (usually posterior)
- mass may have punctate or curvilinear calcifications, which may be visible only with CT

- teratoma

1) **General considerations**
- incidence: patients usually < 30 years old
- location: most chest teratomas in anterior mediastinum
- nature of lesion
  a. germ cell neoplasms (contain mesoderm, endoderm, ectoderm)
  b. unpredictable malignant potential

2) **Radiologic features**
- grow to 10 cm diameter and may contain teeth or hair
- about 25% may show calcifications (good prognostic sign)
- may be predominantly cystic
- CT or MRI helps identify invasion into adjacent tissue

b) Middle mediastinum
- esophageal achalasia

1) **General considerations**
- nature of condition
  a. gastroesophageal sphincter spasm or failure of relaxation
  b. creates obstruction of the esophagus
  c. esophagus is dilated above the diaphragm, and may become elongated, tortuous, or angulated
- incidence: most common between 20 and 40 years old

2) **Clinical features**
- impaired esophageal peristalsis

- dysphagia for both solids and liquids
- chest pain
- regurgitation
- nocturnal cough

3) **Radiologic features**
- usually has significant mediastinal widening
- may demonstrate an air/fluid level
- PA projection: characteristic vertical linear soft tissue density representing the esophageal wall, with lucent right lung on its right and the lucency of gas in the dilated esophagus on its left
- loss of magenblasse (air in fundus of stomach)
- esophagram shows abrupt termination at esophageal/gastric junction

- esophageal carcinoma
  1) **General considerations**
  - increased incidence of esophageal squamous cell carcinoma associated with achalasia, lye stricture, esophageal webs, and squamous cell carcinomas in head and neck
  - smokers and alcoholics at highest risk
  - primary esophageal adenocarcinoma associated with Barrett's metaplasia (with peptic esophagitis, columnar metaplastic epithelium may develop in lower esophagus)
  - chronic gastroesophageal reflux (GER) may predispose patient to Barrett's metaplasia, and thus to adenocarcinoma
  - about 85% are squamous cell carcinoma; 15% are adenocarcinoma

  2) **Clinical features**
  - dysphagia for solids (progressive over several weeks)
  - significant weight loss

  3) **Radiologic features**
  - usually none, but may see subtle alterations of mediastinal contours
  - stricture, mass, or plaque anywhere in the esophagus
  - contrast esophagram may be more diagnostic

  4) **DDX**
  - inflammatory stricture (TB, corrosive agent)

- benign neoplasm (leiomyoma is most common benign tumor of the esophagus)
- esophageal diverticula
  1) **General considerations**
     - Zenker's (pharyngeal) diverticulum: mucosa and submucosa protrude posteriorly through cricopharyngeal muscle
     - traction (mid-esophageal) diverticulum
     - epiphrenic diverticulum: just above the diaphragm
  2) **Clinical features**
     - Zenker's diverticulum
       a. when patient lies down, food that has filled the diverticulum is regurgitated
       b. nocturnal regurgitation may lead to aspiration pneumonitis
       c. enlarging pouch may cause dysphagia
     - traction and epiphrenic diverticula are usually asymptomatic
  3) **Radiologic features**
     - pocket of air in C5/C7 region, with or without fluid level
     - large amount of air may indicate esophageal obstruction
     - usually presents as a mid-line mass
     - barium-swallow is diagnostic

- esophageal varices
  1) nature of condition: varicosities in branches of the azygos vein, which anastomose with branches of the portal vein in the lower esophagus
  2) **Clinical features**
     - seen with portal hypertension, alcoholism
     - may rupture, causing hemoptysis
  3) **Radiologic features:** on barium swallow exam, may form *"snake-like esophageal filling defects,"* especially in lower esophagus (due to portal hypertension)

- thoracic aortic aneurysm (TAA)
  1) **General considerations**
     - vessel diameter > 3.8 cm indicates aneurysm
     - location: ascending aorta, aortic arch, descending aorta
     - fusiform: most common shape; most often in descending aorta

- saccular (eccentric): may occur anywhere in thoracic aorta
- true aneurysm balloons all three layers of vessel wall
- pseudoaneurysm lacks involvement of media, or media and adventitia (predilection for the arch)
- incidence: male predilection (3:1); average age 60 years
- associated variables: hypertension, smoking, advanced age

2) **Etiology**
   - atherosclerosis causes up to 80% of acquired aneurysms in descending thoracic aorta
   - trauma: second most common cause (often causes pseudoaneurysm)
     a. 94% of these are at ligamentum arteriosum in distal arch
     b. may be caused by rapid deceleration injury
     c. penetrating injury: may result from surgery
   - may be congenital
     a. involvement of ascending aorta is suggestive
     b. associated with connective tissue disorders, such as Marfan's syndrome or Ehlers-Danlos syndrome
   - may result from aortitis (e.g., syphilitic aneurysms); also likely to involve ascending aorta

3) **Clinical features**
   - cough, stridor, hoarseness, dyspnea, dysphagia
   - dull, aching pain; usually late in process
   - change in character of pain may herald rupture, dissection, or enlargement
   - treatment: surgical repair

4) **Radiologic features**
   - PA and lateral films may show altered aortic contours
   - diffuse widening of aorta (mediastinal widening)
   - rupture may cause rapid mediastinal widening, or hemothorax
   - optimum assessment is via MRI or CT
   - atherosclerotic aneurysms most common in abdominal aorta; may

occur in thoracic aorta; may show calcification

- aortic arch shadow > 5 mm beyond calcified wall: suggests aneurysm

- hiatal (hiatus) hernia

  1) **General considerations**
     - nature of condition
        a. protrusion of the stomach above the diaphragm
        b. may be congenital or secondary to trauma
     - sliding hiatus hernia
        a. gastroesophageal junction and part of the stomach above the diaphragm
        b. one side of herniated stomach is covered by peritoneum
     - paraesophageal hiatus hernia (rolling type)
        a. gastroesophageal junction is in normal position
        b. portion of the stomach is adjacent to the esophagus
     - location: retrocardiac portion of middle or posterior mediastinum
     - incidence
        a. > 40% of population may have a sliding hiatus hernia
        b. paraesophageal hiatus hernia is less common

  2) **Clinical features**
     - sliding hiatus hernia: often asymptomatic
     - may cause gastroesophageal reflux
     - may cause chest pain, with or without reflux
     - paraesophageal hiatus hernia: usually asymptomatic, but can incarcerate and strangulate
     - either type: can involve occult or massive GI hemorrhage

  3) **Radiologic features**
     - PA: superimposed on cardiac shadow
     - lateral: seen behind heart
     - magenblasse often shifted slightly medial, extending through diaphragm into thorax
     - may contain air only
     - may have air/fluid level interface
     - abdominal compression may be required to show sliding hiatus hernia

- pericardial cyst
  1) **General considerations**
     - most common cause of a middle mediastinal mass
     - usually developmental
     - usually attached to parietal layer of pericardium
  2) **Clinical features**
     - usually asymptomatic
     - may result in dyspnea
  3) **Radiologic features**
     - mainly left-sided thin-walled mass with central fluid density
     - large pericardial cyst may "invert" the left hemidiaphragm (liver prevents this from happening on the right)
     - **DDX:** left ventricular aneurysm
     - pedunculated cyst may show as a teardrop shaped shadow: broad along diaphragm and narrower above
     - may extend into the primary interlobar fissure as "teardrop" shaped mass
     - intrapericardial bronchogenic cyst may show a calcium fluid level, especially on the lateral view

- lymphoid neoplasms (Hodgkin disease)
  1) **General considerations**
     - nature of process
       a. most common subtype, presenting with nodular sclerosis
       b. usually involves the mediastinum, most commonly enlarged mediastinal-hilar nodes
       c. large fibrotic component in neoplasm
       d. tends to be widespread, multicompartmental
       e. shows particular predilection for anterior mediastinum
     - 5-year survival rate between 50 and 75%
     - best prognosis for those with disease only above the diaphragm
     - incidence
       a. two cohorts
          - late teens and 20s (patients with AIDS), with slight male preponderance
          - elderly males
       b. more aggressive disease in elderly patients

  c. 85% of Hodgkin disease patients have mediastinal lymph node involvement at initial presentation

 2) **Clinical features**
- initially, painless lymph node enlargement in neck or groin
- with abdominal involvement: fever, night sweats, weight loss, pruritus
- children may have associated cystic thymic lesions
- massive mediastinal involvement may compress airways when patient is recumbent

 3) **Radiologic features**
- may see bulky widening of mediastinum (by more than one third)
- mass may measure > 10 cm at its widest dimension
- CT is necessary for definitive evaluation of mediastinal involvement
- residual mediastinal mass is common after radiation therapy
  a. calcified nodes and altered mediastinal contours may be expected

- mediastinal cystic hygroma (lymphangioma)
 1) **General considerations**
- fluid-filled cyst
- spongy mass in neck, extending into superior mediastinum

 2) **Clinical features**
- may have palpable, soft, pliable mass in neck
- may be asymptomatic, especially if mediastinal hygroma occurs without mass in neck

 3) **Radiologic features**
- mass of fluid density
- usually a continuation of mass from neck into superior mediastinum
- contour may alter in different phases of respiration

REVIEW—STUDY QUESTIONS

1. What is a teratoma? Is it clinically significant? Describe its radiologic appearance.

2. Name and describe three pneumoconioses. Describe their radiologic appearances.

3. What are the four most common diseases of the anterior mediastinum?

4. What pulmonary pathologies are related to the combined effects of smoking and asbestos exposure?

5. What is TAA, and what are its radiologic features?

6. Describe the radiologic features of asbestosis.

7. Describe the thymoma and its radiologic features. With what condition is it frequently associated?

8. What is the radiologic appearance of a substernal thyroid?

9. Define achalasia. What is the clinical effect of esophageal achalasia? What are its radiologic features?

10. What is Caplan's disease? What are the characteristic locations and behaviors of its lung lesions?

11. What is the "shaggy heart sign" and with what disease is it associated?

12. Name three types of esophageal diverticula, and describe their radiologic appearances.

13. Name and describe four types of silicosis. Contrast and compare their radiologic features.

14. What is the difference between a true aortic aneurysm and a pseudoaneurysm? Is there a radiologic distinction?

15. What are the clinical effects of Zenker's diverticulum? What does it look like on x-ray?

16. What is "rounded atelectasis"? With what process is it associated? What is its radiologic appearance?

17. What is the most common cause of masses in the middle mediastinum? What is its radiologic appearance?

18. What is PMF and what does it look like on plain film? What is its etiology?

19. Name and describe three neoplasms that may be found in the middle mediastinum, and describe their appearance on plain film.

20. What is a "comet tail sign," and with what process is it seen?

c) Posterior mediastinum

- neurofibroma (neurilemoma or neurolemmoma)

  1) **General considerations**
     - benign, neurogenic tumor
     - arises from intercostal nerves and exiting spinal nerve roots
     - very common in mediastinum

  2) **Clinical features**
     - may be manifestation of neurofibromatosis
     - may be asymptomatic, incidental finding until large

  3) **Radiologic features**
     - rounded density; may reach large size
     - forms acute angle with the mediastinum

- has narrow mediastinal base (on PA projection)
- has smooth or lobulated contour
- intraforaminal neurofibroma may extend through IVF, causing "*dumbbell*" tumor (pressure erosions of adjacent pedicles, vertebral body) and extend into posterior mediastinum (oblique views give definitive diagnosis)

4) **DDX:** (for enlarged IVF)
- congenital agenesis of pedicle
- vertebral artery tortuosity with pressure erosion

- ganglioneuroma
  1) **General considerations**
  - benign, neurogenic tumor
  - regarded by many: fully differentiated neuroblastoma
  - arise from sympathetic ganglia
  - very common in mediastinum
  2) **Radiologic features**
  - can become very large
  - mass tends to be elongated vertically rather than round
  - usually has broad mediastinal base (on PA projection)
  - forms obtuse angle with the mediastinum
  - usually smooth; occasionally lobulated

- neurenteric cyst
  1) **General considerations**
  - rare mediastinal cyst
  - formed from remnant of neurenteric canal
  - from the dorsal division of embryonic foregut
  2) **Clinical features**
  - male predilection
  - may be associated with intestinal tract diverticulum or duplication
  - may connect with jejunum via a tube through the diaphragm
  - also associated with anterior vertebral defect
  3) **Radiologic features**
  - cystic mass, connected to meninges by fibrous stalk
  - anterior vertebral defect

- lateral meningocele or anterior meningocele
  1) **General considerations**
  - anterior meningocele: extremely rare, involves significant rib and vertebral anomalies
  - lateral meningocele protrudes

through the intervertebral
foramen

2) **Clinical features**
- lateral meningocele found in
  association with
  neurofibromatosis
- may be isolated and
  asymptomatic

3) **Radiologic features**
- mass seen on PA film as a soft
  tissue density outlined by
  posterior lungs
- may not be seen until quite large

d) Pneumomediastinum
- **General considerations**
  1) air collection in the mediastinum
     outside the bronchial tree
  2) caused by penetrating wound,
     surgery, airway leak, esophageal
     leak, hyperbaric damage to lungs
- **Clinical features**
  1) history of chest trauma or surgery
  2) acute asthma attack or heavy
     coughing (especially with fibrosis
     and/or progressive pulmonary
     fibrosis)
  3) may occur in patients on respirators
- **Radiologic features**
  1) lucent streaks within the
     mediastinum
  2) vertical linear lucencies may outline
     or separate mediastinal structures
  3) on lateral projection, streaks may
     appear anterior to heart and aorta
  4) lucent streaks may extend superiorly,
     dissecting cervical soft tissues
- **DDX:** pneumopericardium
  1) lucent halo around heart, but not
     extending superior to pericardium
  2) pericardial air shifts position when
     patient is filmed upright

e) Lymphadenopathy
- **General considerations**
  1) seen with many pathologies,
     including:
     - malignancy
     - infections, particularly
       mycobacterial and fungal
     - granulomatous diseases
       (sarcoidosis, pneumoconiosis)
  2) anatomical classification (Rouviere's
     classification, as modified by Lien
     and Lund)
     - anterior mediastinal nodes
       a. parietal group
          - internal mammary nodes,

superior diaphragmatic nodes

- drain breasts, liver, anterior chest and abdomen walls, diaphragm, pleura, pericardium

  b. prevascular group
  - prevenous (right anterior) nodes, intermediate anterior nodes, prearterial (left anterior) nodes
  - drain thymus, heart, pericardium, lungs (mainly left upper lobe)
- middle mediastinal nodes
  a. paratracheal group
  - right and left lateral nodes, pretracheal nodes, retrotracheal nodes
  - drain lungs, trachea, bronchi, esophagus, pericardium
  b. subcarinal (intertracheobronchial) group
  c. pulmonary root (tracheobronchial) group
  - drain lungs, trachea, bronchi, esophagus, pericardium
- posterior mediastinal nodes
  a. paraesophageal nodes
  - drain esophagus, pericardium, diaphragm, lower lobes of lungs
  b. paraaortic nodes
  - drain esophagus, pericardium, diaphragm, lower lung lobes
- paravertebral group
  a. prevertebral nodes, laterovertebral nodes
  b. drain posterior chest wall, vertebrae

- **Clinical features**
  1) no clean correlation between pathology and nodal site, but some nodes seem more predilected to certain pathologies
  2) internal mammary nodes may enlarge with Hodgkin disease, breast cancer
  3) superior diaphragmatic nodes may enlarge with lymphomas or liver malignancies (either by metastasis or direct extension)
  4) prevascular nodes involved in

lymphoma, sarcoidosis, metastasis
from bronchogenic carcinoma

5) paratracheal nodes often involved in
lymphoma and metastasis from
bronchogenic carcinoma

6) pulmonary root nodes are commonly
involved with lymphoma, sarcoidosis,
metastasis from bronchogenic
carcinoma

7) posterior mediastinal nodes involved
with lymphoma, metastasis from
esophageal or lung cancer

- **Radiologic features**
    1) evaluation
        - conventional PA projection
        - CT, with bolus injection of
          intravenous contrast
    2) signs of lymphadenopathy:
        - size: no clear parameters, but
          transverse diameter > 1 or 1.5 cm
          is suspect for pathology (best
          evaluated by CT)
        - calcification commonly seen with
          fungal infections (TB,
          histoplasmosis), with silicosis, coal
          worker's pneumoconiosis;
          sometimes with sarcoidosis,
          lymphomas, metastasized
          osteosarcoma; rarely with
          metastasized chondrosarcoma or
          bronchogenic carcinoma
        - lobulated contours (most
          commonly in paratracheal or hilar
          areas)

13. **Vascular and Cardiovascular Diseases**

a) Thoracic aortic dissection
- **General considerations**
    1) nature of condition
        - cleavage of media forming a new
          false lumen through the media
        - when occurring in a preexisting
          aneurysm, this is a dissecting
          aneurysm
    2) etiology
        - may be initiated by intimal
          tearing
        - bleeding from vasa vasorum may
          cause secondary tears
    3) two commonly used classification
       systems for dissections
        - DeBakey system
            a. Type I: involves ascending,
               arch, and descending aorta
            b. Type II: involves ascending
               aorta only
            c. Type III: involves descending
               aorta only

- Stanford system
  a. Type A: involving ascending aorta
  b. Type B: involving only descending aorta

4) acute dissection: (by definition) within 2 weeks of symptom onset
   - these are usually Type A (Type I or II) and are apt to be lethal
   - often associated with Marfan's, so have younger age cohort

5) chronic dissections: typically type B
   - **Clinical features**
     a. male predominance (reported variously as 2:1 or 5:1)
     b. associated (especially Type B) with systemic hypertension
     c. 90% experience tearing, severe, constant pain; pain may be substernal; may radiate: cause left shoulder/upper back pain
     d. may have syncope (with hemopericardium or cardiac tamponade)

6) rare signs: paraparesis or paraplegia (caused by spinal cord ischemia); dyspnea, hoarseness, dysphagia caused by aortic expansion or mediastinal hemorrhage

7) vascular signs: may include angina, renal failure, mesenteric or peripheral ischemia, congestive heart failure

8) hypotension: may indicate shock and imminent rupture
   - differential blood pressures (varying from side to side): in about 50% of patients (considered a reliable indicator of dissection)

9) dissection of ascending aorta: may have acute aortic regurgitation

- **Radiologic features**
  1) optimal imaging: MRI
     - identify intimal flap
     - entry/reentry tears
     - flow in false lumen
  2) CT with bolus infusion: sensitive and quite specific
     - intimal calcification and its displacement
     - false positives caused by pulsation artifact, fluid in superior pericardial recesses
  3) transesophageal echocardiography (TEE): used for initial screening, not

efficient for evaluating arch or descending aorta

   4) dissection may create acute mediastinal widening (without extravascular pooling)

   5) nonspecific findings: displaced intimal calcifications, aortic enlargement, pleural effusions, contour changes

- **DDX**
  - a. contained intramural hematoma
  - b. myocardial infarction
  - c. pericarditis, pleuritis
  - d. mediastinal tumor
  - e. pulmonary embolism

b) Left ventricular aneurysm

- **General considerations**
  1) nature of condition
     - weakened myocardial wall
     - most commonly caused by coronary occlusion, but may result from trauma or inflammation
  2) site: most commonly at left lower cardiac margin, near apex
- **Radiologic features**
  1) bizarre silhouette: diffuse calcific bulge along left lower cardiac border
  2) cinéradiography or fluoroscopy may show paradoxical pulsation
     - **DDX**
       - a. myocardial tumor
       - b. coronary artery aneurysm
       - c. pericardial cyst

c) Rheumatic heart

- **General considerations**
  1) may result in stenotic valves (aortic or mitral stenosis, tricuspid valvular disease)
  2) mitral stenosis and mitral insufficiency
  3) often involves both aortic and mitral valves, resulting in generalized, massive cardiac enlargement
- **Clinical features**
  1) mitral valve insufficiency (incompetence, regurgitation)
     - dyspnea
     - sometimes, hoarseness
     - widely split S_2 on auscultation
     - palpable sustained left parasternal movement
     - palpitations

- sustained, enlarged apical movement, moved slightly to left
- various murmurs: pansystolic or diastolic, depending on location and severity of lesions

2) mitral stenosis
- patients may be asymptomatic for several years before developing symptoms
- exertional dyspnea or fatigue is often earliest symptom
- pulmonary edema
- hemoptysis may follow pulmonary vessel rupture (especially during pregnancy)
- left vocal cord paralysis ("*Ortner's syndrome*") causes hoarseness (seen with mitral stenosis), and is caused by left recurrent laryngeal nerve pressure exerted by dilated pulmonary artery
- when severe, there may be a deep malar flush ("*mitral facies*")
- apical diastolic thrill with left lateral decubitus patient
- may be sustained left parasternal movement
- may be "opening snap" near left lower sternal border, and palpable S_1 and S_2 at the apex

3) aortic insufficiency (aortic incompetence, aortic regurgitation)
- may be asymptomatic for many years
- eventual exertional dyspnea, orthopnea, paroxysmal nocturnal dyspnea
- eventual palpitations, occasionally with nocturnal angina
- slapping pulse (rapid rise with large volume): sometimes called "*water-hammer pulse*" or "*collapsing pulse*"
- auscultation over femoral pulse reveals "*Traube's sign*" ("*pistol-shot sound*")
- "*double Duroziez murmur*": systolic femoral artery murmur heard distal to finger pressure, while a diastolic murmur is heard proximal to finger pressure
- "*Corrigan's pulse*": visible, large carotid pulsations
- "*de Musset's sign*": head nodding, caused by ballistic force of large stroke volume
- "*capillary pulsation*" ("*Quincke's sign*"): pulsatile blanching and

reddening of fingernails under slight pressure

- elevated systolic pressure, with leg systolic pressure > 20 mm Hg higher than brachial systolic pressure (positive "*Hill's sign*")
- visible left parasternal medial retraction
- various murmurs are auscultated, including
  a. "*Cole-Cecil*" murmur: diastolic; heard near axilla or mid left thorax
  b. "*Austin Flint*" murmur: diastolic rumble at apex
  c. "*to-and-fro*" murmur: combined forward ejection and backward regurgitant flow murmur

4) aortic stenosis
  - classic triad: syncope, angina, exertional dyspnea
  - "*bisferiens pulse*": a notch, or dip, in mid-systole
  - "*pulsus parvus*" and "*tardus*": low blood pressure with small pulse pressure
  - mixed-frequency ejection murmur and various other murmurs may be present

5) tricuspid insufficiency (incompetence, or regurgitation)
  - sensation of pulsations in neck (high jugular regurgitant waves)
  - "*Carvallo's sign*": pansystolic, high-pitched murmur best heard at fourth and fifth intercostal spaces, near sternum; or in the epigastrium

6) tricuspid stenosis
  - some fluttering discomfort in the neck, from jugular pulse waves
  - fatigue (symptom of low levels of CO_2)
  - right upper quadrant abdominal discomfort (enlarged liver)
  - giant flickering wave in jugular pulse, or prominent "*v*" wave
  - presystolic murmur at left sternal edge in fourth intercostal space; increases with inspiration

 - **Radiologic features**
  1) mitral stenosis
    - left atrial enlargement alters cardiac silhouette
      a. convex left upper cardiac shadow (enlargement of

posterior heart), below left main bronchus

   b. double contour (double convexity) on right

   c. may increase density of heart shadow below the carina level

   d. elevated main bronchus

   e. esophagus displaced posteriorly, sometimes to the right

   f. possible calcification of mitral valve and mitral annulus

- may ultimately cause left ventricular enlargement or (with pulmonary arterial hypertension) eventual right ventricular enlargement

- size reversal of pulmonary vessels: distention of upper lobe vessels and constriction of lower lobe vessels (without disease, the lower are more prominent)

- *"Kerley's B lines"*: short dense lines extending at right angles to pleural surface in lower lung fields

   a. do not bifurcate

   b. seen best on oblique projections

   c. represent edema and lymphatic distention in interlobular septa

- may also see *"Kerley's A lines"*: straight lines fanning out and up from upper hilar area into upper lung field; about 2–5 inches long

- *"Kerley's C lines"*: transient, fine reticular lines (spider-web) throughout lung

2) mitral insufficiency

- heart enlarged downward and to the left (left ventricular enlargement)

- lower left cardiac contour rounded

- also signs of left atrial enlargement and pulmonary congestion as in mitral stenosis (see above)

3) aortic stenosis

- hypertrophied left ventricle (late in the disease)

- rounding of lower left cardiac contour may be only sign

- convex upper right cardiac margin, caused by normal aortic

knob and enlarged ascending aortic arch
- best seen in left anterior oblique projection
- aortic valve may have calcifications

4) aortic insufficiency
- hypertrophy of left ventricle with dilatation
- left lower cardiac contour elongates, extends below dome of diaphragm
- rounding of left lower contour, and eventual rounding of left upper contour
- aortic knob often prominent
- "*cor bovinum*": massive left ventricular enlargement

5) tricuspid valvular disease
- enlargement (sometimes extreme) of right atrium
- widened cardiac shadow to the right
- increasingly convex lower right cardiac margin
- PA and left anterior oblique projections may show sharp angulation between ascending aorta and projected right auricular appendage (the enlarged right atrium)
- enlarged superior and inferior vena cavae
- lung fields may appear unusually clear, lucent

d) Congestive heart failure (CHF)
- **General considerations**
  1) nature of condition
     - usually refers to left heart failure
     - cardiac output insufficient for body's metabolic needs
     - left heart failure entails pulmonary venous congestion
     - right heart failure involves systemic venous distention
  2) etiology
     - commonly caused by coronary artery disease
     - hypertension
     - less often caused by cardiomyopathies, valvular disorders, shunts
- **Clinical features**
  1) nonspecific symptoms: shortness of breath, dry cough
  2) common in older patients with a history of smoking

3) often found in combination with chronic pulmonary disease

- **Radiologic features**
  1) earliest findings: overdistended pulmonary blood vessels
  2) cephalization of blood flow: upper lobe vessels more distended than lower lobe vessels (the reverse is normal)
  3) interstitial pulmonary edema in lower lung segments (lower lobes appear "veiled"; margins of their vessels less distinct)
  4) distention of interlobular septa ("*Kerley's B lines*")
  5) distended connective tissue between lobes and near hila ("*Kerley's A lines*")
  6) fine reticular lines ("*Kerley's C lines*") (see Radiologic features of mitral stenosis, above, for fuller description)
  7) decreased lung size, even with deep inspiration
  8) rapid development and rapid clearing of pulmonary edema is typical

- **DDX:** with edema secondary to renal disease, see alveolar edema in "*batwing or butterfly pattern*" around hilar regions (much less common with CHF)

e) Left atrial myxoma

- **General considerations**
  1) nature of condition
     - benign primary cardiac tumor
     - primitive connective tissue cells and mesenchyme-like stroma
  2) incidence
     - primary benign or malignant cardiac tumors are rare
     - myxoma: most common primary benign cardiac tumor
     - 50% of all primary myocardial tumors are myxomas
  3) location
     - arises from atrial septum near foramen ovale
     - 75% are in left atrium
     - most others are in right atrium

- **Clinical features**
  1) embolic phenomena
     - especially from gelatinous myxomas
     - from right-sided tumors to lungs; from left-sided tumors to periphery

2) blood flow obstruction
- most commonly at mitral valve
- pulmonary congestion with typical signs of mitral stenosis (murmur, opening snap, accentuated first heart sound)
- may produce "tumor plop" sound

3) constitutional syndromes
- fever, weight loss
- Raynaud's phenomenon, finger clubbing
- anemia (often hemolytic anemia), low platelet count
- elevated ESR and white cell counts
- positive C-reactive protein
- increased gamma globulin (or other abnormal serum proteins)

- **Radiologic features**
  1) echocardiogram for definitive diagnosis
  2) pulmonary congestion visible on chest films
  3) myxoma may contain some calcifications, visible on CT

f) Atherosclerotic ulcers
- **General considerations**
  1) ulceration of atheroma through intima into media
  2) most common in descending aorta

- **Clinical considerations**
  1) often asymptomatic; sometimes back or chest pain, similar to dissection
  2) elderly population, often when hypertension coexists with atherosclerosis
  3) treatment: generally conservative, hypertension management
  4) often associated with saccular aneurysms
  5) may precipitate distal embolization
  6) can lead to intramural hematoma, and eventually to dissection
  7) isolated medial hematoma (with no ulceration) is more ominous and is surgically treated (as an impending dissection)

- **Radiologic features**
  1) effective imaging is via CT, MRI, or transesophageal echocardiography (TEE)
  2) contrast-enhanced CT is sensitive for atherosclerotic ulcers; increased sensitivity with helical CT
  3) MRI: contrast not required to demonstrate ulceration, but contrast

techniques improve differential diagnosis (ulceration vs. dissection)

☞ **g)** Pulseless disease (aortic arch syndrome or *"Takayasu disease"*)

- **General considerations**
  1) incidence
     - most common noninfectious aortitis
     - usually affects young Asian women
     - median age of onset in mid-twenties
     - affects aorta and its branches; particularly vessels of aortic arch
  2) idiopathic, autoimmune process proposed

- **Clinical features**
  1) bruits, diminished or absent pulses, claudication
  2) about half of cases: no systemic symptoms
  3) may cause malaise, myalgia, arthralgia
  4) complications
     - stroke (when aortic arch and its branches are affected)
     - angina or infarction (with ostial coronary stenosis)
     - hypertension (with renal artery involvement)
     - pulmonary hypertension or infarction (pulmonary artery involvement)
     - commonly causes arterial stenosis
     - may cause aneurysms, dissection
     - heart failure caused by aortic regurgitation
  5) treatment
     - corticosteroids
     - surgical bypass
     - balloon angioplasty
     - cytotoxic therapy (used when patients don't respond to steroids)
     - radiologic features
       a. plain film demonstrates vessel wall calcification
       b. traditional imaging has been via angiography
       c. excellent imaging via MRI and MR angiography
     - demonstrate stenosis, occlusion, aneurysm
     - also show inflammatory wall thickening

☞
h) Giant cell arteritis (temporal arteritis)
- **General considerations**
  1) incidence
     - ages 60–80 years
     - slight female predilection
     - large blood vessels, especially those with prominent elastica
       etiology: probably autoimmune
- **Clinical features**
  1) chronic inflammatory disease of large vessels
  2) predilection for temporal arteries, extracranial carotid arteries, brachial arteries in chest, commonly involves arch vessels
  3) can cause aneurysm, stenosis, dissection, rupture of the thoracic aorta (thoracic aorta involved late in process)
  4) headache, tender scalp
  5) polymyalgia rheumatica
  6) fever, malaise
  7) vision loss
  8) jaw claudication with chewing (rather than with speech)
  9) history of other sources of noninfectious aortitis:
     - rheumatoid arthritis (RA)
     - seronegative spondyloarthropathies: e.g., ankylosing spondylitis (AS), Reiter's syndrome
     - rheumatic fever
     - polyarteritis nodosa
     - systemic lupus erythematosus (SLE)
  10) corticosteroid therapy is treatment of choice
- **Radiologic features**
  1) CT or MRI optimal: assess wall thickening, stenosis, aneurysm, periaortic edema
  2) plain film non-contributory

☞
i) Pulmonary embolism
- **General considerations**
  1) mechanisms
     - fatty emboli released from marrow of fractured bones
     - air embolism caused by penetrating chest injury
     - thrombophlebitis
  2) incidence
     - usually young patients with femoral or long bone fractures
     - fairly common, life-threatening complication with trauma

- **Clinical features**
  1) usually 48–72 hours post-injury, but may occur almost immediately
  2) fever, CNS dysfunction, respiratory distress
  3) may be disseminated intravascular coagulation
  4) retinal fat emboli; petechiae
- **Radiologic features**
  1) some not visible on plain film, require ventilation perfusion scan (VQ scan)
  2) diffuse or basilar lung opacities
  3) wedge shaped *"truncated cone"* opacity in lung periphery, base contiguous to visceral pleura, rounded convex apex directed toward hilum (*"Hampton's hump"*)
  4) lung apices frequently spared

REVIEW—STUDY QUESTIONS

1. Describe the radiologic appearance of pneumomediastinum, and compare it with that of pneumopericardium.

2. What complications may arise from temporal arteritis? What is its other name?

3. What are the clinical symptoms and radiologic features of aortic dissection?

4. What is the radiologic appearance of left ventricular aneurysm?

5. Name three disease processes that may result in mediastinal lymphadenopathy.

6. What are the two main effects of rheumatic fever upon the cardiac valves?

7. What are Kerley's B lines, and with what conditions are they associated?

8. Name two common benign tumors of the posterior mediastinum. Contrast their radiologic appearances.

9. How do the radiologic appearances of pulmonary edema caused by CHF and pulmonary edema secondary to renal disease differ?

10. Name five sources of noninfectious aortitis.

11. Where in the heart is a cardiac myxoma most often located?

12. In what area of the aorta is atherosclerotic ulceration most common? What are the most effective imaging modalities for atherosclerotic ulcers?

13. What disease processes commonly cause calcification of mediastinal lymph nodes?

14. List ten clinical signs of rheumatic heart.

15. Describe Takayasu disease. What are its optimal diagnostic imaging modalities?

16. What is the optimal modality to rule out aortic dissection? Are there any plain film signs?

17. What are the clinical signs and symptoms of temporal arteritis? What population often suffers from it?

18. What is cor bovinum and with what condition is it associated?

19. What is Hampton's hump, and with what pathology is it associated?

20. What, if any, plain film findings are indicative of pulseless disease?

14. **Miscellaneous Processes**

    a) *Pneumocystis carinii* pneumonia (PCP)

- **General considerations**
  1) nature of condition
     - pulmonary infection
     - widely varying severity
  2) incidence
     - most common pulmonary infection with patients with AIDS
     - otherwise rare
     - incidence declining with effective prophylactic therapy

- **Clinical features**
  1) if untreated, progresses rapidly, and may cause severe adult respiratory distress syndrome (ARDS) within 24 hours
  2) usually resolves without residual effects
  3) pneumothorax ensues in about 5% of AIDS patients with PCP
  4) pneumatoceles may occur in about 10% of PCP patients

- **Radiologic features**
  1) 10 to 39% of PCP patients have normal chest films
  2) reticulonodular lesions may have symmetric or asymmetric distribution (variable appearance)
  3) mild forms: minimal loss of distinct vascular detail
  4) severe forms: bilateral homogeneous consolidations
  5) resolution may leave parenchymal fibrosis: persistent reticular and linear densities
  6) may present as focal airspace consolidation, or as miliary disease, and occasionally as solitary or multiple nodules (sometimes cavitated)

        7) pneumatoceles appear as thin-walled, air-filled spaces of varied sizes (not specific to PCP)

 b) non-Hodgkin lymphoma (NHL)

- **General considerations**
  1) nature of condition
     - wide variety of classifications and staging formulae
     - high-grade NHL tumors are the most aggressive human malignancies
     - most likely viral etiology (identified as HTLV-I)
  2) incidence
     - most frequent is low-grade, in elderly patients
     - high-grade: predilection for young males, patients with AIDS
     - intrathoracic involvement more common in children than adults
  3) sites
     - cervical or inguinal lymph nodes predilected
     - extranodal sites: CNS, bone, skin, gastric organs, etc.

- **Clinical features**
  1) elderly patient with low-grade NHL may be asymptomatic
  2) high-grade NHL in immunocompromised patients: predilection for the central nervous system

- **Radiologic features**
  1) rib lesions common for young females with NHL:
     - typically small, round cell tumors
     - sometimes: destructive permeative lesion with surrounding soft tissue mass
     - rarely, elliptical pleural plaques
     - mammogram: ill-defined, spiculated mass lesion without calcifications
     - commonly, pleural effusions (secondary to parenchymal involvement)
  2) elderly male patients: parenchymal tumors
     - poorly-defined nodule or mass
     - may show irregular cavitation, without fluid levels
     - mediastinal-hilar node involvement:
       a. more common with Hodgkin lymphoma than with NHL
       b. enlargement of single node group or chain

c. may show explosive, aggressive progression, especially in patient with metastasis of mycosis fungoides (localized cutaneous NHL)

c) Pleural effusion
- **General considerations**
    1) nature of condition
        - accumulation of pleural fluid or exudates
            a. pus
            b. water
            c. blood
            d. fat
            e. proteins
        - due to imbalance of normal fluid exchange
        - caused by pleural disease
    2) etiologies
        - transudative effusion (usually bilateral): disrupted filtering of fluid from microvasculature
            a. pulmonary or systemic venous hypertension
            b. CHF
            c. pulmonary embolism
            d. hepatic cirrhosis
            e. nephrotic syndrome
        - exudative effusion (unilateral or bilateral): pleural disease resulting in increased capillary permeability or impaired lymphatic drainage (exudative effusion with frank pus: empyema)
        - traumatic injury to intrathoracic vessels:
            a. hemothorax
            b. chylothorax
- **Clinical features**
    1) effusion itself usually asymptomatic; a sign of disease
    2) most common symptoms: pleuritic pain; dyspnea (with very large accumulations of fluid)
    3) signs: percussion dullness, decreased thoracic excursion with respiration, decreased or absent breath sounds, absent palpable fremitus
    4) predominantly left-sided effusion: caused by pancreatitis, distal thoracic duct obstruction, Dressler's syndrome (postmyocardial infarction), postpericardiotomy syndrome
    5) predominantly right-sided effusion: caused by proximal thoracic duct obstruction, ascites (with hepatic or

ovarian disease such as carcinoma, endometriosis)

6) *"Meigs' syndrome:"* ovarian fibroma associated with ascites and hydrothorax

7) untreated empyema: may result in inelastic fibrous membrane encasing the lung (*"fibrin peel"*), restricting respiration

8) fibrinopurulent empyema may drain into lungs (*"bronchopleural fistula"*), or through chest wall (*empyema necessitatis, empyema necessitans*)

- **Radiologic features**
    1) free effusion: meniscus sign or subpulmonary fluid
    2) homogenous opacification of dependent portion of thorax
    3) upper border usually meniscus-shaped
    4) lateral decubitus (recumbent) view, with affected side dependent, will demonstrate even small pleural effusions, not visible on upright views
    5) large effusions: may completely opacify the hemithorax
    6) mediastinal shift to the unaffected side
    7) obliteration or "dulling" of costophrenic angle
    8) loculated effusion: fluid collections may simulate soft tissue mass (create an encapsulated pseudotumor within the potential space separating the visceral and parietal pleura)
    9) CT: optimal modality for defining small effusions
    10) imaging modalities cannot differentiate cause of effusion

d) Primary mesothelioma
- **General considerations**
    1) nature of lesions
        - arise from mesothelial cells
        - may be diffuse or localized
        - localized: called *"localized fibrous tumor"*
    2) incidence
        - rare; either benign or malignant
        - no gender predilection
        - usually in 50 years and 60 years of age
- **Clinical features**
    1) about half of patients are asymptomatic
    2) systemic symptoms: symptoms of hypertrophic osteoarthropathy, hypoglycemia

3) may cause straw-colored or
    serosanguineous pleural effusions
4) locally invasive (to chest wall,
    mediastinum, lung parenchyma)
5) occasionally metastasizes
6) diffuse malignant mesothelioma
    usually related to asbestosis; very
    rare

- **Radiologic features**
    1) localized: mass attached to visceral
        or parietal pleura (occasionally to
        the diaphragm or mediastinum)
    2) benign tumor may be pedunculated,
        mobile with positional changes
    3) diffuse: irregular or nodular pleural
        thickening
    4) may cause pleural effusion
    5) may spread over entire lung surface,
        eventually encase lung
    6) may cause hypertrophic
        osteoarthropathy

e) Metastatic tumors
- **General considerations**
    1) 75% are from primary lung, breast,
        and lymphatic tumors
    2) some from ovarian carcinoma
        (fourth most frequent source)
    3) rarely from uterus, cervix,
        gastrointestinal tract, pancreas, bone
- **Clinical features:** depend upon features of
  primary neoplasm
- **Radiologic features**
    1) extrapleural sign (mass adheres to
        pleura)
    2) may be solitary or multiple

f) AIDS
- **General considerations**
    1) nature of condition
        - retrovirus (old name: HTLV-III;
          new name: HIV-I)
        - impairs immune system by
          destroying T lymphocytes
        - depletion of immune competence
          leads to opportunistic infection or
          neoplasm
    2) incidence (1997)
        - cases identified in > 125 countries
        - United States populations most at
          risk: homosexual males, IV drug
          abusers
        - other identified risk groups: blood
          transfusion recipients,
          hemophiliacs, those having
          heterosexual contact with other
          at-risk individuals
- **Clinical features**
    1) *Pneumocystis carinii* pneumonia
        (PCP)

2) various mycobacterial diseases, most often TB or *Mycobacterium avium*

3) less commonly, various fungal infections: histoplasmosis, coccidioidomycosis, cryptococcosis, aspergillosis

4) cytomegalovirus (CMV) pneumonitis

5) pyogenic infections (commonly: *Streptococcus pneumoniae and Hemophilus influenzae*)

6) Kaposi sarcoma (KS): most commonly with cutaneous lesions, but may disseminate, and is variously reported to invade lung parenchyma in 8 to 47% of cases

7) non-Hodgkin lymphoma (about 10% of cases involve intrathoracic structures)

8) bronchogenic carcinoma: may or may not be more frequent in AIDS patients, but when present appears significantly more aggressive

9) lymphocytic interstitial pneumonia (LIP): indolent, benign process usually seen in pediatric AIDS patients

- **Radiologic features**
  1) with PCP: diffuse, fairly symmetric reticular opacifications
  2) with TB
     - initially: heterogeneous reticulonodular opacities, sometimes cavitated, usually in upper lobes and superior segments of lower lobes
     - may be focal alveolar consolidation, with hilar and/or mediastinal adenopathy
     - later: diffuse, symmetric coarse reticular or reticulonodular infiltration
     - occasionally there is a miliary pattern, symmetric or asymmetric
  3) with fungal infections
     - diffuse, coarse nodular infiltrates (histoplasmosis, coccidioidomycosis)
     - diffuse interstitial or alveolar consolidation, pleural effusion, adenopathy, cavitated or non-cavitated nodules (seen with cryptococcosis)
     - aspergillosis may present with single or multiple focal opacities (in the upper lobes, often cavitated); may be tracheal plaques
  4) with CMV pulmonary disease
     - diffuse interstitial prominence,

hazy opacifications, dense
consolidation
- occasionally, discrete nodules

5) with pyogenic pneumonias
- airspace consolidation
- occasionally, cavitation and
sometimes, effusions

6) with Kaposi sarcoma
- ill-defined nodules throughout
lungs
- bilateral, coarse linear opacities
- perihilar peribronchial thickening:
"*tram-tracking*" appearance when
viewed *en face*
- bilateral pleural effusions
- about 10% show hilar adenopathy

7) with non-Hodgkin lymphoma
- pleural effusions, unilateral or
bilateral
- hilar and mediastinal adenopathy
(up to 25% of patients)
- occasionally, interstitial lung
disease; well-defined nodules
(single or multiple, and showing
rapid growth)
- intraluminal mass may obstruct
airway

8) with bronchogenic carcinoma
- effusions
- large central and peripheral
masses

9) with LIP
- appears similar to PCP (diffuse or
local interstitial nodular or linear
densities in a fine pattern,
becoming more coarse over time)
- may include hilar and mediastinal
lymphadenopathy

 g) Pneumothorax
- **General considerations**
1) nature of condition: free air between
visceral and parietal pleura
2) etiologies
- trauma: penetrating injury to
chest wall (open pneumothorax)
or penetration of pleura with
airtight chest wall (closed
pneumothorax) as with fractured
rib or thoracentesis needle;
ruptured bronchus or perforated
esophagus
- pulmonary barotrauma:
mechanical ventilators
- "*spontaneous pneumothorax:*" no
antecedent trauma involved
  a. simple spontaneous
pneumothorax: localized

pulmonary disease in a normally healthy patient; small, local bulla rupture

    b. complicated spontaneous pneumothorax: ruptured bulla in patient with emphysema or other underlying disease

- *"tension pneumothorax"* (positive pressure pneumothorax): air can enter but not leave pleural space unless the pressure within space rises above atmospheric pressure
- induced pneumothorax: air introduced into pleural space for thoracoscopy or to enhance visualization on standard radiographs

- **Clinical features**
    1) vary depending on extent of involvement and etiology
    2) sudden sharp chest pain
    3) dry, hacking cough
    4) may develop severe dyspnea, shock, respiratory failure, and circulatory collapse
    5) referral of pain to shoulder, chest, abdomen
    6) diminished voice and breath sounds (via auscultation)
    7) tympanic percussion sounds
    8) diminished, absent tactile fremitus
    9) diminished chest excursion on affected side
    10) severe cases: hypoxemia, hypercapnia

- **Radiologic features**
    1) mediastinum shifts to unaffected side with large pneumothorax
    2) *"tension pneumothorax"* results in complete lung collapse and contralateral mediastinal shift, with hemidiaphragm depressed or inverted
    3) upright films: visceral pleural line forms border between lucency with lung markings on proximal side and lucency without lung markings on distal side
    4) pneumothorax usually is at lung apex, and lateral to lung; but air may accumulate medially or inferior to lungs
    5) PA film taken on full **expiration** may detect a small pneumothorax
    6) lateral decubitus with affected side uppermost: displays air along lateral borders

15. Review of Some Thoracic Roentgen Signs and Their Significance

a) *air bronchogram sign*: visualization of air in intrapulmonary bronchi; visible only when alveoli are fluid-filled, as in pneumonia, pulmonary edema, pulmonary infarcts, etc.; rarely seen with atelectasis

b) *angel wing sign* (*"spinnaker sail sign"*): elevation of thymic lobes by pneumomediastinal air

c) *bare area sign*: with CT, fluid density posterior to the bare area of the liver is an indication of pleural effusion (helps DDX from subphrenic fluid)

d) *batwing edema* (*"butterfly edema"*): pattern of edema around hilar regions, commonly seen with renal disease but rarely present when edema is caused by CHF

e) *cannonball metastasis*: ill-defined, fluffy, oval or round calcific opacities unevenly distributed over lung fields in metastatic disease (with osteosarcoma as the primary malignancy)

f) *comet-tail sign*: in round atelectasis, curvilinear tail caused by compressed bronchi and vessels between mass and hilum

g) *continuous diaphragm sign*: if diaphragm margin is not obscured by mediastinal structures, it indicates pneumomediastinum

h) *deep sulcus sign*: diaphragmatic sulcus more clearly visible in supine patients in the presence of pneumothorax

i) *double lesion sign*: aids in ruling out bronchogenic carcinoma as cause of atelectasis; collapse of two or more pulmonary lobes or segments that do not share a common or anatomically close airway is usually not caused by a single lesion

j) *dumbbell tumor*: describes shape of erosions of adjacent pedicles and vertebral body caused by a neurofibroma (neurolemmoma, neurilemoma)

k) *eggshell calcification*: thin, distinct rim of calcification around an enlarged node (as seen in lymph nodes with silicosis or sarcoidosis)

l) *finger in glove pattern*: "V" pattern of mucoid impaction with bronchial plugging, characteristic of allergic bronchopulmonary aspergillosis

m) *forward "S" sign*: seen on lateral projection, sign of LLL collapse with marked posterior displacement of major fissure

n) *Garland's Triad*: enlarged hilar, azygos, and right paratracheal lymph nodes, seen in sarcoidosis

o) *mediastinal wedge*: wedge-shaped opacity seen with lower lobe atelectasis (PA projection; or with LLL—right oblique projection)

p) *meniscus sign*: within thoracic cavity, usually at the costophrenic angle, a meniscus pattern in water density differentiates pleural fluid from fibrosis; a sign of free pleural effusion

q) *1-2-3 sign*: lymphadenopathy of bilateral hilar and right paratracheal nodes, suggesting three round balls (see pawnbroker's sign), seen with sarcoidosis

r) *pawnbroker's sign*: bilateral hilar and right paratracheal lymphadenopathy suggests three balls, the symbol of a pawn shop; seen with sarcoidosis

s) *reverse "S" sign of Golden* with atelectasis of right upper lobe: caused by elevation of minor fissure in upper right lateral chest and neoplastic mass restricting its elevation in the medial chest; often indicates bronchogenic carcinoma, but has several other etiologies (see above, atelectasis **Differential considerations**)

t) *shaggy heart sign*: partially obscured border of cardiac shadow, seen in pneumoconioses, especially asbestosis

u) *silhouette sign*: loss of normally visible structural borders, caused by adjacent fluid accumulation or mass; seen with pneumonia

v) *snake-like esophageal filling defects*: indicates esophageal varices (lower esophagus)

w) *split-pleura sign* of empyema: empyema separates parietal and visceral pleura; easily apparent with CT

x) *Swiss cheese pattern (honeycombed pattern)*: indication of pulmonary fibrosis

y) *3 sign*: focal indentation of aorta seen with aortic coarctation

z) *tram-tracking sign*: perihilar peribronchial thickening seen en face; occurs with Kaposi sarcoma

REVIEW—STUDY QUESTIONS

1. What is "middle lobe syndrome"? What is its radiologic appearance?

2. What are radiologic indications of NHL, and in what patient populations is NHL most frequently seen? Describe its differing presentations in the different age cohorts.

3. What is empyema? *Empyema necessitatis*?

4. Name the four most frequent primary sources of metastasis to the pleura.

5. List five conditions associated with the AIDS complex.

6. Explain the different etiologies of transudative and exudative pleural effusion.

7. With what condition is the "tram-tracking sign" produced?

8. What is peripheral atelectasis? List five etiologies for peripheral atelectasis.

9. What is PCP, and in what patient population does it frequently occur?

10. List five radiologic signs of atelectasis. Which are direct signs, and which are indirect signs?

11. What is the significance of a "mediastinal wedge"? Describe its radiologic appearance. What is the optimal projection to demonstrate it?

12. Describe the radiologic signs of pneumothorax.

13. With what disease process is "round atelectasis" associated? Describe its radiologic appearance.

14. What is an "air bronchogram sign," and what is its significance?

15. What is the nature of a "localized fibrous tumor" of the pleura? What might its systemic symptoms be?

16. Name four types of pneumothorax and explain their etiologies.

17. Explain the significance of the "forward "S" sign," and the "reverse "S" sign of Golden": what structures create these appearances, and under what conditions?

18. What is ARDS?

19. What is the "silhouette sign"? What conditions create a positive silhouette sign?

20. What is central atelectasis? Name three of its etiologies.

D.   ABDOMEN: TECHNICAL CONSIDERATIONS

1.   Frontal Projections

a) Kidney, ureter, bladder (**KUB**)
- an AP scout film
- taken at 70 kVp
- demonstrates calcific stones in gallbladder, kidneys, ureters, etc.
- done upright or recumbent

b) Intravenous pyelogram (**IVP**)
- contrast study of kidneys, ureter, and bladder

c) PA abdomen
- for soft tissue detail; liver, gallbladder, spleen
- taken at 100 kVp or higher
- done upright or recumbent

2. Lateral Projections

    a) Lateral abdomen

- used for accurate location of lesions seen on frontal views
- gives visualization of pre-sacral space

E. ABDOMEN: NORMAL ANATOMY

1. **Retroperitoneal organs:** kidneys, ureters, adrenal glands, duodenum, ascending and descending colon, pancreas

2. **Right upper quadrant organs:** liver, gall bladder (in upright position, may move to right lower quadrant), upper portion of ascending colon, hepatic flexure of colon, transverse colon, right kidney and right adrenal gland

3. **Left upper quadrant organs:** spleen, pancreatic tail, stomach, transverse colon, splenic flexure of colon, descending colon, left kidney and left adrenal gland

4. **Right lower quadrant organs:** cecum, appendix, ascending colon, right ovary, right ureter

5. **Left lower quadrant organs:** descending colon, left ovary, left ureter midline abdominal structures: duodenum, pancreatic head and tail, small bowel, aorta

F. PELVIC CAVITY: NORMAL ANATOMY

1. **Right pelvic structures:** lower portion of the cecum, appendix, right ovary, right ureter

2. **Left pelvic structures:** sigmoid colon, left ovary, left ureter

3. **Midline pelvic structures:** uterus, prostate gland, bladder, sigmoid colon, rectum

G. MOBILITY OR STABILITY OF VISUALIZED MASSES

1. Respiration, peristaltic activity may move radiopacities

2. Gravity may cause shift of unattached masses when patient position is changed

3. Calculi in a fluid medium move with position change (e.g., gallbladder or renal stones)

    a) Respiration may cause apparent movement of abdominal lesions

- retroperitoneal calcifications usually do not move with respiration
- upper intraperitoneal calcifications may displace with respiration

    b) Effects of peristalsis

- ureter contractions move urinary calculi
- intraluminal concretions in intestinal tract may move
- may display contour of mass lesion within peritoneal cavity, as mass displaces bowel

H. ABDOMINAL LESIONS

1. **Pneumoperitoneum**

    a) **General considerations**

    - free air within peritoneal cavity visible on plain film
    - may indicate perforation within gastrointestinal tract
    - causes of pneumoperitoneum:
        1) most frequent cause: rupture of peptic ulcer (gastric or duodenal)
        2) perforation of carcinoma of the stomach
        3) ruptured colonic diverticulum
        4) traumatic rupture of intestine or stomach
        5) penetrating injury to abdominal wall
        6) blunt trauma that ruptures a hollow viscus
        7) downward dissection of pneumomediastinum (through parietal peritoneum into peritoneal cavity)
        8) peritoneal septic infection caused by gas-forming organisms
    - idiopathic spontaneous pneumoperitoneum: probably due to rupture of emphysematous gas cysts, perhaps from undiagnosed *"pneumatosis cystoides"*

    ☞ b) **Radiologic features**

    - best seen on AP, supine projection
    - *"air dome"* or *"football sign"*: gas outlines distended peritoneal cavity, with air-outlined falciform ligament suggesting a football seam
    - post-surgical air in peritoneal cavity:
        1) normal finding after abdominal surgery or laparoscopy
        2) visible for a week to 10 days
        3) occasionally visible up to 4 weeks

2. **Stomach Lesions**

    a) Iron or calcium pills

    - may be seen in stomach if taken just before films are made
    - uniform density, characteristic oval or disc shape

    ☞ b) Gastric ulcer

    - **General considerations**
        1) benign or malignant
        2) may cause incisure of stomach opposite the lesion
    - **Clinical findings**
        1) vary from mild dyspepsia to acute illness
        2) occult blood in stools

    3) frank blood in the nasogastric aspirate

- **Radiologic findings**
  1) visible on barium study, in profile as a niche or crater projecting **outside** the lumen
  2) *en face* appears as dense, round, sharply marginated barium pool
  3) *"Hampton's line"*: narrow lucent line across mouth of ulcer (caused by rim of edema at mouth of benign ulcer)
  4) broad-based ulcer that has burrowed under mucosa: *"collar button ulcer"* appearance (more common in colon in ulcerative colitis)
  5) ulcer causing incisure of the stomach: gives stomach an *"hourglass deformity"*

    c) Tumors

- **General considerations**
  1) lymphosarcoma: giant gastric mucosal folds (also may be caused by other pathologies, such as Ménétrier's disease)
  2) gastric leiomyoma: usually uncalcified mass, but possibly contains visible calcifications
  3) stomach hemangiomas (may contain phleboliths)
  4) duplication cyst: at upper lesser curvature of stomach (may contain milk of calcium)
  5) rare: calcified gastric malignancy (most often, adenocarcinoma) known as *"petrified stomach"*

- **Clinical findings**
  1) usually asymptomatic, unless ulcerated
  2) hemorrhage with ulceration
  3) sometimes: sense of "fullness," mild pain after large meal
  4) dysphagia if esophageal inlet is blocked
  5) possibly, eventual weight loss and weakness

- **Radiologic findings**
  1) round, circumscribed filling defect (barium studies)
  2) protrudes into lumen, or creates large exogastric mass, displacing stomach
  3) adenocarcinoma
     - possible ulceration, narrowing gastric air shadow
     - occasional homogeneous calcification, with discrete punctate or faint granular calcifications
     - may grow to huge proportions

4) leiomyoma
   • usually uncalcified, water density mass
   • occasionally streaky or flocculent calcification, projecting away from the gastric lumen

d) Bezoars
   • **General considerations**
      1) concretions of hair and/or fruit and vegetable fibers
      2) do not calcify
   • **Clinical features**
      1) usually asymptomatic
      2) may result in a sense of fullness, nausea, vomiting, pain, bleeding
      3) after gastrectomy: may cause small bowel obstruction
   • **Radiologic features**
      1) seen as densities in stomach only if coated by opaque material (e.g., bismuth)

  e) Pyloric stenosis
   • **General considerations**
      1) may be congenital or acquired
   • **Clinical features**
      1) in infants: projectile vomiting, visible gastric peristalsis (crossing epigastrium from left to right), dehydration, failure to thrive
   • **Radiologic features**
      1) *"umbrella defect"* of the bulb or *"cloverleaf deformity"*
      2) caused by scar tissue deforming mucosal folds (acquired)

3. Small Intestine Lesions

   a) Iron or calcium pills seen anywhere in small bowel
   • characteristic, recognizable shapes: disc or oval
   • homogeneous density

  b) Ileus
   • **General considerations**
      1) two types: mechanical or adynamic
      2) mechanical ileus
         • gross distention caused by mechanical obstruction of bowel by intraluminal or extraluminal pathology
         • most common pathology causing mechanical ileus: neoplasm (carcinoma) or inflammatory disease
         • also caused by volvulus, Crohn's disease, ulcerative colitis

3) adynamic ileus (paralytic ileus)
- decreased tone and loss of propulsion
- gas and fluid accumulations, general distention
- focal inflammations: may cause local ileus
  a. appendicitis, cholecystitis, pancreatitis
- severe trauma to abdomen or spine
  a. occult visceral injury leads to ileus
  b. occult spinal fracture causes ileus

- **Clinical features**
  1) auscultation: high-pitched, tinkling sounds rather than normal bowel tones

- **Radiologic features**
  1) excessive gas distends bowel throughout abdomen ("*stepladder pattern*" with small bowel ileus)

c) Tumors
- **General considerations**
  1) most common tumors in ileum: carcinoid tumors
  2) hemangiomas: most common in distal jejunum and ileum but may occur anywhere in small bowel
  3) enteroliths: form proximal to stenosis, or in diverticula; found in distal small bowel, where pH is more alkaline
  4) lipoma: soft, fatty tumor

- **Clinical features**
  1) carcinoid syndrome
     - due to production of serotonin by malignant ectopic endocrine cells
     - cutaneous flushes, cyanosis, abdominal cramps, diarrhea
     - may cause valvular heart disease, asthma, arthropathy
  2) hemangioma
     - usually asymptomatic, no restricting peristalsis
     - may cause intussusception, become symptomatic
  3) enteroliths: usually asymptomatic
  4) lipoma usually asymptomatic

- **Radiologic features**
  1) carcinoid
     - may develop detectable calcification
     - on plain film: small, well-defined

spheres, slightly larger than phleboliths
- rarely: develop flecks and small arcuate lines of calcification
- fixed calcifications, not moving with peristalsis
- ulcerated tumor: *"bull's eye appearance"* (especially with metastatic lesions from malignant melanoma, breast carcinoma, or Kaposi sarcoma)

2) hemangioma
- about 5% contain phleboliths
- move with peristalsis, may change location in sequential contrast films

3) enteroliths
- various shapes, usually multiple, fairly uniform size
- thin calcified rim, more lucent center
- move freely with peristalsis

4) lipoma
- seen as a fat density on KUB
- may show *"squeeze sign"*: altered shape with peristalsis
- best seen on post-evacuation barium film

5) primary carcinoma and leiomyoma of small bowel
- generally do not calcify
- seen as mass lesion on contrast film
- adenocarcinoma of small bowel may calcify

6) after diagnostic barium filling (normal bowel) may see
- *"snowflake appearance"*: small barium flecks retained by mucosal folds in jejunum
- visible on plain film for a short time, eventually disappear

d) Crohn's disease (regional enteritis)
- **General considerations**
  1) most common in distal ileum, proximal colon
  2) may occur in any part of GI tract
  3) peak incidence: between ages 14 and 24 years
  4) familial tendency noted
  5) no gender predilection
- **Clinical features**
  1) usually displays one of four common patterns of regional enteritis
     - inflammatory
     - obstructive (stenosing)

- combined inflammation and obstruction
- abdominal fistulas and abscesses
2) may cause fistulas between organs
- **Radiologic features**
  1) diagnosed via barium studies
  2) usually shows barium reflux into terminal ileum
  3) irregular, nodular, stiff thickening of ileum wall
  4) narrowed ileal lumen
  5) stenosing type: may have rigid, cast-like terminal ileum ("*String sign of Kantor*")
  6) "*skip lesions*": segments full of barium alternate with empty segments
  7) "*cobblestone appearance*" of lumen, caused by "pseudopolyp" islands of hyperplastic mucosa (seen in other inflammatory GI tract diseases also, e.g., ulcerative colitis)

☞   **e)** Celiac disease (sprue)
- **General considerations**
  1) a malabsorption syndrome
  2) seen in both children and adults
  3) inability to tolerate/absorb gluten
- **Clinical features**
  1) may cause steatorrhea
  2) may be asymptomatic
- **Radiologic features**
  1) demonstrated by barium studies
  2) dilated lumen: most severe in distal jejunum
  3) abnormal mucosal folds: thinned, thickened, or absent
  4) absent folds: "*moulage sign*": a smooth-sided tube with flocculated barium due to excessive secretion
  5) hypersecretion of fluid in lumen: flocculated barium
  6) transient intussusception

☞   **f)** Ascites
- **General considerations**
  1) accumulations of free fluid in the peritoneal cavity
  2) etiologies: liver disease, heart failure, nephrotic syndrome, hypoalbuminemia, constrictive pericarditis, abdominal carcinoma, abdominal TB, hypothyroidism, pancreatitis
- **Clinical features**
  1) small amounts asymptomatic
  2) large amounts: abdominal discomfort, dyspnea

3) shifting dullness on abdominal percussion

4) other symptoms reflect etiology

- **Radiologic features**

    1) "*floating small intestines*": intestines float high in abdomen

    2) hazy, "*ground glass appearance*" to overall abdomen caused by increased water density

    3) "*doggy ears sign*": hazy fluid accumulation in lesser pelvis, around and behind bladder (seen on AP projection)

☞   **g)** Intussusception

- **General considerations**

    1) telescoping of the bowel

    2) in any area of bowel

    3) different causes, e.g., celiac disease

- **Clinical features**

    1) transient may be asymptomatic

    2) may cause general abdominal discomfort

- **Radiologic features**

    1) "*coiled spring appearance*" on barium studies (in some cases)

☞   **h)** Bowel obstructions

- **General considerations**

    1) cause obstructive ileus of varying severity

    2) normal small bowel lumen diameter: 3 cm

    3) duodenal atresia or annular pancreas: may cause near or complete bowel obstruction

    4) newborns: calcified meconium may obstruct bowel; cause perforation, peritonitis (*meconium ileus* and *meconium peritonitis*)

    5) lymphosarcoma in small bowel causes massive dilation

- **Clinical features**

    1) high-pitched, tinkling sounds auscultated

    2) abdominal discomfort with massive dilation, persistent obstruction

- **Radiologic features**

    1) near or complete obstruction of proximal bowel: excessive air trapped in stomach and duodenum ("*double bubble sign*")

    2) "*stacked coin appearance*": gas-filled, distended (> 3 cm) valvulae conniventes

    3) "*step-ladder appearance*": gas-filled bowel traversing abdomen

4) *"aneurysmal dilatation"*: huge dilation of the bowel seen with lymphosarcoma

4. Large Intestine Lesions

a) Colon diverticula

- **General considerations**
  1) most common in sigmoid, descending colons
  2) usually multiple
  3) rare < age 40 years; present in almost 100% of population > age 90 years
  4) complicated by inflammation: result in diverticulitis

- **Clinical features**
  1) usually asymptomatic
  2) may manifest with extensive rectal bleeding
  3) may become inflamed (diverticulitis): cause perforation, abscess, peritonitis, obstruction, fistula formation

- **Radiologic features**
  1) contrast-filled niches or craters on barium studies
  2) may hold barium for days to weeks after study
  3) when ruptured: upright abdominal or chest films will show free air in peritoneal cavity (pneumoperitoneum)

b) Tumors

- **General considerations**
  1) adenocarcinoma
     - slow-growing, common tumor in colon wall
     - most frequently in cecum or rectum
     - most common in elderly population
     - calcified adenocarcinoma shows predilection for patients < 40 years old
  2) hemangioma in colon or rectum

- **Clinical features**
  1) adenocarcinoma
     - may be palpable if large enough
     - usually asymptomatic in ascending colon
     - in descending colon: alternating constipation/diarrhea, pain, obstruction more likely
     - anywhere: may cause occult bleeding, fatigue, severe anemia
  2) hemangioma usually asymptomatic

- **Radiologic features**
  1) calcified adenocarcinoma
     - mottled, speckled, or granular pattern
     - rarely develop peritoneal calcifications in metastases from these tumors
     - carcinoma creates polypoid mass (often in cecum)
     - may create "*apple core appearance*": circumferential stricture caused by infiltration of colonic wall
     - rectal carcinoma may ossify, extend aggressively into pelvic muscles
  2) "*shouldering defect*": barium column terminates abruptly with overhanging edges at distal border of lesion
     - anywhere in GI tract
     - sign of probable malignant lesion
  3) hemangioma: may develop phleboliths

☞ **c)** Ulcerative colitis
- **General considerations**
  1) chronic inflammatory and ulcerative condition of colonic mucosa
- **Clinical features**
  1) crampy abdominal pain
  2) bloody diarrhea
- **Radiologic features**
  1) when complicated by toxicity:
     - paralyzed segment of colon: "*toxic dilation*," or "*acute toxic megacolon*"
     - transverse colon dilated to > 6 cm
  2) "*lead pipe colon*"
     - contracted, shortened colon, without haustrations
     - seen in late stages of disease

☞ **d)** Polyps
- **General considerations**
  1) usually found in sigmoid colon or rectum
  2) sessile or pedunculated
  3) smooth or tubular polyps usually benign
  4) may grow, develop villae: increased risk of malignant degeneration
  5) "*villous adenoma*": polyp with > 80% of glands villous
  6) about 35% of villous adenomas undergo malignant degeneration
- **Clinical features**
  1) usually asymptomatic

2) most frequent complaint: rectal bleeding

3) unusually large polyp: cramps, abdominal pain, obstruction

4) rarely: may prolapse through the anus

5) watery diarrhea may indicate malignant degeneration of villous adenoma

- **Radiologic features**

1) rounded filling defects in barium exam

2) *"frondlike rectal filling defect"*: brush-like border of villous adenoma

☞ e) Volvulus

- **General considerations**

1) twisted bowel

- **Clinical features**

1) gradually increasing constipation, lower abdominal cramping

2) eventual complete obstipation, abdominal distention

- **Radiologic features**

1) *"coffee bean sign"*: adjacent parallel lucencies in twisted bowel loops separated by intestinal walls (seen in sigmoid volvulus)

2) twisted, tapered segment of bowel may show as *"bird's beak* or *crow's beak deformity"*

5. **Lesions in the Appendix**

a) Appendicitis

- **General considerations**

1) appendix may become inflamed, infected

2) appendix may abscess

- **Clinical features**

1) signs vary

2) abdominal pain, usually in right lower quadrant

3) pain may refer to umbilical region or right upper quadrant

4) fever, nausea, vomiting

5) rebound tenderness (sharper pain as palpation pressure is released) at McBurney's point (midway between ASIS and umbilicus)

6) with rupture: clinical findings of peritonitis and adynamic ileus

☞ - **Radiologic features**

1) during barium studies, the normal appendix may not fill, or may remain filled for several days (or longer) after the study

2) *"sentinel loop of appendicitis"*: localized dilated bowel loop around any inflamed area (also seen with

acute pancreatitis and acute cholecystitis)

3) "*appendicolith*": visible concretions present in about 10% of adult appendicitis cases and about 25% of pediatric cases; round or ovoid calcium density shadow, sometimes laminated

4) with severe inflammation: possibly see fluid levels in cecum (upright or *left* lateral decubitus views)

5) with acute appendiceal abscess:
   - "*adynamic ileus*" (massive amounts of gas in bowel)
   - right lower quadrant poorly defined
   - soft tissue mass with normal gas shadows notably absent, but small flocculent gas lucencies within the mass itself
   - possible fecalith

6) appendiceal stump defect: after appendectomy, invaginated stump appears similar to a polyp at the tip of the cecum

b) Tumors or tumorlike processes

☞
- **General considerations**
  1) carcinoid tumors: anywhere within the GI tract, but most frequently in the appendix
  2) other neoplasms found in the appendix: mucoceles (benign or malignant mucoid papillary adenocarcinoma)
  3) very rarely, a colonic type adenocarcinoma

- **Clinical features**
  1) appendiceal carcinoids: produce systemic effects (cutaneous flushes, cyanosis, abdominal cramps, diarrhea)
  2) malignant mucocele: may rupture, causing "*pseudomyxoma peritonaei*" (gelatinous masses on the peritoneal surface, leading to peritonitis, with thickening and fibrosis)

☞
- **Radiologic features**
  1) appendiceal tumors: mobile, round/ ovoid soft-tissue density in right lower quadrant (barium study will show mass attached to cecum, moving with cecum)
  2) mass may laterally or medially displace the cecum
  3) mucoceles: commonly with intramural calcific densities
  4) appendix may be blocked, unable to fill with barium

5) mass may cause a smooth pressure defect in cecal mucosal folds

6) appendiceal carcinoids: tend to be small, not visible on x-ray

6. **Urinary Tract Lesions**

   a) Plain film studies detect:
   - calcific stones
   - abnormal size, shape or number of kidneys
   - abnormal size or shape of bladder shadow

   b) IVP detects filling defects (intrinsic or extrinsic obstruction)

    c) Normal anatomy
   - kidneys: bean-shaped, lie between upper border of T11 and lower border of L3
   - upper pole of kidney tilts medially, axis follows psoas muscle
   - right kidney normally about 2 cm lower than left; both slightly mobile
   - normal sizes: right 13.8 cm; left 14.2 cm
   - difference in size between left and right kidney > 1.5 cm: requires further investigation
   - normal physiologic narrowing of ureters: at ureteropelvic junction, ureterovesical junction, and bifurcation of iliac vessels
   - normal bladder: smooth-walled; rounded or oval

   d) Anomalies
   - single kidney
   - third kidney
   - hypoplastic kidney
   - horseshoe kidney (lower poles fused across midline)
   - prolapsed kidney
   - duplicate renal pelvis and ureter
   - ureterocele (dilatation of ureter proximal to bladder orifice)

   e) Hydronephrosis
   - **General considerations**
     1) dilatation of renal pelvis and calyces, or ureters
     2) caused by obstruction or nonobstructive conditions, e.g., diabetes insipidus, urinary tract infection, chronic constipation
   - **Clinical features**
     1) chronic: asymptomatic, or intermittent dull, aching flank pain
     2) acute: colicky pain (especially in pediatric cases), possibly palpable enlarged kidney mass
   - **Radiologic features**
     1) altered contours, enlarged renal pelvis
     2) enlarged and "clubbed" calyces

3) *"crescent sign"*: accumulated radiopaque dye in damaged parenchyma around dilated calyces

☞ **f)** Nephrocalcinosis
- **General considerations**
  1) parenchymal calcium deposits with:
     - primary hyperparathyroidism
     - hypercalciuria of any etiology
     - hyperchloremic acidosis
     - hypervitaminosis D
     - sarcoidosis
     - milk-alkali syndrome
  2) also with normal calcium levels but damaged renal tissue:
     - chronic pyelonephritis
     - glomerulonephritis
     - lower nephron nephrosis
- **Clinical features**
  1) disturbed renal function may cause polyuria, nocturia, polydipsia
  2) often asymptomatic
- **Radiologic features**
  1) faint, milky, granulations
  2) may develop stippled calcifications of renal cortex and papilla
  3) often, calcifications not visible on plain film

☞ **g)** Renal or ureteric calculi
- **General considerations**
  1) most have enough calcium to be seen on plain film
  2) few pure; most crystalline compounds
  3) most common: calcium phosphate, calcium oxalate, magnesium ammonium phosphate
  4) formation promoted by: urinary stasis, infection
  5) often idiopathic
  6) other factors: metabolic disorders (hypercalcemic conditions, e.g., hyperparathyroidism)
- **Clinical features**
  1) asymptomatic until large enough to cause obstruction, or when passing through ureters
  2) create agonizing ureteral colic
- **Radiologic features**
  1) may fill renal pelvis and calyces like a cast: *"staghorn calculus"*
  2) calcific stones in ureter, usually 1–3 mm, round or oval
  3) those without calcium: located by IVP, seen as filling defects
  4) stones most commonly lodge at ureterovesical junction

h) Infections
- **General considerations**
  1) acute or chronic pyelonephritis
  2) renal abscess
  3) perirenal abscess
  4) xanthogranulomatous pyelonephritis
  5) gestational pyelitis
- **Clinical features**
  1) systemic signs: fever, malaise
  2) dull flank pain
  3) sometimes, rapid or gradual loss of kidney function
  4) xanthogranulomatous pyelonephritis: a severe, chronic process
     - recurrent episodes of low fever
     - fatigue
     - dysuria, frequency
     - flank pain
     - sometimes palpable, fixed, renal mass (usually unilateral, but may present with pyelonephritis in contralateral kidney)

- **Radiologic features**
  1) acute pyelonephritis
     - plain film may show enlarged kidney
  2) emphysematous pyelonephritis: gas in and around the kidney
  3) small abscess: no plain film sign
  4) large renal or perirenal abscess: sometimes visible renal enlargement or altered contour, blurred perirenal fat pad, lack of renal movement with respiration, blurred psoas shadow, possible scoliosis (concave to affected side), and displaced kidney and/or ureter
  5) chronic (atrophic) pyelonephritis
     - visible renal atrophy or size reduction
     - *"clubbed calyces"* (often bilaterally symmetric)
  6) xanthogranulomatous pyelonephritis
     - usually unilateral, without parenchymal calcification
     - IVP may show dilated and blunted calyces, decreased cortical thickness, and deformed ureter

i) Necrotic conditions
- **General considerations**
  1) renal papillary necrosis
     - may be iatrogenic (from prolonged phenacetin use)
  2) bilateral renal cortical necrosis
- **Clinical features**
  1) papillary necrosis

- female predilection
- usually bilateral
- may create a concretion from sloughed necrotic tissue
- often, pyuria
- hematuria: common if sickle-cell disease is involved

2) cortical necrosis
- bilateral, symmetric
- spares the medullary kidney and a thin subcapsular cortical rim
- causes fatal acute renal failure
- associated with severe trauma, infection, incompatible blood transfusion, pregnancy

 • **Radiologic features**
1) papillary necrosis
- medullary cavities within papilla
- sloughs entire papilla, leaving a cavity extending into adjacent pyramid
- *"ring shadow"*: triangular lucencies with dense opaque border caused by necrotic papilla within the calyx
- dense concretion
- calcific shell with lucent center

2) cortical necrosis
- kidneys first enlarge, then shrink
- within about 2 months: develop a faint shell-like calcified rim around the cortical periphery (may require CT to demonstrate this)
- renal contour sometimes altered

j) Inflammatory conditions, chronic low-grade infections
- **General considerations**
1) renal tuberculosis
2) pyeloureteritis cystica
3) pyelitis cystica
4) ureteritis cystica
- **Clinical features**
1) parenchymal cavitation and destruction
2) may eventually lead to obstruction and complete kidney destruction
3) *"putty kidney"*: normal tissue replaced with caseous material and calcium
4) markedly shrunken kidney
5) with obstructed ureter: hydronephrosis
- **Radiologic features**
1) renal tuberculosis
- cloudy flocculent calcifications

throughout a progressively shrinking kidney

- IVP shows ulcerative papillary lesions in the calyx; loss of papilla and formation of an irregular, ragged cavity; sometimes local constriction caused by fibrosis
- ureters show strictures or local nodules
- eventually an unusually straight ureter ("*pipe stem ureter*") from renal pelvis to pelvic brim

k) Cystic diseases of the kidney
- **General considerations**
  1) dysplasias
  2) polycystic disease
  3) cortical cysts
  4) medullary cysts
  5) intrarenal or extraparenchymal renal cysts
- **Clinical features**
  1) remain asymptomatic for years
  2) with enlarged cysts: lumbar pain, hematuria, infection, colic, loss of renal function

- **Radiologic features**
  1) may see enlarged kidneys (asymmetric)
  2) depending on the specific condition
     - elongated infundibula and calyces
     - irregular calyx enlargement, with multiple crescent-shaped contours
     - indistinct kidney on plain film
  3) smooth, local enlargement within the kidney
  4) sometimes: cyst wall rimmed with a thin shell of calcium
  5) cyst may become much larger than kidney
  6) renal angiogram may have a "*claw sign*": triangular claw-like projections of renal parenchyma (indicative of cyst rather than neoplasm)
  7) medullary cysts
     - small, multiple renal calculi sometimes visible on plain film in fanlike pattern clusters in the renal pyramids
     - tubules dilated
  8) hydatid cysts often calcify; may produce clusters of "*daughter cysts*"

l) Vascular abnormalities
- **General considerations**
  1) renal artery aneurysm
  2) polyarteritis nodosa

        3) renal artery occlusion

        4) renal vein thrombosis

        5) renovascular hypertension

- **Clinical features**
  1) may result in aneurysm rupture, thrombosis, renal infarction (causing pain and hematuria), loss of kidney function
  2) thrombosis: caused by extrinsic pressure of tumors, or from ileocolitis (chief cause in pediatric patients)
  3) renovascular hypertension caused by renal artery stenosis
     - hypertension
     - upper abdominal bruit
     - flank pain

- **Radiologic features**
  1) 25–30% of renal artery aneurysms: ring-like calcification, visible on plain film
  2) renal angiography: required to display multiple microaneurysms of polyarteritis nodosa
  3) renal artery occlusion
     - IVP to show a nonfunctioning kidney
     - arteriography used for definitive diagnosis
  4) renovascular hypertension
     - diagnosed via urogram
     - shows change of renal size, delayed or decreased volume of excreted contrast medium, vascular indentations on upper ureter and/or renal pelvis
     - later films show hyperconcentration, areas of local atrophy, decreased concentration in parenchyma

m) Renal neoplasms

- **General considerations**
  1) benign renal tumors: adenoma, fibroma, lipoma, leiomyoma, hemangioma, or hamartoma
  2) pseudotumor: renal hypertrophy or hyperplasia
  3) renal cysts
  4) malignant tumors: adenocarcinoma or hypernephroma (Grawitz tumor, or renal cell carcinoma), embryoma or Wilms' tumor, renal pelvis carcinoma, sarcoma, malignant lymphoma

- **Clinical features**
  1) may be asymptomatic until enlarged

2) may cause signs of infection (pain, hematuria)

3) may impair renal function

4) may cause noticeable tissue or gritty material in urine (along with hematuria)

5) may create a palpable abdominal mass

- **Radiologic features**

    1) angiomyolipoma (hamartoma)
        - solitary or multiple masses
        - may enlarge the kidney, distort the renal pelvis and calyces
        - angiography: multiple microaneurysms of interlobar and interlobular arteries

    2) lipomas (fibrolipomatosis)
        - may show fatty deposition similar to one or more cysts

    3) adenocarcinoma
        - seen via excretory urography as kidney enlargement
        - indistinct mass contiguous with the kidney
        - central, eccentric or peripheral curvilinear or amorphous calcifications
        - renal pelvis may be compressed, displaced, or invaded
        - calyx may be elongated, compressed, separated or amputated

    4) renal cell carcinoma (Grawitz tumor, hypernephroma, adenocarcinoma of the kidney)
        - local or general kidney enlargement (varies with size of tumor)
        - perirenal fat planes preserved but sometimes lobulated, distorted and irregular
        - visible calcifications in 15% of cases: scattered, irregular calcification, or curvilinear
        - possible renal axis rotation caused by large medially-placed mass in upper or lower pole
        - tumors enlarge significantly: may displace kidney or nearby organs

    5) Wilms' tumor
        - on scout film: may be huge mass displacing adjacent structures
        - rarely with calcifications

    6) squamous metaplasia of renal pelvis
        - sometimes large, laminated masses
        - sometimes irregular plaques with linear striations

- sometimes roughened, wrinkled renal pelvis
    7) malignant lymphoma or leukemia
        - enlarge the kidneys, usually bilaterally
        - show no dilatation or obstructions
        - may involve single or multiple nodules

n) Ureteric neoplasms
- **General considerations**
    1) most common in distal third of ureters
    2) benign tumors: papilloma, hemangioma, epithelial carcinoma
- **Clinical features**
    1) epithelial carcinoma in renal pelvis: may seed proximal ureter
    2) ureteric masses usually distal
    3) cause hydronephrosis, other signs of ureter obstruction
- **Radiologic features**
    1) usually in lower one-third of ureter
    2) contrast may outline an intraluminal mass
    3) may be signs of ureteral obstruction
        - carcinoma may narrow lumen locally
        - may cause tip of catheter to coil when it abuts the mass

o) Bladder anomalies
- **General considerations**
    1) bladder exstrophy
    2) bladder duplication
    3) congenital bladder enlargement
    4) extraperitoneal herniations
- **Clinical features**
    1) bladder exstrophy: may obstruct ureters
    2) extraperitoneal bladder herniations: associated with clinical inguinal hernia

- **Radiologic features**
    1) bladder exstrophy: wide separation at symphysis pubis (diastasis is approximately the width of the sacrum)
    2) extraperitoneal herniation: *"bladder ears"*: lateral protrusions through internal inguinal ring that disappear when bladder is filled completely

p) Bladder calculi (vesicle calculi)
- **General considerations:** usually caused by obstruction and infection
- **Clinical features**
    1) usually asymptomatic

       2) when caused by infection: clinical signs of infection are present

 • **Radiologic features**

    1) may be calcified and visible on plain film

    2) may be noncalcific, not visible without contrast medium (air or contrast cystography)

    3) single or multiple midline concretions

    4) calcific stones: usually very dense, laminated, may be faceted

    5) *"jackstone calculus"*: large calculus with irregular, serrated margins

q) Bladder infections

• **General considerations**

    1) acute cystitis

    2) chronic cystitis

    3) emphysematous cystitis

       • 50% of cases in diabetics

       • develops gas in the bladder wall

    4) *"Schistosomiasis"*: caused by blood flukes

• **Clinical features**

    1) urinary urgency

    2) pain

    3) hematuria

 • **Radiologic features**

    1) diagnostic imaging via cystography

    2) bladder wall may be serrated

    3) contraction greatest at the dome (*"Christmas tree bladder"*)

    4) emphysematous cystitis

       • gas in the vesicle wall (transient)

       • shows on film as a lucent ring outlining the bladder wall

       • sometimes gas within the bladder

    5) *"schistosomiasis"*

       • thickened, ulcerated wall and papillomas

       • wall may calcify with chronic infection

          a. empty bladder: thin, parallel densities

          b. contrast-filled bladder: lamination, with a thin lucent line between the medium and the submucosal calcification

          d. calculi form in bladder, ureters, and kidneys

          e. distal ureter walls may calcify

 r) Bladder obstruction

• **General considerations**

    1) usually caused by prostatic enlargement (benign prostatic hypertrophy, or prostatic carcinoma)

      2)   other causes: acquired urethral stenosis, urethral valves, cord bladder (neurogenic)

- **Clinical features**
  1) gradually reduced flow from bladder
  2) reflux into ureters
  3) abdominal distention and discomfort
  4) hydronephrosis, and eventual total inability to void
- **Radiologic features** (via cystography)
  1) with benign prostatic hypertrophy
     - bladder floor elevation
     - "*j-shaped*" (or "*hockey-stick*", or "*fish-hook*") appearance of distal ureters
  2) with obstruction of any origin
     - bladder wall hypertrophy: enough to cause a visible soft-tissue shadow
     - interlacing bands of hypertrophied muscle: form "trabeculae" with intervening cellules or even deeper diverticula
     - medium refluxes into ureters
     - bladder enlarges, retains increasing amounts of urine
     - may show on scout film as large, soft-tissue mass
  3) with neurogenic bladder: bladder wall thin and smooth

s) Bladder diverticulum

- **General considerations**
  1) single or multiple localized mucosal herniations
  2) some congenital, some caused by chronic obstruction
- **Clinical features**
  1) reflect etiology: congenital silent
  2) acquired show clinical signs of obstruction or infection
- **Radiologic features**
  1) rounded calcific density, similar to phlebolith but outside normal bladder margin
  2) calculus in neck of diverticulum: "*dumbbell calculus*"
  3) very large diverticulum: may create mass shadow on plain film, clearly outlined by contrast medium on IVP

t) Bladder tumors

- **General considerations**
  1) usually in the trigone region
  2) usually benign papilloma
  3) bladder carcinoma: primary, or

direct extension from prostate, rectum, or uterus
- **Clinical features**
  1) create features of ureteric obstruction: gradual loss of function, reflux into ureters, hydronephrosis and eventual total inability to void
  2) may see hematuria
- **Radiologic features**
  1) cystography: small tumors visible as filling defects in trigone region
  2) carcinoma: usually at base of bladder
  3) rhabdomyosarcoma
     - ureters laterally displaced
     - lobulated filling defect in bladder
     - may send nodules into urethra: create cone of dilatation

u) Bladder trauma
- **General considerations**
  1) rupture (intraperitoneal or extraperitoneal)
  2) perivesical hematoma
- **Radiologic features**
  1) cystography: contrast material extravasated into peritoneal cavity
  2) extraperitoneal rupture: extravasated contrast outlines tissue planes of pelvic floor

v) Prostatic calculi
- clinically asymptomatic
- radiologic features
  1) small, mottled densities
  2) clustered above symphysis pubis

REVIEW—STUDY QUESTIONS

1. What are bezoars? What are their clinical symptoms?
2. What causes the "collar button appearance" in an ulcer?
3. What is celiac disease? Give five of its radiologic signs.
4. What is a "pipe stem ureter" and with what pathology is it associated?
5. What is intussusception? What are its radiologic features?
6. Describe the differing radiologic appearances of acute, chronic, and xanthogranulomatous pyelonephritis.
7. What causes the "bull's eye appearance" of some carcinoids?
8. What is a "petrified stomach"?
9. Explain why or how a bladder infection creates the appearance of a "Christmas tree bladder" on a contrast study or IVP.
10. What is the "string sign of Kantor," and with what condition is it associated?
11. What are the symptoms of carcinoids?

12. What causes aneurysmal dilatation of the small bowel?

13. What is a villous adenoma? Where does it most often occur? What is its radiologic appearance?

14. What causes a mass with an "apple core" appearance?

15. What is Hampton's line and when is it visible?

16. What is the significance of a "shouldering defect"?

17. What is "lead pipe colon" and with what condition is it associated?

18. Describe the four common clinical patterns seen in patients with Crohn's disease.

19. What is "staghorn calculus"?

20. Name at least three radiologic indications of gastric tumors.

7. **Gallbladder**

   a) Normal location
   - on recumbent films: upper right quadrant
   - on upright films: may descend into mid-abdomen or upper pelvic basin

   b) Cholelithiasis
   - **General considerations**
     1) stones of cholesterol salts (radiolucent)
     2) stones of bilirubin pigments with calcium carbonate (about 10% of all stones)
     3) "milk of calcium" or limy bile: with cystic duct obstruction
   - **Clinical features**
     1) most frequent in elderly and obese
     2) female predilection, especially gravid or multiparous women
     3) increased incidence with chronic hemolytic anemias, sickle cell anemia
     4) variable presentation
        - often asymptomatic
        - duct obstruction with colicky pain (epigastric, right upper quadrant, or referred to right inferior scapula)
     5) pain: constant with periodic peaks
     6) nausea, vomiting
     7) if stone obstructs biliary or pancreatic ducts: pain, jaundice, pancreatitis, infection
     8) pass through cystic duct into small intestine: may obstruct ileocecal valve, cause gallstone ileus
   - **Radiologic features**
     1) about 10% calcified; visible on plain film

    2) *"Mercedes Benz sign"* (or *"crow-foot sign"*): gas pockets in fissures in a gallstone

    3) triad of findings typical of *"gallstone ileus"* caused by cholelithiasis:
- *"stepladder appearance"* of small bowel obstruction
- gallstones found in small bowel
- air seen in the biliary tree

    4) varied appearance of stones
- often concentrically laminated, with alternating opacity and lucency
- may have mottled matrix
- rarely an amorphous, spiculated calcification: stone calcified on only one surface (usually in the cystic duct)

    5) stones in gallbladder move with position changes and over time

    6) stones in cystic duct are fixed

c) *"Porcelain gallbladder"*
- **General considerations**
  1) calcified wall, vulnerable to fracture
  2) may predispose to carcinoma
- **Clinical features**
  1) involves obstructed cystic duct
  2) sometimes caused by chronic inflammation, hemorrhage
  3) usually between ages 40–70 years
  4) clear female predilection (5:1)
  5) despite its effects, usually asymptomatic
- **Radiologic features**
  1) pear-shaped or ovoid aggregation of calcium plaques or flakes in right upper quadrant (or lower in right abdomen)
  2) cystic duct may be visible: opaque tube superomedial to gallbladder
  3) possible double border of calcium: both mucosa and muscularis calcify
  4) shape conformed to *"Phrygian cap"* or any deformation of the gallbladder

d) Gallbladder carcinoma
- *General considerations*: fifth most common gastrointestinal malignancy in females, following colon, pancreas, stomach, and esophagus
- **Clinical features**
  1) invasive, aggressive tumors
  2) patients have low five-year survival rate
  3) usually asymptomatic until advanced
- **Radiologic features**
  1) usually undetectable on plain film
  2) may calcify—usually with punctate pattern

e) Cholecystitis

- **General considerations**
  1) usually accompanies obstructed duct
  2) *"emphysematous cholecystitis"*: usually caused by *Clostridium welchii* or *Escherichia coli*
- **Clinical features**
  1) infection: pain, nausea, vomiting, fever
  2) *"emphysematous cholecystitis"*: associated with uncontrolled diabetes
  3) gas in gallbladder or biliary ducts also caused by fistula from GI tract (most often duodenum); sometimes spontaneous; sometimes caused by ulceration of a gallstone into duodenum, or perforating duodenal ulcer
- **Radiologic features**
  1) *"emphysematous cholecystitis"*
     - may have gas within gallbladder (visible on plain film)
     - gas in the gallbladder wall (rim of bubbles or lucent streaks parallel to the gallbladder lumen) or adjacent tissues
     - sometimes see a fluid level on upright films
     - late in process, gas in ducts
  2) gas in biliary duct: *"Y"*-shaped lucency in the right upper quadrant

8. Liver

a) Normal location: upper right quadrant

b) Normal size:
- upper margin defined by right hemidiaphragm
- may cross midline, with left lobe slightly to left of spine
- in thin person, liver may be vertically oriented: inferior margin may extend almost to the level of the iliac crest

      c) Hepatic infections

- **General considerations**
  1) granulomatous infection (TB or histoplasmosis)
  2) usually multiple lesions, very rarely a solitary lesion
- **Clinical features**
  1) fever, malaise
  2) very little jaundice
  3) only slight hepatomegaly
- **Radiologic features**
  1) histoplasmosis: multiple, well-defined calcifications (about the size of a

match head) in the liver (also in lungs and spleen)

2) TB: small round hepatic calcifications
   - homogeneously dense or laminated or mottled
   - quite small, or up to 1 cm diameter
   - may have shaggy borders

3) *Brucellosis suis*: multiple, 1–2 cm diameter, round calcifications in liver and spleen

4) *Armillifer armillatus* (parasite from West Africa and Philippines): pathognomonic *"C-shaped"* calcifications and calcific *"dash marks"* in the liver

d) Hepatic malignancies
- **General considerations**
  1) metastatic or (rarely) primary
  2) solitary lesions more often than multiple
  3) metastatic tumors from ovary and colon most often, sometimes from pancreas, breast, melanoma or mesothelioma
  4) primary hepatocellular carcinoma, cholangiocarcinoma or mixed malignant tumor
- **Clinical features**
  1) abdominal pain
  2) weight loss
  3) palpable right upper quadrant mass
  4) sometimes fever
  5) if the tumor ruptures or hemorrhages: acute abdomen
  6) if ducts are blocked: jaundice
- **Radiologic features**
  1) metastatic ovarian and colon carcinomas
     - calcify in the liver
     - calcifications faint, amorphous masses with punctate or stippled patterns
     - may be so close together the liver appears granular
     - with colonic metastasis, calcification may occur only in the liver
     - ovarian metastases almost always with simultaneous calcifications in the peritoneum or in the primary tumor
  2) most common primary lesion
     - mixed malignant tumor
     - slow-growing, calcified globular mass

- coarse, dense, punctate calcification (single or multiple)

e) Benign hepatic tumors or cysts
- **General considerations**
  1) benign tumors: most often, cavernous hemangioma, rarely calcify
  2) hepatic cysts: most often hydatid disease (caused by a parasitic larva)
  3) noninflammatory cysts rarely calcify
- **Clinical features**
  1) may obstruct ducts, cause jaundice, palpable mass
  2) often totally asymptomatic
- **Radiologic features**
  1) cavernous hemangioma (most common primary benign neoplasm)
     - usually not visible on plain film
     - may calcify as a dense mass, or irregular projections from central mass
  2) cysts
     - hepatomegaly with oval, irregular, or round lesions with calcific rims
     - densely calcified, or mottled with lucent areas
     - hydatid cyst: usually smooth outer wall, but sometimes irregularly calcified
     - with calcifications in "*daughter cysts*": polyhedral lesion

f) Hemochromatosis
- **General considerations**
  1) called "*bronze diabetes*"
  2) excess of iron deposited in the liver
- **Clinical features**
  1) middle-aged patients
  2) causes cirrhosis of the liver, bronzed skin, cardiomegaly, heart failure, abdominal pain, arthritis
  3) strong association with hepatoma
  4) strong association with diabetes mellitus (50–60% of cases)
- **Radiologic features**
  1) homogeneous opacification of the liver (and spleen)

g) Hepatomegaly
- **General considerations**
  1) enlargement of the liver
  2) various causes, including cysts, neoplasms, infections
- **Clinical features** reflect origin of enlargement
- **Radiologic features**
  1) may displace the colon's hepatic

flexure and the right kidney
downward

   2) may displace stomach backward and
to the left (if left lobe of liver is
enlarging)

   3) generalized enlargement: may
elevate diaphragm

9. **Spleen**

  a) Normal location: posterior left upper
quadrant, lateral to stomach

  b) Splenomegaly

   • **General considerations**

    1) occurs with hemochromatosis

    2) with cirrhosis of the liver

    3) with blocked splenic or portal veins

    4) with infections

    5) with lymphoproliferative or
myeloproliferative processes

    6) with chronic hemolytic anemias

    7) with storage diseases

    8) with splenic cysts

   • **Clinical features**

    1) sometimes palpable

    2) causes feelings of fullness when
eating

    3) upper left quadrant abdominal pain

    4) sometimes splenic friction rub

    5) sometimes epigastric or splenic
bruits

   • **Radiologic features**

    1) spleen may encroach on stomach

    2) may depress splenic flexure

    3) may elevate diaphragm

  c) Rupture of spleen

   • **General considerations**

    1) usually caused by trauma

    2) diseased spleen may rupture
spontaneously (e.g., otherwise
asymptomatic TB in spleen)

   • **Clinical features**

    1) severe pain

    2) rapid blood loss into the abdominal
cavity

    3) with slow blood loss, radiologic
examination helpful in diagnosis

   • **Radiologic features**

    1) diseased spleen may be enlarged

    2) prominent mucosal folds of
stomach's greater curvature

    3) gastric dilatation

    4) stomach displaced inferior and to
the right

    5) intestinal loops separated by
intraperitoneal blood

    6) pleural effusion at left lung base

☞   **d)** Splenic calcifications
            • **General considerations**
                1) seen with granulomatous infections, cysts, splenic artery aneurysms, metastatic carcinoma from the ovary, or calcification of the splenic capsule
                2) possible opacification with hemochromatosis, sickle cell disease, or retained contrast material (Thorotrast)
            • **Clinical features**
                1) calcification itself, asymptomatic
                2) hemosiderosis
                    • usually middle-aged patients
                    • causes liver cirrhosis
                    • bronzed skin
                    • cardiomegaly, heart failure
                    • abdominal pain
                    • arthritis
                    • association with hepatoma and diabetes mellitus (50–60% of cases)
            • **Radiologic features**
                1) with sickle cell anemia
                    • spleen may be diffusely opaque
                    • may have multiple granular or punctate calcifications
                    • spleen shrinks over time, usually becoming more opaque
                    • usually with concomitant aseptic necrosis of humeral heads, gallstones, cardiomegaly
                2) with *bronze diabetes* (hemochromatosis)
                    • spleen usually enlarged and homogeneously opacified
                3) retained thorotrast
                    • first: a homogeneously dense spleen
                    • over several years: acquires a mottled appearance
                    • peripancreatic lymph nodes sometimes opacified
                    • liver may have "feathery," fine density

        e) Splenic tumors, cysts
            • **General considerations**
                1) very rare: usually benign hemangioma, occasionally hamartoma
                2) splenic tumors almost always benign
                3) exception: metastasized ovarian carcinoma
                4) splenic cysts common
                    • congenital, parasitic, or traumatic

- about two-thirds of acquired cysts: caused by *Echinococcus granulosus*
- trauma: hemorrhagic or serous cysts

- **Clinical features**
    1) most cysts usually asymptomatic
    2) hydatid disease may cause splenomegaly
    3) no splenomegaly with hemangioma

- **Radiologic features**
    1) splenic hemangioma (most common splenic tumor)
        - phleboliths possible, but rare
        - tumor usually > 5 mm in diameter
        - central lucencies
        - no splenomegaly, despite large tumors
    2) hydatid disease (*Echinococcosis*)
        - most frequent cause of splenic cysts
        - heavily calcified walls of cysts
    3) serous or hemorrhagic cysts
        - usually fibrous walls
        - resemble hydatid cysts with circumferential calcifications
        - smooth outer and more irregular inner wall
        - larger cysts: sometimes intermittent calcification of the wall

10. **Pancreas**

    a) Normal location
        - pancreatic head: midline in posterior superior epigastrium, surrounded by duodenal loop
        - body: usually posterior to the stomach's antrum and body
        - tail reaches medial border of spleen

    b) Carcinoma of pancreas
        - **General considerations**
            1) may invade duodenum or stomach
            2) almost never calcific
            3) seen with alcoholism
        - **Clinical features**
            1) exocrine tumors
                - ductal adenocarcinoma
                    a. possible jaundice, splenic vein obstruction, splenomegaly, gastric or esophageal varices, and hemorrhage
                    b. patients more often male (2:1) in their 50s
                    c. weight loss

d. abdominal pain that radiates
    to the back and is relieved in
    the fetal position (symptoms
    are late in the disease
    process)

• cystadenocarcinoma

a. earlier symptoms of upper
    abdominal pain

b. palpable mass

c. more hopeful prognosis

2) endocrine tumors

• may be nonfunctioning

a. obstruct the biliary tract or
    duodenum

b. cause GI bleeding and
    palpable masses

• functioning tumors

a. produce various hormones

b. cause various syndromes

• insulinoma

a. hypoglycemia, with
    headache, confusion, visual
    and motor disturbances,
    personality changes

• gastrinoma

a. Zollinger-Ellison Syndrome:
    aggressive peptic ulceration

b. about 50% are malignant

• WDHA

a. caused by tumors of non-β
    islet cells

b. **W**atery **D**iarrhea,
    Hypokalemia, **A**chlorhydria

c. known as "*Vipoma
    Syndrome*"

• glucagonoma

a. predilection for females: 80%
    of cases

b. 80% malignant

c. weight loss

d. necrolytic migratory
    erythema (exfoliating,
    brown-red lesions of the
    extremities), smooth, shiny,
    vermilion tongue; cheilitis

• **Radiologic features**

1) pancreatic carcinoma

• may create a "*pad sign*" (or
   Case's pad sign): extrinsic
   pressure defect on antrum and
   greater curve of the stomach, and
   third and fourth portions of
   duodenum

• may efface and indent the
   margins above and below the
   papilla of Vater, creating
   "*Frostberg's inverted 3 sign*"
   (same sign may be caused by
   cystic inflammation)

2) cystadenoma or cystadenocarcinoma
  - may calcify, with dense, irregular, widely-scattered clumps of calcification; "*sunburst*" or "*radial*" pattern
3) islet tumors (benign or malignant)
  - rarely calcify
  - when calcified, appear coarse, irregular, and poorly defined
4) pancreatic adenocarcinoma
  - rarely calcifies
  - more common in patients with chronic calcifying pancreatitis

c) Inflammations and infections
  - **General considerations**
    1) chronic inflammation
      - most often caused by alcoholism
      - rarely caused by hyperparathyroidism, pancreatic duct obstruction (stenosis, stones, carcinoma), or hereditary pancreatitis
    2) acute pancreatitis
      - caused by biliary tract calculi, alcoholism, drug reactions, infections, hyperlipidemia, ductal anomalies or obstructions, vascular disease, trauma, hyperparathyroidism, hypercalcemia, kidney transplants
  - **Clinical features**
    1) chronic pancreatitis
      - periodic episodes of severe epigastric pain
      - eventually: steatorrhea and creatorrhea (greasy stools or oil droplets)
      - may develop glucose intolerance
    2) acute pancreatitis
      - usually severe, intractable, steady, boring abdominal pain
      - pain may radiate into the back
      - pain intensified by coughing, deep breathing
      - nausea and vomiting
      - profuse sweating
      - may develop fever
      - may produce plate-like atelectasis, gastric ileus, ascites
  - **Radiologic features**
    1) chronic calcifying pancreatitis
      - multiple discrete densities across the midline at L1-L2 level
      - densities throughout the pancreas, from midline into the left upper quadrant in a continuous chain of opacities

- in some, only the head of the pancreas contains calcifications
- densities of varied shapes and sizes
- well-defined and dense
- laminated or mottled

2) acute pancreatitis
- "*colon cut-off sign*": either complete absence of gas in transverse colon, or a gas-filled transverse colon with complete absence of gas in the descending colon

d) Pancreatic cysts
- **General considerations**
  1) rare
  2) pseudocysts occur in pancreatic tail
- **Clinical features**
  1) pseudocysts: most common form
  2) usually asymptomatic unless blocking a duct, or infected
  3) then:
     - may cause abdominal pain
     - rarely burrow into mediastinum (via aortic or esophageal hiatus)
     - may rupture into pleural space, causing pleural effusion
- **Radiologic features**
  1) calcify with opaque rims, complete or incomplete, and thick or thin
  2) most often in the pancreatic tail
  3) may contain milk of calcium

11. Adrenal Glands

☞ **a)** Neonatal hemorrhage
- may result in unilateral or asymmetric bilateral calcifications
- mottled calcifications
- faint or dense
- localized or distributed throughout gland
- may appear as triangular clump of opacities

☞ **b)** Addison's disease
- *General considerations*: condition of adrenal insufficiency
- **Clinical findings**
  1) weakness, fatigue
  2) orthostatic hypotension
  3) pigmentation changes (usually darkening)
  4) dark freckles
  5) later: weight loss, hypotension, dehydration, anorexia, nausea, vomiting, diarrhea, syncope, decreased tolerance for cold
- **Radiologic findings**
  1) sometimes mottled calcification of entire gland

2) sometimes homogeneous density increase throughout gland

3) sometimes multiple, discrete calcifications throughout gland

c) Granulomatous infections
- include tuberculosis, histoplasmosis
- may result in Addison's disease
- detectable on plain film only when calcifications of Addison's disease occur

 d) Adrenal cysts
- usually asymptomatic (except for cystic pheochromocytoma)
- **Radiologic features**
  1) may enlarge enough to alter gland contour
  2) some types calcify
  3) "*pseudocyst*": due to hemorrhage or necrosis
     - most frequently calcified adrenal cystic lesions
     - walls totally or partially calcified
     - may simulate primary or metastatic neoplasm (usually melanoma)
  4) epithelial- or endothelial-lined cyst
     - may contain milk of calcium
     - shows as faint, diffuse opacity
  5) cystic pheochromocytoma
     - arclike, "*eggshell*" circumferential calcification
     - often 3–4 cm in diameter

e) Adrenal neoplasms
- may show speckled or mottled calcification, with no indication of nature of tumor or its size
- malignant tumor: tendency toward greater enlargement of gland than with benign lesions
- nonfunctional, benign adrenal tumors usually asymptomatic
- benign pheochromocytoma
  1) most common adrenal medullary tumor
  2) **Clinical features**
     - hypertension (paroxysmal or persistent)
     - tachycardia
     - diaphoresis
     - postural hypotension
     - tachypnea, dyspnea
     - flushing
     - headache
     - cold and clammy skin
     - angina
     - palpitation

- nausea, vomiting, epigastric pain
- visual disturbances
- paresthesias
- constipation
- sense of impending doom

3) **Radiologic features**
- may have cyst-like calcifications
- may have punctate or mottled calcifications
- benign ganglioneuroma: infrequent medullary neoplasm
- adrenal adenoma: medullary neoplasm
- myelolipoma (choristoma): medullary neoplasm, may have small mottled or punctate calcifications
- large hemangioma: may contain phleboliths
- malignant neuroblastoma: medullary tumor, usually in patients < 3 years old
- adrenal cortical carcinoma
  a. metastasizes; presents as a metastatic process
  b. sometimes shows amorphous solid calcification
  c. sometimes a conglomerate mottled or punctate mass
- adrenal hematoma: may contain calcifications

12. **Uterus and Cervix**

    a) Leiomyoma (uterine fibroid)
- **General considerations**
  1) commonly calcified
  2) when large, may extend from pelvis up into abdomen
  3) leiomyosarcoma is rare; malignant
- **Clinical features**
  1) usually asymptomatic
  2) may cause pain or bleeding
- **Radiologic features**
  1) mottled calcification
  2) "*popcorn ball*" appearance within irregularly rounded, rimless mass
  3) may be solitary or multiple
  4) multiple tumors: sometimes not all of them calcify
  5) sometimes only a small part of tumor calcifies
  6) leiomyosarcoma: may look identical to benign fibroid

    b) Endometrial adenocarcinoma and cervical squamous cell carcinoma
- rarely calcified

- **Clinical features**
    1) cardinal symptom: inappropriate uterine bleeding
    2) often preceded by several months of watery or mucoid discharge
- **Radiologic features**
    1) uncalcified soft tissue mass in pelvis
    2) may go undetected until very large
    3) may be demonstrated via contrast CT exam

c) Malignant mixed uterine tumors
- comprise about 6% of all uterine primary malignancies
- some have calcifications
- contain elements of both sarcoma and carcinoma

☞ **13. Lithopedion ("stone baby")**

a) General considerations
- result of untreated ectopic pregnancy
- dead fetus retained >3 months may petrify

b) Clinical features
- severe cramping and spotting (ectopic pregnancy signs)
- usually treated surgically
- maternal death common, if untreated
- occasionally: dead fetus retained
- after petrifaction, mother may be asymptomatic

c) Radiologic features
- three classes of lithopedions
    1) lithokelyphos
        - normal fetal skeleton
        - surrounded by rigid shell of calcified membranes
    2) lithokelyphopedion
        - calcified fetal skeleton
        - surrounded by calcified membrane shell
    3) lithopedion
        - fetal skeleton calcified
        - surrounding membrane uncalcified
        - may be anywhere in abdomen or pelvis
        - quite mobile when implanted on omentum

14. Fallopian Tubes

a) Fallopian tube lesions
- **General considerations**
    1) involve calcification of tubal lumen, or stone formation within tubes
    2) rarely: malignant tumor: carcinoma of the oviduct

- **Clinical features**
  1) usually asymptomatic, but may cause infertility
  2) ectopic pregnancy: may implant in tube, create severe pain
  3) primary carcinoma of the oviduct:
  4) vague symptoms of bladder or rectal pressure as the tumor enlarges
  5) may cause ascites or a palpable mass

15. **Ovarian Lesions**

   a) Ovarian cysts (dermoid cyst, cystic teratoma)
   - **General considerations**
     1) about 10% of all ovarian tumors
     2) bilateral in about 20% of cases
     3) may be multiple
     4) rarely undergo malignant degeneration
   - **Clinical features**
     1) may be asymptomatic
     2) may create a sensation of fullness, achy heaviness
     3) with rupture: sharp pain, fever, signs of shock
     4) twisted cyst: intermittent colicky pain
   - **Radiologic features**
     1) cystic teratoma
        - usually 5–15 cm in diameter
        - sometimes soft tissue mass with no calcification
        - up to 60%: identifiable, rudimentary tooth (or teeth)
        - wall of cyst: sometimes visible as a thin, curvilinear calcification (10% of cases)
        - cyst seen as lucent, smoothly rounded mass
        - other patterns of calcification occur

   b) Ovarian neoplasms
   - **General considerations**
     1) 80% of are papillary cystadenoma, or cystadenocarcinoma
     2) gonadoblastoma: rare, sometimes bilateral, usually benign
   - **Clinical features**
     1) remain asymptomatic for a long while
     2) eventually: vague abdominal discomfort, digestive complaints
     3) late: abdominal swelling, pelvic pain, ascites, anemia, cachexia
     4) cystadenocarcinoma
        - most common ovarian malignancy

- most often in patients 30–60
    years old
  5) gonadoblastoma
     - most common < 25 years old
     - hormonally active
     - causes amenorrhea, virilization,
       hirsutism, clitoral hypertrophy,
       infantilism of the uterus
  - **Radiologic features**
    1) cystadenocarcinoma
       - often bilateral
       - primary and metastatic forms:
         both with discrete, small,
         uniformly distributed
         calcifications ("*psammoma
         bodies*," "*corpora amylacea*," or
         "*calcospherites*")
    2) benign serous cystadenoma
       - may rarely develop curvilinear
         wall calcification
       - mucinous lesions do not calcify
    3) gonadoblastoma
       - sometimes bilateral
       - circumscribed punctate or mottled
         calcifications within a soft-tissue
         mass

  c) Granulomatous infection
     - usually tuberculosis, may affect ovaries
     - clinically: ovarian tuberculosis: usually
       silent
     - **Radiologic features**
       1) unilateral or bilateral mottled
          calcification
       2) similar to calcified lymph nodes, but
          larger

  d) Ovarian autoamputation
     - may leave a calcified, mobile residual
       mass
     - **Clinical features:** asymptomatic; calcified
       remnant is an incidental radiologic finding
     - **Radiologic features**
       1) oval, coarsely stippled mass
       2) freely mobile in the pelvis or lower
          abdomen
       3) usually only a few centimeters in
          diameter

  e) Idiopathic calcification of the corpora
     albicantia (rare)

16. **Vas Deferens**

  a) **General considerations**
     - vessel wall calcification
     - intramural calcification with diabetes
     - intraluminal calcification with infection

    b) Clinical features

- in elderly, normal calcifications: asymptomatic
- clinical signs of diabetes, or infection

    c) Radiologic features

- appears tortuous, with conduit-like calcification
- coursing medial and inferior toward the urethra
- may extend into the scrotum

17. Seminal Vesicle

    a) Seminal vesicle calcification: with TB or gonorrhea

    b) Usually asymptomatic

    c) Radiologic features

- sometimes: entire seminal vesicles filled with a cloud of concretions
- sometimes: small, intraluminal concretions behind the bladder, above the prostate

18. Scrotum

    a) Hydrocele or spermatocele

- clinically: painless, will transilluminate
- **Radiologic features**
  1) lucent mass in the scrotum
  2) may have cystic curvilinear calcification of the wall

    b) Scrotal tuberculosis

- **Clinical features:** painful swelling characteristic of epididymo-orchitis (with any scrotal infection)
- **Radiologic features:** dense oval calcifications (with any scrotal inflammation)

    c) Testicular infarction

- **Clinical features**
  1) seen in normal or in undescended testicle
  2) usually caused by torsion
  3) more often in the newborn
  4) may cause local pain and edema, nausea and vomiting, fever
- **Radiologic features**
  1) at first: a soft-tissue mass
  2) may calcify, causing a roughly rounded or oval, dense opacity
  3) occasionally in an undescended testicle, so may be in the abdomen
  4) hematoma in the scrotum
     - may require surgical treatment if it is large and fails to resorb

d) Testicular tumor
- **General considerations**
    1) benign or malignant
    2) malignancies include seminoma, teratoma, embryonal carcinoma, teratocarcinoma, and choriocarcinoma
    3) benign lesions include fibromas, fibroadenomas, adenomatoid tumors, and lipomas
- **Clinical features:** create firm mass, sometimes painful
- **Radiologic features**
    1) rarely calcify; usually a soft-tissue mass
    2) teratoma may present fine, punctate calcifications
    3) Leydig cell tumor: sometimes lacy or streaked calcifications

19. Retroperitoneal Lesions

a) Tumors
- **General considerations**
    1) rare
    2) benign or malignant teratoma
    3) mesenchymoma: a sarcoma
    4) ectopic pheochromocytoma
    5) lymphoma
- **Clinical features**
    1) often asymptomatic
    2) may cause back pain

- **Radiologic features**
    1) teratoma most characteristic appearance
        - large mass anterior between adrenal and kidney
        - contains bone or teeth
    2) mesenchymoma
        - diffuse, poorly-defined calcifications; only faintly visible on plain film
        - may have cystic rim of calcification
    3) pheochromocytoma: ring of calcification (cystic appearance)

20. Aneurysms: see chapter 7; section B-7

21. Review of Named Abdominal Roentgen Signs and their Significance

a) *acute toxic megacolon*: with ulcerative colitis, paralyzed transverse or descending colon may dilate to > 6 cm in diameter

b) *air dome*: gas outlining distended peritoneum with pneumoperitoneum, seen in cross-table lateral projection

c) *aneurysmal dilatation*: extreme distention of the small bowel seen with lymphosarcoma

d) *apple core appearance*: carcinoma forms a polypoid mass, commonly in the cecum; rarely seen with inflammatory processes

e) *bird's beak*: tapered, twisted bowel segment affected by volvulus

f) *bladder ears*: lateral protrusions of an extraperitoneal bladder herniation through the inguinal ring; disappear when bladder fills

g) *bull's eye appearance*: ulcerated carcinoid tumor in small bowel

h) *Case's pad sign*: extrinsic pressure defect on portions of stomach and duodenum, caused by pancreatic carcinoma

i) *Christmas tree bladder*: with cystography, serrated bladder wall is visible, showing greatest contractions at the dome

j) *claw sign*: on KUB, renal cysts may produce an appearance of triangular, claw-like projections of normal parenchyma

k) *cobblestone appearance*: regions of hyperplastic mucosa, forming "pseudopolyps," in gastrointestinal inflammatory conditions (e.g., Crohn's disease, ulcerative colitis)

l) *coffee bean sign*: adjacent parallel lucencies with intestinal walls between them, seen in twisted large bowel loops with sigmoid volvulus

m) *coiled spring appearance*: suggests intussusception of the small intestine

n) *collar button ulcer*: appearance of broad-based ulceration, where ulcer has burrowed under the mucosa; especially common in the colon with ulcerative colitis

o) *colon cut-off sign*: acute pancreatitis may be indicated by either complete absence of gas in the transverse colon, or a gas-filled transverse colon

p) *crescent sign*: in IVP, dye accumulates in damaged parenchyma around dilated calyces in crescent patterns

q) *crow-foot sign*: gallstone with gas-filled fissures

r) *crow's beak deformity*: volvulus may create a tapered, twisted bowel segment

s) *doggy ears*: ascites accumulated around and behind the bladder, giving hazy fluid appearance

t) *double bubble sign*: obstruction of the proximal bowel traps excessive air in the stomach and duodenum (caused by duodenal atresia or an annular pancreas)

u) *dumbbell calculus*: calculus formed in the neck of a calyceal diverticulum

v) *fish-hook bladder*: characteristic appearance of bladder obstructed by benign prostatic hypertrophy

w) *floating small intestines*: small bowel is raised high in abdominal cavity by ascites

x) *football sign*: pneumoperitoneum may outline the falciform ligament, so it looks like a football seam across the lucent peritoneum (see "air dome")

y) *frondlike rectal filling defect*: caused by brush-border of villous adenoma

z) *Frostberg's inverted 3 sign*: indentations in margins above and below papilla of Vater, may indicate carcinoma or cystic inflammation of the pancreas

aa) *giant gastric mucosal folds*: indicate stomach pathology, such as lymphosarcoma

bb) *ground glass appearance*: increased water density in abdomen caused by ascites

cc) *Hampton's line*: narrow line of lucency across the mouth of a barium-filled ulcer seen in profile; indicates benign ulcer with edematous rim

dd) *hockey-stick bladder*: characteristic appearance of bladder obstructed by benign prostatic hypertrophy

ee) *hourglass deformity* of the stomach: incisure of the stomach opposite an ulcer

ff) *"j"-shaped bladder*: characteristic appearance of bladder obstructed by benign prostatic hypertrophy

gg) *lead pipe colon*: contracted, shortened colon, without haustra, indicates late stages of ulcerative colitis

hh) *meconium ileus*: small bowel obstruction in a newborn, caused by calcified meconium

ii) *meconium peritonitis*: newborn; bowel perforation caused by calcified meconium

jj) *Mercedes Benz sign*: gallstone with gas-filled fissures

kk) *moulage sign*: barium has flocculated appearance caused by hypersecretion of fluid in the intestinal lumen, walls of lumen are smooth; seen with celiac disease

ll) *pad sign*: extrinsic pressure defect on portions of stomach and duodenum, caused by pancreatic carcinoma

mm) *pipe stem ureter*: straight ureter from renal pelvis to pelvic brim, seen in advanced tuberculosis affecting the urinary tract

nn) *putty kidney*: dense, amorphous appearance of destroyed kidney in which normal parenchyma has been replaced by calcium and caseous material; seen with chronic infections like tuberculosis

oo) *ring shadow*: with renal necrosis, dense opacity forms a border around triangular lucencies, indicating necrotic papilla within the calyx

pp) *sentinel loop*: focal dilatation of bowel adjacent to an area of abdominal inflammation (e.g., acute pancreatitis, cholecystitis, or appendicitis)

qq) *shouldering defect*: abrupt termination of barium column with overhanging edges as distal border of the lesion, indicates probable malignant lesion anywhere in GI tract

rr) *skip lesions*: barium-filled segments of bowel affected by inflammatory bowel disease; areas of bowel uninvolved or skipped by the disease (celiac disease, ulcerative colitis, Crohn's disease, granulomatous colitis)

ss) *snowflake appearance*: retained flecks of barium on jejunal mucosal folds

tt) *squeeze sign*: soft lipoma will show altered contours with peristalsis, as tumor is squeezed

uu) *stacked coin appearance*: distended valvulae conniventes caused by gas filling when the small bowel is obstructed

vv) *staghorn calculus*: cast-like filling of renal pelvis and calyces by renal calculi

ww) *step-ladder appearance*: obstructed, gas-filled small bowel traversing the abdomen

xx) *Stierlin's sign*: inflamed cecum and terminal ileum do not fill with barium, remain empty (intestinal tuberculosis may create this sign on a barium study)

yy) *string sign of Kantor*: narrow, straight, rigid terminal ileum of Crohn's disease

zz) *target sign*: a pedunculated polyp seen *en face*, the wider circle is the polyp head, and the smaller concentric ring represents the stalk

aaa) *toxic dilation* (*toxic megacolon*): transverse or descending colon dilates to > 6 cm diameter with ulcerative colitis

bbb) *umbrella defect of the bulb*: seen in pyloric bulb when there is pyloric stenosis

REVIEW—STUDY QUESTIONS

1. What is a teratoma, what is its radiologic appearance?
2. What is the most common cause of hepatic cysts?
3. What is Case's pad sign, and what lesion does it indicate?
4. Name three causes of emphysematous cholecystitis.
5. What is the radiologic appearance of a testicular infarction and where might it be seen?
6. Name five etiologies of calcifications in the liver.
7. The radiologic appearance of a Y-shaped lucency in the upper right quadrant should cause the clinician to suspect what condition?
8. Describe the radiologic appearance of a calcified vas deferens. What clinical condition is associated with it?
9. What liver lesions are most often apt to cause jaundice, and why?
10. What is WDHA? What lesions produce these effects?
11. What are radiologic indicators of hepatomegaly?
12. Name three radiologic signs or features of splenic rupture.
13. What might be the radiologic appearance of the adrenal glands in a patient with Addison's disease?
14. What is the most commonly calcified uterine neoplasm? Describe its typical appearance.
15. Describe the radiologic signs in the chest and abdomen of sickle cell anemia.
16. What is the pathognomonic radiologic appearance of infestation by *Armillifer armillatus*?
17. What is the most common benign tumor of the spleen?
18. What is the Mercedes Benz sign?
19. What are "skip lesions"?
20. Describe the radiologic appearance of the liver in the presence of hemochromatosis.
21. What are two radiologic appearances of the colon cut-off sign that results from acute pancreatitis?
22. What triad of radiologic findings is typically seen with gallstone ileus?
23. What adrenal neoplasm may create an "eggshell calcification" pattern?
24. What may choleliths be composed of? Which are radiopaque, and which are radiolucent?
25. Name three etiologies for the radiologic appearance of an opacified spleen.

1. The peripheral margin of a parenchymal lung mass may be smooth or jagged:
   a) but this is not a useful factor in differentiation of lung lesions.
   b) and this helps differentiate between primary and metastatic lesions.
   c) and this helps differentiate between benign or malignant lesions.
   d) and this helps differentiate between neoplastic and inflammatory lesions.

2. Esophageal achalasia is:
   a) a benign tumor.
   b) a vascular inflammation leading to esophageal varices.
   c) an obstruction caused by a mass lesion impinging on the esophagus.
   d) a gastroesophageal sphincter spasm or failure of relaxation.

3. Neurofibroma is frequently diagnosed via oblique radiographs, as it:
   a) extends like a "teardrop" from the neck into the mediastinum.
   b) exerts mass pressure, inverting the left hemidiaphragm.
   c) creates massive widening of the mediastinum.
   d) becomes a "dumbbell" tumor, extending through the IVF.

4. Patients with AIDS who develop Kaposi sarcoma may show radiologic signs, such as:
   a) a tram-tracking appearance caused by peribronchial thickening.
   b) cavitated opacities in the upper lobes.
   c) symmetric, coarse reticulonodular infiltration.
   d) airspace consolidation with an air bronchogram sign.

5. Plain films of a patient with esophageal achalasia may show:
   a) a significantly enlarged and distended magenblasse.
   b) loss of the magenblasse.
   c) mediastinal shift to the right.
   d) tracheal deviation.

6. On an upright view, subpulmonary fluid presents all of the following signs except:
   a) meniscus sign.
   b) shallow costophrenic angles.
   c) separation of gastric air bubble from diaphragm.
   d) high hemidiaphragm.

7. Lymphangitic metastases in the lung are most often from:
   a) the prostate.
   b) the breast.
   c) the colon.
   d) the liver.

8. Kerley's A, B, and C lines are indicative of:
   a) bullous emphysema.
   b) lymphatic dilation.
   c) pulmonary edema.
   d) pneumonic infiltrates.

9. The residual fibrosis of varicella pneumonia must be differentiated radiologically from the similar-appearing "snowstorm" calcifications of:
   a) histoplasmosis.
   b) enteroviruses.
   c) Epstein-Barr virus.
   d) schistosomiasis.

10. With full inhalation, a PA projection should demonstrate (in most normal patients):
    a) the anterior end of the right 8th rib visible above the right hemidiaphragm.
    b) the posterior end of 11 ribs visible above the right hemidiaphragm.
    c) the anterior end of the right 9th rib visible above the right hemidiaphragm.
    d) the posterior end of 10 ribs visible above the right hemidiaphragm.

11. Meconium ileus is:
    a) an intussusception.
    b) a small bowel obstruction in a newborn.
    c) a bowel perforation caused by calcified meconium.
    d) a skip lesion.

12. Sub-sternal thyroid is an synonym for:
    a) lymphoma.
    b) intrathoracic goiter.
    c) thymoma.
    d) teratoma.

13. A mediastinal cystic hygroma is:
    a) a lymphangioma.
    b) a teratoma.
    c) a pericardial cyst.
    d) a thymoma.

14. A lucent mass in the scrotum, with or without calcification of its wall, is probably:
    a) a hydrocele or spermatocele.
    b) scrotal tuberculosis.
    c) scrotal lipoma.
    d) a hematoma.

15. The most common benign cardiac tumor is:
    a) leiomyoma.
    b) cystic hygroma.
    c) myxoma.
    d) neurilemoma.

16. Fluid trapped between the lung and diaphragm creates (on an upright view) the appearance of:

    a) a meniscus sign.
    b) an elevated hemidiaphragm.
    c) a shift of mediastinal structures.
    d) an air bronchogram sign.

17. In the lungs, the most common source of solitary metastatic lesions is:

    a) the ovaries.
    b) the colon.
    c) the pancreas.
    d) the kidney.

18. The most common cause of extrapleural sign is:

    a) extrapleural hematoma.
    b) neurofibroma.
    c) metastatic lesions in the ribs.
    d) multiple myeloma of the ribs.

19. A tortuous curvilinear calcification, coursing medial and inferior in the lower pelvic basin, may be:

    a) prostatic calcifications.
    b) a calcified vas deferens.
    c) a calcified internal iliac artery.
    d) seminal vesicle calcification.

20. An air/fluid level seen behind the heart on a PA & lateral chest X ray is probably:

    a) esophageal diverticula
    b) hiatus hernia
    c) esophageal carcinoma
    d) cascade stomach

21. "Lumpy jaw" is a cervicofacial form of:

    a) sarcoidosis.
    b) coccidioidomycosis.
    c) aspergillosis
    d) actinomycosis.

22. The radiographic appearance of substernal thyroid requires differentiation from:

    a) esophageal varices.
    b) thymoma.
    c) hiatus hernia.
    d) aortic coarctation.

23. A thin-walled mass with central fluid density that appears to extend into the primary interlobar fissure like a "teardrop" is probably:

    a) a carcinoid.
    b) a teratoma.
    c) a pericardial cyst.
    d) round atelectasis.

24. A cystic teratoma is also called:

    a) a lithopedion.
    b) a uterine fibroid.
    c) a dermoid cyst.
    d) a gonadoblastoma.

25. *Cor bovinum* is:

    a) enlargement of the right atrium, seen with tricuspid valvular disease.
    b) massive elongation of the heart, seen with Marfan's syndrome.
    c) massive left ventricular enlargement, seen with aortic insufficiency.
    d) a "pancake heart," seen with cardiac tamponade.

26. A meniscus sign may indicate:

    a) middle lobe syndrome.
    b) atelectasis of a lower lobe.
    c) free pleural effusion.
    d) interstitial infiltrates.

27. Calcification of a pulmonary nodule indicates that it is most likely:

    a) a primary malignant tumor.
    b) a benign lesion.
    c) a metastatic lesion.
    d) a cystic lesion.

28. An air bronchogram sign is:

    a) a normal finding caused by air-filled bronchi.
    b) an abnormal finding indicating atelectasis.
    c) an abnormal finding indicating bronchial displacement.
    d) an abnormal finding indicating dense infiltrate within the lung parenchyma.

29. A "popcorn ball" appearance in the medial pelvic bowl is characteristic of:

    a) a uterine leiomyoma.
    b) endometrial adenocarcinoma.
    c) cervical squamous cell carcinoma.
    d) a malignant mixed tumor of the uterus.

30. The right lateral decubitus projection is made with the patient:

    a) lying on the right side with the x-ray beam perpendicular to the floor.
    b) lying on the left side with the x-ray beam perpendicular to the floor.
    c) lying on the left side with the x-ray beam parallel to the floor.
    d) lying on the right side with the x-ray beam parallel to the floor.

31. Actinomycosis is often contracted via:

    a) spread from a dental infection.
    b) inhaled dust in an area where the organism is endemic.
    c) air-borne droplets from the cough or sneeze of an infected person.
    d) hematogenous spread from a primary gastrointestinal infestation.

32. A thymoma may be seen on a lateral projection as a small mass:

    a) at the level of the aortic knob.
    b) at the base of the heart.
    c) at the apex of the heart.
    d) at the level of C7/T1.

33. The small, intraluminal concretions within the seminal vesicle usually are seen:
    a) lateral to the prostate.
    b) below the prostate.
    c) above the prostate.
    d) behind the cecum.

34. With large amounts of free pleural effusion:
    a) the affected hemithorax appears excessively lucent.
    b) there may be a mediastinal shift to the affected side.
    c) there may be a mediastinal shift to the unaffected side.
    d) there is no mediastinal shift, but there may be tracheal deviation.

35. Mitral stenosis may produce the radiographic appearance of:
    a) a silhouette sign.
    b) an air bronchogram sign.
    c) an extrapleural sign.
    d) Kerley's B lines.

36. Lower lobe collapse may be indicated on plain film by:
    a) a comet-tail sign.
    b) a mediastinal wedge.
    c) obliteration of the adjacent heart border.
    d) scoliosis, convex to the affected side.

37. Specific radiologic signs of traumatic rupture of the aorta include:
    a) increased mediastinal width.
    b) tracheal shift to the right.
    c) right displacement of superior vena cava.
    d) aortic arch distorted, indistinct.

38. The adrenal "pseudocyst" is caused by:
    a) emphysematous infection.
    b) hemorrhage or necrosis.
    c) hypercalcemia.
    d) Addison's disease.

39. The majority of lobar pneumonia cases are caused by:
    a) *Hemophilus influenzae.*
    b) *Mycoplasma pneumoniae.*
    c) *Streptococcus pneumoniae.*
    d) *Klebsiella.*

40. The major radiologic finding with Addison's disease is:
    a) hypertrophic arthropathy.
    b) gross enlargement of the adrenal glands.
    c) calcification of the adrenals, either mottled, discrete, or homogeneous.
    d) cystic lesions in the adrenals, with lucent centers.

41. Acute pancreatitis may be seen radiographically to cause:
    a) "Frostberg's inverted 3 sign."
    b) a "ring shadow."
    c) a "colon cut-off sign."
    d) a "moulage sign."

42. The "pseudopolyps" of hyperplastic mucosa, seen with inflammatory conditions of the gastrointestinal tract, give a radiologic sign known as:
    a) "coffee bean sign."
    b) "floating small intestines."
    c) "stacked coin appearance."
    d) "cobblestone appearance."

43. A patient who is experiencing both dyspnea and dysphagia, and has a hoarse-sounding voice, may be suspected to have:
    a) a thoracic aortic aneurysm.
    b) an intrathoracic goiter.
    c) esophageal varices.
    d) atelectasis.

44. Free pleural effusion is best demonstrated on plain film by:
    a) an upright PA projection.
    b) a lateral decubitus view, with affected side dependent.
    c) a lateral decubitus view, with affected side up.
    d) a cross-table lateral projection.

45. Left atrial enlargement with a double convexity on the right side of the heart shadow, with posterior displacement of the esophagus may indicate:
    a) mitral stenosis.
    b) aortic stenosis.
    c) aortic insufficiency.
    d) tricuspid valvular disease.

46. The comet-tail sign is a roentgen indication of:
    a) round atelectasis.
    b) upper lobe atelectasis.
    c) plate-like atelectasis.
    d) sudden, rapid atelectasis.

47. Intercostal muscle splinting, shallow breathing, or inactivated lung surfactant may cause:
    a) bronchospasms.
    b) tachycardia.
    c) atelectasis.
    d) bradycardia.

48. The lung apices are predilected to:
    a) abscess.
    b) pneumonia.
    c) carcinoma.
    d) silicosis.

49. Bronchial adenoma usually:
    a) occurs near a hilum, and contains calcifications.
    b) occurs in the periphery of the lung, and contains calcifications.
    c) occurs in the periphery of the lung, and does not calcify.
    d) occurs near a hilum, and does not calcify.

50. A calcified fetal skeleton surrounded by an uncalcified membrane is a:

    a) uterine fibroid.
    b) lithokelyphos.
    c) lithokelyphopedion.
    d) lithopedion.

51. Bilateral transudative pleural effusion is a common finding with all of the following except:

    a) pulmonary embolism.
    b) congestive heart failure.
    c) nephrotic syndrome.
    d) impaired lymphatic drainage.

52. The most common form of thoracic aortic aneurysm is:

    a) a berry aneurysm.
    b) a fusiform aneurysm.
    c) a saccular aneurysm.
    d) an eccentric aneurysm.

53. An adrenal tumor with an arclike, "eggshell" circumferential calcification is:

    a) a cystic pheochromocytoma.
    b) an adrenal pseudocyst.
    c) a benign ganglioneuroma.
    d) a myelolipoma (choristoma).

54. "Case's pad sign" is:

    a) indentation in the cecum caused by extrinsic pressure.
    b) an extrinsic pressure defect on portions of the stomach and duodenum.
    c) excessive thickening of the bladder walls.
    d) lateral displacement of a kidney.

55. Hypertrophic osteoarthropathy is most often a clinical indication of:

    a) atelectasis.
    b) previous pulmonary tubercular infection.
    c) pleurisy.
    d) bronchogenic carcinoma.

56. The KUB is:

    a) an AP "scout film."
    b) a contrast study.
    c) a time-sequence study.
    d) an MRI setting.

57. Indirect roentgen signs of lung collapse include all of the following except:

    a) vascular or bronchial crowding.
    b) herniation of lung tissue.
    c) tracheal deviation.
    d) narrowed rib cage on collapsed side.

58. The radiographic appearance of a left ventricular aneurysm may be misdiagnosed as:

    a) a pericardial cyst.
    b) a lymphoma.
    c) a bronchogenic carcinoma.
    d) round atelectasis.

59. The right lung normally has three segmental bronchi to the upper lobe, two segmental bronchi to the middle lobe, and:

    a) "5" segmental bronchi to the lower lobe.
    b) "4" segmental bronchi to the lower lobe.
    c) "3" segmental bronchi to the lower lobe.
    d) "2" segmental bronchi to the lower lobe.

60. An endocrine tumor of the pancreas that is malignant in 80% of cases is:

    a) insulinoma.
    b) gastrinoma.
    c) glucagonoma.
    d) non-islet cell tumor.

61. An ovarian cyst appears as:

    a) a small, densely calcified, oval opacity.
    b) a smooth, thin curvilinear, calcified rim around a lucent mass.
    c) a "popcorn-ball" calcification.
    d) an opaque, lobulated mass.

62. An aortic aneurysm should be suspected any time the vessel diameter is seen to measure:

    a) > 2 cm.
    b) > 3 cm.
    c) >3.2 cm.
    d) >3.8 cm.

63. The ascending colon, hepatic flexure, and right kidney all are located anatomically in the:

    a) left upper quadrant of the abdomen.
    b) left lower quadrant of the abdomen.
    c) right upper quadrant of the abdomen.
    d) right lower quadrant of the abdomen.

64. The term "potato nodes" describes the appearance of hilar lymph nodes in the presence of:

    a) schistosomiasis.
    b) tuberculosis.
    c) actinomycosis.
    d) sarcoidosis.

65. The Pancoast syndrome consists of an apical pulmonary mass, pain down the arm, possible rib or vertebra destruction, and:

    a) localized emphysema.
    b) obstructive pneumonitis.
    c) Horner's syndrome.
    d) bloody sputum.

66. Aortic coarctation usually **does not** create the radiographic appearance of:

    a) the "1–2–3 sign."
    b) rib notching.
    c) esophageal indentation.
    d) poststenotic and prestenotic dilatation.

67. Three direct signs of lung collapse, seen on plain film, are:

    a) increased lung lucency, displaced fissures, and hilar elevation.

b) increased lung opacity, displaced fissures, and vascular or bronchial crowding.

c) unilateral hemidiaphragm elevation, tracheal deviation, displaced fissures.

d) hilar displacement, displaced fissures, hyperlucency of unaffected lung.

68. The normal anatomic location of the pancreatic head is:

a) posterior to the antrum of the stomach.

b) posterior to the body of the stomach.

c) surrounded by the duodenal loop.

d) immediately inferior to the duodenal loop.

69. Pneumoperitoneum is considered "normal" when seen:

a) in a patient with diverticulitis.

b) in a patient with Crohn's disease.

c) after laparoscopy.

d) in a patient with a duodenal ulcer.

70. The "angel wing sign" is a radiologic indication of:

a) hemothorax.

b) pneumomediastinum.

c) non-Hodgkin lymphoma.

d) Hodgkin disease.

71. Non-Hodgkin lymphoma (NHL), as a high-grade malignancy in immunocompromised patients, shows a predilection for:

a) the kidneys.

b) the liver.

c) the central nervous system.

d) bone.

72. The indication of the presence of esophageal varices (on a barium swallow exam) is:

a) dilation of the distal esophagus.

b) constriction of the distal esophagus.

c) out-pouchings in the esophageal walls.

d) "snake-like" filling defects.

73. An "angel wing" pattern of fibrosis, lung scarring with hilar elevation, and a straight stretched lower lobe, are radiologic signs typical of:

a) progressive massive fibrosis (complicated CWP).

b) advanced silicosis.

c) advanced asbestosis.

d) simple pneumoconiosis.

74. The most common splenic tumor is hemangioma, which is seen radiographically as:

a) a densely calcified tumor.

b) a huge soft tissue mass, creating massive splenomegaly.

c) a large tumor with central lucencies, but without splenomegaly.

d) a small soft tissue mass with no calcifications.

75. The Pancoast tumor is:

a) a form of bronchogenic carcinoma in the superior pulmonary sulcus.

b) an apical argentaffinoma.

c) a carcinoid located in the lung apex.

d) apical alveolar cell carcinoma.

76. The "3 sign" is:

a) an indication of bronchogenic carcinoma.

b) an indication of old, healed tuberculosis.

c) an indication of hiatus hernia.

d) an indication of aortic coarctation.

77. The most common cause of mechanical ileus is:

a) volvulus.

b) ulcerative colitis.

c) Crohn's disease.

d) neoplasm.

78. Although normal lymph node size may vary, pathology should be ruled out when the transverse diameter of a node is:

a) > 5 mm.

b) > 3 mm.

c) > 8 mm.

d) > 10 mm.

79. Tumors in the spleen usually are:

a) metastasized ovarian carcinoma.

b) benign hamartoma.

c) benign hemangioma.

d) parasitic cysts.

80. A good diagnostic film for pneumothorax would be:

a) PA with full inhalation.

b) cross-table lateral.

c) lateral decubitus with affected side down.

d) lateral decubitus with affected side up.

81. "Petrified stomach" is most often caused by:

a) hypercalcemia.

b) gastric hemangioma.

c) duplication cyst.

d) gastric adenocarcinoma.

82. Adenocarcinoma in the lower esophagus may develop as a sequel to:

a) excessive consumption of caffeine.

b) drinking excessively hot liquids.

c) eating excessively hot (spicy) foods.

d) chronic gastroesophageal reflux.

83. The "comet tail sign" is created by:

a) bowel intussusception.

b) paralytic ileus.

c) compression of bronchi and vessels between a mass lesion and the hilum.

d) volvulus.

84. Adynamic ileus may be caused by:

a) Crohn's disease.

b) carcinoma.

c) occult spinal fracture.

d) volvulus

85. "Bronze diabetes" is caused by:
    a) cardiomegaly.
    b) pancreatitis.
    c) cirrhosis of the liver.
    d) excessive iron deposited in the liver.

86. The "vanishing tumor," or "phantom tumor" of the lung is really:
    a) resorption of encapsulated pleural effusion.
    b) shifting of free effusion with the change of position of the patient.
    c) resolution of interstitial edema.
    d) re-inflation of a collapsed lobe.

87. Retroperitoneal organs include:
    a) the spleen, pancreatic head, and kidneys.
    b) the liver, kidneys, and pancreas.
    c) the spleen, gall bladder, and pancreatic tail.
    d) the duodenum, pancreas, and kidneys.

88. Posterior mediastinal lymph nodes include:
    a) subcarinal nodes.
    b) pulmonary root nodes.
    c) paraesophageal nodes.
    d) parietal nodes.

89. The "aortic window" is created by:
    a) the trachea and the aortic arch.
    b) the aortic arch.
    c) the bronchi at the carina, and the aortic arch.
    d) the aorta and the esophagus, at the diaphragmatic hiatus.

90. With large pneumothorax one might see:
    a) accentuated lung markings on the side distal to the lesion.
    b) a shift of the mediastinum to the unaffected side.
    c) a "pancake" heart.
    d) absence of lung markings on the side proximal to the lesion.

91. An elderly woman who complains of headache and jaw claudication with chewing (but not with speech) should be examined to rule out:
    a) osteoma.
    b) giant cell arteritis.
    c) Horner's syndrome.
    d) encephalitis.

92. The most common tumors in the ileum are:
    a) hemangiomas.
    b) leiomyomas.
    c) carcinoid tumors.
    d) carcinomas.

93. Multiple small, round calcifications in the liver may represent:
    a) metastatic carcinoma from the ovaries.
    b) granulomatous infection.
    c) mixed malignant tumor.
    d) cavernous hemangioma.

94. The Ghon tubercle is:
    a) the azygos lobe (created by an anomalous azygos vein).
    b) a coin lesion, caused by a calcified tubercular granuloma.
    c) an apical lung tumor.
    d) a lung abscess.

95. Metastases from the thyroid to the lung are usually:
    a) fairly evenly distributed, small, sharply defined nodules.
    b) solitary, round to oval lesions, > 5 cm diameter.
    c) solitary, cavitating lesions.
    d) multiple, round, cavitating lesions.

96. Encapsulated fluid does not present a radiographic appearance of:
    a) "lava" (no shift of fluid with position change).
    b) pleural thickening elsewhere in the same hemithorax.
    c) an air bronchogram sign.
    d) a "pseudotumor" with convex borders.

97. Carcinoid syndrome is caused by:
    a) irritation of the parasympathetic nerves by a tumor in the gastrointestinal wall.
    b) production of serotonin by malignant, ectopic endocrine cells.
    c) production of corticosteroids by an active tumor in the adrenal cortex.
    d) irritation of the adrenal gland caused by pressure of an adjacent, enlarging tumor.

98. Pneumomediastinum may be seen radiologically as:
    a) a lucent halo around the heart.
    b) an excessively lucent lung area.
    c) round or oval lucent "bubbles" overlying the heart.
    d) vertical linear lucent streaks, outlining or separating mediastinal structures.

99. With normal lungs, PA films performed at full exhalation:
    a) show a heart that appears "pancaked," and lungs that appear less lucent.
    b) show a heart that appears elongated, and lungs that appear less lucent.
    c) show a heart that appears "pancaked," and lungs that appear more lucent.
    d) show a heart that appears elongated, and lungs that appear more lucent.

100. Air-space disease may be indicated on plain film by:
    a) Kerley's lines.
    b) "honeycomb lung".
    c) a "bat-wing" pattern of dense infiltrates, with an air bronchogram sign.
    d) a meniscus sign.

PRACTICE TEST CHAPTER 9—ANSWER KEY

1. a	11. b	21. d	31. a	41. c	51. d	61. b	71. c	81. d	91. b
2. d	12. b	22. b	32. b	42. d	52. b	62. d	72. d	82. d	92. c
3. d	13. a	23. c	33. c	43. a	53. a	63. c	73. a	83. c	93. b
4. a	14. a	24. c	34. c	44. b	54. b	64. d	74. c	84. c	94. b
5. b	15. c	25. c	35. d	45. a	55. d	65. c	75. a	85. d	95. a
6. a	16. b	26. c	36. b	46. a	56. a	66. a	76. d	86. a	96. c
7. b	17. d	27. b	37. c	47. c	57. a	67. b	77. d	87. d	97. b
8. b	18. c	28. d	38. b	48. d	58. a	68. c	78. d	88. c	98. d
9. a	19. c	29. a	39. c	49. d	59. a	69. c	79. c	89. b	99. a
10. d	20. b	30. d	40. c	50. d	60. c	70. b	80. d	90. b	100. c

Test 1

FINAL TEST

The following 600 multiple choice questions are provided as a self-test that covers the material concerning the nine chapters of this study guide. The number of questions concerning the various pathologies is consistent with what we feel may be the weighting most likely to be encountered in your board examinations. These will assist you as you prepare for state and national board examinations in the area of radiology.

1. The symphysis pubis is an example of:
    a) a synarthrosis.
    b) an amphiarthrosis.
    c) a fibrous joint.
    d) an essentially immobile joint.

2. Synovial joints are essentially:
    a) diarthroses.
    b) fibrous.
    c) cartilaginous.
    d) immobile.

3. Inflammation at the site of tendon or ligament insertion into periarticular bone is called:
    a) osteitis.
    b) tendinitis.
    c) enthesopathy.
    d) periostitis.

4. The radiologic hallmark of rheumatoid arthritis at the knee is:
    a) the development of large, subchondral cysts.
    b) peripheral erosions of the intraarticular tibia and femur.
    c) uniform, bicompartmental loss of joint space.
    d) suprapatellar synovial effusion.

5. 75% of cardiac myxomas are:
    a) in the left ventricle.
    b) in the right ventricle.
    c) in the left atrium.
    d) in the right atrium.

6. An x-ray sign that aids in differentiation of parosteal sarcoma from a sessile osteochondroma is:

   a) the parosteal sarcoma is usually diaphyseal.
   b) the parosteal sarcoma points toward the joint.
   c) the parosteal sarcoma points away from the joint.
   d) the parosteal sarcoma has a "cleavage plane" between the normal bone and the neoplasm.

7. Hereditary multiple exostosis (HME):

   a) spares the knees.
   b) spares the hands.
   c) spares the elbows.
   d) spares the shoulders.

8. The most common skeletal locations for hemangiomas are in the:

   a) neural arch of the spine and occiput.
   b) vertebral body and the frontal bone.
   c) neural arch of the spine and the frontal bone.
   d) vertebral body and the occiput.

9. An "open fracture" is the term now used for the injury that was once called:

   a) a comminuted fracture.
   b) a butterfly fragment.
   c) a compound fracture.
   d) a simple fracture.

10. The hematoma at a fracture site:

    a) is normally resorbed during the first two or three days of healing.
    b) is gradually replaced by granulation tissue.
    c) hastens necrosis at the site and may delay healing.
    d) may be expected to continue increasing in size for up to ten days.

11. Inhalation of airborne fragments of hyphae is the usual route of infection with:

    a) actinomycosis.
    b) coccidioidomycosis.
    c) schistosomiasis.
    d) aspergillosis.

12. A minimum radiographic study after cervical trauma should include:

    a) an AP open mouth, AP lower cervical, and a lateral projection.
    b) an AP open mouth, AP lower cervical, lateral and swimmer's lateral projections.
    c) an AP cervical, left and right obliques, and a lateral projection.
    d) an AP open mouth, AP lower cervical, left and right obliques, and a lateral projection.

13. An infection that mimics osteoid osteoma, with pain worse at night and relieved by aspirin, is:

    a) Pott's puffy tumor.
    b) Garré's sclerosing osteomyelitis.
    c) Brodie's abscess.
    d) childhood inflammatory discitis.

14. The majority of metastatic tumors in the lungs are from:

    a) gastrointestinal tract.
    b) ovarian carcinoma.
    c) primary lung, breast or lymphatic tumors.
    d) primary uterine, cervical, or pancreatic tumors.

15. A male in his late teens with back pain, radiologically evident spondyloarthritis and "pear-shaped" vertebrae, is likely to have a diagnosis of:

    a) spondyloepiphyseal dysplasia tarda.
    b) Ehlers-Danlos syndrome.
    c) Hurler's syndrome.
    d) osteopetrosis.

16. A patient with pectus excavatum, agenesis of the radius, and Sprengel's deformity may be suspected to have:

    a) achondroplasia.
    b) Morquio's syndrome.
    c) Holt-Oram syndrome.
    d) massive osteolysis of Gorham.

17. The dense zone of provisional calcification seen in the metaphysis of long bones of patients with scurvy is called:

    a) Wimberger's sign of scurvy.
    b) scorbutic zone.
    c) the white line of Frankel.
    d) the Trummerfeld zone.

18. For optimal viewing of the heart and great vessels, the oblique projection to use is:

    a) an LAO with the patient rotated 45°.
    b) an RAO with the patient rotated 45°.
    c) an LAO with the patient rotated 30°.
    d) an LPO with the patient rotated 30°.

19. Cytomegalovirus may cause:

    a) lesions similar to shingles in adult patients.
    b) cardiomegaly in neonates.
    c) interstitial pneumonia in neonates and immunosuppressed adults.
    d) lesions similar to "cannon ball metastasis" in immunosuppressed adults.

20. Eisenstein's method is:

    a) used for evaluating lumbosacral instability.
    b) a means of evaluating lumbar stenosis.
    c) used with frontal films to evaluate interpediculate distance.
    d) significant in determining facet imbrication.

21. Pauciarticular lesions refer specifically to those involving:

    a) a single joint.
    b) two or more joints.
    c) two to four joints.
    d) more than four joints.

22. Rheumatoid arthritis, ankylosing spondylitis, psoriatic arthritis, and scleroderma are all:

    a) seronegative arthritides.
    b) inflammatory arthritides.
    c) positive for RA factor.
    d) degenerative arthritides.

23. Osteophytes at the hip, caused by osteoarthritis, usually are found:

    a) at the superolateral surface of the greater trochanter.
    b) at the superolateral acetabular rim.
    c) at the superomedial surface of the lesser trochanter.
    d) at the inferolateral acetabular rim.

24. An encapsulated pseudotumor within the potential space between viseral and parietal pleura is caused by:
    a) transudative effusion.
    b) exudative effusion.
    c) free pleural effusion.
    d) loculated effusion.

25. The most significant feature of hereditary multiple exostosis (HME) is:
    a) the incidence of cord compression with neurologic symptoms.
    b) the incidence of fracture of the lesions.
    c) the incidence of subluxation of the radioulnar joints.
    d) the incidence of malignant degeneration.

26. Distinctive multiple osteomas, which appear as dense, protuberant, oval masses attached to bone cortices, are seen in:
    a) Ollier's disease.
    b) Gardner's syndrome.
    c) Maffucci's syndrome.
    d) Kahler's disease.

27. In the appendicular skeleton, osteoblastoma is most often seen:
    a) in the small, tubular bones of the hands and feet.
    b) in the shoulder girdle.
    c) in the distal tibia and fibula and in the calcaneous.
    d) around the knee and the hip.

28. The clinical significance of a non-ossifying fibroma (NOF) or a fibrous cortical defect (FCD) lies in:
    a) their propensity for malignant degeneration.
    b) their tendency to produce vague systemic effects, such as malaise and low-grade fever.
    c) their tendency to produce painful, warm, local swelling.
    d) their tendency to weaken bone, making it vulnerable to pathologic fracture.

29. Lobar enlargement, an air bronchogram sign, and a bulged fissure (away from the involved lobe), are radiologic indications of:
    a) atelectasis.
    b) lymphangitic spread of metastatic lesions.
    c) lobar pneumonia.
    d) interstitial bacterial pneumonia.

30. In fracture healing, there is a cellular phase during which:
    a) a vascular spindle forms in the vascular "swamp" of the injured area.
    b) the hematoma at the injury site should not be disturbed.
    c) the primary callus develops.
    d) cartilage begins to form within the primary callus.

31. Potentially fatal pulmonary emboli caused by deep vein thrombosis is facilitated by:
    a) inadequate stabilization of the fracture.
    b) early weight-bearing after fracture.
    c) immobilization and bed rest after fracture.
    d) inappropriate casting after fracture.

32. In the thoracic spine, the most frequent fracture site is:
    a) T1.
    b) T4–6.
    c) T9.
    d) T11–12.

33. The most common cause of a mass in the middle mediastinum is:
    a) a lymphoma.
    b) a teratoma.
    c) a pericardial cyst.
    d) a substernal thyroid.

34. Bilateral, painless joint swellings in children with congenital syphilis are called:
    a) Charcot's joints.
    b) Chopart's joints.
    c) Clutton's joints.
    d) Cruveilhier's joints.

35. Infantile cortical hyperostosis tends to:
    a) spare the epiphyses.
    b) affect the tarsals.
    c) affect the phalanges.
    d) be asymptomatic until the child begins weight bearing.

36. Occipital vertebrae that tend to limit upper cervical lateral flexion are:
    a) paracondylar process.
    b) epitransverse process.
    c) condylus tertius.
    d) os odontoideum.

37. The radiographic appearance of scurvy includes a lucent band immediately beneath the white line of Frankel. This lucency is called:
    a) a growth arrest line.
    b) the scorbutic zone.
    c) the zone of provisional calcification.
    d) umbau zonen.

38. The trachea and esophagus are considered to be structures of:
    a) the anterior mediastinum.
    b) the middle mediastinum.
    c) the posterior mediastinum.
    d) the inferior mediastinum.

39. The anode heel effect causes:
    a) the beam to be weaker at the cathode end.
    b) the beam to be weaker at the anode end.
    c) the beam to be stronger at the anode end.
    d) both a and c are correct.

40. To visualize the extreme apex of the lungs:
    a) use an apical lordotic view.
    b) use an overpenetrated PA projection.
    c) use an underpenetrated PA projection.
    d) use an overpenetrated AP projection.

41. Actinomycosis, though classed as a fungal infection, is caused by:
    a) a virus.
    b) a parasite.
    c) Gram-positive bacteria.
    d) inflammatory inhalants.

42. There is a clear correlation between thymomas and:
    a) rheumatoid arthritis.
    b) Grave's disease.
    c) myasthenia gravis.
    d) Horner's syndrome.

43. In cases of systemic lupus erythematosus, osteonecrosis occurs most commonly:

    a) in the proximal tibia.
    b) at the talar dome.
    c) in the distal femur.
    d) in the femoral and humeral heads.

44. The "dagger sign" seen with ankylosing spondylitis is caused by:

    a) ossification of the posterior longitudinal ligament.
    b) ossification of the anterior longitudinal ligament.
    c) ossification of the supraspinous and interspinous ligaments.
    d) ossification of the outer annular fibers of the disc.

45. With focal giantism caused by elephantiasis neuromatosa occurring with neurofibromatosis, the affected bone:

    a) becomes deformed and symmetrically enlarged.
    b) undergoes fusiform enlargement.
    c) retains its normal shape.
    d) becomes deformed and asymmetrically enlarged.

46. Polyostotic fibrous dysplasia with endocrinopathy causing precocious sexual development is called:

    a) Turner's syndrome.
    b) Gardner's syndrome.
    c) Maffucci's syndrome.
    d) McCune-Albright syndrome.

47. The primary neuroblastoma lesion is most frequently located:

    a) in the adrenal gland.
    b) in the posterior mediastinum.
    c) in the pituitary gland.
    d) in the paravertebral sympathetic ganglionic chain.

48. The radiographic appearance of fibrosarcoma usually includes:

    a) thickened, expanded cortices.
    b) fluffy, punctate, or broken-ring calcifications in the lesion matrix.
    c) an associated huge soft tissue mass.
    d) spiculated or onion-skin periosteal reaction.

49. Prussian's disease is an example of:

    a) stress fracture.
    b) post-traumatic myositis ossificans.
    c) CPPD.
    d) hypertrophic callus formation.

50. When performing chest films for soft tissue imaging:

    a) mAs settings should be raised for better lung detail.
    b) kVp settings should be lower than for skeletal imaging.
    c) kVp settings should be the same as for skeletal imaging.
    d) kVp should be 120 or higher.

51. A stroke or a brachial plexus lesion might result in:

    a) inferior glenohumeral joint dislocation.
    b) partial inferior displacement of the glenohumeral joint.
    c) elevation of the shoulder caused by unopposed force of the trapezius.
    d) internal rotation of the humerus caused by unopposed force of the pectoralis major.

52. Osgood-Schlatter's disease may predispose a young athlete to:

    a) avulsion of the inferior pole of the patella.
    b) tibial tuberosity avulsion.
    c) osteochondritis dissecans.
    d) Pelligrini-Stieda disease.

53. A radiologic sign typical of simple silicosis is:

   a) enlarged hilar and mediastinal nodes with "eggshell calcification."
   b) confluent nodules, > 1 cm in diameter.
   c) an emphysematous area of lung surrounding nodules.
   d) "ground glass" appearance of diffuse airspace disease.

54. Patients with sarcoidosis frequently show "Garland's Triad":

   a) involvement of the lung apices, the lingula, and the right middle lobe.
   b) enlargement of hilar, azygos, and right paratracheal lymph nodes.
   c) right paratracheal node enlargement, right middle lobe involvement, and right hilar node involvement.
   d) symmetric bilateral hilar node enlargement, right middle lobe involvement, and bilateral paratracheal node enlargement.

55. A fabella is:

   a) an ununited chip fracture from the lateral femoral condyle.
   b) a sesamoid bone in the lateral tendon of the gastrocnemius.
   c) a small sesamoid bone in the gracilis tendon.
   d) a sesamoid bone in the semitendinosus tendon.

56. The most common consequence of blunt chest injury is:

   a) pneumothorax.
   b) rib fracture.
   c) atelectasis.
   d) lung contusion.

57. In infants, the radiologic signs of "small epiphyses," "sail vertebra," and wormian bones are indicative of:

   a) a hyperactive thyroid.
   b) a hypoactive thyroid.
   c) an anterior pituitary tumor.
   d) severe renal pathology.

58. Lung abscess shows a predilection for:

   a) upper lobe anterior segments.
   b) the right lower lobe superior segment.
   c) the lung apices.
   d) the lower lung fields.

59. The zone of provisional calcification:

   a) is at the junction of the physis and metaphysis.
   b) contains layers of cartilage in the process of maturation.
   c) produces lengthwise bone growth.
   d) is seen on x-ray as a lucent band.

60. The "forward S" sign (on a lateral chest projection) is caused by:

   a) aortic coarctation.
   b) a substernal thyroid.
   c) major fissure posterior displacement with left lower lobe collapse.
   d) aortic aneurysm.

61. Young females with non-Hodgkin lymphoma commonly develop:

   a) rib lesions.
   b) prominent mediastinal-hilar node involvement.
   c) localized, cutaneous lymphomas.
   d) elliptical pleural plaques.

62. Late radiologic signs of lumbar degenerative joint disease include:

   a) vacuum cleft of Knuttson.
   b) retrolisthesis.
   c) loss of intersegmental motion.
   d) anterior lipping.

63. Groups of dense, round nodules in the periphery of the apical lungs is a typical radiologic sign of:

    a) silicosis.
    b) coccidioidomycosis.
    c) Caplan's disease.
    d) asbestosis.

64. A "button hole" rupture at the proximal interphalangeal joint (seen with RA) causes:

    a) flexion of the PIP in a "swan-neck" deformity.
    b) extension of the PIP in a "swan-neck" deformity.
    c) flexion of the PIP in a "boutonniere" deformity.
    d) extension of the PIP in a "boutonniere" deformity.

65. Hemangiomas in the spine are usually:

    a) in thoracolumbar vertebral bodies.
    b) in the cervical vertebral bodies.
    c) in the neural arch of the upper lumbar vertebrae.
    d) in the cervicothoracic vertebral bodies.

66. A "target calcification" is:

    a) an area of sequestered bone in a Brodie's abscess.
    b) the nidus of an osteoid osteoma.
    c) a secondary ossification center in a vertebra, such as an apophysis.
    d) a fleck of calcium within a mature nidus in an osteoid osteoma.

67. In the ilium, chondroblastoma has a marked predilection for:

    a) the iliac crest apophysis.
    b) the posterior superior iliac spine apophysis.
    c) the anterior superior iliac spine apophysis.
    d) the triradiate cartilage.

68. Thoracic aortic dissection:

    a) shows a predilection for hypertensive females.
    b) shows a predilection for hypertensive males.
    c) shows a predilection for athletes who engage in strenuous contact sports.
    d) shows no gender predilection, but is associated with hypertension.

69. The horizontal fissure:

    a) separates the right lower lobe from the middle and upper lobes.
    b) separates the left upper lobe from the lingula and lower lobe.
    c) separates the right upper lobe from the middle lobe.
    d) separates the left lower lobe from the lingula and upper lobe.

70. Three sub-phases of fracture healing included in the inflammatory or circulatory phase are:

    a) the exudative phase, the circulatory phase, and the callus phase.
    b) the hematoma phase, the clot phase, and the callus phase.
    c) the cellular phase, the vascular phase, and the primary callus phase.
    d) the cellular phase, the granulation tissue phase, and the primary callus phase.

71. A vertebral body "burst fracture" is:

    a) an unstable fracture.
    b) the result of extreme lateral flexion forces.
    c) a pathologic fracture.
    d) indicative of osteoporosis.

72. In the lumbar spine, a posterior limbus bone:
    a) is frequently seen in osteoporotic, geriatric patients.
    b) is most commonly caused by traction avulsion during traumatic hyperflexion.
    c) is usually caused by gymnastics, weight lifting, or significant trauma in a young person.
    d) is almost always an asymptomatic, incidental finding.

73. Chronic osteomyelitis appears on x-ray as:
    a) sclerotic bone with thickened cortex, periosteal new bone, and lytic destruction with dense sequestra.
    b) dense, sclerotic lesions in cancellous bone.
    c) lytic cortical lesions with laminated periosteal new bone and a dense sclerotic rind.
    d) aggressively expansile lytic lesions, which do not disrupt the cortex nor cause formation of periosteal new bone.

74. In Stage II of sarcoidosis, one might expect the radiologic appearance of:
    a) hilar lymphadenopathy with normal lung fields.
    b) pulmonary lesions without hilar lymphadenopathy.
    c) pulmonary lesions and hilar lymphadenopathy.
    d) normal-appearing plain films.

75. Atlantoaxial instability often is a feature of:
    a) Marfan's syndrome.
    b) cleidocranial dysplasia.
    c) achondroplasia.
    d) spondyloepiphyseal dysplasia tarda.

76. The flowing candle wax appearance of melorheostosis is:
    a) seen only in adult patients.
    b) usually periosteal in adult patients.
    c) the cause of increased limb length in young patients.
    d) most frequently seen in the upper limbs.

77. "Plate-like atelectasis" is described as:
    a) Fleischner lines.
    b) round atelectasis.
    c) middle lobe syndrome.
    d) central atelectasis.

78. The silhouette sign is caused by:
    a) a lesion of water density in anatomic contact with the heart, aorta, or diaphragm.
    b) an enlarged heart.
    c) atelectasis.
    d) pneumothorax.

79. The oblique fissure is:
    a) the minor fissure of the left lung.
    b) the major fissure of the right lung.
    c) the horizontal fissure of the right lung.
    d) the minor fissure of the right lung.

80. A lateral skull projection enables the clinician to use all of the following except:
    a) Macrae's line.
    b) biventor line.
    c) Chamberlain's line.
    d) sphenobasilar angle.

81. Pulmonary embolism:

    a) has no radiologic signs, and requires a VQ scan to demonstrate it.

    b) is seen as a "truncated cone" opacity, usually in the lung apex.

    c) is seen as "Hampton's hump" in the peripheral lung.

    d) is seen as a round or ovoid opacity near the hilum.

82. The clinical presentations of CPPD vary widely, but the most common is designated:

    a) Type A, pseudogout.

    b) Type B, pseudorheumatoid.

    c) Type C, pseudoosteoarthritis.

    d) Type F, pseudoneuropathy.

83. Thin, faint lines about 1–3 cm long that form a "stepladder" pattern in the lateral lung bases, are called:

    a) "spiderweb" lung.

    b) Kerley's A lines.

    c) "honeycomb" lung.

    d) Kerley's B lines.

84. The appearance of an enlarged hilar lymph node with an ipsilateral peripheral Ghon tubercle is called:

    a) a tubercular granuloma.

    b) a Pancoast syndrome.

    c) a Rhanke complex.

    d) Kerley's complex.

85. The most common primary malignancy of the lungs is:

    a) alveolar cell carcinoma.

    b) argentaffinoma (carcinoid).

    c) bronchoalveolar carcinoma

    d) bronchogenic carcinoma.

86. The typical radiologic appearance of polyostotic fibrous dysplasia in the ribs is:

    a) a mildly expansile, lesion < 3 cm or less in length.

    b) a nonexpansile, long, loculated lucency.

    c) a grossly expansile, loculated, lesion > 4 cm in length.

    d) a mildly expansile, short, (< 3 cm) "ground glass" lesion.

87. Atelectasis is:

    a) a punctured lung.

    b) a lung with fluid-filled air spaces.

    c) a collapsed, airless lung.

    d) a lung shifted out of its normal position.

88. The great majority of bone lesions of Hodgkin lymphoma are:

    a) lytic.

    b) sclerotic, with no periosteal response.

    c) sclerotic, with an "onion-skin" periosteal response.

    d) mixed lytic/sclerotic lesions with a periosteal response.

89. Clinical signs such as retinal hemorrhages and localized traumatic alopecia may indicate:

    a) drug abuse.

    b) Münchausen's disease.

    c) nonaccidental trauma.

    d) subdural hemorrhage.

90. The most commonly fractured carpal bone is:

    a) the lunate.

    b) the scaphoid.

    c) the capitate.

    d) the hamate.

91. SLAP lesions are:

    a) facial bone fractures.
    b) anterior to posterior tears of the glenoid labrum.
    c) perilunate dislocations.
    d) tears of the metacarpophalangeal ligaments.

92. Barrett's metaplasia is:

    a) development of metaplastic epithelium around the cervix.
    b) development of metaplastic epithelium in the ileum.
    c) development of metaplastic epithelium in the lower esophagus.
    d) development of metaplastic epithelium in the bladder.

93. Bilateral, symmetric pleural plaques up to 10 mm thick may be seen in the lower thorax of patients with:

    a) pleurisy.
    b) lobar pneumonia.
    c) hemothorax (TB).
    d) asbestosis.

94. The radiologic appearance of Osgood-Schlatter's disease may be simulated by:

    a) an aneurysmal bone cyst.
    b) a nonossifying fibroma.
    c) a normal immature tibial tuberosity.
    d) Ewing's sarcoma.

95. Pitt's pits appear on x-ray as:

    a) lucencies in the proximal humeral head.
    b) lucencies in the greater tuberosity of the humerus.
    c) lucencies in the greater trochanter of the femur.
    d) lucencies in the femoral neck.

96. The most common anomaly of the chest wall is:

    a) pectus excavatum.
    b) pectus carinatum.
    c) Srb's anomaly.
    d) Luschka's bifurcated rib.

97. A "coin lesion" is:

    a) an eosinophilic granuloma.
    b) a "silver dollar vertebra."
    c) a form of histiocytosis X.
    d) a solitary pulmonary nodule.

98. Peripheral atelectasis may be caused by all of the following except:

    a) aortic aneurysm.
    b) chest wall trauma.
    c) emphysema.
    d) loss of surfactant.

99. Parathormone:

    a) induces protein anabolism.
    b) serum levels drop with increased osteoclastic activity.
    c) is produced in the anterior pituitary gland.
    d) promotes calcium resorption from bone.

100. The apical lordotic projection is made:

    a) with the patient leaning backwards to press head, neck, and upper thoracic spine against the bucky.
    b) with the patient standing upright, and a 45° cephalic tube tilt.
    c) with the patient standing upright, and a 15° cephalic tube tilt.
    d) with the patient leaning forward, pressing the anterior shoulders and upper chest to the bucky, and the head turned away from the side of interest.

101. Typical lesions of metabolic arthritides appear on radiographs as:

    a) poorly defined erosions with osteopenic subarticular bone.
    b) sclerotic subarticular bone with poorly defined erosions.
    c) symmetrically distributed, poorly defined erosions with osteophytic growth.
    d) sharply defined erosions in asymmetric distribution.

102. Early radiologic signs of lumbar degenerative joint disease include:

    a) the vacuum cleft of Knuttson.
    b) loss of intersegmental motion.
    c) severe disc space diminution.
    d) vertebral body displacement.

103. A radiographic sign typically seen in cases of erosive osteoarthritis (EOA) is:

    a) the overhanging margin sign.
    b) the gull wings sign.
    c) the mouse ears sign.
    d) the pencil in cup sign.

104. The spinal area most commonly affected by diffuse idiopathic skeletal hyperostosis is:

    a) the cervical spine.
    b) the upper thoracic area.
    c) the lower thoracic area.
    d) the lumbar spine.

105. The "spotty carpal sign," "zig-zag deformity," and ulnar styloid erosion are radiologic signs all associated with:

    a) erosive osteoarthritis (EOA).
    b) rheumatoid arthritis (RA).
    c) Reiter's syndrome.
    d) gout.

106. Cavernous hemangiomas are most commonly found in:

    a) flat bones.
    b) metaphyses of long bones.
    c) epiphyses of long bones.
    d) the spine and skull.

107. The classic clinical picture for osteoid osteoma is:

    a) an elderly female with spinal pain that is worse at night and is relieved by aspirin.
    b) an adolescent male with anterior knee pain that is worse after strenuous athletic activity.
    c) a young male (< 25 years) with a painful, tender swelling that is worse at night and relieved by aspirin.
    d) a young, obese female, with hip pain that is worse with weight-bearing activity.

108. Codman's tumor is the eponym given to:

    a) an osteoblastoma.
    b) a periosteal chondroma.
    c) a chondroblastoma.
    d) a fibrous xanthoma of bone.

109. The most common cause of death in multiple myeloma patients is:

    a) kidney failure.
    b) respiratory failure (with pneumonia).
    c) cardiac failure.
    d) pulmonary embolism.

110. Depressed fractures and compression fractures are sub-types of:

    a) occult fractures.
    b) stress fractures.
    c) comminuted fractures.
    d) impaction fractures.

111. Volkmann's contracture may ensue if the pressure of edema and hemorrhage after fracture become too great in the:

    a) anterior tibial compartment.
    b) anterior forearm.
    c) adductor canal.
    d) inguinal canal.

112. Avulsion of the anteroinferior vertebral body of a cervical vertebra results in:

    a) a nuchal bone.
    b) an intercalary bone.
    c) a teardrop fracture.
    d) narrowed interlaminar and interspinous spaces, as shown on a lateral view.

113. A dysplastic spondylolisthesis is distinguished from other spondylolistheses by the fact that it:

    a) never involves progressive slippage.
    b) usually exists as a solitary, isolated anomaly.
    c) does not involve pars defects.
    d) is usually identified in newborns.

114. Periostitis caused by osteomyelitis is especially exuberant in:

    a) neonates.
    b) toddlers and young school-aged children.
    c) children entering puberty.
    d) young adults who have just attained full bone growth.

115. Tuberculous dactylitis gives a characteristic radiographic appearance described as:

    a) Pott's puffy tumor.
    b) Pitt's pits.
    c) spina ventosa.
    d) caries sicca.

116. The "thumb sign" is sometimes used to suggest a diagnosis of:

    a) achondroplasia.
    b) Morquio's syndrome.
    c) Marfan's syndrome.
    d) nail-patella syndrome.

117. Albers-Schönberg's disease is an eponym for:

    a) osteopoikilosis.
    b) osteogenesis imperfecta.
    c) osteopetrosis.
    d) osteopathia striata.

118. Menopause accelerates bone loss in the female lumbar spine to a rate of as much as:

    a) 3% per year.
    b) 4% per year.
    c) 5% per year.
    d) 6% per year.

119. The amount of radiation a patient receives:

    a) varies directly with the distance from the beam source.
    b) varies inversely with the distance from the beam source.
    c) varies inversely with the square of the distance from the beam source.
    d) varies inversely with the square of the time of exposure.

120. Water's projection is taken:

    a) anteroposterior.
    b) with the forehead and nose tip against the bucky.
    c) with a 15° caudal tube tilt.
    d) with slight cervical extension.

121. Pigmented villonodular synovitis (PVNS) is essentially:

    a) a hereditary condition.
    b) an idiopathic degeneration of hyaline cartilage.
    c) an idiopathic degeneration of fibrocartilage.
    d) an idiopathic inflammation of synovium.

122. The Kayser-Fleischer ring, hematuria, psychoses, incoordination, and grossly inappropriate behaviors are seen in the clinical presentation of:

    a) hemochromatosis.
    b) Wilson's disease.
    c) tuberous sclerosis.
    d) Ehlers-Danlos syndrome.

123. The most common site of spinal involvement in gouty arthritis is:

    a) the cervical spine.
    b) the upper thoracic spine.
    c) the thoracolumbar spine.
    d) the lumbosacral spine.

124. Spinal involvement in Reiter's syndrome may result in the formation of:

    a) asymmetrically distributed thick, nonmarginal syndesmophytes.
    b) symmetrical, bilateral non-marginal syndesmophytes.
    c) symmetrical, bilateral marginal syndesmophytes.
    d) asymmetrical, often unilateral, marginal syndesmophytes.

125. The most common distribution of polyostotic fibrous dysplasia is:

    a) bilateral but asymmetric.
    b) cranial-facial, with monomelic limb involvement.
    c) spinal with limb involvement.
    d) cranial-facial with spinal involvement.

126. "Hourglass" enlargement of a cervical intervertebral foramina is likely caused by:

    a) an anomalous, tortuous vertebral artery.
    b) fibroma molluscum of neurofibromatosis.
    c) CSF pulsations with dural ectasia.
    d) a dumbbell neurofibroma from a spinal nerve root.

127. Malignant degeneration of pagetic bone most commonly involves:

    a) chondrosarcoma.
    b) giant cell tumor.
    c) osteosarcoma.
    d) fibrosarcoma.

128. The most consistent symptom of a spheno-occipital chordoma is:

    a) ataxia.
    b) hemiparesis.
    c) headache.
    d) blurred vision, dizziness, and tinnitus.

129. A very sensitive, but not specific, means of imaging occult stress fractures is:

    a) MRI.
    b) contrast CT.
    c) scintigraphy.
    d) underpenetrated plain films.

130. The "pie sign" is a radiologic indication of:

    a) scaphoid fracture.
    b) pisiform fracture.
    c) lunate dislocation.
    d) perilunate dislocation.

131. One of the best radiographic indications of an occult elbow fracture is:

    a) the FBI sign.
    b) a positive fat-pad sign.
    c) articular distention and increased width of joint spaces.
    d) malalignment.

132. Healing of a middle clavicle fracture often features extensive callus formation caused by:

    a) hyperemia due to extensive soft tissue damage in the area.
    b) malalignment and/or overlap of the proximal and distal fragments.
    c) avascular necrosis of the distal fragment.
    d) inadequate stabilization of the fracture.

133. Van Neck's disease, which radiographically simulates expansile destruction of bone, is really:

    a) ischemic necrosis.
    b) a nonossifying fibroma.
    c) a fibrous cortical defect.
    d) a normal developmental variant.

134. The major differential concern in cases of suspected osteochondritis dissecans is:

    a) avulsion fracture.
    b) degenerative joint disease.
    c) normal growth variants and ossification variations.
    d) infection.

135. A variant called the "third leg syndrome" involves:

    a) an incomplete ilium.
    b) rudimentary femoral head and neck that articulates with the superior pubic ramus.
    c) a rudimentary femoral head and neck that articulates with the inferior pubic ramus.
    d) an incomplete inferior pubic ramus.

136. The appearance of a horizontally oriented lucency at the base of the dens may be caused by:

    a) the central incisor gap.
    b) the Mach effect.
    c) a tongue shadow.
    d) the anterior arch of the atlas.

137. The gouged-out lesions at articular margins, called "bite signs," are typical of:

    a) osteoarthritis.
    b) erosive osteoarthritis.
    c) corticosteroid arthropathy.
    d) psoriatic arthropathy.

138. Psammoma bodies are:

    a) small adrenal cysts.
    b) small ovarian cysts.
    c) discrete calcifications in cystadenocarcinomas.
    d) ovoid lucencies in the bladder wall, seen with neurogenic bladder.

139. An inverted A/G ratio and the presence of Bence Jones proteinuria suggests a diagnosis of:

    a) gout.
    b) RA.
    c) prostate metastasis.
    d) multiple myeloma.

140. Frontal chest films normally are taken:

    a) AP with full inspiration.
    b) PA with full inspiration.
    c) PA with full exhalation.
    d) AP with full exhalation.

141. Periosteum is not present:

    a) at the site of a newly healed fracture.
    b) on intracapsular bone.
    c) on neonatal bone.
    d) at entheses.

142. Irregular loss of acetabular joint space and large supraacetabular subchondral cysts typify:

    a) radiographic findings of early Paget's disease.
    b) radiographic findings of rheumatoid arthritis.
    c) radiographic findings of neurotrophic arthritis.
    d) radiographic findings of osteoarthritis.

143. The best modality for diagnostic imaging of early osteoarthritis of the knee is:

    a) scintigraphy.
    b) arthrography.
    c) MRI.
    d) CT.

144. A diagnosis of Forestier's disease requires flowing hyperostosis at the anterior portions of at least:

    a) two contiguous vertebrae.
    b) three contiguous vertebrae.
    c) four contiguous vertebrae.
    d) five contiguous vertebrae.

145. Hemangioma in the spine as seen on plain film radiographs is most often:

    a) multiple, in contiguous vertebrae.
    b) solitary, and non-expansile.
    c) multiple, in non-contiguous vertebrae.
    d) a single, markedly expansile lesion.

146. Osteoblastoma in the spine is most often found:

    a) in the lumbar vertebral bodies.
    b) in the thoracolumbar neural arches.
    c) in the upper cervical articular processes.
    d) in the thoracic vertebral bodies.

147. Caffey's defect is the eponym for:

    a) a fibrous cortical defect (FCD).
    b) a nonossifying fibroma (NOF).
    c) a periosteal chondroma.
    d) a Hills Sach defect.

148. The most common patellar neoplasm is:

    a) a malignant giant cell tumor.
    b) a benign giant cell tumor.
    c) a benign chondroblastoma.
    d) a benign enchondroma.

149. Greenstick (hickory stick) fractures and torus (buckling) fractures are types of:

   a) incomplete fractures.
   b) stress fractures.
   c) open fractures.
   d) occult fractures.

150. The final stage of healing after the fracture of a long bone is:

   a) the sealing of the marrow cavity from the fractured cortex.
   b) restoration of the medullary cavity and bone marrow.
   c) the remodeling of the callus along stress lines.
   d) buttressing of the cortical ends of the fractured bone by the thickened callus.

151. Among delayed complications of fracture healing, avascular necrosis is most often seen at the:

   a) distal clavicle.
   b) proximal humerus.
   c) proximal tibia.
   d) proximal femur (femoral head).

152. Anatomic composition of the spine at the level of the atlas is described by:

   a) Wolff's law.
   b) Eisenstein's method of sagittal canal measurement.
   c) Steele's Rule of Thirds.
   d) the Hueter-Volkmann principle.

153. The terms *sequestrum, involucrum,* and *cloaca* are commonly used to describe the features of:

   a) parosteal sarcoma.
   b) Paget's disease.
   c) suppurative osteomyelitis.
   d) fibrosarcoma.

154. Calcifications in a paravertebral abscess, sometimes seen with Pott's disease, have the radiographic appearance of:

   a) rings and broken rings.
   b) cotton-wool.
   c) linear streaks.
   d) snowflake pattern.

155. Marfan's syndrome might be expected to affect:

   a) the gastrointestinal, cardiovascular, and auditory systems.
   b) the skeletal, ocular, and cardiovascular systems.
   c) the skeletal, urinary, and central nervous systems.
   d) mentation, reproduction, and circulation.

156. Hurler's syndrome is a mucopolysaccharidosis that is also known as:

   a) chondrodystrophy.
   b) gargoylism.
   c) familial osteodystrophy.
   d) eccentro-osteochondrodysplasia.

157. Generalized osteoporosis may be the result of:

   a) lower limb casting after a long bone fracture.
   b) long-term NSAID therapy.
   c) long-term hormone replacement therapy.
   d) heparin therapy

158. A triangular clump of opacities near the spine at the thoracolumbar junction in a newborn may indicate:

   a) congenital adrenal hydatid cyst.
   b) cystic pheochromocytoma.
   c) Wilms' tumor.
   d) neonatal adrenal hemorrhage.

159. A longer scale on a film:

   a) is related to lower contrast.
   b) is related to higher contrast.
   c) is related to lower kVp settings.
   d) is primarily a function of the mAs setting.

160. When positioned for a cervical flexion lateral projection, the patient should:

   a) first lift the chin, then flex the neck.
   b) first flex the neck, then lift the chin.
   c) first flex the neck, then tuck the chin.
   d) first tuck the chin, then flex the neck.

161. In geriatric patients, the intervertebral discs may have become:

   a) increasingly gelatinous.
   b) fibrocartilaginous medially as well as peripherally.
   c) peripherally less fibrocartilaginous.
   d) peripherally increasingly collagenous.

162. Rheumatoid arthritis is a connective tissue disorder that selectively targets:

   a) synovial tissue.
   b) highly vascularized tissue.
   c) articular cartilage.
   d) fibrocartilage.

163. The most common form of Still's disease is:

   a) polyarticular Still's disease, with a clear male predilection and severe systemic symptoms.
   b) pauciarticular Still's disease, with a slight male predilection and few or no systemic symptoms.
   c) polyarticular Still's disease, with a female predilection and mild systemic manifestations.
   d) classic systemic Still's disease, with no gender predilection and severe systemic manifestations.

164. Dural ectasia with ankylosing spondylitis is linked with:

   a) early ankylosis of the sacroiliac joints.
   b) upper cervical involvement.
   c) cauda equina syndrome.
   d) increased peripheral joint involvement.

165. Osteoma is characterized as:

   a) a benign tumor of cartilaginous bone.
   b) a malignant tumor of cartilaginous bone.
   c) a benign tumor of membranous bone.
   d) a malignant tumor of membranous bone.

166. The margins of a bone island:

   a) usually are smooth and well-defined.
   b) usually are indistinct.
   c) may have a "brush border" of radiating spicules.
   d) usually are incomplete.

167. The typical radiologic appearance of a simple bone cyst (SBC) is:

   a) a bubbly, lucent, long, geographic lesion, wider at its metaphyseal end.
   b) a purely lucent, oval geographic, metadiaphyseal lesion.
   c) a lucent, truncated cone, narrower at its metaphyseal end.
   d) an eccentric, bubbly, lucent lesion with laminated periosteal response.

168. The most frequent skeletal site for primary central osteosarcoma is:

   a) the distal metaphysis of the femur.
   b) the proximal diaphysis of the humerus.

    c) the distal metaphysis of the humerus.
    d) the proximal metaphysis of the femur.

169. A "banana fracture" is:

    a) the bent torus fracture with no cortical disruption.
    b) the transverse pathologic fracture seen in Paget's disease.
    c) the fracture of the distal digits of the hands or feet.
    d) a fracture at the distal femoral condyle, seen in fibrous dysplasia.

170. Arterial rupture accompanying a fracture is most commonly seen at the:

    a) femoral artery.
    b) popliteal artery.
    c) radial artery.
    d) brachial artery.

171. Films performed after a head injury should, at a minimum, include:

    a) a lateral skull projection, an AP Towne's, and a PA Caldwell.
    b) a lateral skull projection, an AP Towne's, and an APOM (AP open mouth projection).
    c) a lateral skull projection and a PA Caldwell.
    d) right and left lateral skull projections, an AP Towne's, and a PA Caldwell.

172. Compression fractures at T4–8 are most commonly the result of:

    a) landing shock to parachute jumpers.
    b) high diving injuries.
    c) convulsions or strong electric shocks.
    d) excessive weight lifting.

173. Marjolin's ulcer is a squamous cell carcinoma that develops:

    a) from a duodenal ulcer.
    b) in esophageal varices.
    c) in a colonic diverticula.
    d) in a cloaca, usually in the femur or tibia.

174. Parenchymatous neurosyphilis gives rise to gradual behavior changes, emotional instability, and:

    a) granulomatous lesions called "gummata."
    b) Argyll Robertson pupil.
    c) endarteritis obliterans.
    d) tabes dorsalis.

175. Erlenmeyer flask deformity is common to all of the following except:

    a) Pyle's disease.
    b) sickle cell anemia.
    c) Gaucher's disease.
    d) thalassemia.

176. The "elastic lady" suffers from:

    a) Fong's syndrome.
    b) Ehlers-Danlos syndrome.
    c) tuberous sclerosis.
    d) Marfan's syndrome.

177. General osteoporosis may be seen on plain film characterized by:

    a) endosteal scalloping.
    b) "dot-and-dash" cortical lesions.
    c) thin cortices with reduced marrow cavity size.
    d) onion-skin laminated periosteal response.

178. When the right middle lobe is collapsed:

    a) the silhouette of the left cardiac border is usually obliterated.
    b) the silhouette of the ascending aorta is usually obliterated.
    c) the silhouette of the right hemidiaphragm is usually obliterated.
    d) the silhouette of the right cardiac border is usually obliterated.

179. MRI is the optimal imaging modality for detecting all of the following except:

    a) IVD lesions.
    b) occult cranial fractures.
    c) osseous spinal metastasis.
    d) TMJ derangements.

180. An AP thoracic spine film is preferably taken:

    a) on full expiration.
    b) during respiration.
    c) on full inspiration.
    d) without regard to respiratory phase, but with respiration halted.

181. Intraosseous granulomas of sarcoidosis may create:

    a) both diffuse reticular lesions and localized, well-circumscribed lytic lesions.
    b) a laminated periosteal response.
    c) subchondral sclerosis.
    d) fluffy, ill-defined opacities.

182. deQuervain's disease (stenosing tenosynovitis at the radial styloid) may be related to:

    a) scleroderma.
    b) CPPD.
    c) ochronosis.
    d) HADD.

183. CPPD (calcium pyrophosphate dihydrate crystal deposition disease) has its peak incidence in:

    a) neonates.
    b) adolescents.
    c) adults aged 40 years.
    d) adults aged 60 years.

184. In hypertrophic osteoarthropathy, radionuclide studies show a characteristic:

    a) trolley track sign.
    b) star sign.
    c) thickened cortex sign.
    d) double stripe sign.

185. An asymptomatic posterior mediastinal mass in a patient with neurofibromatosis is most likely to be:

    a) elephantiasis neuromatosa.
    b) intrathoracic meningocele.
    c) fibroma molluscum.
    d) intrathoracic lipoma.

186. Hemangioma may be differentiated radiographically from Paget's disease in the spine because Paget's, and not hemangioma, commonly causes:

    a) squaring of vertebral bodies.
    b) pathologic fractures.
    c) endplate cortical thickening.
    d) vertically striated appearance.

187. Metastatic lesions that are most likely to cause a periosteal response are:

    a) neuroblastoma metastasis in children.
    b) metastases from the kidney into the pelvis.
    c) metastases from the lungs into the hands.
    d) metastases from the cecum into the feet.

188. In most cases, nuclear scanning does not detect:

    a) infection lesions.
    b) osteoblastic lesions.

c) osteoclastic lesions.
d) myeloma lesions.

189. For stress fractures to be detectable on plain films, one should delay filming during a latent period of:

a) 3 to 7 days.
b) 2 to 5 weeks.
c) 10 days to 3 weeks.
d) 2 to 3 months.

190. A radiologic study for possible wrist fracture should, at a minimum, include:

a) neutral PA wrist, PA wrist with ulnar flexion, and lateral wrist projections.
b) neutral PA wrist and lateral wrist projections.
c) neutral PA wrist, oblique wrist, and lateral wrist projections.
d) neutral and ulnar flexion PA wrist, oblique wrist, and lateral wrist projections.

191. A "chisel fracture" is:

a) a comminuted fracture of the humeral head.
b) a comminuted fracture of the radial head.
c) an impaction fracture of the talar dome.
d) an incomplete fracture of the radial head.

192. Dupuytren's fracture differs from Pott's fracture in that:

a) it does not involve diastasis.
b) it involves fracture of the lateral malleolus.
c) it involves fracture of the medial malleolus.
d) it does not involve malleolar fracture.

193. The "silver dollar" ("coin-on-end" or "wafer thin") vertebra of Calvé's disease is a manifestation of:

a) Histiocytosis X.
b) leukemia.
c) Hand-Schüller-Christian disease.
d) Cushing's syndrome.

194. Two major age cohorts subject to Blount's disease are:

a) infants (1–3 years), and geriatric patients (> 70 years).
b) young adults (15–20 years), and geriatric patients (> 70 years).
c) children (3–7 years), and young adults (20–35 years).
d) infants (1–3 years) and adolescents (8–15 years).

195. A calcified Cooper's ligament may be seen:

a) between a supracondylar process and the humeral condyle.
b) between the inferior sacrum and the ischial tuberosity.
c) parallel to the superior line of the pubic bones.
d) between the transverse process of the fifth lumbar vertebra and the posterior superior iliac spine.

196. The "bayonette" appearance caused by a prominent ulnar styloid and posterior subluxation of the distal ulna is characteristic of:

a) a negative ulnar variance.
b) Kirner's deformity.
c) Madelung's deformity.
d) a positive ulnar variance.

197. Cushing's syndrome creates a characteristic radiologic sign in the spine called:

a) the "ghost vertebra."
b) the "marginal condensation" sign.
c) the "empty vertebra."
d) the "butterfly vertebra."

198. Pancreatic carcinoma is associated with:

    a) alcoholism.
    b) diabetes mellitus.
    c) hemosiderosis.
    d) Crohn's disease.

199. The thinning of the cortex is typical of the following processes, except for:

    a) an eccentric, benign tumor.
    b) osteoporosis.
    c) osteoid osteoma.
    d) Brodie's abscess.

200. The lateral wrist projection is optimal for displaying:

    a) the lateral ulnar angle.
    b) lunate malalignment.
    c) the radioulnar angle.
    d) the medial ulnar angle.

201. Rheumatoid arthritis (RA) has a recognized predilection for:

    a) females over the age of 50.
    b) males over the age of 50.
    c) females below the age of 45.
    d) males below the age of 45.

202. Osteoarthritis of the shoulder often is accompanied by calcific tendinitis, most commonly at:

    a) the long head of the biceps insertion into the supraglenoid tuberosity.
    b) the short head of the biceps insertion into the coracoid process.
    c) the supraspinatus insertion into the greater tuberosity.
    d) the infraspinatus insertion into the greater tuberosity.

203. In the lower thoracic spine, DISH does not affect the:

    a) costovertebral joints.
    b) right lateral paravertebral ligaments.
    c) apophyseal joints.
    d) costotransverse joints.

204. The "six Ds" of neurotrophic arthropathy are radiologic signs:

    a) common in non-weight-bearing joints during the atrophic stage of the disease.
    b) common in non-weight-bearing joints during the hypertrophic stage of the disease.
    c) common in weight-bearing joints during the atrophic stage of the disease.
    d) common in weight-bearing joints during the hypertrophic stage of the disease.

205. Osteoma usually is found:

    a) in the small tubular bones of the hands.
    b) in the bones of the face.
    c) in the bones of the pelvis.
    d) in the bones of the spine.

206. About 10% of osteoid osteomas occur in the spine, where they may create the x-ray appearance of:

    a) a "winking owl" sign.
    b) a sclerotic pedicle.
    c) a "soap bubble" spinous process.
    d) a "double spinous" sign.

207. A frequent sign of spinal osteoblastoma, present in more than 50% of cases, is:

    a) loss of the lumbar curve.
    b) loss of the cervical curve.
    c) a gibbus deformity.
    d) a painful scoliosis.

208. The most common skeletal site for solitary enchondroma is in the:

    a) mandible.
    b) hands or feet.
    c) proximal or distal femur and proximal tibia.
    d) humerus.

209. When assessing a fracture, discussion of "alignment" refers to:

    a) the distance between fragments.
    b) the angulation of the proximal fragment in relation to the distal fragment.
    c) the angulation of the distal fragment in relation to the proximal fragment.
    d) the amount of rotation the distal fragment has undergone.

210. Open reduction usually is required to prevent deformity after a:

    a) Salter-Harris Type I fracture.
    b) Salter-Harris Type II fracture.
    c) Salter-Harris Type IV fracture.
    d) Salter-Harris Type V fracture.

211. A luxated joint is one that has:

    a) been dislocated.
    b) suffered a fracture/dislocation.
    c) suffered a diastatic fracture.
    d) suffered an intracapsular fracture.

212. During the metabolic phase of fracture healing, callus performs all of the following functions except:

    a) buttressing the outer cortex of the fractured bone ends.
    b) sealing the marrow from the fracture site.
    c) connecting the cortical ends of the fractured bone.
    d) serving as a template for remodeling of the bone.

213. The earliest radiologic signs of osteomyelitis usually are:

    a) elevation of the adjacent fat pad caused by soft tissue swelling.
    b) periosteal response.
    c) permeative destruction of medullary bone.
    d) cortical erosion or scalloping.

214. Males up to 16 years of age are particularly vulnerable to:

    a) spinal osteomyelitis, especially in the cervical spine.
    b) childhood inflammatory discitis, especially in the lumbar spine.
    c) chronic osteomyelitis, especially in the axial "S" joints (spine, sacroiliac, etc.).
    d) Maduromycosis, especially in the bones of the feet.

215. Massive osteolysis is also known as:

    a) pyknodysostosis.
    b) arthrochalasis multiplex congenita.
    c) vanishing bone disease.
    d) tuberous sclerosis.

216. "Saturn's ring" is normal, white sclera around the cornea in:

    a) the blue sclera of Marfan's disease.
    b) pyknodysostosis.
    c) the blue sclera of osteogenesis imperfecta.
    d) Morquio's disease.

217. Ward's triangle is:

  a) a relatively lucent area in the iliac wing, bounded by weight-bearing and tensile trabeculae.
  b) a relatively lucent area in the femoral neck, bounded by weight-bearing and tensile trabeculae.
  c) a relatively opaque area in the humeral head where the major stress-bearing trabeculae converge.
  d) a relatively opaque area just medial to Kohler's teardrop, where weight-bearing trabeculae converge.

218. The spleen may be homogeneously opacified by:

  a) hemochromatosis.
  b) granulomatous infections.
  c) metastatic carcinoma from the ovary.
  d) *Echinococcus granulosus* cysts.

219. Myelography:

  a) indicates the specific location of a lesion within the spinal canal.
  b) indicates the specific nature of a spinal lesion.
  c) indicates whether a spinal tumor is benign or malignant.
  d) indicates clinically significant activity of a spinal lesion.

220. Hadley's "S" curve may be used when evaluating:

  a) a lateral lumbar spine projection.
  b) both AP lumbar and oblique lumbar projections.
  c) only an AP lumbar projection.
  d) only an oblique lumbar projection.

221. The relative probability of facet imbrication may be evaluated with:

  a) Shenton's line.
  b) Macnab's line.
  c) McGregor's line.
  d) Macrae's line.

222. Arc and ring calcification is most characteristic of:

  a) lesions with a fatty matrix.
  b) lesions with a cartilaginous matrix.
  c) lesions with an osseous matrix.
  d) lesions with a fibrous matrix.

223. The development of a scoliosis may indicate:

  a) collapse of an entire lung.
  b) middle lobe syndrome.
  c) left upper lobe collapse.
  d) left lower lobe collapse.

224. An anterior pituitary neoplasm may cause:

  a) primary Cushing's disease.
  b) secondary Cushing's disease.
  c) Grave's disease.
  d) secondary hyperparathyroidism.

225. Limbus bones:

  a) usually are imbedded within the nuchal ligament.
  b) represent nonunion of secondary ossification centers from vertebral endplates.
  c) are ossicles seen near posterior vertebral body margins.
  d) are ossicles seen near the zygapophyseal joints.

226. The "thumbnail sign" in the aortic arch is an indication of:

  a) anomalous arterial formation.
  b) a dissecting aneurysm.
  c) a saccular aneurysm.
  d) atherosclerosis.

227. Calvé's disease is:

    a) an avascular necrosis.
    b) an eosinophilic granuloma.
    c) a bacterial infection in the vertebral body.
    d) erosion of the vertebral body by a neuroma.

228. Hawkin's sign is:

    a) a curvilinear subchondral lucency indicating collapse of the articular surface of the femoral head.
    b) a ADI that increases > 5 mm with anterior cervical flexion.
    c) a subarticular lucent band in the talar dome.
    d) a sclerotic transverse metaphyseal line in the distal tibia.

229. The most common site of stress fracture in the entire skeleton is:

    a) the calcaneous.
    b) the second and third metatarsals.
    c) the tibial metaphysis (proximal).
    d) the pars interarticularis.

230. The "Terry Thomas sign" may be indicative of:

    a) a scaphoid fracture with avascular necrosis.
    b) a scaphoid fracture with nonunion.
    c) a scaphoid fracture with scapholunate dissociation.
    d) a perilunate dislocation.

231. The optimal view for evaluation of the scaphoid is:

    a) the oblique wrist.
    b) the neutral PA wrist.
    c) the lateral wrist.
    d) the PA wrist with ulnar deviation.

232. Radiologic indications of posterior glenohumeral joint dislocation include:

    a) altered humeral head shape, hatchet defect, and Bankart lesion.
    b) Hill-Sachs lesion, altered humeral head shape, and vacant glenoid sign.
    c) trough sign, rim sign, and vacant glenoid sign.
    d) inferior humeral displacement, Bankart lesion, and "tennis racquet" appearance of the humeral head.

233. With neurofibromatosis in the spine, vertebral body scalloping is:

    a) caused by a dumbbell neurofibroma usually is posterocentral, and at multiple levels.
    b) caused by dural ectasia usually is unilateral and eccentric, at multiple levels.
    c) caused by dural ectasia usually is unilateral and eccentric, at a single level.
    d) caused by dural ectasia usually is posterocentral and at multiple levels.

234. When pagetic bone is seen on an x-ray, the skeleton is best surveyed for additional sites of involvement:

    a) by a series of 10 plain films.
    b) by bone scan.
    c) by CT scan.
    d) by MRI.

235. There is a clear geographic pattern in the incidence of Paget's disease, with occurrence most prevalent in:

    a) Canada and the northern United States.
    b) Asia and Africa.
    c) Scandinavia and South America.
    d) the United Kingdom, Australia, and New Zealand.

236. The most common cause of the radiographic "extrapleural sign" is:
    a) bronchogenic carcinoma.
    b) occult rib fracture.
    c) sessile osteochondroma.
    d) metastatic tumor.

237. Perivascular granulomas of sarcoidosis, infiltrating the Haversian canals, give:
    a) the radiographic appearance of geographic lesions.
    b) the radiographic appearance of blastic metastases.
    c) the radiographic appearance of a "lacelike" trabecular pattern.
    d) the radiographic appearance of an aggressive malignancy.

238. Young adult females are predilected by:
    a) gout.
    b) scleroderma.
    c) pseudogout (CPPD).
    d) Reiter's syndrome.

239. The most common skeletal site of arthritis caused by ochronosis is:
    a) the hips and knees.
    b) the shoulders and elbows.
    c) the spine.
    d) the wrists and hands.

240. One of the earliest radiographic signs of osteoarthritis of the knee is:
    a) sharpening of the tibial eminences.
    b) erosion of the tibial eminences.
    c) joint mice.
    d) chondrocalcinosis.

241. Possibly related to calcifying tendinitis, Pellegrini-Stieda disease is:
    a) the formation of a fabella.
    b) a post-traumatic calcification in the iliotibial band.
    c) calcification in the quadriceps tendon at the patella.
    d) post-traumatic calcification in the medial collateral ligament of the knee.

242. Baastrup's syndrome is a synonym for:
    a) anterolisthesis.
    b) hemispheric spondylosclerosis.
    c) Napoleon hat sign.
    d) kissing spinous sign.

243. A "SLAC deformity" refers to:
    a) hypermobility of the shoulder girdle in cleidocranial dysplasia.
    b) hypermobility of the wrists in Holt-Oram syndrome.
    c) genu recurvatum (knee hyperextension) with Ehlers-Danlos syndrome.
    d) advanced collapse of the scaphoid and lunate with CPPD.

244. Knees most at risk for chondromalacia patellae are:
    a) those of sedentary, obese patients.
    b) those of geriatric patients with a decreased Q angle ($< 15°$).
    c) those of adolescent patients with a decreased Q angle ($< 15°$).
    d) those of adolescent patients with an increased Q angle ($> 20°$).

245. Hydroxyapatite deposition disease (HADD) may result in intervertebral disc calcifications:
    a) in the annular fibers of pediatric male patients, most commonly.
    b) in the nucleus pulposus of pediatric male patients, most commonly.
    c) in multiple nucleus pulposus of pediatric female patients, most commonly.
    d) in single nucleus pulposus of pediatric female patients, most commonly.

246. A typical radiologic appearance for an osteoma is:
    a) a lucent, loculated, soap-bubble appearance.
    b) a lobulated, lucent lesion with thin, well-defined cortices.
    c) a well-circumscribed, round or oval opacity, usually < 2 cm in diameter.
    d) a well-circumscribed, oval lucency with an opaque nidus within it.

247. Multiple enchondromatosis combined with cavernous hemangiomas in the soft tissues is called:
    a) Gardner's syndrome.
    b) Ollier's disease.
    c) Maffucci's syndrome.
    d) Caffey's disease.

248. Both "active" and "latent" simple bone cysts:
    a) have the potential to grow.
    b) are adjacent to the immature growth plate.
    c) are displaced from the growth plate.
    d) are neoplasms in immature bone.

249. The term "traumatic determinism" describes:
    a) the ability of an organism to respond to treatment after trauma.
    b) the development of pathology at the site of an antecedent trauma.
    c) the discovery of a pathologic lesion because a trauma renders it symptomatic.
    d) the development of terminal pathology following an emotional trauma.

250. Diastasis, or a diastatic fracture, is commonly seen at:
    a) the acetabular joint.
    b) the glenohumeral joint.
    c) the acromioclavicular joint.
    d) the pubic symphysis.

251. The danger of fat embolism following a fracture is greatest:
    a) during the first 24 hours after the injury.
    b) during the first month after the injury.
    c) during the first 48 hours after the injury.
    d) during the first 5 days after the injury.

252. A linear skull fracture may be differentiated radiologically from a vascular groove because the fracture:
    a) involves both inner and outer tables of the skull.
    b) often is serrated.
    c) does not cross suture lines.
    d) usually is depressed.

253. A spondylolisthesis is defined correctly as:
    a) bilateral pars defects.
    b) unilateral or bilateral pars defects.
    c) a "slipping" of the vertebral body in any direction.
    d) an anterior slippage of the vertebral body.

254. Patients with adult suppurative spondylitis usually develop the earliest sign of infection:
    a) in the intervertebral disc.
    b) in the anterior subchondral endplate.
    c) in the neural arch structures.
    d) in the meninges.

255. A very specific test for syphilitic infection is:
    a) VDRL.
    b) CIE.
    c) FTA-ABS.
    d) STS.

256. Hurler's syndrome, achondroplasia, and Morquio's syndrome are all:
    a) forms of dwarfism.
    b) frequently accompanied by epilepsy.
    c) causes of mental retardation.
    d) recognizable and diagnosed at birth.

257. The x-ray signs of "Erlenmeyer flask deformity" and spinal "sandwich vertebrae" or "endobones" may all be present in a patient with:
    a) osteopoikilosis.
    b) osteopetrosis.
    c) fibrous dysplasia.
    d) osteopathia striata.

258. With osteoporosis there is:
    a) a huge increase in the incidence and severity of hip degenerative joint disease.
    b) no change in the incidence and severity of hip DJD as compared with non-osteoporotic patients.
    c) a low incidence of hip DJD (< 5% of osteoporosis cases).
    d) a moderately increased incidence of hip DJD (approximately 18% of osteoporosis cases).

259. Asymmetry of lesion distribution might suggest a diagnosis of:
    a) rheumatoid arthritis.
    b) psoriasis.
    c) leukemia.
    d) hyperparathyroidism.

260. Eisenstein's sagittal canal measurement assesses the distance between the posterior vertebral body margin and:
    a) the spinous/lamina junction.
    b) a line connecting the tips of the articulating superior and inferior facet joints.
    c) the tip of the spinous process.
    d) a line connecting the tips of the spinous processes.

261. The front leg of the "Scotty dog" seen on a lumbar oblique projection is formed by:
    a) the contralateral pedicle.
    b) the superior articular process.
    c) the inferior articular process.
    d) the pedicle.

262. The neural arch of the spine is a preferred site for:
    a) chondrosarcoma.
    b) multiple myeloma.
    c) osteoid osteoma.
    d) Ewing's sarcoma.

263. Loculation (encapsulation) of pleural effusion is caused by:
    a) a penetrating chest wound.
    b) a growing mass lesion.
    c) pleural adhesions.
    d) atelectasis.

264. All of the following are radiologic manifestations typical of fluorosis except:
    a) growth arrest lines.
    b) exuberant vertebral hyperostosis.
    c) periostitis.
    d) sclerotic, irregular vertebral endplates

265. All of the following are features of progressive diaphyseal dysplasia except:

 a) it may elongate the long bones.
 b) it involves laminated periosteal response.
 c) expands the diameter of long bones.
 d) spares the metaphyses of long bones.

266. There is a female predilection for a more common type of Arnold-Chiari malformation:

 a) Type I, which is tonsilar ectopia.
 b) Type II, which is tonsilar herniation.
 c) Type II, which involves a dorsally kinked medulla and displaced cervical nerves.
 d) Type I, which is the least common type.

267. The three phases of congenital syphilis appear consecutively as:

 a) metaphysitis, periostitis, and osteitis.
 b) metaphysitis, osteitis, and periostitis.
 c) periostitis, metaphysitis, and osteitis.
 d) osteitis, metaphysitis, and periostitis.

268. The "bone within a bone" radiographic appearance caused by cortical splitting is characteristic of:

 a) rickets.
 b) sickle-cell anemia.
 c) thalassemia.
 d) tuberculous dactylitis.

269. The type of spondylolisthesis most commonly found at L4 is:

 a) isthmic.
 b) pathologic.
 c) degenerative.
 b) traumatic.

270. Clinically, slipped femoral capital epiphysis (SFCE) typically involves:

 a) an obese teen-aged woman with bilateral hip pain.
 b) an obese teen-aged male with bilateral hip pain.
 c) an obese young teen with knee pain and a limp.
 d) a young teen-aged athlete with increasing pain after field sports.

271. A fat, blood, interface (FBI) sign in the suprapatellar bursa is best demonstrated radiographically with:

 a) a lateral projection done horizontally.
 b) a weight-bearing lateral projection.
 c) a "sunrise" projection.
 d) a tangential knee projection.

272. A Jones' fracture is defined as:

 a) a horizontal fracture of the proximal fifth metatarsal.
 b) a transverse fracture of the cuboid.
 c) a transverse fracture of the proximal fifth metacarpal.
 d) a transverse fracture of the proximal fifth metatarsal.

273. Bone islands usually are:

 a) intramedullary lesions aligned with the long axis of trabeculae.
 b) diaphyseal lesions aligned along the long axis of the bone.
 c) intramedullary lesions aligned at right angles to the long axis of the trabeculae.
 d) cortical lesions aligned at right angles to the long axis of the bone.

274. A lucent metadiaphyseal lesion with a truncated cone appearance is likely to be:

    a) an aneurysmal bone cyst.
    b) a nonossifying fibroma.
    c) a simple bone cyst.
    d) an osteoblastoma.

275. The most common primary malignant bone tumor is:

    a) multiple myeloma.
    b) central osteosarcoma.
    c) Ewing's sarcoma.
    d) chondrosarcoma.

276. Ewing's sarcoma has a predilection for:

    a) middle-aged males.
    b) pregnant females.
    c) young females.
    d) young males.

277. Gouty arthritis in the sacroiliac joint is:

    a) common, and usually bilateral and symmetric.
    b) present in less than 20% of cases, and usually bilateral and asymmetric.
    c) almost always unilateral, and present in almost all cases.
    d) almost always unilateral, but present in less than 20% of cases.

278. Bilaterally symmetric triangular sclerotic areas on the lower half of the ilium of a female patient are usually:

    a) blastic metastasis.
    b) hyperostosis triangularis ilii.
    c) preauricular sulci.
    d) early Paget's disease.

279. Jaccoud's syndrome primarily affects:

    a) the hands.
    b) the thoracic spine and the shoulders.
    c) the lower extremities.
    d) the sacroiliac joints.

280. "Lover's heels" refers to:

    a) the x-ray sign of "whiskering" at the plantar surface of the calcaneus.
    b) the x-ray sign of "whiskering" at the Achilles tendon insertion into the calcaneus.
    c) the clinical sign of pain caused by an occult stress fracture of the calcaneus.
    d) the clinical sign of pain at the Achilles insertion seen with Reiter's syndrome.

281. The "cocktail sausage digit" is a clinical manifestation characteristic of early:

    a) gout.
    b) psoriatic arthritis.
    c) erosive osteoarthritis.
    d) rheumatoid arthritis.

282. The paraspinal ossifications typical of ankylosing spondylitis are:

    a) marginal osteophytes.
    b) non-marginal osteophytes.
    c) marginal syndesmophytes.
    d) non-marginal syndesmophytes.

283. An x-ray sign of juvenile rheumatoid arthritis, antegonal notching is:
    a) apparent obturator foramen enlargement, seen with JRA in the hip.
    b) erosion of the anterosuperior odontoid, seen with JRA lesions at the transverse ligament.
    c) multiple lesions of the carpal bones, seen with JRA in the wrists and hands.
    d) a concave lesion anterior to the angle of the mandible, seen with JRA in the mandible.

284. Radiographic signs of the atrophic stage of neurotrophic arthropathy include:
    a) a tapered bone end at the joint space.
    b) joint debris.
    c) joint distention.
    d) subchondral sclerosis.

285. Fusiform expansion of the metadiaphyseal shaft of the proximal femur with cortical thickening and endosteal scalloping, and a large lucent, oval lesion with scattered calcifications within its matrix would cause the radiologist to consider:
    a) osteoblastoma.
    b) Ewing's sarcoma.
    c) osteosarcoma.
    d) chondrosarcoma.

286. A significant laboratory finding when central osteosarcoma is suspected is:
    a) elevated PSA.
    b) elevated serum calcium.
    c) elevated alkaline phosphatase.
    d) elevated acid phosphatase.

287. A solitary plasmacytoma is a localized plasma cell proliferation that:
    a) has a 70% chance of eventually developing diffuse multiple myeloma.
    b) has a 50% chance of eventually developing diffuse multiple myeloma.
    c) has a 10% chance of eventually developing diffuse multiple myeloma.
    d) has no recognized correlation with diffuse multiple myeloma.

288. Approximately half of the simple bone cysts are found in young patients (more often male):
    a) in the proximal tibia.
    b) in the distal femur.
    c) in the proximal femur.
    d) in the proximal humerus.

289. Nonunion in an ankle fracture is most frequently seen:
    a) when the talus is fractured.
    b) when the lateral malleolus is fractured.
    c) when a medial malleolar fracture is not treated with internal fixation.
    d) when two or more bones are affected.

290. Segond's fracture is usually associated with:
    a) rupture of the posterior cruciate ligament.
    b) the "unhappy triad" injury to the medial knee.
    c) sartorius tendon rupture.
    d) a damaged anterior cruciate ligament.

291. Current thought favors the view of spondylolysis as:
    a) a congenital condition.
    b) a traumatic fracture.

c)   an hereditary condition.
d)   a stress fracture.

292.   The "Davis series" of cervical views:

a)   consists of six views.
b)   consists of an AP open mouth, an AP lower cervical, a lateral, and two oblique films.
c)   should be done for a whiplash victim if no contraindications are present.
d)   consists of an AP open mouth, an AP lower cervical, and three lateral views.

293.   Trauma may be responsible for aneurysm formation at:

a)   the junction of the aorta and the common iliac arteries.
b)   the junction of the aorta and the splenic arteries.
c)   the junction of the aorta and the renal arteries.
d)   the ligamentum arteriosum attachment to the aorta.

294.   Mycotic osteomyelitis infections are most often secondary to primary:

a)   HIV infection.
b)   septic osteomyelitis.
c)   respiratory system infection.
d)   gastrointestinal infestation.

295.   The "classic triad" of Klippel-Feil syndrome consists of:

a)   a short, webbed neck, a low hairline, and an omovertebral bone.
b)   a low hairline, an omo-hyoid bone, and a torticollis.
c)   a torticollis, neck webbing, and scoliosis.
d)   a short, webbed neck, a low hairline, and decreased cervical range of motion.

296.   Putti's triad includes all of the following except:

a)   small or absent proximal femoral epiphysis.
b)   hypoplastic greater trochanter.
c)   laterally displaced femur.
d)   increased inclination of acetabular roof.

297.   "Fish vertebrae" describes the radiologic appearance of the vertebrae that may appear in all of the following except:

a)   osteomalacia.
b)   osteoporosis.
c)   Schmorl's nodes.
d)   sickle cell anemia.

298.   The "Mercedes Benz sign" is an image of:

a)   air in the biliary tree.
b)   pneumoperitoneum.
c)   an air-distended duodenal-jejunal junction.
d)   gas pockets in gallstone fissures.

299.   Which one of the following is an intradural intramedullary lesion?

a)   neurofibroma.
b)   IVD herniation.
c)   meningioma.
d)   syrinx.

300.   A posteroanterior wrist projection would not show a relatively smooth arc at:

a)   the proximal scaphoid, lunate, and triquetrum surfaces.
b)   the distal scaphoid, lunate, and triquetrum surfaces.
c)   the proximal capitate and hamate surfaces.
d)   the distal metacarpal surfaces.

301.   The Risser-Ferguson method of evaluating scoliosis:

a)   generally is preferred over the Cobb method.
b)   often yields values up to 25% greater than those indicated by the Cobb method.

c) may yield values up to 25% lower than those indicated by the Cobb method.

d) measures the angle formed by the intersection of lines perpendicular to the endplates of the vertebrae at the upper and lower limits of the scoliotic curve.

302. Nuclear scanning is contraindicated for:

   a) patients who suffer from claustrophobia.
   b) patients who are pregnant or lactating.
   c) patients who have a history of seizures.
   d) patients who have an iodine sensitivity.

303. Cystography on a patient with a neurogenic bladder will show a bladder wall that is:

   a) hypertrophied enough to create a visible soft-tissue shadow.
   b) thin and smooth.
   c) interlaced by bands of hypertrophied muscle that form "trabeculae."
   d) pocked with diverticula.

304. The pseudofractures of osteomalacia usually appear on plain film as:

   a) bilaterally symmetrical linear lucencies, widening over time.
   b) bilateral, asymmetrical linear lucencies, closed over time by thickening sclerosis.
   c) unilateral linear lucencies, lengthening over time to invade the medullary bone.
   d) bilateral, sclerotic densities extending from the cortex well into the medullary bone.

305. A broad, short, hypoplastic scapula with its glenoid process directed inferiorly is called:

   a) Klippel-Feil syndrome.
   b) an omovertebral bone.
   c) Sprengel's deformity.
   d) *pterygium coli.*

306. A "rocker bottom" foot may be a clinical indication of:

   a) a tarsal bar.
   b) a congenital talonavicular dislocation.
   c) a rigid pes cavus.
   d) Morton's syndrome.

307. Mycotic osteomyelitis caused by actinomycosis is most commonly secondary to:

   a) respiratory system infection.
   b) chronic bowel disease.
   c) recent oral surgery or infection.
   d) HIV infection.

308. The two most commonly visualized arterial calcification sites are the aorta and:

   a) the carotid arteries.
   b) the renal arteries.
   c) the splenic artery.
   d) the iliac arteries.

309. The "empty vertebra sign" on a frontal lumbar film indicates the presence of:

   a) lytic metastatic disease.
   b) congenital absence of both pedicles.
   c) a fulcrum fracture.
   d) spina bifida occulta.

310. Although progressive displacement with spondylolisthesis is a controversial topic, it is generally agreed that:
    a) strenuous activities should be curtailed in patients with a radiographically demonstrable spondylolisthesis.
    b) risk of displacement is greater if there is an associated spina bifida occulta.
    c) risk of displacement is greater for males, because of their affinity for contact sports.
    d) instability of the lesion is always present, although it may not be radiographically demonstrable.

311. Ipsilateral vertical fractures of the superior pubic and ischiopubic rami with fracture or dislocation of the ipsilateral sacroiliac joint is called:
    a) a Malgaigne fracture.
    b) a saddle fracture.
    c) a bucket-handle fracture.
    d) a straddle fracture.

312. A basicervical fracture of the proximal femur may be described as:
    a) subtrochanteric.
    b) intertrochanteric.
    c) intracapsular.
    d) extracapsular.

313. An axial projection of the calcaneus usually will show a simple bone cyst as:
    a) a lesion lateral to the midline.
    b) a lesion medial to the midline.
    c) a central lesion.
    d) an elongated, ovoid, midline lesion.

314. Giant cell tumors may be eccentric, metaphyseal lesions, or may occur as:
    a) epiphyseal lesions in children and adolescents.
    b) subarticular lesions in adults.
    c) central, uniformly expansile metaphyseal lesions.
    d) central, uniformly expansile diaphyseal lesions.

315. The radiologic hallmark of multiple myeloma:
    a) is the pathologic vertebral collapse known as "vertebra plana" or "wrinkled vertebra" of myeloma.
    b) is the generalized osteopenia, most prominent in the thoracic and lumbar vertebrae.
    c) is the appearance of "punched out lesions" in the skull, pelvis, long bones, clavicles, and ribs.
    d) is the appearance of a solitary "ivory vertebra" in the presence of generalized osteopenia.

316. Extraosseous osteosarcoma most frequently develops in:
    a) the cranial dura.
    b) the breast.
    c) the soft tissues of the buttocks.
    d) the soft tissues of the thigh.

317. Non-articular symptoms of rheumatoid arthritis may include any of the following except:
    a) Raynaud's phenomenon.
    b) generalized osteopenia.
    c) pneumonia that occurs, clears, and recurs.
    d) fatigue and general muscle weakness.

318. The first articular radiologic sign of rheumatoid arthritis in the hands is usually:

    a) subchondral sclerosis.
    b) an osteophyte.
    c) marginal erosions.
    d) periarticular periostitis.

319. In the absence of a history of trauma, bilateral protrusio acetabuli may be the result of:

    a) ischemic necrosis.
    b) congenital hip dislocation.
    c) neurotrophic arthropathy.
    d) rheumatoid arthritis.

320. Ocular, genitourinary, pulmonary, and cardiovascular problems may accompany articular effects of:

    a) erosive osteoarthritis.
    b) ankylosing spondylitis.
    c) rheumatoid arthritis.
    d) enteropathic arthritis.

321. Numerous acute attacks of gout:

    a) posed no danger of neurologic effects.
    b) deposited gouty tophi in the more highly vascularized tissues.
    c) caused deposits of tophi if the attacks continued over two to six months.
    d) could result in renal disorders, hypertension, and vascular disturbances.

322. The main radiologic feature of CPPD is:

    a) chondrocalcinosis, in hyaline cartilage only.
    b) chondrocalcinosis, in fibrocartilage only.
    c) chondrocalcinosis in both hyaline cartilage and fibrocartilage.
    d) ligamentous, tendinous, and vascular calcifications.

323. Wilson's disease primarily is:

    a) an abnormality of collagen synthesis and organization.
    b) a genetic disorder involving the absorption of iron in the gastrointestinal tract.
    c) a disturbance in copper metabolism.
    d) a disturbance in calcium metabolism.

324. Spinal changes associated with ochronosis feature:

    a) vacuum phenomenon simultaneously present at multiple levels.
    b) thin, marginal syndesmophytes.
    c) non-marginal syndesmophytes.
    d) sparing of facet joints.

325. The most frequently seen chordoma is:

    a) a lesion in the C2 vertebral body.
    b) a spheno-occipital lesion (in the clivus of Blumenbach).
    c) an "hourglass" lesion in a cervical intervertebral foramen.
    d) a sacrococcygeal lesion.

326. Synovioma is most likely to occur:

    a) in the femoral metaphyses.
    b) in the metaphyses of the long bones of the upper extremities.
    c) in the diaphyses of the long bones of the lower extremities.
    d) in the juxtaarticular bone of the lower extremities.

327. Acral metastasis is rare, and when it occurs in the hands it is usually from:

    a) the kidneys.
    b) the breast.
    c) the lung.
    d) the colon.

328. Most metastatic lesions in the skull are:
    a) blastic lesions from the thyroid or breast.
    b) lytic lesions from the thyroid or breast.
    c) lytic lesions from the prostate or gastrointestinal tract.
    d) lytic lesions from the kidneys or thyroid.

329. George's line and Ulmann's line are both useful in the evaluation of:
    a) lumbar disc degeneration.
    b) lumbar facet imbrication.
    c) spinal stenosis.
    d) spondylolisthesis.

330. Recent lumbar compression fractures often show:
    a) contiguous disc degeneration.
    b) syndesmophyte development.
    c) a zone of impaction.
    d) osteophyte development.

331. The ''horizontal facet'' sign on an AP cervical projection may indicate the presence of:
    a) spinal DJD.
    b) facet dislocation.
    c) articular pillar fracture.
    d) spondylolisthesis.

332. The slowest healing bone in the body is the:
    a) clavicle.
    b) mandible.
    c) carpal navicular (scaphoid).
    d) patella.

333. A poor prognosis accompanies Legg-Calvé-Perthes disease that displays:
    a) Waldenstrom's sign.
    b) a crescent sign in the superior weight-bearing surface of the femoral head.
    c) an extensive metaphyseal lucent defect.
    d) a reduced femoral head size.

334. Bones undergo endosteal thickening and periostitis in:
    a) hemophilia.
    b) myelofibrosis.
    c) sickle-cell anemia.
    d) thalassemia.

335. Paraspinal abscesses (often in the psoas) that tend to calcify are common to:
    a) actinomycosis and tuberculosis.
    b) childhood inflammatory discitis and tuberculosis.
    c) Coccidioidomycosis and tuberculosis.
    d) suppurative osteomyelitis and Actinomycosis.

336. Skeletal manifestations of hemophilia are most likely to include:
    a) Erlenmeyer flask deformity, pathologic fracture of weight-bearing long tubular bones.
    b) spinal osteoporosis with marked loss of disc space, thin marginal syndesmophytes.
    c) expansile, geographic bone lesions, growth arrest lines, solid periosteal new bone formation.
    d) ''pseudotumors'' (expansile lesions), ballooned epiphyses, severe arthropathy at knee, ankle and elbow joints.

337. Transient regional osteoporosis is an idiopathic, self-limiting condition that:

    a) most commonly occurs in the spine.
    b) affects periarticular bone.
    c) occurs only at the hip.
    d) occurs only at the knee.

338. The most common anomaly of the aortic arch is:

    a) mirror-image branching.
    b) double aortic arch.
    c) aberrant right subclavian artery.
    d) a retroesophageal circumflex left ligamentum arteriosum.

339. A trauma patient whose chest films show focal bulging of a lung border with focal consolidation of the lung may be suspected to have:

    a) a fractured rib.
    b) a punctured lung.
    c) a "coin lesion."
    d) a lung contusion.

340. The Jones projection is also called:

    a) the abduction projection.
    b) the medial oblique elbow projection.
    c) the tangential elbow projection.
    d) the medial oblique wrist projection.

341. Heel pad thickness greater than 2.5 cm may indicate:

    a) acromegaly.
    b) achondroplasia.
    c) Down's syndrome.
    d) heel spurs.

342. The renal tumor that is the most common malignancy of pediatric patients is:

    a) malignant lymphoma.
    b) sarcoma.
    c) adenocarcinoma.
    d) Wilms' tumor.

343. Sensitive, but not specific, radiologic signs of traumatic rupture of the aorta include:

    a) depressed left mainstem bronchus.
    b) prominent left apical cap.
    c) widened right paraspinal stripe.
    d) right displacement of a nasogastric tube.

344. Osteomalacia may be secondary to:

    a) osteoporosis.
    b) scurvy.
    c) neurofibromatosis.
    d) Paget's disease.

345. Coxa vara may be defined as an angle of incidence:

    a) $< 120°$.
    b) $< 145°$.
    c) $> 120°$.
    d) $> 145°$.

346. All of the following are true of Sprengel's deformity except:

    a) it is often associated with Klippel-Feil syndrome.
    b) it has a demonstrated female predilection of about 2:1.
    c) it may be unilateral or bilateral.
    d) clinically, it limits humeral flexion and internal rotation.

347. The patella of a patient with hemophilia shows a characteristic:
    a) superolateral dislocation.
    b) multipartite appearance.
    c) attenuated, squared inferior pole.
    d) roughened, spiculated posterior surface.

348. The most common peripheral aneurysm occurs in:
    a) the brachial artery.
    b) the profunda femoris artery.
    c) the radial artery.
    d) the popliteal artery.

349. Lytic metastasis, most often in the lower thoracic or lumbar vertebrae, may result in the x-ray appearance of the:
    a) winking owl sign.
    b) ghost vertebra.
    c) "H" vertebra.
    d) corduroy cloth vertebra.

350. Spinal metastasis is usually polyostotic and most commonly involves:
    a) cervical vertebral bodies.
    b) the sacrum.
    c) thoracic or lumbar vertebral bodies and pedicles.
    d) thoracic or lumbar articular processes.

351. The most common skeletal site of Hodgkin lymphoma is:
    a) the pelvis.
    b) the ribs and sternum.
    c) the vertebral body.
    d) the skull.

352. Lichtenstein's rule of thumb concerns:
    a) diagnosis of fibrosarcoma.
    b) evaluation for spinal stenosis.
    c) evaluation of spondylolisthesis.
    d) diagnosis of fibrous dysplasia.

353. When there is clinical evidence of neurologic deficits with cervical trauma:
    a) a full Davis series of radiographs should be taken.
    b) pillar projections must be taken.
    c) fracture should be presumed to exist.
    d) an MR study should be considered.

354. Severe traumatic hyperflexion may cause bilateral interfacetal dislocation (BID), which most often occurs at:
    a) C4–C7.
    b) C1–C2.
    c) C2–C4.
    d) C7–T2.

355. A "suicide jumper's fracture," caused by falling from great height, is:
    a) a crush fracture of the calcaneus.
    b) bilateral fracture of the femoral necks.
    c) bilateral fractures of the posterosuperior acetabular roofs.
    d) horizontal fracture of the upper sacrum.

356. A "floating knee" is a term used to describe:
    a) a comminuted patellar fracture.
    b) a fracture through both the proximal fibula and the proximal tibia.
    c) supracondylar femoral fracture with superolateral patellar avulsion fracture.
    d) supracondylar femoral fracture with tibial shaft fracture.

357. Urinary homogentisic acid is a laboratory finding common in the diagnosis of:

    a) gout.
    b) Wilson's disease.
    c) CPPD.
    d) ochronosis.

358. Calcifying tendinitis of the supraspinatus is radiographically visible:

    a) on an external rotation view, superimposed over the greater tuberosity promontory.
    b) on an external rotation view, seen in profile, adjacent to the greater tuberosity promontory.
    c) on an internal rotation view, seen in profile, superimposed over the greater tuberosity promontory.
    d) on an internal rotation view, seen in profile, adjacent to the greater tuberosity promontory.

359. Primary hemochromatosis is attributed to:

    a) alcoholism (cirrhosis of the liver).
    b) overingestion of iron.
    c) a genetic defect in absorption in the gastrointestinal tract.
    d) anemia.

360. A patient with x-ray signs that include "spotty carpal sign" and periarticular erosions with prominent "overhanging margins" is likely to have a diagnosis of:

    a) Reiter's syndrome.
    b) psoriatic arthritis.
    c) gout.
    d) rheumatoid arthritis.

361. Scleroderma is commonly associated with:

    a) reflex sympathetic dystrophy.
    b) rheumatic fever.
    c) erosive osteoarthritis.
    d) Raynaud's phenomenon.

362. Nonmarginal syndesmophytes may form in both:

    a) psoriatic arthritis and Reiter's syndrome.
    b) psoriatic arthritis and ankylosing spondylitis.
    c) psoriatic arthritis and enteropathic arthropathy.
    d) ankylosing spondylitis and enteropathic arthropathy.

363. A psoriasis patient is markedly more likely to develop psoriatic arthritis when (s)he has clinical lesions:

    a) at the extensor forearm.
    b) at the scalp.
    c) at the nails.
    d) at the pubic area.

364. The spinal segments most frequently (and earliest) affected by juvenile rheumatoid arthritis are:

    a) C1–C4.
    b) C6–T2.
    c) T10–L2.
    d) L4–S1.

365. An intraosseous lipoma is characterized radiographically as:

    a) an ovoid lytic lesion with punctate calcifications.
    b) an ovoid, sclerotic lesion, with a central lucent nidus.
    c) an ovoid, lobulated lytic lesion, with "target" or "doughnut-shaped" calcific sequestrum.
    d) a diaphyseal, expansile, purely lytic lesion.

366. In the spine, aneurysmal bone cysts are most likely to form:
    a) in the cervical spinous processes.
    b) in thoracic vertebral bodies.
    c) in thoracic or lumbar neural arch structures.
    d) in lumbar vertebral bodies.

367. A clear lytic lesion at the base of the neck of the calcaneus, with a straight, vertical anterior margin and a curvilinear posterior border is typical of the radiologic appearance of:
    a) an aneurysmal bone cyst (ABC).
    b) a fibrous cortical defect (FCD).
    c) a simple bone cyst (SBC).
    d) a nonossifying fibroma (NOF).

368. Approximately half of all chondromyxoid fibromas occur:
    a) in the radius.
    b) in the femur.
    c) in the tibia.
    d) in the humerus.

369. In the most common hip dislocation, the flexed and abducted femur usually fractures:
    a) the medial lip of the acetabulum.
    b) the posterior lip of the acetabulum.
    c) the central acetabular roof.
    d) the anterior lip of the acetabulum.

370. "Herndon's hump," "Capener's sign," and a "pistol-grip deformity" are all x-ray signs associated with:
    a) SFCE.
    b) occult subcapital femoral fracture.
    c) Legg-Calvé-Perthes disease.
    d) Paget's disease.

371. When geriatric patients suffer fractures of the proximal femur, they often die from:
    a) exposure and hypothermia.
    b) the predisposing pathology (e.g., malignancies).
    c) stroke caused by emboli from the fracture.
    d) ensuing pulmonary or cardiac complications.

372. Wilkinson's syndrome is:
    a) stress hypertrophy of a pedicle opposite a congenitally absent pedicle.
    b) an osteoid osteoma in a pedicle.
    c) congenital agenesis of a lumbar pedicle.
    d) stress hypertrophy of a pedicle opposite a unilateral pars defect.

373. The diagnostic imaging modality of choice for evaluating and monitoring aneurysms is:
    a) angiography.
    b) scintigraphy.
    c) contrast CT
    d) ultrasonography.

374. Avascular necrosis at the carpal lunate is called "lunate malacia" or:
    a) Freiberg's disease.
    b) Kienboch's disease.
    c) Kohler's number 2 disease.
    d) Preiser's disease.

375. Madelung's deformity:
    a) is more often bilateral than unilateral.
    b) has a clear male predilection.
    c) is most often diagnosed at birth.
    d) is always seen as part of a condition known as dyschondrosteosis.

376. Os odontoideum has an association with:

    a) Morquio's syndrome.
    b) osteogenesis imperfecta.
    c) Marfan's syndrome.
    d) Arnold-Chiari malformation.

377. "Moon face" and "buffalo hump" are clinical descriptions characteristic of patients with:

    a) Grave's disease.
    b) Cushing's disease.
    c) Gaucher's disease.
    d) Hand-Schüller-Christian disease.

378. Renal tuberculosis eventually leads to:

    a) "pipe stem ureter."
    b) "staghorn calcification."
    c) "ring shadows."
    d) progressive renal enlargement.

379. Bone may actually be produced in the lung parenchyma due to:

    a) lymphangitic metastasis from the breast.
    b) hematogenous metastasis from the prostate.
    c) hematogenous metastasis from a primary osteosarcoma.
    d) lymphangitic metastasis from a primary melanoma.

380. An angle formed by the intersection of a line drawn from the anterior superior iliac spine to the center of the patella, and a line drawn from the tibial tubercle to the center of the patella, is the:

    a) "Q" angle.
    b) tibial angle.
    c) femoral angle of the knee.
    d) condylar angle.

381. A frog-leg projection is helpful in early detection of:

    a) coxa vara.
    b) slipped femoral capital epiphysis (SFCE).
    c) coxa valga.
    d) protrusio acetabulae.

382. A radiologic sign of appendicitis is:

    a) a "crow's beak" sign.
    b) a "coiled spring" sign.
    c) a "sentinel loop."
    d) a "string sign."

383. Squamous cell carcinoma, oat cell cancer, undifferentiated large cell carcinoma, and adenocarcinoma are all:

    a) primary tumors of the large bowel.
    b) histologic types of bronchogenic carcinoma.
    c) productive endocrine tumors.
    d) dermatologic malignancies.

384. Plain films of the hands of a patient with acromegaly might be expected to show:

    a) acroosteolysis.
    b) "licked candy stick" appearance of distal ends of the small tubular bones.
    c) coned ungual tufts.
    d) spade-like ungual tufts.

385. A supracondylar process must be differentiated from:

    a) an osteochondroma.
    b) an osteoid osteoma.
    c) a large osteophyte.
    d) an osteoblastoma.

386. The term "synpolydactyly" refers to:
    a) syndactyly involving the third and fourth fingers and/or second and third toes.
    b) syndactyly of third and fourth fingers with partial or complete duplication of fingers three and four in the web; or fourth and fifth toes with duplication of toes four or five in the web.
    c) middle phalanx of the fifth finger rudimentary or absent.
    d) syndactyly with metacarpal or metatarsal synostosis, usually on the medial side of the hand.

387. Preiser's disease is now recognized as caused by:
    a) repetitive trauma to the flexor tendons, as with golf swings that are abruptly terminated by striking the ground, affecting the carpal lunate.
    b) ununited fracture of the scaphoid.
    c) ischemic necrosis of the scaphoid, not associated with fracture.
    d) repetitive trauma to the lateral foot, as with professional dancing or marching with heavy packs, affecting the tarsal navicular.

388. Typical x-ray appearance of the thoracic spine of a patient with Scheuermann's disease may include:
    a) trapezoidal, anteriorly wedged vertebral bodies, multiple Schmorl's nodes.
    b) normal disc heights, but severe reduction of anterior vertebral body height.
    c) slightly reduced disc heights with moderate anterior vertebral body wedging.
    d) occasional Schmorl's nodes, normal disc heights, irregular endplates with occasional compression fractures.

389. An "explosion fracture" is:
    a) a central acetabular fracture.
    b) a posterior acetabular fracture, separating the ilioischial line from the teardrop.
    c) also called a "dashboard fracture."
    d) a simple fracture of the anterior acetabulum, interrupting the iliopubic line.

390. Subcapital femoral fractures:
    a) are the most common femoral fractures.
    b) are missed frequently because they may involve impaction and no displacement or angulation.
    c) usually are pathologic fractures.
    d) usually are comminuted fractures.

391. Common complications of hip dislocation include:
    a) trigonal rupture of the ureters, femoral artery rupture, and rupture of the hemidiaphragm.
    b) damage to the femoral nerve, loss of the patellar reflex, and deep vein thrombosis.
    c) inguinal ligament disruption, femoral artery rupture, and femoral nerve damage.
    d) sciatic nerve paralysis, femoral head avascular necrosis, and myositis ossificans.

392. In a significantly traumatized ankle, stability evaluation should be made for:
    a) the lateral collateral, deltoid, and tibiofibular ligaments.
    b) the medial collateral, deltoid, and tibiofibular ligaments.
    c) only the lateral and medial collateral ligaments.
    d) only the medial collateral and deltoid ligaments.

393. Radiologic signs which indicate that the lesion is a simple bone cyst (SBC) include:

    a) cortical disruption.
    b) a truncated cone appearance.
    c) a laminated periosteal response.
    d) a fluid/fluid level.

394. All of the following may be present with multiple myeloma except:

    a) Bence Jones protein in the urine.
    b) reversed A/G ratio.
    c) reduced serum calcium.
    d) rouleaux formation.

395. When central osteosarcoma has metastasized, lung resection with chemotherapy may give a 5-year survival rate of up to:

    a) 80%.
    b) 50%.
    c) 20%.
    d) 5%.

396. The clinical presentation of peripheral Ewing's sarcoma often mimics:

    a) eosinophilic granuloma.
    b) infection.
    c) non-Hodgkin lymphoma.
    d) leukemia.

397. A common eponym for ankylosing spondylitis (AS) is:

    a) Still's disease.
    b) Marie-Strümpell's disease.
    c) Forestier's disease.
    d) Von Bechterew's disease.

398. Psoriatic arthropathy may be almost impossible to differentiate from:

    a) systemic lupus erythematosus.
    b) rheumatoid arthritis.
    c) erosive osteoarthritis.
    d) Reiter's syndrome.

399. The early signs of axial involvement with ankylosing spondylitis:

    a) is early, unilateral or asymmetric sacroiliac involvement, and thoracolumbar lesions.
    b) involves the lower cervical spine first, progressing upward.
    c) involves the mid-lumbar vertebra, progressing down to the lumbosacral junction.
    d) involves the thoracolumbar junction, and bilateral sacroiliac joints.

400. Arthritic manifestations with systemic lupus erythematosus are:

    a) invariably present, and almost always in a bilateral distribution.
    b) present in up to 90% of cases, and usually bilateral but asymmetric.
    c) present in up to 90% of cases, in bilateral, symmetric distribution.
    d) present almost exclusively in the spine.

401. Clinically, the most commonly seen arthritis is:

    a) rheumatoid arthritis.
    b) gout.
    c) osteoarthritis.
    d) scleroderma.

402. Radiographic evidence of sarcoidosis in the distal extremities is most frequently seen:

    a) bilaterally, in the middle and distal phalanges of the hands.
    b) bilaterally, in the tarsus.
    c) unilaterally, in the distal radius and ulna.
    d) unilaterally, in the carpus.

403. The postulated process for the development of osteitis condensans ilii is:

    a) stress caused by added weight on the pelvis during pregnancy.
    b) trauma during parturition.
    c) stress caused by ligamentous laxity of pregnancy or within menstrual cycles.
    d) low-grade infection that invades during parturition.

404. Complications of Reiter's syndrome include all of the following except:

    a) aortitis.
    b) cranial nerve palsy.
    c) pancreatitis.
    d) urinary tract obstructions.

405. An expansile, lytic lesion with a thin cortex is likely to be:

    a) an osteoblastoma.
    b) an osteoma.
    c) an osteoid osteoma.
    d) an intraosseous lipoma.

406. The definitive diagnosis of multiple myeloma is made with:

    a) MRI.
    b) bone marrow biopsy.
    c) serum analysis and urinalysis.
    d) CT.

407. The most common cause of secondary chondrosarcoma is:

    a) Paget's disease.
    b) multiple osteochondroma (HME).
    c) fibrous dysplasia.
    d) enchondromatosis (Ollier's disease).

408. Metastatic spread of a tumor is rare:

    a) in the brain.
    b) in the skull.
    c) distal to the knees or elbows.
    d) in the cervical spine.

409. Osteomyelitis is most likely to become a complication:

    a) after surgical reduction of a fracture.
    b) after a comminuted fracture.
    c) after a stress fracture.
    d) after a pathologic fracture.

410. A leptomeningeal cyst is caused by:

    a) CSF pulsations eroding bone in a "pocket" of torn dura adhering to a bone fragment.
    b) pulsations from a ruptured cerebral artery eroding the bone.
    c) pressure of a small aneurysm against bone.
    d) pressure from a slowly enlarging epidural hematoma.

411. The most common odontoid process fracture is:

    a) a Type 2 (Anderson/Dalonzo classification) fracture.
    b) a Type 3 (Anderson/Dalonzo classification) fracture.
    c) a Type 1 (Anderson/Dalonzo classification) fracture.
    d) a fracture at the dentocentral synchondrosis.

412. Of those listed below, the optimal radiograph for visualizing pars defects above L5 is:

    a) a lateral lumbar spot, with the side of interest adjacent to the film.
    b) an upright anterior oblique projection.
    c) an upright posterior oblique projection.
    d) a Ferguson's view.

413. The term nonsuppurative osteomyelitis refers to:

    a) the osseous lesions of tuberculosis.
    b) Tom Smith's arthritis.
    c) chronic osteomyelitis.
    d) syphilitic osteomyelitis.

414. "Lues" is a term that is synonymous with:

    a) Pott's disease.
    b) tubercular arthritis.
    c) syphilitic osteomyelitis.
    d) tuberous sclerosis.

415. The radiologic appearance of multiple Wormian bones, basilar impression, a thin calvarium, and pencil-thin cortices is typical of:

    a) osteoporosis.
    b) osteogenesis imperfecta.
    c) osteomalacia.
    d) osteopoikilosis.

416. An enlarged head with a prognathic jaw and a beaked nose, and koilonychia are all signs of:

    a) pyknodysostosis.
    b) osteopetrosis.
    c) osteopoikilosis.
    d) Paget's disease.

417. Sudeck's atrophy shows a predilection for:

    a) males.
    b) females.
    c) patients > 50 years of age.
    d) pediatric patients.

418. Small bowl obstruction may show on x-ray as:

    a) a "coiled spring sign."
    b) a "coffee bean sign."
    c) a "double bubble sign."
    d) a "crow's beak deformity."

419. The most common benign tumor of the lung is:

    a) bronchial adenoma.
    b) pulmonary hamartoma.
    c) hemangioma.
    d) laryngeal papilloma.

420. With infants, the acetabular angle, iliac angle, diaphyseal interval, and iliac index are determined with reference to:

    a) the parallelogram of Kopitz.
    b) the Y-Y line.
    c) the vertical line of Ombredanne.
    d) the pivot point interval.

421. The Angle of Wiberg should measure approximately:

    a) 20°.
    b) 15°.
    c) 36°.
    d) 10°.

422. The carcinoid tumor may develop a "bull's eye" appearance on plain film if:

    a) it becomes ulcerated.
    b) it becomes productive (producing serotonin).
    c) it ceases producing serotonin.
    d) it begins to regress and atrophy.

423. A poorly-defined oval mass of water density, in which CT may demonstrate a thickened, irregular wall, is most likely:

    a) a primary malignant tumor.
    b) an abscess.
    c) a primary benign tumor.
    d) a metastatic tumor.

424. Hydroxyapatite deposition disease (HADD) is essentially:

    a) calcifying tendinitis.
    b) arterial calcification.
    c) costochondral calcification.
    d) chondrocalcinosis.

425. The most common developmental anomaly of the hands is:

    a) syndactyly.
    b) polydactyly.
    c) trident hand.
    d) dystelephalangy.

426. Calcification of the basal ganglia is:

    a) never seen as a normal variant.
    b) sometimes associated with early onset diabetes.
    c) sometimes associated with pseudopseudohypoparathyroidism.
    d) sometimes associated with renal dystrophy.

427. The most common skeletal site for congenital syphilitic osteomyelitis is:

    a) the skull.
    b) the sternum.
    c) vertebral bodies.
    d) long bone metaphyses.

428. Patients who have sickle cell anemia suffer from "hand-foot syndrome," which may be caused by their predisposition for:

    a) mycotic osteomyelitis.
    b) *Salmonella* osteomyelitis.
    c) Tom Smith's arthritis.
    d) chronic osteomyelitis.

429. An unstable, comminuted fracture of the pubic arches is called:

    a) a straddle fracture.
    b) a bucket-handle fracture.
    c) an explosion fracture.
    d) a Malgaigne fracture.

430. Tibial plateau fractures most commonly:

    a) involve both lateral and medial plateaus.
    b) involve the lateral plateau.
    c) involve plateau avulsions by the cruciate ligaments.
    d) involve the medial plateau.

431. A fracture of the medial malleolus is unstable if it is:

    a) proximal to the tibiotalar joint line.
    b) distal to the plafond of the talus.
    c) distal to the tibiotalar joint line.
    d) associated with rupture of the tibiofibular ligament.

432. The vast majority of shoulder girdle dislocations are:

    a)   sternoclavicular joint dislocations.
    b)   posterior glenohumeral dislocations.
    c)   anterior glenohumeral dislocations.
    d)   acromioclavicular joint dislocations.

433. The most frequent sources of skeletal metastases are primary tumors in the:

    a)   breast, prostate, lung, and kidney.
    b)   lung, prostate, colon, and thyroid.
    c)   breast, uterus, ovaries, and colon.
    d)   breast, skin, thyroid, and uterus.

434. All of the following must be considered in differential diagnosis of lytic metastasis except:

    a)   osteomalacia.
    b)   Gorham's angiomatosis.
    c)   neurofibromatosis.
    d)   hyperparathyroidism (brown tumors).

435. All of the following could be effects of Paget's disease except:

    a)   basilar invagination.
    b)   moon face.
    c)   leontiasis ossea.
    d)   "saber shin" deformity.

436. Malignant degeneration of fibrous dysplasia is:

    a)   a frequent complication with the polyostotic forms of the disease.
    b)   a frequent complication of all forms of the disease.
    c)   a rare complication of any form of the disease.
    d)   not known to occur.

437. Reiter's syndrome is believed to have:

    a)   a genetic etiology.
    b)   a familial predisposition.
    c)   an etiology of venereal or enteric infection.
    d)   an etiology including predisposing trauma.

438. Metatarsophalangeal joint involvement with rheumatoid arthritis:

    a)   rarely occurs.
    b)   characteristically involves the first MTP joint initially, and progresses laterally to the fifth.
    c)   characteristically involves the fifth MTP joint initially, progressing medially to the first.
    d)   is the only manifestation of rheumatoid arthritis in the feet.

439. Forestier's disease is an eponym for:

    a)   ankylosing spondylitis.
    b)   sarcoidosis.
    c)   diffuse idiopathic skeletal hyperostosis.
    d)   von Becterew's disease.

440. Maigne's syndrome, sometimes seen with osteoarthritis, is described as:

    a)   sciatic pattern pain referred from thoracic facet arthrosis.
    b)   sciatic pattern pain referred from sacroiliac arthrosis.
    c)   lower lumbar pain referred from thoracic facet arthrosis.
    d)   thoracic pain referred from thoracolumbar facet arthrosis.

441. Clinical signs of ostephytes in the cervical spine may include:

    a)   long tract neurologic deficits in the lower limbs.
    b)   abnormal deep tendon reflexes.
    c)   cervical hyperlordosis.
    d)   dysphagia.

442. Intra-articular loose bodies, subchondral cysts, subchondral sclerosis, and osteophytes are all signs of:

    a) enteropathic arthritis.
    b) psoriatic arthritis.
    c) degenerative arthritis.
    d) hydroxyapatite deposition disease (HADD).

443. Synoviochondrometaplasia is most commonly seen:

    a) in the hips of elderly patients.
    b) in the knees of elderly patients.
    c) in the knees of young and middle-aged adults.
    d) in the elbows of adolescent patients.

444. Cervical involvement with rheumatoid arthritis typically includes all of the following effects except:

    a) upper cervical instability.
    b) loss of up to 50% of the length of the neck.
    c) osteophyte development.
    d) "sharpened pencil" radiologic appearance of lower cervical spinous processes.

445. The most common form (approximately 70% of cases) of fibrous dysplasia is:

    a) cherubism.
    b) monostotic.
    c) polyostotic.
    d) polyostotic with endocrine abnormalities.

446. All of the following may present with increment fractures except:

    a) osteoporosis.
    b) osteomalacia.
    c) hyperphosphatasia.
    d) florid rickets.

447. Paget's coxopathy is:

    a) pseudofractures at the femoral neck.
    b) increment fractures at the subtrochanteric region.
    c) protrusio acetabuli with concentric joint narrowing from both acetabulum and femur.
    d) neurologic dysfunction in the hip flexors and extensors caused by spinal stenosis.

448. Ivory vertebra may result from any of the following except:

    a) Paget's disease.
    b) Hodgkin lymphoma.
    c) neurofibromatosis.
    d) blastic metastasis.

449. A Hill-Sachs defect is:

    a) a chip fracture acquired during posterior shoulder dislocation.
    b) a Bankart lesion.
    c) an impaction fracture usually acquired during anterior shoulder dislocation.
    d) an impaction fracture usually acquired during posterior shoulder dislocation.

450. The most frequently fractured proximal humeral structure is:

    a) the anatomic neck.
    b) the greater tuberosity.
    c) the lesser tuberosity.
    d) the surgical neck.

451. A "skyline" (tangential) knee projection is the best radiographic study for displaying:

    a) a horizontal patellar fracture.
    b) a vertical patellar fracture.
    c) a stellate patellar fracture.
    d) a multipartite patella.

452. A step defect is:

    a) a disruption of the anterior cortical line of a vertebra by an anteriorly displaced superior corner (indicative of a compression fracture).
    b) the inferiorly displaced portion of the superior vertebral body endplate with a Schmorl's node.
    c) disruption of the cervical posterior vertebral body margin line with anterolisthesis.
    d) disruption of the smooth Hadley's curve line with facet imbrication.

453. Sickle cell anemia causes widened medullary cavities of the long bones, thinning the cortices, and:

    a) chronic endosteal appositional new bone that creates a sclerotic skeleton.
    b) chronic, repetitive pathologic fractures.
    c) thinned or "wiped out" trabeculae.
    d) medullary geographic, purely lytic lesions.

454. Bilateral lower extremity bone thickening by successive thick, undulating solid periosteal new bone may be due to:

    a) venous insufficiency.
    b) lymphocytic leukemia.
    c) myelocytic leukemia.
    d) reaction to radiation therapy.

455. Neurofibromatosis and tuberous sclerosis are related in that they both:

    a) involve epilepsy in a classic triad of symptoms.
    b) show a clear male predilection.
    c) are phakomatoses.
    d) usually result in mental retardation.

456. Kidney involvement occurs with tuberous sclerosis:

    a) extremely rarely.
    b) in up to 80% of cases.
    c) in almost 50% of cases.
    d) in 20% of cases.

457. Gaucher's disease creates vertebral radiologic appearances which are similar to those created by:

    a) Morquio's syndrome.
    b) sickle cell anemia.
    c) spondyloepiphyseal dysplasia tarda.
    d) Marfan's syndrome.

458. The "umbrella defect of the bulb" is a radiologic sign also known as:

    a) "cloverleaf deformity."
    b) "football sign."
    c) "air dome sign."
    d "hourglass deformity."

459. The most common pattern of lung infection with tuberculosis is:

    a) primary infection of the apices with spread to the lower lobes.
    b) primary infection of the middle lobe with spread to the apex.
    c) primary infection of the lower lobes, with spread to the apices.
    d) primary infection of the apices, with spread to the middle lobes.

460. A measurement used to evaluate the possibility of protrusio acetabuli is:

    a) Shenton's line.
    b) Kohler's line.
    c) Klein's line.
    d) Ferguson's line.

461. The femoral angle is also known as:

    a) the angle of incidence.
    b) the "Q" angle.
    c) the carrying angle.
    d) the Angle of Wiberg.

462. The "collar button ulcer" that burrows beneath the mucosa, is most commonly seen:

    a) in a colon affected by ulcerative colitis.
    b) in a stomach affected by hypochlorhydria.
    c) in a duodenum affected by hypochlorhydria.
    d) in the colon of a diabetic patient.

463. Sarcoidosis is:

    a) a non-caseating granulomatous disease.
    b) a caseating granulomatous disease.
    c) a fungal infection.
    d) a viral infection.

464. The radiographic appearance of osseous lesions caused by Hand-Schüller-Christian disease is described as:

    a) "hole within a hole" appearance.
    b) multiple small (< 2 mm in diameter) lytic lesions.
    c) multiple small sclerotic lesions.
    d) large (5–10 mm in diameter) sclerotic lesions.

465. At birth, over 50% of patients with tuberous sclerosis have detectable:

    a) myolipomas.
    b) rhabdomyomas.
    c) retinal phakomas.
    d) hematuria.

466. A patient with pyknodysostosis may have:

    a) "heaped-up" vertebrae.
    b) "spool-shaped" vertebrae.
    c) "bullet-nosed" vertebrae.
    d) inferior "beaking" of vertebrae.

467. The late stages of myelofibrosis cause bone changes that appear on x-ray as:

    a) diffuse osteoporosis.
    b) lucent, geographic lesions.
    c) "ground glass" or "wiped out trabeculae" appearance.
    d) homogeneously dense bone with no delineation between cortex and marrow cavity.

468. The most common malignant disease of childhood is:

    a) Wilm's tumor.
    b) acute lymphocytic leukemia.
    c) cystic fibrosis.
    d) neuroblastoma.

469. Lumbar compression fractures are usually stable, but are considered unstable if:

    a) the middle column (mid-vertebral body to posterior longitudinal ligament) is disrupted.
    b) the posterior column (posterior longitudinal ligament to supraspinous ligament) is disrupted.

c) any two or more "columns" are disrupted.

d) the anterior column (anterior longitudinal ligament to mid-vertebral body) is disrupted.

470. A barroom fracture is:

a) a chip fracture of the first metacarpal.

b) fracture of the fourth or fifth metacarpal neck.

c) fracture of the second or third metacarpal neck.

d) fracture of the proximal phalanx of the fourth or fifth digits of the hand.

471. The joint most often dislocated in adults is:

a) the knee.

b) the shoulder.

c) the elbow.

d) the interphalangeal joints of the fingers.

472. When elbow fracture is suspected, a minimum radiologic study should include:

a) AP and lateral views with the elbow in full extension.

b) AP and lateral views with the elbow in 90° flexion.

c) AP with full elbow extension, lateral, medial oblique, and axial olecranon views.

d) AP and lateral views in full extension, a medial oblique, and a "baby elbow."

473. Pagetic lesions in the skull:

a) usually start in the temporal and parietal bones.

b) do not cross the sutures.

c) spare the inner table, but destroy the outer table from within.

d) are uniformly small and round, creating a "raindrop skull."

474. With lytic metastatic disease in the spine, one may expect to see:

a) picture frame vertebrae.

b) vertebra plana.

c) sandwich vertebra.

d) rugger jersey vertebra.

475. Metastasis to the bone is most likely to be from:

a) melanoma of the skin.

b) a primary tumor in the brain.

c) a primary tumor in the breast.

d) a primary tumor in the spinal cord.

476. Chondrosarcoma and chordoma both are seen on x-ray to create:

a) ivory vertebrae.

b) lesions crossing the joint space.

c) solid or laminated periosteal response.

d) bone destruction with an associated large soft tissue mass.

477. The hips are affected by rheumatoid arthritis:

a) in one-third of the cases.

b) in about half the cases.

c) in virtually all cases.

d) in less that 10% of the cases.

478. HLA-B27 is frequently present in cases of all of the following arthritides except:

a) rheumatoid arthritis.

b) psoriatic arthritis.

c) ankylosing spondylitis.

d) Reiter's syndrome.

479. Periosteal "whiskering" seen with ankylosing spondylitis is an x-ray sign of:

    a) malignant degeneration.
    b) a healing pathologic fracture.
    c) enthesopathy.
    d) reaction to carrot-stick fracture.

480. Systemic lupus erythematosus commonly effects the joints of:

    a) the lower extremities.
    b) the upper extremities.
    c) the cervical spine.
    d) the lumbosacral spine.

481. Cortical erosion of the anterior femur, about 2–3 cm proximal to the superior margin of the patella, usually indicates:

    a) hyperparathyroidism.
    b) medial patellofemoral joint osteoarthritis.
    c) patellar osteophyte development.
    d) patellar subluxation or dislocation.

482. OPLL is most likely to involve neurologic symptoms when it:

    a) involves the upper thoracic spine.
    b) involves the lower thoracic spine.
    c) involves the cervical spine.
    d) involves the lumbar spine.

483. Rheumatoid arthritis shows a clear predilection (3:1) for:

    a) men over 40 years of age.
    b) men under 40 years of age.
    c) women under 40 years of age.
    d) women over 40 years of age.

484. The ESR (erythrocyte sedimentation rate) is:

    a) specific to inflammatory arthritides.
    b) constantly elevated in any patient with an inflammatory arthritide.
    c) apt to be elevated only during episodes of active inflammation (regardless of its etiology).
    d) rarely elevated in arthritis patients.

485. The most common skeletal site, overall, of fibrosarcoma is:

    a) in the ilium.
    b) in the humeral epicondyles.
    c) around the knee.
    d) in the skull.

486. Ewing's tumor most commonly occurs in:

    a) the metaphysis of the humerus.
    b) the metaphysis of the femur or tibia.
    c) the diaphysis of the femur or tibia.
    d) the diaphysis of the humerus.

487. Chondrosarcoma can metastasize, usually via venous channels, and most often to the:

    a) brain.
    b) skeleton.
    c) lungs.
    d) colon.

488. A 45-year-old patient with a tender, opaque, slowly growing juxtacortical mass on the popliteal surface of the distal femur, may be suspected to have:

    a) a parosteal sarcoma.
    b) a solitary osteochondroma.
    c) post-traumatic myositis ossificans.
    d) chondrosarcoma.

489. The majority of elbow fractures in children:
    a) involve the radial head and neck.
    b) involve the olecranon.
    c) are impaction fractures.
    d) are supracondylar.

490. Acromioclavicular joint separations that may require open fixation are:
    a) types II and III.
    b) type III only.
    c) type II only.
    d) Open fixation is not usually required for AC joint separations.

491. Nonunion and osteonecrosis are common complications of:
    a) a scaphoid fracture.
    b) a Colles' fracture.
    c) a Barton's fracture.
    d) a Smith's fracture.

492. A "ping-pong" fracture is:
    a) a fracture of the carpal navicular.
    b) a fracture of the pliable skull of a pediatric patient.
    c) a fracture of the ulnar styloid.
    d) a fracture of the maxilla (also called "LeFort I").

493. Radiologically, the effects of sickle-cell anemia on the small tubular bones of the hands and feet may simulate:
    a) osteomyelitis.
    b) hypertrophic arthropathy.
    c) neurotrophic arthropathy.
    d) Tom Smith's arthritis.

494. Phemister's triad comprises:
    a) joint space narrowing, peripheral erosions, and laminated periostitis.
    b) sudden, rapid joint space narrowing, "rat bite" cortical erosions, and solid reactive new bone deposition.
    c) subchondral cortical destruction, juxtaarticular osteoporosis, and laminated periostitis.
    d) slowly progressive joint space loss, juxtaarticular osteoporosis, and peripheral erosive defects.

495. "Periosteal warts," or cortical excrescences, occur on the tibia in patients with:
    a) tuberous sclerosis.
    b) osteopoikilosis.
    c) pyknodysostosis.
    d) neurofibromatosis.

496. Venous clefts of Hahn are most often found:
    a) in the lower thoracic vertebral bodies.
    b) in the lumbar vertebral bodies.
    c) on the upper thoracic vertebral bodies.
    d) in the lower cervical vertebral bodies.

497. Eosinophilic granuloma may occur in the mandible, causing:
    a) massive bone expansion.
    b) a prognathic jaw.
    c) a receding jaw.
    d) a "floating teeth sign."

498. When pneumoperitoneum results in air outlining the falciform ligament, it shows on plain film as:
    a) the "football sign."
    b) the inverted hemidiaphragm.

c) the "stepladder sign."
d) the "Mercedes Benz sign."

499. In the normal infant hip, the iliac angle should average between:

a) 10 to 20°.
b) 20 to 30°.
c) 45 to 55°.
d) 15 to 30°.

500. The 1-2-3 sign denotes:

a) the contours created by aortic coarctation.
b) the involvement, unilaterally, of all three lobes of the lung.
c) the bilateral involvement of all three lung lobes.
d) symmetric bilateral hilar node enlargement with right paratracheal node enlargement.

501. Although the "double lesion sign" is not specific for any pathology, it is an aid in ruling out:

a) bronchogenic carcinoma.
b) substernal thyroid.
c) pulmonary tuberculosis.
d) Kaposi sarcoma.

502. The acetabular angle of an infant is derived from an AP pelvis projection, using the intersection of:

a) the Y-Y line and a line connecting the lateral and medial acetabular margins.
b) the vertical line of Ombredanne and a line connecting the lateral and medial acetabular margins.
c) the vertical line of Ombredanne and a line tangential to the lateral iliac body margin.
d) the Y-Y line and a line tangential to the lateral iliac body margin.

503. A mycetoma is a ball of matted fungal hyphae, which may be seen in the apical lung of a patient with:

a) actinomycosis.
b) aspergillosis.
c) blastomycosis.
d) coccidioidomycosis.

504. The incidence of hyperparathyroidism:

a) shows no gender predilection, but is greatest in people < 25 years old.
b) shows a predilection for women (3:1) between 30 and 50 years old.
c) shows a male predilection, and is most common before the age of 30.
d) shows a female predilection (5:1) for patients > 60 years old.

505. A conoid tubercle:

a) is a protuberance from the sternum.
b) is a protuberance from the sacrum.
c) is a protuberance from the clavicle.
d) is a protuberance from the scapula.

506. Conditions often associated with melorheostosis include all of the following except:

a) osteogenesis imperfecta.
b) tuberous sclerosis.
c) hemangiomas.
d) neurofibromatosis.

507. Radiologically apparent skull lesions caused by acquired syphilis usually are:

    a) sclerotic reactive new bone excrescences in the frontal bone.
    b) permeative, geographic lesions in the temporal and parietal bones.
    c) gummatous lytic lesions through both tables of the parietal bones.
    d) gummatous lytic lesions through the outer table of the frontal bone.

508. In addition to "sickle-shaped" erythrocytes, laboratory tests of sickle-cell patients typically show:

    a) small numbers of RBCs with reduced HB, elevated serum bilirubin, and leukocytosis.
    b) normal numbers of very small RBCs, elevated serum bilirubin, and lymphocytosis.
    c) erythrocytosis, elevated serum bilirubin, and leukocytopenia.
    d) small numbers of RBCs, elevated serum bilirubin, and lymphocytopenia.

509. The most common fracture of the atlas is:

    a) a posterior arch fracture.
    b) a Jefferson fracture.
    c) an atlas lateral mass fracture.
    d) an atlas anterior arch avulsion.

510. Paralysis often accompanies fracture dislocations at T4–7 because of:

    a) small canal diameter.
    b) heavily vascularized structures.
    c) its location at the apex of the kyphosis.
    d) associated damage by splintered rib fragments.

511. A vertically shortened epiphysis, a widened physis with irregular margins, and a frayed metaphyseal/growth plate margin are all radiologic signs of:

    a) Legg-Calvé-Perthe's disease.
    b) ischemic necrosis of the femoral head.
    c) slipped femoral capital epiphysis.
    d) a Salter-Harris Type V fracture.

512. Stress fracture of the first rib occurs as a:

    a) result of violent coughing.
    b) result of "bear hugs," especially in the presence of osteopenia.
    c) result of strenuous or repetitive throwing movements.
    d) result of severe muscle spasms during seizures.

513. Ewing's sarcoma:

    a) rarely metastasizes.
    b) usually metastasizes to bone and lungs late in the disease process.
    c) usually metastasizes to the brain late in the disease process.
    d) usually metastasizes to bone and lungs early in the disease process.

514. The most common radiologic appearance of non-Hodgkin lymphoma is:

    a) a permeative, lytic lesion with marked cortical destruction and spiculated periosteal response.
    b) a metaphyseal or diaphyseal permeative, lytic lesion, with onion skin periosteal response and large soft tissue mass.
    c) lytic cortical destruction with a "hair-on-end" periosteal response.
    d) a permeative, lytic medullary lesion, later with patchy cortical destruction and soft tissue mass.

515. The most common skeletal site for metastasis (40%) is:

    a) the ribs.
    b) the shoulder.
    c) the spine.
    d) the skull.

516. The patients for whom Paget's disease has a predilection are:

    a) perimenopausal females.
    b) osteoporotic females > 60 years of age.
    c) males > 55 years of age.
    d) males between 35 and 50 years of age.

517. Necrobiotic pulmonary nodules and diffuse interstitial fibrosis are commonly concomitants of:

    a) enteropathic arthritis.
    b) rheumatoid arthritis.
    c) Paget's disease.
    d) neurofibromatosis.

518. Five to ten percent of ulcerative colitis patients develop:

    a) rheumatoid arthritis.
    b) ankylosing spondylitis.
    c) Reiter's syndrome.
    d) systemic lupus erythematosus.

519. Psoriatic arthritis in the foot:

    a) leads to osteoporosis and stress fractures.
    b) is not known to lead to intertarsal ankylosis.
    c) involves characteristic early changes at the great toe interphalangeal joint.
    d) usually causes solid or single lamination periostitis.

520. The hallmarks of Jaccoud's syndrome are:

    a) involvement of both sacroiliac joints and the thoracolumbar spine.
    b) bilateral, irreversible deformations of the hands.
    c) severe periostitis with subchondral erosions.
    d) ulnar deviation, and flexion of the metacarpophalangeal joints.

521. Gout is a metabolic arthritide that involves:

    a) sodium monourate deposits within joints.
    b) noncaseating granulomas within joints.
    c) homogentisic acid deposited within joints.
    d) hydroxyapatite deposits within joints.

522. Pyrophosphate arthropathy most frequently:

    a) resembles gouty arthritis, with overhanging margins and sparing of joint space.
    b) resembles rheumatoid arthritis, with uniform loss of joint space and marginal erosions.
    c) resembles osteoarthritis, with osteophytes, subchondral sclerosis, and loss of joint space.
    d) resembles psoriatic arthritis, with extensive periostitis.

523. The definitive triad of Reiter's syndrome includes:

    a) urethritis, polyarthritis, and Bell's palsy.
    b) intermittent neurogenic claudication, prostatitis, and polyarthritis.
    c) prostatitis, conjunctivitis, and polyarthritis.
    d) urethritis, conjunctivitis, and polyarthritis.

524. Common radiologic evidence of rotator cuff rupture caused by rheumatoid arthritis includes:

    a) resorption of the humeral head.
    b) increased glenohumeral joint space.

c) glenoid rim sclerosis.
d) a concavity on the inferior acromion.

525. Blastic metastasis are most often from primary tumors in the:

a) lung, kidneys, or breast.
b) lung, breast, or prostate.
c) prostate, cecum, bronchi, or breast.
d) kidneys, uterus, or lung.

526. When prostatic carcinoma spreads to the skeleton, laboratory investigation is likely to show:

a) markedly elevated serum calcium levels.
b) elevated potassium levels.
c) normal ESR.
d) elevated acid phosphatase.

527. In female patients, the primary source of skeletal metastasis is a primary tumor in the:

a) ovary.
b) kidney.
c) breast.
d) uterus.

528. The ivory vertebra of Hodgkin lymphoma of bone may be distinguished from ivory vertebrae of other etiologies by:

a) the "squaring" of the vertebral body.
b) the posterior scalloping of the vertebral body.
c) the anterior or lateral scalloping of the vertebral body.
d) the "barrel-shaped" expansion of the vertebral body.

529. The "extrapleural sign," which may be caused by such lesions as a hematoma adjacent to a rib fracture:

a) is seen as a clear lucency with its convex border directed into the lung.
b) is seen as a radiopacity with its convex border directed into the lung.
c) is seen as a clear lucency convex away from the lung.
d) is seen as a radiopacity convex away from the lung.

530. Hallux rigidus is often a sequela of:

a) gout.
b) Lisfranc's injury.
c) a phalangeal fracture of the great toe.
d) rheumatoid arthritis.

531. The Laug-Hansen method classifies ankle fractures according to:

a) the location of the lesions.
b) the number of fragments involved.
c) the forces that produced the fracture(s).
d) the fibular fracture position.

532. Rounding and sclerosis of fracture margins are radiographic signs of:

a) early callus formation.
b) nonunion.
c) malunion.
d) posttraumatic degenerative joint disease.

533. Signs of thalassemia that are visible on plain film include:

a) bone expansion, thickened cortices, and narrowed medullary cavities.
b) periosteal new bone, thickened cortices, and widened medullary cavities.
c) widened, purely lucent medullary cavities, and thinned cortices.
d) widened medullary cavities with "honeycomb" trabeculation, and bone expansion with thinned cortices.

534. The "sagging rope sign" is a residual deformity of Legg-Calvé-Perthes disease, describing the radiologic appearance of:

    a) a flattened, widened femoral head.
    b) a concavity in the superior articular surface of the femoral head.
    c) a curvilinear concave opacity superimposed over the metaphysis.
    d) an increased concavity of the lateral margin of the narrowed femoral neck.

535. Although osteopoikilosis itself is usually asymptomatic, about 25% of cases have associated:

    a) genu vara or genu valgum.
    b) scoliosis.
    c) cutaneous abnormalities.
    d) ocular defects.

536. A persistent metopic suture may be an indication of:

    a) cleidocranial dysplasia.
    b) osteogenesis imperfecta.
    c) osteopetrosis.
    d) epiphyseal dysplasia multiplex.

537. With primary hyperparathyroidism, laboratory tests may show:

    a) hypercalcemia and hyperphosphatemia.
    b) hypercalcemia and hypophosphatemia.
    c) hypocalcemia and hypophosphatemia.
    d) hypocalcemia and hyperphosphatemia.

538. One would not expect to see an "air bronchogram sign" in a patient with diagnosed:

    a) pulmonary edema.
    b) pulmonary infarct.
    c) atelectasis.
    d) lobar pneumonia.

539. The "shaggy heart sign" (partially obscured heart border) is a radiologic feature of:

    a) honeycomb lung.
    b) asbestosis.
    c) coccidioidomycosis.
    d) bronchogenic carcinoma.

540. For an AP hip projection:

    a) the foot is internally rotated 15°.
    b) the thigh is flexed 90° and abducted as far as possible.
    c) the foot is externally rotated 15°.
    d) there is no foot or thigh rotation.

541. Positive pressure pneumothorax is a synonym for:

    a) induced pneumothorax.
    b) complicated spontaneous pneumothorax.
    c) tension pneumothorax.
    d) simple spontaneous pneumothorax.

542. Caplan's disease is:

    a) asbestosis with rheumatoid arthritis.
    b) silicosis with pulmonary arthropathy.
    c) pneumoconiosis with pulmonary arthropathy.
    d) rheumatoid pneumoconiosis.

543. A tumor that may spread over the lung surface, encasing the lung entirely, is:

    a) myxoma.
    b) cystic hygroma.
    c) thymoma.
    d) mesothelioma.

544. The characteristic radiographic appearance of lesions caused by hyperparathyroidism can be described as:

    a) "lace-like" margination of irregular, frayed cortical lesions.
    b) beveled margination of cortical lesions.
    c) jagged, "saw-tooth" margination of cortical lesions.
    d) smooth, heavily sclerotic margins on ovoid lesions in subperiosteal cortical bone.

545. A normal variant that has the appearance of "horns" protruding laterally from the odontoid process is sometimes called the:

    a) ossiculum terminale persistens of Bergman.
    b) Mach effect.
    c) Viking helmet sign.
    d) os odontoideum.

546. The preauricular sulcus:

    a) shows a predilection for males.
    b) is usually bilateral and symmetrical.
    c) is also called the paraglenoid sulcus.
    d) has been correlated with pudendal nerve anomalies.

547. Radiographic signs of Legg-Calvé-Perthes disease include all of the following except:

    a) Herndon's hump (lateral femoral neck buttressing).
    b) "head-within-a-head" femoral head appearance.
    c) "snowcap" femoral head appearance.
    d) Gage's sign (lucent defect at lateral epiphysis and adjacent metaphysis).

548. The age group predilected for myelofibrosis is:

    a) 2–5 years old.
    b) 12–18 years old.
    c) 30–50 years old.
    d) 50–70 years old.

549. All of the following statements are true of an occult fracture except:

    a) it is initially evident clinically but not radiologically.
    b) it may become radiologically visible a week or two after it is clinically evident.
    c) it often occurs at the carpal navicular (scaphoid) or in the ribs.
    d) it is most commonly seen in pediatric patients.

550. A slipped capital femoral epiphysis is a classic example of a:

    a) Torus fracture.
    b) occult fracture.
    c) Salter-Harris Type V fracture.
    d) Salter-Harris Type I fracture.

551. A fracture caused by normal stress on weakened bone is called:

    a) a march fracture.
    b) an insufficiency fracture.
    c) a fatigue fracture.
    d) an occult fracture.

552. Bennett's fracture:

    a) is an intraarticular fracture through the base of the first metacarpal.
    b) is a chip fracture of the head of the first metacarpal.
    c) is a chip fracture of the trapezium.
    d) is a transverse fracture through the shaft of the first metacarpal.

553. All of the following bone disorders may cause benign polyostotic tumorlike lesions except:

    a) histiocytosis "X."
    b) Paget's disease.

c) hereditary multiple exostoses (HME).
d) sickle cell anemia.

554. The likelihood of malignant degeneration of a neurofibroma is:

a) very high (approximately 92%).
b) moderately high (approximately 68%).
c) moderately low (approximately 27%).
d) very low (approximately 5%).

555. An enchondroma is the result of:

a) residual cartilage in the metaphysis.
b) a genetic defect in the ossification process.
c) post-traumatic alteration of stress patterns in bone.
d) exuberant subcortical osteoblastic activity.

556. A cartilaginous lesion beneath the metaphyseal periosteum of a tubular bone is likely to be:

a) a chondromyxoid fibroma.
b) a solitary enchondroma.
c) a periosteal chondroma.
d) a periosteal osteochondroma.

557. A frontal chest film of a patient with sarcoidosis might show the radiographic signs:

a) silhouette sign, honeycomb lung, and tracheal deviation.
b) rib notching, air bronchogram, and silhouette sign.
c) honeycomb lung, pawnbroker's sign (1-2-3 sign), and "potato nodes."
d) air bronchogram, tracheal deviation, and 1-2-3 sign.

558. The hallmark lesion of sarcoidosis is:

a) noncaseating granuloma.
b) fibroma molluscum.
c) peau chagrin.
d) vitiligo.

559. Nonuniform loss of joint space is typical of:

a) enteropathic arthritis.
b) systemic lupus erythematosus.
c) rheumatoid arthritis.
d) degenerative joint disease.

560. Caplan's syndrome, Felty's syndrome, and Sjögren's syndrome may all be concomitants of:

a) Reiter's syndrome.
b) synoviochondrometaplasia.
c) scleroderma.
d) rheumatoid arthritis.

561. A discrete rash of red and purple nodules associated with sarcoidosis is called:

a) a butterfly rash.
b) lupus pernio.
c) Lofgren's syndrome.
d) erythema nodosum.

562. A hereditary amino acid metabolism disorder causing a lack of homogentisic acid oxidase is responsible for:

a) ochronosis.
b) sarcoidosis.
c) Wilson's disease.
d) hemochromatosis.

563. Hydroxyapatite deposition disease (HADD) at the hip may be misdiagnosed as:

   a) early Paget's disease changes.
   b) phleboliths.
   c) calcification of the internal iliac artery.
   d) a calcified lymph node.

564. Hemochromatosis is known to have:

   a) no gender predilection.
   b) a 20:1 female predilection.
   c) a 20:1 male predilection.
   d) a 2:1 male predilection.

565. A periosteal chondroma:

   a) is a benign lesion that shows no response in periosteal new bone formation.
   b) is a benign lesion, but may have a laminated periosteal bone response.
   c) is a malignant lesion with a laminated periosteal bone response.
   d) is a benign lesion that often has a buttress of periosteal bone at its proximal margin.

566. An oval, lytic, medullary lesion in the epiphysis of a young patient, showing stippled or fluffy calcifications within a slight marginal rim of sclerosis is most likely to be:

   a) a chondromyxoid fibroma.
   b) a solitary enchondroma.
   c) a chondroblastoma.
   d) an eosinophilic granuloma.

567. Aneurysmal bone cysts in long bones are most often:

   a) eccentric metaphyseal lesions.
   b) subperiosteal metadiaphyseal lesions.
   c) centrally located diaphyseal lesions.
   d) centrally located metadiaphyseal lesions.

568. Fibroma molluscum are:

   a) tumors on the nerve roots, which may erode the intervertebral foramina, especially in the cervical spine.
   b) subcutaneous nodules that may become painful and undergo malignant degeneration.
   c) pedunculated, nipplelike, or sessile cutaneous nodules of varying sizes.
   d) large soft tissue masses that may cause focal giantism.

569. Fracture of the second or third metacarpal neck is called:

   a) barroom fracture.
   b) boxer's fracture.
   c) Barton's fracture.
   d) Bennett's fracture.

570. Ischemic necrosis most often ensues in a scaphoid fracture located:

   a) at the distal pole.
   b) at the proximal pole.
   c) at the distal waist.
   d) at the proximal waist.

571. Half of the diagnosed Salter-Harris Type II fractures occur at the:

   a) distal radius.
   b) distal femur.
   c) proximal tibia.
   d) distal fibula.

572. Osteochondritis dissecans represents a common type of:

    a) occult fracture.
    b) chondral fracture.
    c) osteochondral fracture.
    d) impaction fracture.

573. Traction-avulsion of the ossification center of the inferior patellar pole and posttraumatic patellar ligament ossification are causative factors in:

    a) spontaneous osteonecrosis of the knee (SONK).
    b) tripartite patella.
    c) Blount's disease.
    d) Sinding-Larsen-Johansson disease.

574. Infections caused by brucellosis are most commonly seeded into:

    a) the distal lower extremities.
    b) the shoulder girdle.
    c) the spine and sacroiliac joints.
    d) the carpal and metacarpal bones.

575. Chondrocalcinosis is a feature of all of the following except:

    a) Wilson's disease.
    b) neurotrophic arthropathy.
    c) hemochromatosis.
    d) CPPD.

576. The "jelling phenomenon" typical of rheumatoid arthritis causes:

    a) erosion of cortical bone in the "bare areas."
    b) increased arthritic stiffness after extended rest (e.g., in the morning).
    c) relatively more severe symptoms in weight-bearing joints.
    d) increased symptoms after moist heat is applied to affected joints.

577. The "brown tumors of hyperparathyroidism" are:

    a) exuberantly expansile, egg-shell marginated peripheral lucencies.
    b) non-expansile, distinctly marginated peripheral lucencies.
    c) densely sclerotic, non-expansile peripheral masses.
    d) slightly expansile, lightly septated, central geographic lucencies.

578. The most common skin manifestation of neurofibromatosis (NF) is:

    a) smoothly marginated (Coast of California) café au lait spots.
    b) irregularly marginated (Coast of Maine) café au lait spots.
    c) fibroma molluscum.
    d) elephantiasis neuromatosa.

579. Lesions of the anterior mediastinum typically include:

    a) leukemia, thymoma, tamponade, and teratoma.
    b) thymoma, tamponade, teratoma, and lymphoma.
    c) thymoma, intrathoracic goiter, teratoma, and lymphoma.
    d) intrathoracic goiter, teratoma, thymic hypoplasia, and leukemia.

580. Nonunion or delayed union at a fracture site is most commonly caused by:

    a) adjacent soft tissue damage.
    b) inadequate immobilization.
    c) disturbance of the hematoma.
    d) delayed weight-bearing.

581. The hangman's fracture may be described as:

    a) a traumatic spondylolisthesis.
    b) a burst fracture of the axis.
    c) a compression fracture.
    d) an avulsion fracture.

582. The "fibrin peel" is:
    a) an uncalcified membrane around a cyst.
    b) a fibrous membrane encasing an abscess.
    c) a fibrous membrane encasing the lung.
    d) an uncalcified plaque sloughed from a pleural membrane.

583. A notable feature of the distribution of polyostotic fibrous dysplasia is that:
    a) unilateral involvement of the pelvis invariably is accompanied by ipsilateral proximal femoral involvement.
    b) unilateral pelvic involvement frequently is accompanied by contralateral proximal femoral involvement.
    c) the pelvis is invariably involved bilaterally.
    d) pelvic involvement is invariably accompanied by contralateral involvement of the shoulder girdle.

584. The subperiosteal resorption of hyperparathyroidism is notably prominent at:
    a) the radial margins of proximal and middle phalanges in second and third fingers.
    b) the ulnar styloid and the ulnar side of the proximal row of carpal bones.
    c) the radial styloid and the radial side of the proximal row of carpals.
    d) the entheses of the small tubular bones of the feet.

585. Rheumatoid involvement of the hands may result in the extensor digitorum tendon rupturing at the base of the distal phalanx, producing a deformity known as:
    a) "swan-neck" deformity.
    b) "mallet finger."
    c) "boutonniere" deformity.
    d) "Lanois deformity."

586. A patient whose x-ray findings include a "star sign," "Romanus lesions," and "Andersson lesions" may be expected to have a diagnosis of:
    a) gout.
    b) rheumatoid arthritis.
    c) ankylosing spondylitis.
    d) psoriatic arthritis.

587. The earliest radiologic sign of childhood inflammatory discitis, usually visible 3 to 4 weeks after the onset of symptoms, is:
    a) subchondral sclerosis.
    b) subchondral endplate fragmentation.
    c) disc space narrowing.
    d) soft tissue swelling (paravertebral abscess).

588. Joint effusion in the hip (regardless of etiology) increases the distance between the lateral margin of Kohler's teardrop and the medial margin of the femoral head, creating:
    a) Capener's sign.
    b) Waldenstrom's sign.
    c) Hawkin's sign.
    d) Pelkin's sign.

589. The second most common fracture in the lumbar spine is:
    a) a Chance fracture.
    b) a burst fracture.
    c) a vertebral body compression fracture.
    d) a transverse process fracture.

590. Severe pelvic trauma, with significant pelvic fractures, is most likely to be associated with:

    a) rupture of the right hemidiaphragm.
    b) rupture of the left hemidiaphragm.
    c) rupture of the spleen.
    d) pelvic and abdominal organ injury, but rarely with injury to the thoracic organs.

591. Slipped femoral capital epiphysis (SFCE) has a recognized association with:

    a) rickets, renal osteodystrophy, and Frölich's syndrome.
    b) familial history of osteoporosis and avascular necrosis.
    c) familial history of juvenile rheumatoid arthritis.
    d) familial history of rheumatoid arthritis.

592. The proximal tibial metaphysis is commonly fractured:

    a) when the femoral condyles are forced into the tibia as the knee is in flexion.
    b) when a young child jumps on a trampoline with a much heavier person.
    c) when a young child falls from a bicycle.
    d) when a pedestrian is struck by an automobile bumper.

593. With fibrous dysplasia the medullary canal of an affected long tubular bone:

    a) is completely occluded.
    b) is markedly narrowed.
    c) is widened, as the endosteum is thinned and scalloped.
    d) loses its trabeculation, but its dimensions are not altered.

594. When differentiating between metastatic carcinoma and Paget's disease, the doctor should remember that all of the following are common to Paget's disease, not to metastasis, except:

    a) cortical disruption.
    b) cortical thickening.
    c) significant bone expansion.
    d) long bone subarticular lesions.

595. A "shepherd's crook deformity" is:

    a) a slipped femoral capital epiphysis.
    b) an increment fracture at the femoral neck.
    c) a varus deformity of the hip with bowing of the femur.
    d) a elongated lucent defect in the femoral neck and proximal diaphysis.

596. Malignant degeneration of pagetic bone is most likely to occur in:

    a) the spine.
    b) the skull.
    c) the femur.
    d) the pelvis.

597. The "bare area" is:

    a) subchondral bone, which is devoid of periosteum.
    b) hyaline cartilage covered by pannus.
    c) hyaline cartilage not covered by pannus.
    d) intraarticular bone that is devoid of periosteum or hyaline cartilage.

598. Severe atlantoaxial instability is a common complication of:

    a) crystalline arthropathy.
    b) inflammatory arthritis.
    c) neurotrophic arthropathy.
    d) erosive osteoarthritis.

599. Ankylosing spondylitis in the lumbar spine may ossify ligamentum flavum and interspinous ligaments, resulting in the appearance on frontal films of:
    a) the "dagger sign."
    b) the "bamboo spine."
    c) the "poker spine."
    d) the "trolley track sign."

600. All of the following are x-ray signs typical of psoriatic arthritis in the hands except:
    a) ivory phalanx.
    b) pencil-in-cup deformity.
    c) rat bite erosions.
    d) mouse ears erosions.

FINAL TEST 1—ANSWER KEY

#	Ans	#	Ans	#	Ans	#	Ans	#	Ans	#	Ans	#	Ans	#	Ans	#	Ans	#	Ans
1.	b	49.	b	97.	d	145.	b	193.	a	241.	d	289.	c	337.	b	385.	a	433.	a
2.	a	50.	d	98.	a	146.	b	194.	d	242.	d	290.	d	338.	c	386.	b	434.	a
3.	c	51.	b	99.	d	147.	a	195.	c	243.	d	291.	d	339.	d	387.	b	435.	b
4.	c	52.	b	100.	a	148.	c	196.	c	244.	d	292.	c	340.	c	388.	a	436.	c
5.	c	53.	a	101.	d	149.	a	197.	b	245.	b	293.	d	341.	a	389.	a	437.	c
6.	d	54.	b	102.	a	150.	b	198.	a	246.	c	294.	c	342.	d	390.	b	438.	c
7.	c	55.	b	103.	b	151.	d	199.	c	247.	c	295.	d	343.	b	391.	d	439.	c
8.	b	56.	d	104.	c	152.	c	200.	b	248.	a	296.	b	344.	c	392.	a	440.	c
9.	c	57.	b	105.	b	153.	c	201.	c	249.	c	297.	c	345.	a	393.	b	441.	d
10.	b	58.	b	106.	d	154.	d	202.	c	250.	d	298.	d	346.	d	394.	c	442.	c
11.	b	59.	a	107.	c	155.	b	203.	c	251.	d	299.	d	347.	c	395.	a	443.	c
12.	d	60.	c	108.	c	156.	b	204.	d	252.	a	300.	d	348.	d	396.	b	444.	c
13.	c	61.	a	109.	b	157.	d	205.	b	253.	c	301.	c	349.	a	397.	b	445.	b
14.	c	62.	c	110.	d	158.	d	206.	b	254.	b	302.	b	350.	c	398.	d	446.	a
15.	a	63.	c	111.	b	159.	a	207.	d	255.	c	303.	b	351.	c	399.	d	447.	c
16.	c	64.	c	112.	c	160.	d	208.	b	256.	a	304.	a	352.	a	400.	c	448.	c
17.	c	65.	a	113.	c	161.	b	209.	c	257.	b	305.	c	353.	d	401.	c	449.	c
18.	a	66.	d	114.	a	162.	a	210.	c	258.	c	306.	b	354.	a	402.	a	450.	d
19.	c	67.	d	115.	c	163.	c	211.	a	259.	b	307.	c	355.	d	403.	c	451.	b
20.	b	68.	b	116.	c	164.	c	212.	d	260.	b	308.	d	356.	d	404.	c	452.	a
21.	c	69.	c	117.	c	165.	c	213.	a	261.	c	309.	c	357.	d	405.	a	453.	a
22.	b	70.	c	118.	d	166.	c	214.	b	262.	c	310.	b	358.	b	406.	b	454.	a
23.	b	71.	a	119.	c	167.	a	215.	c	263.	c	311.	a	359.	c	407.	d	455.	c
24.	d	72.	c	120.	d	168.	a	216.	c	264.	d	312.	c	360.	c	408.	c	456.	b
25.	d	73.	a	121.	d	169.	b	217.	b	265.	b	313.	a	361.	d	409.	a	457.	b
26.	b	74.	c	122.	b	170.	b	218.	a	266.	a	314.	b	362.	a	410.	a	458.	a
27.	d	75.	a	123.	a	171.	d	219.	a	267.	a	315.	c	363.	c	411.	a	459.	c
28.	d	76.	b	124.	a	172.	c	220.	b	268.	b	316.	d	364.	a	412.	b	460.	b
29.	c	77.	a	125.	b	173.	d	221.	b	269.	c	317.	c	365.	c	413.	a	461.	a
30.	b	78.	a	126.	d	174.	a	222.	b	270.	c	318.	c	366.	c	414.	c	462.	a
31.	c	79.	b	127.	c	175.	b	223.	a	271.	a	319.	d	367.	c	415.	b	463.	a
32.	d	80.	b	128.	c	176.	b	224.	b	272.	d	320.	b	368.	c	416.	a	464.	a
33.	c	81.	c	129.	c	177.	a	225.	b	273.	a	321.	d	369.	b	417.	c	465.	c
34.	c	82.	c	130.	c	178.	d	226.	d	274.	c	322.	c	370.	a	418.	c	466.	b
35.	a	83.	d	131.	b	179.	b	227.	b	275.	a	323.	c	371.	d	419.	a	467.	d
36.	a	84.	c	132.	b	180.	c	228.	c	276.	d	324.	a	372.	d	420.	b	468.	b
37.	b	85.	d	133.	d	181.	a	229.	d	277.	b	325.	d	373.	d	421.	c	469.	c
38.	b	86.	c	134.	c	182.	d	230.	c	278.	b	326.	d	374.	b	422.	a	470.	b
39.	b	87.	c	135.	c	183.	d	231.	d	279.	a	327.	c	375.	a	423.	b	471.	b
40.	b	88.	a	136.	b	184.	d	232.	c	280.	d	328.	b	376.	a	424.	a	472.	c
41.	c	89.	c	137.	c	185.	b	233.	d	281.	b	329.	d	377.	b	425.	a	473.	c
42.	c	90.	b	138.	c	186.	c	234.	b	282.	c	330.	c	378.	a	426.	c	474.	b
43.	d	91.	b	139.	d	187.	a	235.	d	283.	d	331.	c	379.	c	427.	d	475.	c
44.	c	92.	c	140.	b	188.	d	236.	d	284.	a	332.	b	380.	a	428.	b	476.	d
45.	c	93.	d	141.	b	189.	c	237.	c	285.	d	333.	c	381.	b	429.	a	477.	a
46.	d	94.	c	142.	d	190.	d	238.	b	286.	c	334.	b	382.	c	430.	b	478.	a
47.	a	95.	d	143.	c	191.	d	239.	c	287.	a	335.	c	383.	b	431.	a	479.	c
48.	c	96.	a	144.	c	192.	b	240.	a	288.	d	336.	d	384.	d	432.	c	480.	b

FINAL TEST 1—ANSWER KEY

481.	b	493.	a	505.	c	517.	b	529.	b	541.	c	553.	d	565.	d	577.	d	589.	d
482.	c	494.	d	506.	a	518.	b	530.	c	542.	d	554.	d	566.	c	578.	c	590.	b
483.	c	495.	a	507.	d	519.	c	531.	c	543.	d	555.	a	567.	a	579.	c	591.	a
484.	c	496.	a	508.	a	520.	d	532.	b	544.	a	556.	c	568.	c	580.	b	592.	b
485.	c	497.	d	509.	a	521.	a	533.	d	545.	c	557.	c	569.	b	581.	a	593.	c
486.	c	498.	a	510.	a	522.	c	534.	c	546.	c	558.	a	570.	d	582.	c	594.	a
487.	c	499.	c	511.	c	523.	d	535.	c	547.	a	559.	d	571.	a	583.	a	595.	c
488.	a	500.	d	512.	c	524.	d	536.	a	548.	d	560.	d	572.	c	584.	a	596.	c
489.	d	501.	a	513.	d	525.	c	537.	b	549.	d	561.	b	573.	d	585.	b	597.	d
490.	a	502.	a	514.	d	526.	d	538.	c	550.	d	562.	a	574.	c	586.	c	598.	b
491.	a	503.	b	515.	c	527.	c	539.	b	551.	b	563.	d	575.	b	587.	c	599.	d
492.	b	504.	b	516.	c	528.	c	540.	a	552.	a	564.	c	576.	b	588.	b	600.	c

Test 2

SUPPLEMENTARY TEST

Just when you thought your final exam was over, here is your *final* final examination. In the process of determining which questions to include in the "600 question test," we accumulated a surplus of good questions ... too good to not include in this guide. Here are an additional 225 questions to test your diagnostic acumen in preparation for your upcoming board examinations. Good luck—we hope this study guide will adequately serve its intended purpose.

1. During the self-limiting course of Legg-Calvé-Perthes disease, the articular cartilage of the affected hip:

   a) becomes thinned and fragmented.
   b) hypertrophies in pannus-like response.
   c) becomes softened and deformed.
   d) remains unaffected.

2. When the proximal fibula is fractured, there is high possibility of:

   a) distal tibiofibular diastasis.
   b) popliteal artery rupture.
   c) peroneal nerve damage.
   d) sural nerve damage.

3. The most common site for osteoarthritis in the foot is:

   a) the second and third metatarsal heads.
   b) the talonavicular joint.
   c) the first metatarsophalangeal joint.
   d) the base of the fifth metatarsal.

4. With solitary enchondroma, the cortex of the host bone:

   a) is expanded and thickened by reactive sclerosis.
   b) may show laminated or solid periosteal new bone.
   c) is expanded and thinned, and may show endosteal scalloping.
   d) is thinned and interrupted, but shows no periosteal reaction.

5. The "cauliflower spine" appearance in the vertebral neural arch is an x-ray sign of:

   a) osteoid osteoma.
   b) osteoblastoma.
   c) aneurysmal bone cyst.
   d) osteochondroma.

6. Fibrous dysplasia:

   a) expands bone and usually disrupts the cortex.
   b) is not an expansive lesion, but softens and deforms the bone.
   c) expands bone and thins, but usually does not disrupt the cortex.
   d) expands the bone and thickens the cortex.

7. Sarcoidosis has systemic effects including all the following except:

   a) iritis and uveitis.
   b) lymphadenopathy.
   c) renal failure.
   d) hepatosplenomegaly.

8. The most commonly fractured metacarpal is:

   a) the fifth.
   b) the fourth.
   c) the second.
   d) the first.

9. The most common cause of acquired thoracic aortic aneurysms is:

   a) trauma.
   b) atherosclerosis.
   c) hypertension.
   d) connective tissue disorders, e.g., rheumatoid disease.

10. DRSA (dialysis-related spondyloarthropathy) creates radiologic appearances of:

    a) vertebral erosions in endplates, facets, and vertebral bodies.
    b) "picture frame" vertebra.
    c) "ghost" vertebra.
    d) ivory vertebra.

11. Osteoporosis may become a post-fracture complication if:

    a) the hematoma is disturbed during early fracture healing.
    b) early weight-bearing is attempted.
    c) functional weight-bearing is delayed.
    d) the patient is more than 35 years of age.

12. The radiographic latent period for radiation-induced bone changes is:

    a) 2 years.
    b) 2 to 6 months.
    c) 1 to 2 months.
    d) 3 to 12 months.

13. Hodgkin disease may create a radiologic appearance of:

    a) "cannon-ball" lesions in the hilar areas.
    b) bulky mediastinal widening.
    c) extrapleural sign.
    d) silhouette sign.

14. Pott's paraplegia is:

    a) syphilitic neuropathy.
    b) intermittent paraplegia caused by soft tissue swellings with suppurative spinal osteomyelitis.
    c) sudden lower limb paraplegia with spinal tubercular infection.
    d) insidious onset, gradually increasing lower limb neurologic deficit, resulting ultimately in paraplegia, seen with ankylosing spondylitis.

15. Patellar dislocation is usually:

    a) inferomedial.
    b) vertical.
    c) superolateral.
    d) horizontal.

16. In rheumatoid arthritis, pannus destroys:

    a) subchondral bone.
    b) hyaline cartilage.
    c) fibrocartilage.
    d) periosteum.

17. Codman's tumor is the eponym given to:

    a) an osteoblastoma.
    b) a periosteal chondroma.
    c) a chondroblastoma.
    d) a fibrous xanthoma of bone.

18. An eroded or enlarged appearance of an IVF causes the radiologist to consider a tortuous vertebral artery, congenital agenesis of a pedicle, or:

    a) Hodgkin lymphoma.
    b) non-Hodgkin lymphoma.
    c) neurilemoma.
    d) cystic hygroma.

19. In an x-ray tube:

    a) the positive cathode ejects electrons toward the negative anode.
    b) the negative anode ejects electrons toward the positive cathode.
    c) the positive anode ejects electrons toward the negative cathode.
    d) the negative cathode ejects electrons toward the positive anode.

20. The most frequently dislocated carpal bone is:

    a) the lunate.
    b) the scaphoid.
    c) the capitate.
    d) the pisiform.

21. The best prognosis with sarcoidosis is associated with:

    a) insidious onset in a patient > 40 years of age.
    b) insidious onset in a patient < 40 years of age.
    c) bone lesions and skin lesions in a young patient.
    d) erythema nodosum over the anterior tibia in a young patient with acute onset.

22. The typical radiologic appearance of polyostotic fibrous dysplasia lesions is described as:

    a) a purely lucent lesion.
    b) a ground glass, or wipe out of trabecular patterns.
    c) a cumulus cloud.
    d) a granular, punctate stippling.

23. Stenotic heart valves and mitral insufficiency are common results of:

    a) rheumatoid arthritis.
    b) rheumatic heart disease.
    c) German measles.
    d) varicella pneumonia.

24. Heberden's nodes are located:

    a) at distal interphalangeal joints.
    b) at the first metatarsophalangeal joints.
    c) at the metacarpophalangeal joints.
    d) at proximal interphalangeal joints.

25. The clinical significance of the FBI sign is that it indicates:

    a) arterial rupture.
    b) neurologic injury.
    c) articular soft tissue damage.
    d) occult intraarticular fracture.

26. Radiographic indications of rheumatoid arthritis may include any of the following except:

    a) uniform loss of joint space.
    b) asymmetrical distribution.
    c) juxtaarticular osteoporosis.
    d) periarticular soft tissue swelling.

27. Legg-Calvé-Perthes disease has:

    a) a 3:1 female predilection.
    b) a 2:1 male predilection.
    c) a 5:1 male predilection.
    d) no gender predilection.

28. Benign cysts or neoplasms that may be characterized by periosteal buttressing include all of the following except:

    a) aneurysmal bone cyst.
    b) simple bone cyst.
    c) periosteal chondroma.
    d) chondroblastoma.

29. A butterfly fragment is:

    a) a triangular fragment of cortical bone.
    b) an avulsed cortical fragment.
    c) the exposed portion of an open fracture.
    d) a cortical fragment which has migrated distal to the fracture site.

30. *Pneumocystis carinii* pneumonia (PCP) is a pulmonary infection:

    a) most commonly seen in patients with AIDS.
    b) caused by a parasite found in South Asia.
    c) that occurs in newborns with inactivated surfactant.
    d) that commonly complicates comatose or quadriplegic patients.

31. The "1-2-3 sign" seen with sarcoidosis is also called:

    a) the reverse "S" sign of Golden.
    b) the "3" sign.
    c) the "butterfly" sign.
    d) the "pawnbroker's" sign.

32. Posttraumatic necrosis of the body of the talus is called:

    a) Hass's disease.
    b) Diaz's disease.
    c) Kohler's disease.
    d) Sever's disease.

33. Within a tubular bone, Brodie's abscess is most frequently located:

    a) in subarticular cancellous bone.
    b) in the metaphysis.
    c) in the diaphysis.
    d) in the physis of a preadolescent child.

34. Pulseless disease (aortic arch syndrome) is:

    a) caused by aortic coarctation.
    b) caused by situs inversus.
    c) a noninfectious aortitis.
    d) caused by excessive cholesterol deposits.

35. Rheumatoid arthritis most often:

    a) affects the wrists more severely than it does the hands.
    b) affects the hands more severely than it does the wrists.
    c) spares the wrists.
    d) spares the ulnar articulations of the wrists.

36. Polyostotic fibrous dysplasia:

    a) is progressive in only a minority of cases ($< 30\%$).
    b) typically features recurrent pathologic fracture and severe deformity.

c) is infrequently disfiguring, although it may result in pathologic fracture.

d) typically affects a single bone in each limb, but is bilateral and symmetrical.

37. Fischer's fracture is:

a) the second most common carpal fracture (triquetrum).
b) the most common carpal fracture (scaphoid).
c) a fracture of the lunate.
d) a fracture of the hook of the hamate.

38. The normal tracheal bifurcation, at the carina, is usually at the spinal level of:

a) T4.
b) T2.
c) T6.
d) C7.

39. The pneumoconioses, and especially asbestosis, is likely to create the roentgen finding known as:

a) the 1-2-3 sign.
b) the split pleura sign.
c) the shaggy heart sign.
d) the extrapleural sign.

40. In children, the normal atlantodental interspace may be as great as:

a) 8 mm.
b) 3 mm.
c) 5 mm.
d) 10 mm.

41. Pigmented villonodular synovitis (PVNS) in the hip may create the x-ray sign known as:

a) shepherd's crook.
b) coxa vara.
c) pistol grip deformity.
d) apple core deformity.

42. There is a predilection for gouty tophi to form in such sites as:

a) the helix of the ear.
b) the popliteal fossa.
c) the antecubital region.
d) the axilla.

43. Tuberculous spondylitis in young patients may create a "gibbus" deformity, which eventually causes development of:

a) vertebra plana.
b) kyphoscoliosis.
c) "long vertebra."
d) "bullet-nosed vertebra."

44. The "split-pleura sign," easily identified on CT scans, is caused by:

a) loculated pleural effusions.
b) free pleural effusions.
c) atelectasis, with the lung pulled away from the chest wall.
d) empyema separating parietal and visceral pleura.

45. Toddlers, usually around 3 years of age or younger, are most likely to suffer:

a) a trimalleolar fracture.
b) an undisplaced spiral fracture of the tibia.
c) a Lisfranc's injury.
d) a Jones' fracture.

46. With rheumatoid arthritis, sacroiliac joint involvement:
    a) is usually asymmetric or unilateral.
    b) is almost always present and is an early manifestation of RA.
    c) involves extensive sclerosis of the inferior ⅓ of the joint.
    d) frequently results in fibrous or osseous ankylosis.

47. The gender predilection for giant cell tumors is characterized as follows:
    a) 3:2 female predilection in benign tumors, and 3:1 male predilection in malignant tumors.
    b) 3:2 female predilection in benign tumors, and 3:1 female predilection in malignant tumors.
    c) 3:2 male predilection in benign tumors, and 3:1 female predilection in malignant tumors.
    d) 3:2 male predilection in benign tumors, and 3:1 male predilection in malignant tumors.

48. A frequent complication of Osgood-Schlatter's disease is:
    a) localized infection.
    b) stress fracture.
    c) complete rupture of the patellar tendon.
    d) chondro-osseous avulsion with persistent osseous fragments.

49. The most common reasons for mediastinal lymph node calcifications include:
    a) sarcoidosis and metastasized osteosarcoma.
    b) bronchogenic carcinoma and lymphoma.
    c) fungal infections and pneumoconiosis.
    d) metastasized chondrosarcoma and neurofibroma.

50. The joint most frequently dislocated in children is:
    a) the elbow.
    b) the shoulder.
    c) the hip.
    d) the knee.

51. The postural presentation most typical of a patient with Scheuermann's disease is:
    a) a marked double scoliosis.
    b) an increase of cervical lordosis, thoracic kyphosis, and lumbar lordosis, with protuberant abdomen and increased pelvic tilt.
    c) an increased thoracic kyphosis in an otherwise "military spine."
    d) a long "C-curve" scoliosis with a sharp gibbus deformity in the thoracic spine.

52. The combined findings of Kerley's A, B, and C lines; interstitial pulmonary edema in the lower lung lobes; and cephalization of blood flow in the lungs indicates a diagnosis of:
    a) congestive heart failure (CHF).
    b) aortic stenosis.
    c) mitral valve insufficiency.
    d) tricuspid valvular disease.

53. Blount's disease usually presents:
    a) unilaterally.
    b) bilaterally.
    c) unilaterally in the younger cohort, and bilaterally in the older cohort of patients.
    d) bilaterally in the younger cohort, but unilaterally in the older cohort of patients.

54. Spontaneous osteonecrosis of the knee (SONK) is most likely to affect:
    a) a perimenopausal female.
    b) a young male athlete.

    c) a female > 60 years old.
    d) children who have not reached puberty.

55. The lesions typical of osteopoikilosis:

    a) may change size (become larger or smaller), disappear, or
        reappear.
    b) usually are diaphyseal in long bones.
    c) are most often found in the skull and spine.
    d) usually are monostotic.

56. The radiologic hallmark of congenital agenesis of a pedicle in the
    lumbar spine is:

    a) contralateral pedicle hypertrophy and sclerosis.
    b) bilaterally dysplastic transverse processes.
    c) malformed articular processes.
    d) posteriorly displaced articular processes.

57. Sir James Paget's original discussion of the pathology of Paget's
    disease:

    a) occurred with the help of x-ray findings.
    b) occurred at the same time as Roentgen's discovery of X-ray.
    c) occurred before the discovery of X-ray.
    d) occurred 20 years after Roentgen's discovery of X-ray.

58. Both black and Scandinavian populations are at increased risk for:

    a) gout.
    b) CPPD.
    c) sarcoidosis.
    d) tumoral calcinosis.

59. The effects of Paget's disease on vertebral bodies include:

    a) scalloping of the anterior and lateral vertebral bodies.
    b) enlarging the vertebral body and accentuating the vertical
        trabeculae.
    c) causing "step defects" at the anterosuperior vertebral body
        margins.
    d) creating "wasp waist" vertebrae caused by expansion of the
        superior and inferior portions of the vertebral body.

60. All of the following are true of the KUB study except:

    a) it is usually done as a PA projection.
    b) it is a scout film, often used when renal stone formation is
        suspected.
    c) it is usually done as an AP projection.
    d) the PA projection is helpful with obese patients.

61. Inflammatory arthritides include all of the following except:

    a) psoriatic arthritis.
    b) erosive osteoarthritis.
    c) ankylosing spondylitis
    d) Reiter's syndrome.

62. Degenerative joint disease of the knee secondary to osteochondritis
    dissecans usually:

    a) involves all three joint compartments.
    b) involves the patellofemoral joint.
    c) involves the lateral joint.
    d) involves the medial joint.

63. Synovial fluid leaking into subchondral bone may create:

    a) geodes.
    b) synovial metaplasia.
    c) joint mice.
    d) eburnation.

64. An eponym for a "dancer's fracture" is:

    a) Dupuytren's fracture.
    b) Smith's fracture.
    c) Jones' fracture.
    d) Pott's fracture.

65. Acromegaly is usually the result of:

    a) hyperthyroidism.
    b) productive ectopic adrenal tissue.
    c) pituitary eosinophilic adenoma.
    d) excessive growth hormone produced during adolescence.

66. Rheumatoid arthritis at the elbow:

    a) may progress to severe osteolysis resembling neurotrophic arthropathy.
    b) usually involves pressure erosions from rheumatoid nodules.
    c) usually involves rheumatoid nodules on the flexor surface of the forearm.
    d) usually is too mild to produce definitive radiologic signs.

67. Although central osteosarcoma is a primary malignant bone tumor, it has a recognized association with:

    a) primary bronchogenic carcinoma.
    b) fibrous dysplasia.
    c) Paget's disease.
    d) Ollier's disease.

68. The majority of patients who develop osteosarcoma are young men who:

    a) are obese.
    b) are taller than average for their age.
    c) participate in contact sports.
    d) are exceptionally sedentary.

69. A radiopaque line across a long bone of a trauma patient may indicate:

    a) an avulsion fracture.
    b) a comminuted fracture.
    c) an impaction fracture.
    d) an open fracture.

70. The radiopharmaceutical agent for nuclear scanning is introduced into the body via all of the following routes except:

    a) ingestion.
    b) injection.
    c) inhalation.
    d) absorption.

71. The Hutchinson's fracture (chauffeur's fracture) consists of:

    a) fracture of the distal radius and ulnar styloid.
    b) fracture of the distal ulna and radial styloid.
    c) fracture of the radial styloid.
    d) fracture of the ulnar styloid.

72. In tumoral calcinosis, calcium carbonate and calcium triphosphate salts fill multiloculated cysts:

    a) in subarticular bone.
    b) in the medullary canal.
    c) in intraarticular sites.
    d) in extracapsular, periarticular sites.

73. The thickened cortex of the pelvic rim, seen in Paget's disease, with the obliteration of Kohler's teardrop, is called:

    a) protrusio acetabulae.
    b) the "tear drop sign."

    c) the "twisted ribbon appearance."
    d) the "brim sign."

74. "Mainliners' syndrome" has a predilection to implant osteomyelitis in:

    a) the small tubular bones of the hands and feet.
    b) the tarsal bones.
    c) the carpal bones.
    d) the axial skeleton's "S" joints (spine, sternoclavicular joints, etc.).

75. Rheumatoid arthritis commonly has significant visceral effects on:

    a) the liver and spleen.
    b) the liver and kidneys.
    c) the heart, lungs and pleura.
    d) the spleen and pancreas.

76. Paget's disease in the spine may create the radiographic appearance of:

    a) cod-fish vertebra and ivory vertebra.
    b) rugger jersey vertebra and vertebra plana.
    c) ivory vertebra and picture frame vertebra.
    d) corduroy cloth vertebra and vertebra plana.

77. Fluorosis may involve negative effects if the rate of ingestion of fluorine is:

    a) < 2 ppm.
    b) < 1 ppm.
    c) > 2 ppm.
    d) > 1 ppm.

78. Clavicle fracture is frequently complicated by:

    a) damage to the brachial plexus, the jugular vein, and the external carotid artery.
    b) damage to the long thoracic nerve, the subclavian artery, and the innominate vein.
    c) damage to the brachial plexus, the sympathetic chain, and the jugular vein.
    d) damage to the subclavian artery, the brachial plexus, and/or the sympathetic chain.

79. The thickness of material (usually lead) that will absorb 90% of the energy of the x-ray beam is expressed as:

    a) half-value layer (HVL).
    b) tenth-value layer (TVL).
    c) as low as reasonably achievable (ALARA).
    d) maximum permissible dose (MPD).

80. With forceful wrist hyperextension, proximal carpal dislocation with posterior fracture of the articular surface of the radius may occur, creating:

    a) a reversed Barton's fracture.
    b) a rim fracture.
    c) a Bennett's fracture.
    d) a reversed Colles' fracture.

81. Hemosiderin deposits in synovial tissue, and a brown or serosanguinous synovial fluid aspirate would indicate a probable diagnosis of:

    a) Wilson's disease.
    b) hemochromatosis.
    c) pigmented villonodular synovitis (PVNS).
    d) ochronosis.

82. The treatment of choice for tumoral calcinosis is:
    a) dietary control of the disease.
    b) surgical excision.
    c) chemotherapy.
    d) radiation therapy.

83. Primary central osteosarcoma is commonly associated with:
    a) metastasis to the brain.
    b) cannonball metastases to the lungs.
    c) colon metastases.
    d) metastasis to the breast.

84. Reiter's syndrome primarily involves:
    a) peripheral joints of the lower extremity.
    b) peripheral joints of the upper extremity.
    c) the lower lumbar spine and sacroiliac joints.
    d) the joints of the upper cervical spine.

85. Pseudoarthrosis after pathologic fracture due to neurofibromatosis is most common in the:
    a) lower two-thirds of the tibia.
    b) proximal third of the femur.
    c) lower third of the femur.
    d) proximal third of the humerus.

86. Widened diploe, "hair-on-end" periostitis, well-circumscribed large lytic lesions and granular osteoporosis are radiologic characteristics of the skull in a patient with:
    a) neuroblastoma.
    b) thalassemia.
    c) Caisson disease.
    d) Paget's disease.

87. The majority (80%) of neuroblastomas are found in:
    a) adolescents.
    b) children between 5 and 12 years of age.
    c) children < 3 years of age.
    d) pregnant females.

88. In a middle clavicle fracture, malalignment is a common problem because:
    a) the deltoid tends to elevate the distal fragment while the SCM elevates the proximal fragment.
    b) the trapezius and deltoid elevate the distal fragment, and the clavicular head of the pectoralis depresses the proximal fragment.
    c) the weight of the shoulder depresses the lateral fragment as the SCM elevates the medial fragment.
    d) the shoulder weight depresses the lateral fragment and the pectoralis major depresses the medial fragment.

89. Which type of arthritide produces a radiographic appearance of "osteoarthritis with a vengeance?"
    a) gout
    b) rheumatoid arthritis
    c) neurotrophic arthropathy
    d) psoriatic arthritis

90. The most common skeletal site for osteochondritis dissecans is:
    a) the talar dome.
    b) the medial aspect of the medial femoral condyle.
    c) the medial aspect of the lateral femoral condyle.
    d) the lateral aspect of the medial femoral condyle.

91. Periosteal reactions:

    a) do not occur with Paget's disease.
    b) invariably occur with Paget's disease.
    c) occur early in the process of Paget's disease.
    d) occur with aggressive pagetic lesions.

92. Both Pott's fracture and Maisonneuve's fracture:

    a) are fractures of the proximal fibula.
    b) involve bimalleolar fracture.
    c) feature tibiofibular diastasis with no malleolar fracture.
    d) are fractures of the distal fibula.

93. Sever's disease is not a disease at all, but rather a normal developmental variant at:

    a) the ischio-pubic junction.
    b) the calcaneal apophysis.
    c) the carpal navicular.
    d) the tarsal navicular.

94. A "dinner fork deformity" is the clinical appearance characteristic of:

    a) a Galeazzi fracture.
    b) a Smith's fracture.
    c) a Colles' fracture.
    d) a Barton's fracture.

95. Tumoral calcinosis targets the age group:

    a) over 60 years of age.
    b) 40–60 years of age.
    c) 6–25 years of age.
    d) neonatal and toddler.

96. When osteosarcoma metastasizes to the lungs, it may lead to:

    a) spontaneous pneumothorax and hypertrophic osteoarthropathy.
    b) pneumonia that clears and recurs.
    c) calcified "coin lesions."
    d) massive pleural effusions.

97. A widened pulse pressure, hypersensitivity to heat, and tachycardia are clinical signs that may indicate:

    a) a cortical adrenal malfunction.
    b) a pituitary condition.
    c) a parathyroid condition.
    d) a hyperthyroid condition.

98. The three most common abdominal malignancies in females, in order of decreasing incidence, are:

    a) gallbladder, colon, and stomach carcinoma.
    b) pancreas, colon, and gallbladder carcinoma.
    c) stomach, colon, and esophageal carcinoma.
    d) colon, pancreas, and stomach carcinoma.

99. Neer classification is a system used for categorizing:

    a) ankle fractures.
    b) fractures involving the physis.
    c) wrist fracture/dislocations.
    d) fractures of the proximal humerus.

100. The poorest prognosis of any form of juvenile rheumatoid arthritis (JRA) is associated with:

    a) seropositive JRA.
    b) classic systemic Still's disease.
    c) polyarticular Still's disease.
    d) mono- or pauciarticular Still's disease.

101. The most common complication of Paget's disease is:

    a) bananalike fractures.
    b) third cranial nerve palsy.
    c) malignant degeneration.
    d) anemia.

102. An intestinal mass lesion that shows a "squeeze sign" is most likely:

    a) carcinoid.
    b) an enterolith.
    c) lipoma.
    d) hemangioma.

103. Complete collapse of the vertebral body is common to:

    a) Kummel's disease and Panner's disease.
    b) Scheuermann's disease and Calvé's disease.
    c) Calvé's disease and Kummel's disease.
    d) Scheuermann's disease and Panner's disease.

104. Gallstone ileus caused by cholelithiasis typically presents with a triad of radiologic findings, including:

    a) air in the biliary tree, gallstones in the small bowel, and "stepladder appearance."
    b) gallstones in the small bowel, a "Mercedes Benz sign," and volvulus.
    c) mechanical ileus, gallstones in the small bowel, and "crow-foot sign."
    d) volvulus, "crow-foot sign," and mechanical ileus.

105. A Smith's fracture is:

    a) a distal radius fracture with the distal fragment angulated posteriorly.
    b) a distal radius fracture and ulnar styloid fracture with the distal fragments angulated posteriorly.
    c) a distal radius fracture with the distal fragment angulated anteriorly.
    d) a distal radius fracture and ulnar styloid fracture with the distal fragments angulated anteriorly.

106. The most commonly affected articulation with hydroxyapatite deposition disease (HADD) is:

    a) the wrist.
    b) the knee.
    c) the shoulder.
    d) the cervical spine.

107. Cortical disruption, a large soft tissue mass, and periosteal "sunburst" or "Codman's reactive triangle" are x-ray findings typical of:

    a) Brodie's abscess.
    b) solitary plasmacytoma.
    c) osteosarcoma.
    d) osteoblastoma.

108. Crohn's disease (regional enteritis) most commonly affects:

    a) the distal ileum and proximal colon.
    b) the descending colon and sigmoid colon.
    c) the distal duodenum and proximal jejunum.
    d) the distal jejunum and proximal ileum.

109. Cholelithiasis patients report constant pain with periodic peaks, and sometimes pain referred to:

    a) the left shoulder and arm.
    b) the mid-scapular region.
    c) the lumbosacral spine.
    d) the right inferior scapula.

110. The vast majority of fractures in the Neer classification are:

    a) one-part fractures.
    b) two-part fractures.
    c) three-part fractures.
    d) four-part fractures.

111. Idiopathic chondrolysis of the hip:

    a) is most common in obese adolescent males.
    b) is most common in young male athletes.
    c) has a 6:1 female predilection, and is usually seen in patients in their second decade.
    d) has a 2:1 female predilection, and is usually seen in girls ages 4–10 years.

112. Neurologic effects of Paget's disease may include:

    a) peripheral neuropathy.
    b) hot flashes.
    c) nerve deafness.
    d) Raynaud's phenomenon.

113. Monostotic fibrous dysplasia is most commonly seen:

    a) in the clavicle, pelvis, or ribs.
    b) in the scapula, mandible, and pelvis.
    c) in the lower extremities, ribs, or skull.
    d) in the pelvis, lower extremities, or mandible.

114. The esophageal diverticulum protruding through the cricopharyngeal muscle is called:

    a) a traction diverticulum.
    b) Zenker's diverticulum.
    c) Meckel's diverticulum.
    d) Ganser's diverticulum.

115. Resolution of the residual deformity following osteonecrosis is caused by:

    a) creeping substitution.
    b) Salter-Harris Type I fracture of the physis.
    c) phagocytotic resorption of necrotic bone.
    d) biological plasticity of new bone.

116. The most frequent cause of pneumoperitoneum is:

    a) perforation of a stomach carcinoma.
    b) rupture of colonic diverticulum.
    c) ruptured gastric or duodenal peptic ulcer.
    d) ruptured emphysematous gas cysts.

117. *Echinococcosis*, or hydatid disease, causes splenic cysts that appear radiographically:

    a) with "eggshell" calcific rims.
    b) with heavily calcified cyst walls.
    c) with lucent matrices, and often an air/fluid level.
    d) with amorphous, streaked calcifications.

118. A mature medullary infarct in metaphyseal or diaphyseal bone presents a characteristic radiologic appearance of:

    a) an "eggshell" rim of calcification around a lucent, elongated lesion.
    b) a dense serpiginous rim of calcification around an elongated lesion filled with areas of patchy sclerosis.
    c) thickened cortical bone around a wide and short, sclerotic medullary lesion.
    d) a dense central sequestrum in a lucent lesion, surrounded by a wide, poorly delineated rim of calcification.

119. A rigid, cast-like terminal ileum, occurring with Crohn's disease, may be seen on barium studies as:

    a) a cobblestone appearance.
    b) the String sign of Kantor.
    c) a skip lesion.
    d) a pseudotumor.

120. Colles' fracture is defined as:

    a) a distal radius fracture (20–35 mm proximal to the joint), with the distal fragment angulated posteriorly.
    b) a distal radius fracture and ulnar styloid fracture (10–20 mm proximal to the joint), distal fragments angulated posteriorly.
    c) a distal radius fracture and ulnar styloid fracture, distal fragments angulated anteriorly.
    d) a distal radius fracture with the distal fragment angulated anteriorly.

121. Synonyms for a renal adenocarcinoma include all of the following except:

    a) Grawitz tumor.
    b) renal cell carcinoma.
    c) renal pelvis carcinoma.
    d) hypernephroma.

122. Even with a history of deep sea diving, differential considerations for Caisson's disease should include spontaneous osteonecrosis, steroid therapy, posttraumatic infarction, and:

    a) renal osteodystrophy.
    b) hyperphosphatasia.
    c) leukemia.
    d) hemoglobinopathies.

123. The most frequent site of clinical and radiologic signs of CPPD is:

    a) the knee.
    b) the carpus.
    c) the elbow.
    d) the shoulder.

124. The rare multicentric osteosarcoma:

    a) consists of multiple, simultaneous, slow-growing sarcomas, usually in geriatric males.
    b) is a polyostotic form of osteosarcoma, which responds favorably to chemotherapy.
    c) is a rapidly fatal form of osteosarcoma, with early pulmonary metastasis, seen in pediatric patients.
    d) is a rapidly fatal form of osteosarcoma, with early pulmonary metastasis, seen in elderly patients.

125. One radiologic indication of sprue is the absence of luminal folds, called:

    a) the string sign.
    b) the lead pipe sign.
    c) the smooth bowel sign.
    d) the moulage sign.

126. A flap fracture is:

    a) a fracture of the tibial tubercle.
    b) a chip fracture of the anterior talar dome.
    c) a fracture of the hook of the hamate.
    d) a fracture of the greater tuberosity of the humeral head.

127. An uncalcified mass lesion in the small bowel must be suspected to be:

    a) a carcinoid.
    b) hemangioma.

    c) primary carcinoma.
    d) an enterolith.

128. Giant gastric mucosal folds may indicate the presence of:

    a) gastric leiomyoma.
    b) gastric hemangioma.
    c) gastric lymphosarcoma.
    d) gastric adenocarcinoma.

129. Tumorous nodules extending from the bladder into the urethra, creating a cone of dilatation, indicate:

    a) primary bladder carcinoma.
    b) direct extension of carcinoma from the rectum.
    c) rhabdomyosarcoma.
    d) benign papilloma.

130. A patient with a diagnosis of idiopathic chondrolysis of the hip should be advised to:

    a) exercise by using a treadmill.
    b) exercise by using a stationary bicycle.
    c) exercise with regular swimming.
    d) exercise by using a walking machine such as a "Nordic Track."

131. The great majority (about 90%) of cases of Paget's disease are:

    a) subject to constant, slowly-increasing pain.
    b) subject to pain that is present day and night, but is relieved by aspirin.
    c) asymptomatic, often for many years.
    d) subject to mild pain, aggravated by exertion.

132. A "coiled spring appearance" describes the radiographic image of:

    a) volvulus.
    b) intussusception.
    c) adynamic ileus.
    d) hiatal hernia.

133. The most common bladder tumor is:

    a) benign papilloma.
    b) primary bladder carcinoma.
    c) transitional cell carcinoma.
    d) rhabdomyosarcoma.

134. Fracture of the distal radial shaft with associated distal radioulnar diastasis is called:

    a) a Monteggia fracture.
    b) a reverse Colles' fracture.
    c) a Galeazzi fracture.
    d) a "B-B" fracture.

135. X-ray signs of gout include:

    a) laminated periostitis in the long bones.
    b) subchondral periarticular lucent erosions.
    c) generalized osteopenia.
    d) "gull wings" erosions at interphalangeal joints.

136. Chondrosarcoma most commonly occurs in patients:

    a) < 10 years of age.
    b) < 25 years of age.
    c) between 40 and 60 years of age.
    d) > 60 years of age.

137. Diverticula may rupture, creating radiologic signs of:

    a) ascites.
    b) pneumoperitoneum.
    c) empyema.
    d) intussusception.

138. Fracture of the proximal humerus carries the risk of injury to:
    a) the brachial plexus.
    b) the subclavian artery.
    c) the axillary nerve.
    d) the brachiocephalic artery.

139. A "Christmas tree bladder" is indicative of:
    a) a hydatid cyst of the bladder.
    b) adenocarcinoma of the bladder.
    c) benign cystitis.
    d) schistosomiasis of the bladder.

140. X-rays of a patient with idiopathic chondrolysis of the hip are likely to show:
    a) osteophytes.
    b) periarticular osteopenia and subchondral cysts.
    c) widened joint space.
    d) subchondral sclerosis.

141. An obstructed cystic duct may result in the formation of:
    a) a staghorn calculus.
    b) a jackstone calculus.
    c) a porcelain gallbladder.
    d) an accessory gallbladder.

142. Hass's disease is avascular necrosis, usually caused by interruption of the:
    a) rotator cuff arterial supply to the humeral head.
    b) dorsalis pedis arterial supply to the tarsal navicular.
    c) dorsalis pedis arterial supply to the talus.
    d) posterior tibial arterial supply to the calcaneus.

143. In hemochromatosis, the liver may appear:
    a) homogeneously opacified.
    b) filled with stippled or punctate calcifications.
    c) sprinkled with calcifications in "rings and broken rings."
    d) filled with streaky, amorphous calcification.

144. Gallstone ileus is caused by:
    a) a stone-filled, spastic gallbladder.
    b) a gallstone lodged at the ileocecal valve.
    c) a gallstone lodged in the pancreatic duct.
    d) a gallstone lodged in the biliary duct.

145. Ascites may result from any of the following except:
    a) hyperthyroidism.
    b) liver disease.
    c) nephrotic syndrome.
    d) pancreatitis.

146. The "doggy ears sign" indicates:
    a) an accumulation of free pleural effusions around the heart.
    b) an accumulation of pus (empyema) between the layers of the pleura.
    c) an accumulation of fluid around and behind the bladder.
    d) an occult fracture of an articular process.

147. Current treatment for Paget's disease may include supportive braces to minimize deformity in weight-bearing bones, and:
    a) calcitonin (both salmon and human).
    b) nonsteroid anti-inflammatory drugs.
    c) steroid anti-inflammatory drugs.
    d) surgical excision of smaller, symptomatic lesions.

148. The "apple core appearance" in a barium-filled colon is a sign of:

    a) colonic wall strictures caused by adenocarcinoma.
    b) an ulcerated diverticulum.
    c) malignant degeneration of a colonic polyp.
    d) twisted bowel loops caused by volvulus.

149. One indication of a probable malignant lesion, seen on barium studies, is:

    a) the "stacked coins" appearance.
    b) the "squeeze sign."
    c) the "snowflake appearance."
    d) the shouldering defect.

150. Emphysematous cystitis is strongly association with:

    a) smoking.
    b) diabetes.
    c) alcoholism.
    d) hypertension.

151. The Galeazzi fracture is also called:

    a) a reversed Monteggia fracture.
    b) a reverse Colles' fracture.
    c) an Essex–Lopresti fracture.
    d) a Dupuytren's fracture.

152. Articular effects in gout:

    a) include early, asymmetric loss of joint space.
    b) include early, uniform loss of joint space.
    c) commonly result in ankylosis.
    d) usually result in late, uniform loss of joint space.

153. The location of a tumor in the leptomeninges is most accurately described as:

    a) intradural extramedullary.
    b) intramedullary.
    c) intradural intramedullary.
    d) extradural.

154. The "snowflake appearance" describes:

    a) normal retention of barium flecks on jejunal mucosal folds.
    b) the usual appearance of prostate calcifications.
    c) the calcifications seen in colonic adenocarcinoma.
    d) the radiologic appearance of villous adenoma.

155. Uncontrolled diabetes has a strong association with:

    a) emphysematous cholecystitis.
    b) porcelain gallbladder.
    c) gallbladder carcinoma.
    d) cholelithiasis.

156. Valvular heart disease, asthma, and arthropathy may all result from:

    a) rheumatoid arthritis.
    b) rheumatic heart disease.
    c) carcinoid syndrome.
    d) bronchogenic carcinoma.

157. Primary hemochromatosis has a strong association with:

    a) sickle cell disease.
    b) thalassemia minor.
    c) diabetes mellitus.
    d) alcoholism.

158. The "String sign of Kantor" is associated with:

    a) abdominal fistulas caused by Crohn's disease.
    b) adynamic ileus.

c) stenosing regional enteritis.
d) volvulus.

159. The small fragment seen with osteochondritis dissecans:

a) is a bony fragment.
b) is a cartilage fragment.
c) is an osteochondral fragment.
d) may be either cartilage or cartilage and bone.

160. What two disorders produce "giant gastric folds"?

a) Menetriers disease and Chrohn's disease.
b) Lymphosarcoma and granulomatous gastritis.
c) Lymphosarcoma and Menetrier's disease.
d) Menetrier's disease and adenocarcinoma of the stomach.

161. Gastrointestinal hemangiomas are most frequently found:

a) in the distal jejunum and ileum.
b) in the stomach.
c) in the proximal jejunum.
d) in the duodenum.

162. The majority of splenic cysts are:

a) traumatic.
b) pyogenic infections.
c) congenital.
d) parasitic.

163. Mechanical ileus may be caused by:

a) inflammatory bowel disease.
b) spinal fracture.
c) focal inflammation, such as appendicitis.
d) occult visceral injury.

164. In the bladder, tumors are most commonly found:

a) at the ureterovesical junction.
b) within bladder diverticula.
c) in the trigone region.
d) at the uvula of the bladder.

165. The most common tumor of the large bowel is:

a) carcinoid.
b) leiomyoma.
c) adenocarcinoma.
d) hemangioma.

166. When cystography is done on a patient with bladder obstruction, and the distal ureters appear to have a "fish-hook" configuration, the bladder obstruction is likely caused by:

a) benign prostatic hypertrophy.
b) urethral stenosis.
c) urethral valves.
d) neurogenic bladder.

167. Two radiologic signs commonly seen in patients with ulcerative colitis are:

a) "apple core appearance" and toxic dilation.
b) "lead pipe colon" and "apple core appearance."
c) "frondlike rectal filling defect" and "moulage sign."
d) "lead pipe colon" and toxic dilation.

168. A "jackstone calculus" is:

a) complete filling of the renal pelvis and calyces with renal stones.
b) a ureteric stone that is lodged at the ureterovesical junction.
c) a large, symptomatic but non-calcific (and therefor not visible without contrast medium) stone in the bladder.
d) a large bladder stone with irregular, serrated margins.

169. "Case's pad sign" and "Frostberg's inverted 3 sign" are both indicative of:

    a) duodenal atresia.
    b) gallstone ileus.
    c) sprue.
    d) pancreatic carcinoma.

170. Carcinoid syndrome entails all of the following clinical features except:

    a) cutaneous flushes.
    b) diarrhea.
    c) syncope.
    d) cyanosis.

171. Lateral protrusions through the internal inguinal ring (with extraperitoneal bladder herniation) that disappear as the bladder is completely filled, may be seen on contrast studies, and are termed:

    a) "doggy ears."
    b) "bladder ears."
    c) "pooch pouches."
    d) "disappearing ears."

172. A normal measurement of the lumen diameter in the small bowel is approximately:

    a) 1 cm.
    b) 3 cm.
    c) 5 cm.
    d) 8 cm.

173. Sprue (celiac disease) is:

    a) an inflammatory disease.
    b) a parasitic infestation.
    c) a malabsorption syndrome.
    d) a yeast infection.

174. Sinding-Larsen-Johansson disease is sometimes a concomitant of:

    a) SONK.
    b) Blount's disease.
    c) Osgood-Schlatter's disease.
    d) osteochondritis dissecans.

175. Calcifications within the liver are likely to be caused by any of the following except:

    a) a primary, mixed malignant tumor.
    b) a metastatic lesion from the ovaries.
    c) histoplasmosis.
    d) cavernous hemangioma.

176. There is an increased incidence of cholelithiasis in patients with:

    a) Marfan's syndrome.
    b) diabetes mellitus.
    c) sickle cell anemia.
    d) neurofibromatosis.

177. "Hampton's line" indicates:

    a) a good prognosis after a talar dome fracture.
    b) an ulcer is probably not malignant.
    c) the probability of facet imbrication.
    d) the probability of basilar impression.

178. Ureteric neoplasms most frequently develop in:

    a) the distal third of ureters.
    b) the middle third of ureters.
    c) the proximal third of ureters.
    d) the ureterovesical junction.

179. Radiologic signs of scleroderma are most prevalent in:
    a) the larger peripheral joints.
    b) the spine.
    c) the hands.
    d) the pelvis.

180. The most common childhood abdominal neoplasm is:
    a) neurofibroma.
    b) Wilms' tumor.
    c) hemangioma.
    d) neuroblastoma.

181. An indication of increased risk of malignant degeneration in a patient with colonic polyps is:
    a) > 50% of the polyps are pedunculated.
    b) the development of villae on a growing polyp.
    c) the ulceration of a large polyp.
    d) the preponderance of the polyps are tubular.

182. Non-islet cell tumors may cause the "Vipoma syndrome," which consists of:
    a) mucoid diarrhea, hyperglycemia, achlorhydria.
    b) constipation, hypoglycemia, hyperchlorhydria.
    c) irritable bowel syndrome, diabetes mellitus, hypochlorhydria.
    d) watery diarrhea, hypokalemia, achlorhydria.

183. A comminuted radial head fracture coupled with distal radioulnar dislocation is called a:
    a) "baby car" fracture.
    b) Galeazzi fracture.
    c) Essex-Lopresti fracture.
    d) Monteggia fracture.

184. Pannus formation is involved in the pathologic process of all the following arthritides except:
    a) gout.
    b) hypertrophic osteoarthropathy.
    c) psoriatic arthritis.
    d) seropositive JRA.

185. Chondrosarcoma is most frequently seen:
    a) in the spine.
    b) in the pelvis and proximal femur.
    c) in the distal femur and proximal tibia.
    d) in the scapula and proximal humerus.

186. Appendicitis may be clinically indicated by:
    a) pain referred to the inferior angle of the right scapula.
    b) rebound tenderness at McBurney's point.
    c) pulsating low back pain, more pronounced when the patient is supine.
    d) a tearing sensation between the scapulae.

187. The chief cause of renal thrombosis in pediatric patients is:
    a) pressure from a Wilms' tumor.
    b) pressure from a hydatid cyst.
    c) ileocolitis.
    d) renal arterial anomalies.

188. A comminuted distal humeral fracture with associated ulnar and radial fractures often occurs:
    a) when a child falls from a bicycle.
    b) when an elbow is impacted as it protrudes from a car window.
    c) when an osteoporotic patient falls backwards.
    d) when a child is the victim of non-accidental trauma.

189. The spinal level at which kidneys normally lie is:

   a) L1-L4.
   b) T11-L3.
   c) T10-L1.
   d) T12-L5.

190. Ureteric calculi most commonly lodge:

   a) in the renal pelvis.
   b) in the proximal third of the ureter.
   c) in the middle third of the ureter.
   d) at the ureterovesical junction.

191. A sympathicoblastoma (neuroblastoma) usually occurs as:

   a) a primary tumor of the midbrain that metastasizes to bone.
   b) a primary tumor of the spinal cord or nerve root that spreads by direct extension to bone.
   c) a primary pituitary tumor that metastasizes to bone.
   d) a primary abdominal tumor that metastasizes to the brain and to bone.

192. The "claw sign" on a renal angiogram indicates that the lesion is probably:

   a) a benign adenoma.
   b) a Grawitz tumor.
   c) a renal cyst.
   d) malignant lymphoma.

193. Clusters of "daughter cysts" may be produced by:

   a) renal hydatid cysts.
   b) benign medullary cysts.
   c) renal polycystic disease.
   d) extraparenchymal renal cysts.

194. A villous adenoma is:

   a) a colonic polyp with > 80% of the mucosal glands villous.
   b) a malignant tumor of the jejunal villae.
   c) a villae-covered tumor of the proximal ileum.
   d) a rapidly growing bladder polyp, covered with villae.

195. Significant enlargement, with displacement of a kidney, and (in 15% of cases) curvilinear or irregular calcifications are radiologic signs of:

   a) angiomyolipoma.
   b) fibrolipomatosis.
   c) Grawitz tumor.
   d) Wilms' tumor.

196. The "frondlike rectal filling defect" in a barium examination is an indication of:

   a) ulcerative colitis.
   b) fistulous Crohn's disease.
   c) villous adenoma.
   d) an ulcerated diverticulum.

197. Polyarteritis nodosa causes the renal arteries:

   a) to develop multiple microaneurysms.
   b) to become occluded.
   c) to become narrowed and tortuous.
   d) to become rigid.

198. A "crescent sign" in the kidney, seen on an IVP study, might indicate:

   a) hydronephrosis.
   b) nephrocalcinosis.
   c) pyelonephritis.
   d) renal papillary necrosis.

199. Abnormal self-destructive or aggressive behavior in a mentally retarded patient with hyperuricemia is descriptive of:

    a) Caplan's syndrome.
    b) Lesch-Nyhan syndrome.
    c) Felty's syndrome.
    d) Sjögren's syndrome.

200. When the humeral shaft is fractured between the deltoid and pectoralis major insertions, the humeral head:

    a) is adducted.
    b) is rotated and abducted.
    c) is abducted but not rotated.
    d) is rotated but not abducted.

201. Renal medullary cysts may sometimes be visible on plain film as:

    a) "eggshell" curvilinear calcifications.
    b) aneurysmal swelling of the kidney.
    c) punctate calcifications within rimless ovoid masses.
    d) fanlike pattern clusters in the renal pyramids.

202. Osteolysis at the terminal tufts, progressing to complete osteolysis of a phalanx, is a characteristic of:

    a) psoriatic arthritis.
    b) erosive osteoarthritis.
    c) scleroderma.
    d) gout.

203. The majority of epicondylar fractures are:

    a) avulsions.
    b) chip fractures.
    c) comminuted fractures.
    d) pathologic fractures.

204. The "ring shadow" (triangular lucencies with dense opaque borders) is a radiographic sign that may indicate:

    a) a renal pelvis and calyces packed with renal stones.
    b) acute pyelonephritis.
    c) renal papillary necrosis.
    d) nephrocalcinosis.

205. Traumatic flexion at the elbow may result in:

    a) an avulsion fracture of the medial epicondyle.
    b) an avulsion fracture at the radial insertion of the biceps.
    c) an avulsion fracture of the olecranon.
    d) an avulsion fracture of the lateral epicondyle.

206. Hypertrophic osteoarthropathy resolves with:

    a) surgical excision of the primary lesion and vagal resection.
    b) surgical excision of the primary lesion and irradiation.
    c) surgical excision of the primary lesion and chemotherapy.
    d) vagal resection and steroid therapy.

207. The incidence of gout is particularly high among:

    a) British men.
    b) natives of Polynesia and New Zealand.
    c) Native Americans.
    d) Eskimos.

208. All of the following must be considered in the differential diagnosis of thymoma except:

    a) teratoma.
    b) substernal thyroid.
    c) lymphoma.
    d) neurofibroma.

209. The "classic triad" of hypertrophic osteoarthropathy signs includes:

    a) conjunctivitis, uveitis, and arthropathy.
    b) Raynaud's phenomenon, periostitis, and arthropathy.
    c) periostitis, symmetric arthritis, and digital clubbing.
    d) periostitis, tuftal osteolysis, and symmetric arthritis.

210. Mechanisms that may predispose a site to deposition of tophi include all of the following except:

    a) proteoglycan levels in the tissue.
    b) microtrauma.
    c) hypervascularity.
    d) comparatively lower temperatures.

211. "Putty kidney" is a condition caused by:

    a) necrotic changes following traumatic injury to the kidney.
    b) renal lipoma.
    c) chronic infection, such as renal tuberculosis.
    d) congenital malformation of the kidneys.

212. The pain of Hodgkin's lymphoma lesions:

    a) is noticed only when there is pathologic fracture.
    b) is noticed only when there is cord compression caused by vertebral body collapse.
    c) is rarely a presenting symptom.
    d) is brought on or intensified by alcohol consumption.

213. Acute attacks of gouty arthritis:

    a) are most common in the upper extremity.
    b) usually last only a few hours.
    c) are most likely to occur in the early morning hours.
    d) seldom recur.

214. The most common radial neck fracture is:

    a) a torus fracture.
    b) an avulsion fracture.
    c) an impaction fracture.
    d) a spiral fracture/dislocation.

215. A lytic subarticular lesion with granular calcification specks and a nodular soft tissue mass near a joint is likely to represent:

    a) osteochondroma.
    b) chondrosarcoma.
    c) synovioma.
    d) giant cell tumor.

216. A kidney that first swells, then shrinks and develops a faint rim of calcification, is undergoing:

    a) papillary necrosis.
    b) nephrocalcinosis.
    c) formation of an abscess.
    d) cortical necrosis.

217. Hydroxyapatite deposition disease (HADD) is essentially:

    a) chondrocalcification.
    b) arterial calcinosis.
    c) costochondral calcinosis.
    d) calcifying tendinitis.

218. The peak age of incidence of Ewing's sarcoma is:

    a) 5 years.
    b) 15 years.
    c) 22 years.
    d) 30 years.

219. Dietary purine should be eliminated or minimized in patients with:

    a) calcium pyrophosphate dihydrate crystal deposition disease.
    b) Wilson's disease.
    c) ochronosis.
    d) gout.

220. "Staghorn calculus" is:

    a) a calcified villous adenoma.
    b) calcification of the iliac arteries at their bifurcation.
    c) renal stones, filling the renal pelvis and calyces.
    d) extensive costochondral calcification.

221. A major limitation of nuclear bone scans is that they:

    a) are not specific.
    b) are not sensitive.
    c) render a high radiation dose to the patient.
    d) are excessively expensive.

222. Osteolytic metastasis is most common, constituting:

    a) 40% of metastatic lesions.
    b) 75% of metastatic lesions.
    c) 50% of metastatic lesions.
    d) 65% of metastatic lesions.

223. Skeletal lesions of Hodgkin's lymphoma usually are:

    a) primary malignant bone tumors.
    b) secondary to systemic Hodgkin's lymphoma.
    c) secondary to osteosarcoma.
    d) secondary to degeneration of Paget's disease.

224. With Paget's disease, laboratory findings usually include:

    a) markedly increased serum calcium.
    b) markedly decreased serum calcium.
    c) decreased alkaline phosphatase.
    d) normal serum calcium.

225. Pseudofractures, such as those seen in Paget's disease, are also common to:

    a) metastatic carcinoma.
    b) fibrosarcoma.
    c) fibrous xanthoma.
    d) fibrous dysplasia.

SUPPLEMENTARY TEST 2—ANSWER KEY

1.	d	24.	a	47.	a	70.	d	93.	b	116.	c	139.	c	162.	d	185.	b	208.	d
2.	c	25.	d	48.	d	71.	c	94.	c	117.	b	140.	b	163.	a	186.	b	209.	c
3.	c	26.	b	49.	c	72.	d	95.	c	118.	b	141.	c	164.	c	187.	c	210.	c
4.	c	27.	c	50.	a	73.	d	96.	a	119.	b	142.	a	165.	c	188.	b	211.	c
5.	d	28.	c	51.	b	74.	d	97.	d	120.	a	143.	a	166.	a	189.	b	212.	d
6.	c	29.	a	52.	a	75.	c	98.	d	121.	c	144.	b	167.	d	190.	d	213.	c
7.	c	30.	a	53.	d	76.	c	99.	d	122.	d	145.	a	168.	d	191.	d	214.	c
8.	a	31.	d	54.	c	77.	c	100.	a	123.	a	146.	c	169.	d	192.	c	215.	c
9.	b	32.	b	55.	a	78.	d	101.	a	124.	c	147.	a	170.	c	193.	a	216.	d
10.	a	33.	b	56.	a	79.	b	102.	c	125.	d	148.	a	171.	b	194.	a	217.	d
11.	c	34.	c	57.	c	80.	b	103.	c	126.	d	149.	d	172.	b	195.	c	218.	b
12.	d	35.	a	58.	c	81.	c	104.	a	127.	c	150.	b	173.	c	196.	c	219.	d
13.	b	36.	b	59.	b	82.	b	105.	c	128.	c	151.	a	174.	c	197.	a	220.	c
14.	c	37.	a	60.	a	83.	b	106.	c	129.	c	152.	d	175.	d	198.	a	221.	a
15.	c	38.	a	61.	b	84.	a	107.	c	130.	c	153.	a	176.	c	199.	b	222.	b
16.	b	39.	c	62.	a	85.	a	108.	a	131.	c	154.	a	177.	b	200.	a	223.	b
17.	c	40.	c	63.	a	86.	b	109.	d	132.	b	155.	a	178.	a	201.	d	224.	d
18.	c	41.	d	64.	c	87.	c	110.	a	133.	a	156.	c	179.	c	202.	c	225.	d
19.	d	42.	a	65.	c	88.	c	111.	c	134.	c	157.	c	180.	b	203.	a		
20.	a	43.	c	66.	a	89.	c	112.	c	135.	b	158.	c	181.	b	204.	c		
21.	d	44.	d	67.	c	90.	d	113.	c	136.	c	159.	d	182.	d	205.	c		
22.	b	45.	b	68.	b	91.	d	114.	b	137.	b	160.	c	183.	c	206.	a		
23.	b	46.	a	69.	c	92.	c	115.	d	138.	c	161.	a	184.	b	207.	b		

Index

Page numbers followed by *t* and *f* indicate tables and figures, respectively.